HEARING SCIENCE

Editor in chief, Speech, Language, and Hearing Science Series
Raymond G. Daniloff, PhD

HEARING SCIENCE
Recent Advances

Edited by

Charles I. Berlin, PhD

Department of Otolaryngology and Biocommunication
Kresge Hearing Institute Laboratory of the South
Louisiana State University Medical Center

 COLLEGE-HILL PRESS, San Diego, California

College-Hill Press
4284 41st Street
San Diego, California 92105

© 1984 by College-Hill Press, Inc.

Library of Congress Cataloging in Publication Data
Main entry under title:

Hearing science: Recent advances.

  Bibliography: p.
  Includes index.
  1. Audiology. I. Berlin, Charles I. [DNLM:
1. Hearing. WV 270 H4356]
RF290.H433 1984   617.7   84-11424

ISBN 0-933014-96-1

Printed in the United States of America

Publisher's Note

These volumes were developed under the supervision of a group of leading scientists charged with the responsibility of assessing the most critical book needs of the speech-language-hearing profession. In consultation with William H. Perkins and Raymond G. Daniloff, serving as editors in chief of the ensuing volumes on speech, language, and hearing disorders (Perkins) and speech, language, and hearing science (Daniloff), the publisher planned a series of nine mutually independent texts covering the entirety of state-of-the-art knowledge in these disciplines, with contributions by respected, productive, and current scholars known for their expertise as specialists in key areas.

Each contribution has been stringently refereed for content, pedagogy, and practical value for students and practitioners by the individual volume editors, Charles Berlin, Janis Costello, Raymond Daniloff, Audrey Holland, James Jerger, Rita Naremore, and their designated reviewers, in close consultation throughout with the editors in chief and the publisher. Users are thus assured that their needs for accurate, timely information, reflecting the highest standards of scholarship and professionalism, have been faithfully met.

On behalf of the speech-language-hearing profession, its researchers, teachers, practitioners, and students, present and future, the publisher thanks the more than 100 authors and editors who have given generously of their time and knowledge to produce this magnificent contribution to the literature.

Hearing Science, edited by Charles I. Berlin, is one of nine state-of-the-art volumes comprising the College-Hill Press series covering the current body of knowledge in speech, language, and hearing.

Volume Titles:	Editors:
Speech Disorders in Children	Janis M. Costello
Speech Disorders in Adults	Janis M. Costello
Speech Science	Raymond G. Daniloff
Language Disorders in Children	Audrey L. Holland
Language Disorders in Adults	Audrey L. Holland
Language Science	Rita C. Naremore
Pediatric Audiology	James Jerger
Hearing Disorders in Adults	James Jerger
Recent Advances: Hearing Science	Charles I. Berlin

Editor in chief, Speech, Language, and Hearing Disorders Series: William H. Perkins

Editor in chief, Speech, Language, and Hearing Science Series: Raymond G. Daniloff

CONTENTS

Contributors

Preface

1 Comparative Psychoacoustics:
New Directions 1
WILLIAM C. STEBBINS, SHERYL COOMBS, CYNTHIA PROSEN

2 Developmental Mechanisms of Mammalian
Inner Ear Formation 49
THOMAS R. VAN DE WATER

3 Recent Advances Toward Understanding
Auditory System Development 109
EDWIN W RUBEL, DONALD E. BORN, JEFFREY S. DEITCH,
DIANNE DURHAM

4 Neurotransmitters of the Cochlea and
Lateral Line Organ 159
RICHARD P. BOBBIN, SANFORD C. BLEDSOE, JR.,
GARY L. JENISON

5 Anatomical Measures of Physiological
Parameters in the Cochlea 181
ALLEN F. RYAN

6 Inner Ear Function Based on the
Mechanical Tuning of the Hair Cells . . . 213
SHYAM M. KHANNA

7 Functional Roles of the Inner- and
Outer-Hair-Cell Subsystems in the Cochlea
and Brainstem 241
D.O. KIM

8   Speech Encoding in the
    Auditory Nerve 263
    MURRAY B. SACHS

9   Cochlear Implants 309
    JOSEF M. MILLER, BRYAN E. PFINGST

10 Neurotransmitters of the Auditory Nerve
    and Central Auditory System 341
    ROBERT J. WENTHOLD, MICHAEL R. MARTIN

11 The Structural Basis for Stimulus Coding
    in the Cochlear Nucleus of the Cat 371
    NELL B. CANT, D.K. MOREST

12 Response Characteristics of Neurons
    of the Cochlear Nuclei 423
    ERIC D. YOUNG

13 Asymmetries in Evoked Potentials 461
    CHARLES I. BERLIN, LINDA J. HOOD, PRUDENCE ALLEN

    Author Index 479

    Subject Index 491

Contributors

Prudence Allen, MA, Department of Otolaryngology and Biocommunication, Kresge Hearing Research Laboratory of the South, Louisiana State University Medical Center, New Orleans, LA 70119

Charles I. Berlin, PhD, Kresge Hearing Research Laboratory of the South, Louisiana State University Medical Center, New Orleans, LA 70119

Sanford C. Bledsoe, Jr., PhD, Kresge Hearing Research Institute, University of Michigan Medical School, Ann Arbor, MI 48109

Richard P. Bobbin, PhD, Department of Otolaryngology and Biocommunication, Kresge Hearing Research Laboratory of the South, Louisiana State University Medical Center, New Orleans, LA 70119

Donald E. Born, BA, Neuroscience Program, University of Virginia Medical Center, Charlottesville, VA 22908

Nell B. Cant, PhD, Department of Anatomy, Duke University Medical Center, Durham, NC 27710

Sheryl Coombs, PhD, Parmly Hearing Institute, Loyola University of Chicago, Chicago, IL 60626

Jeffrey S. Deitch, BA, Neuroscience Program, University of Virginia Medical Center, Charlottesville, VA 22908

Dianne Durham, PhD, Department of Otolaryngology, University of Virginia Medical Center, Charlottesville, VA 22908

Linda J. Hood, PhD, Department of Otolaryngology and Biocommunication, Kresge Hearing Research Laboratory of the South, Louisiana State University Medical Center, New Orleans, LA 70119

Gary L. Jenison, PhD, Department of Otolaryngology and Biocommunication, Kresge Hearing Research Laboratory of the South, Louisiana State University Medical Center, New Orleans, LA 70119

Shyam M. Khanna, PhD, Columbia University College of Physicians and Surgeons, New York, NY 10032

D.O. Kim, DSc, Departments of Physiology and Biophysics, Biomedical Engineering Program, Washington University, St. Louis, MO 63110

Michael R. Martin, PhD, Laboratory of Neuro-otolaryngology, National Institute of Neurological and Communicative Disorders and Stroke, National Institutes of Health, Bethesda, MD 20205

Josef M. Miller, PhD, Department of Otolaryngology, University of Washington School of Medicine, Seattle, WA 98195

D.K. Morest, MD, Department of Anatomy, University of Connecticut Health Center, Farmington, CT 06032

Bryan E. Pfingst, PhD, Department of Otolaryngology, University of Washington, Seattle, WA 98195

Cynthia Prosen, PhD, Department of Biology, Michigan Technological University, Houghton, MI 49931

Edwin W Rubel, PhD, Departments of Otolaryngology and Physiology, University of Virginia Medical Center, Charlottesville, VA 22908

Allen F. Ryan, PhD, Division of Otolaryngology, Department of Surgery, University of California, San Diego Medical School, La Jolla, CA 92093

Murray B. Sachs, PhD, Biomedical Engineering, The Johns Hopkins University School of Medicine, Baltimore, MD 21205

William C. Stebbins, PhD, Department of Psychology and Kresge Hearing Research Institute, University of Michigan, Ann Arbor, MI 48109

Thomas R. Van De Water, PhD, Kennedy Center, Box 27, Laboratory of Developmental Otobiology, Departments of Otolaryngology and Neuroscience, South Bronx, NY 10461

Robert J. Wenthold, PhD, Department of Neurophysiology, 607 Waisman Center, University of Wisconsin, Madison, WI 53705

Eric D. Young, PhD, Biomedical Engineering, The Johns Hopkins University School of Medicine, Baltimore, MD 21205

PREFACE

Eleven years ago Dallos closed his now-classic text *The Auditory Periphery* (Academic Press, 1973, p. 524) with these comments:

> "Rapid development can be expected in the near future in a number of areas that are directly revelant to our subject. Among these are studies of nonlinear processes in the cochlea, which have been shown by a variety of current experimentation to be much more important to the normal functioning of the ear than hitherto assumed. Other areas of active interest are the development of correlations between gross and elementary potentials and the concomitant study of cochlear electroanatomy. The identification and description of the elusive generator potential can also be anticipated to happen in the near future. Much interest will be attached to the delineation of the respective roles and the interaction between inner and outer hair cells. Of great and enduring interest is the mode of functioning of the efferent system with natural sound stimulation. Finally, an important chapter in the investigation of the cochlea has just barely begun with the growing interest in the biochemical mechanisms in hearing. We can all look forward to exciting times."

Some of the work Dallos anticipated is summarized in this volume. The first chapter sets the tone for the book, giving us an overview of the importance of areas as distantly related as hair cell rigidity and lateral dominance, themes which are covered in various chapters in this volume.

Stebbins and his colleagues review and catalogue hearing capabilities for various species; the review shows that frequency ranges of hearing in most land-based animals are related to middle ear characteristics and basilar membrane dimensions, and the extent to which certain calls seem to be frequency-modulated appears to contribute to the accuracy with which those sounds can be localized.

They review the recent work suggesting that a loss of stereocilia rigidity may result in temporary threshold shift by disrupting the structure of actin filaments within the stereocilia. The importance of actin and the rigidity of the filaments and mechanical sharpening of frequency analysis by the filaments recurs in a number of places in this book, especially in the work of Rubel (chap. 3) and colleagues, Ryan (chap. 5), Khanna (chap. 6) and Kim (chap. 7).

The data they cite also stress that psychophysical tuning curves and lateral suppression data are more sensitive indices of an impaired auditory system than any shift in the pure-tone audiogram. There is even a point made that guinea pigs, whose absolute thresholds increase following noise exposure, demonstrate signs of loudness recruitment just like monkeys and humans.

Stebbins and colleagues' review of comparative psychoacoustics points out that many animals have qualities of both cerebral dominance and lateral asymmetry in their auditory systems similar to those seen in humans. They also show that some animals have more difficulty than would be predicted from their sensitivity curves in learning calls that are not common to their species.

They suggest very wisely that neither a strict phonetic processing model nor a strict psychoacoustic model leaves room for species-specific neural feature detectors, which probably play an important part in animal communication.

In a remarkable tour de force, Van De Water takes us through the in vitro development of the otic capsule. Otocysts between 9.5 and 10 days old require interaction with brainstem tissues for continuing development; 10.5-day-old otocysts are capable of limited vestibular development in the absence of brainstem interaction, but development of any auditory sensory structures requires continuing inductive influence of the rhombencephalon. Results using filters of average pore diameters less than 0.2 μm demonstrate that cellular contact is not required for the passage of the brainstem inductive message but that molecular exchange is essential. His work illustrates the importance of tissue interactions between the epithelial cells in the otocysts and their surrounding periotic mesenchyme; disruptions of these interactions result in maldevelopment of the labryinth. Coiling of the cochlea seems to be a result of the interaction at the tissue interface between the developing otocysts and their surrounding periotic mesenchyme, or even possibly by the presence of the physical barrier provided by the cartilage in the immediate area of the developing cochlea. Van De Water goes on to give data which support the hypothesis that there may be a limited period where sensory structures like hair cells generate a chemotrophic gradient field such that inward chemotaxis is the mechanism for the establishment of the pattern of innervation of the inner ear receptors.

By presenting a map describing the ultimate fate of individual cells in the otocysts Van De Water provides two important pieces of information. He shows that cell determination has already occurred at or before the 11th day after gestation; secondly the fate map of a normal mouse otocyst can be used to generate a model for normal structural development of the inner ear. It was intriguing to find that if one were to culture the otocysts of a genetically abnormal mouse (homozygotic kreisler kr/kr), the otocysts raised in vitro produce results similar to what would have occurred if the otocysts were left in the developing tissue instead of in the glass culture dish. Homozygotic kreisler otocysts developed abnormally while heterozygotic kreisler otocysts (+ /kr) developed according to the fate map of a normal mouse.

Van De Water further suggests that some genetic abnormalities may not directly affect the inner ear, but may be the result of abnormalities interfering with the normal sequence of tissue interactions that direct the formation of the inner ear. He suggests that this mechanism may operate in the genetic syndromes such as Waardenburg's disease, Pendred's syndrome, etc. He rightly suggests that investigators might focus attention on common mechanisms which could result in heterogeneous final results, instead of focusing on just the inner ear abnormalities.

Van De Water discusses in vitro development. In an equally powerful and important chapter, Rubel and associates carry on with important new data on in vivo ontogeny. In chap. 3, Rubel and his colleagues report that in developing chick inner ears, the sensitivity to low tones develops *at the base* and moves toward the apex with maturation. This startling and paradoxical report has been confirmed and supported in other laboratories and forms one of the main underpinnings of the New Biology of the inner ear. Stebbins's work helped to outline the initial and final ranges of hearing for various species cited in Table 1 of chap. 3; Rubel and his group use this table as a springboard to outline the ontogeny of the auditory system in a unique manner interweaving the themes of both the Van De Water and Stebbins and associates chapters with this one. The base-to-apex functional change is different from the well-known and accepted *gradient of differentiation* which extends in both directions from the midbasal region. This latter gradient is morphologically recognizable as a maturation of elements; the newly reported base-to-apex shift is a physicomechanical or perhaps physiological shift of sensitivity to tones of various frequencies. Rubel and his group present compelling evidence that the middle ear is not the mediating first-order filter in the shift of cochlear susceptibility to noise damage, and that the transduction properties of the cochlea are changing with maturation. Their model suggests that only low or mid-low frequencies are transduced by the cochlea and that the transduction is mediated by relatively basal regions of the cochlea. The common themes of Kim's chap. 7 with Khanna's chap. 6 and Rubel's chap. 3 will be even more cogent if it is ultimately shown that the shift in basilar membrane tuning is secondary to developmental changes in stiffness and/or electromechanical properties of the hair tufts and hair cells.

In extensive additional work these authors also address issues of deafferentation, environmental isolation, drug effects, and so forth on the developing auditory system. They complement Van De Water's predictions that cellular morphology can be altered by almost any chronically abnormal activity but the abnormality must occur at a critical period to have any major effects.

In the broad fields of neurophysiology and neurochemistry an extremely small subset of the great many neurotransmitters currently under study have been conclusively identified. The evidence supporting, for instance, the role of acetylcholine in neuromuscular transmission is extremely persuasive, and a modicum of progress has been made in the determination of several invertebrate neurotransmitters. This is far from the case for vertebrate sensory transmitters, particularly those of the auditory system. Bobbin, Bledsoe, and Jenison review the current data characterizing the afferent and efferent neurotransmitters of the cochlea. Wenthold and Martin concentrate on those entailing the cochlear nuclei. Both groups of investigators have consistently provided insight to this field and each, within the context of their reviews, freely expresses their inclinations and biases.

Since many endogenous neurotransmitters can potentially be mimicked by a number of exogenously applied compounds, it has become traditional (if not universally accepted) to set up a highly arbitrary set of criteria against which to measure the validity of the "proof" supporting any putative neurotransmitters. These criteria are listed in both the Bobbin and associates and Wenthold and Martin chapters in slightly different form; however, both chapters complement one another to give a solid description of current studies in the biochemistry of auditory neurotransmission. This readership may especially appreciate the relevance to the *auditory* system; but if new chemical systems of neurotransmission are uncovered by this work, neurophysiology as a whole stands to benefit. Clinically, major improvement in the management of sensorineural loss and/or genetic deafness, as well as in the management of tinnitus and fluctuant hearing loss, will follow our more complete understanding of the biochemistry of the auditory system.

Chapter 5 presents Ryan's important summary of his findings in the auditory system using four new techniques. Using energy dispersive X-ray analysis [(EDXA), the so-called electron microprobe] he was able to demonstrate that the fluids underlying the subsurface of the tectorial membrane are endolymphatic in nature. Autoradiographic demonstrations of amino acid uptake, 2-deoxy-D-glucose and the aforementioned electron microprobe technique helped to outline active portions of the cochlea and central nervous system during various types of stimulation and shed light on uptake of various amino acids in the cochlea and organ of Corti. His work suggests that an amino acid might serve as a cotransmitter or modulator of *efferent* as well as afferent synaptic activity. Marked differences between inner and outer hair cell functions and support for the aspartic and glutamic acid hypotheses of transmitter substances is also reported. The careful reader will note the important links between Ryan's reports on marked differences between inner and outer hair cell functions and the mechanoelectrical theories propounded by Kim (chap. 7) and Khanna (chap. 6), as well as the support for and interrelationships between this work and the two chapters on biochemistry by Bobbin and associates and Wenthold and Martin.

Soon after von Békésy won the Nobel Prize in physiology for his work on cochlear partition mechanics, scientists have had to postulate a "second filter" to account for the sharpness of tuning of single nerve fibers. Khanna and Kim both show that the sharply tuned nonlinear response originates at the hair cells and is primarily determined by the mechanical parameters of its own stereocilia. The stimulation of the hair cells by the tectorial membrane attachment to the tallest row of stereocilia is transmitted to the basilar membrane and therefore part of the sharply tuned response of the hair cell is seen in the basilar membrane response. Trauma seems to reduce the stiffness of the tallest stereocilia and the loss of stiffness lowers their resonant frequency, while the loss of coupling is said to reduce their sensitivity. Khanna attributes the loss of sharpness of tuning in the basilar membrane after damage to the *loss of coupling* between the stereocilia, the tectorial membrane, and the basilar membrane itself. In contrast, Kim ascribes the loss of sharpness to the *loss of an electromechanical gain control system.*

Khanna's work is especially cogent in the view of the introductory comments of Stebbins and his colleagues. Comparative biologists starting with E.G. Wever have pointed out that many species lack tectorial membranes or their equivalents yet seem to have tuning properties similar to, if not identical to, those seen in the mammalian species. The chapters of Khanna and Kim, coupled with the overview given by Stebbins and his colleagues, highlight the importance to hearing science of bringing together comparative biology, experimental physiology, and biomechanics to unravel the mysteries of cochlear transduction.

In a creative and adventuresome chapter, Kim contrasts with Khanna in that he proposes an *active* electromechanical tuning of the cochlea mediated primarily by outer hair cells. Kim's chap. 7 brings together the exciting work of Kemp on active mechanical tones generated by the cochlea and postulates two distinct parallel auditory subsystems using the outer hair cells as modulators and inner hair cells as carriers of auditory information. He suggests that there is an active *bidirectional* transduction mechanism in the stereocilia and cuticular plate region where the electrochemical energy of the endolymphatic potential and the outer hair cell membrane potential can also be used to drive the hair bundles mechanically. He suggests this property of the outer hair cell gives rise to an active nonlinear biomechanical gain control system in the cochlea that is highly vulnerable physiologically and had been overlooked because of its susceptibility to physiological insult. He also points out that the endocochlear potential is present only in the cochlea and not in the vestibular system despite the contiguity of the fluid sources. He ascribes this paradox to the need of the outer hair cells for an energy source to drive the motor action of the outer hair cells in modulating the mechanical responses of the cochlear partition.

Future applications of these important ideas, if they are corroborated, should include direct current stimulation of the damaged cochlea as a possible treatment for both tinnitus and/or some of the symptoms of outer hair cell loss, electromechanical modulation of the cochlea to make up for the loss of outer hair cells, and modification of hearing instruments which can modulate not only sound pressure but also Dc current throughout the cochlea.

Sachs in chap. 8 presents unique and lucidly organized data showing the eighth nerve response from stimuli ranging from vowels to stop consonants and fricatives as they contribute to the peripheral encoding of speech. He addresses two theoretical issues: whether rate-place versus temporal or phase-place dominates the encoding of speech. He ultimately shows that vowel formant frequencies and stop-consonants are well preserved in temporal-place encoding schemes. Fricatives are more effectively represented in a rate-place system; as is voice pitch. Thus he concludes that the CNS needs both systems to decode speech well, a conclusion which presages the reports of Miller and Pfingst (chap. 9) on speech perception with the phase-place type of cochlear implants.

In chap. 9, Miller and Pfingst give an excellent review of the current state of cochlear implants in humans and animals. Their work dovetails with the chapter by Sachs on the response of the auditory nerve to speech. They address the issues of single- versus multi-channel implants and conclude that most workers believe that ultimately a multi-channel implant will be more useful in carrying speech code. Among the more important clinically relevant findings is their report that there is greater risk of damage with molded versus tubular scala tympani implants.

The authors discuss the superior safety of middle ear implants and/or round window implants as compared to intracochlear implants, and show that something other than a simple electrochemical mechanism underlies any intracochlear damage related to electrical stimulation. If simple electrochemical mechanisms were at the basis of damage to the cochlea, the threshold current for damage would vary at 6 dB per octave, keeping the charge density constant; these authors report that a change in the damage threshold is closer to 6 dB per *decade*. They suggest that an investigation of pH changes, toxic by-products, and other biochemical changes in the fluid and tissues surrounding the electrode should be evaluated at high frequencies of stimulation.

The authors rightfully conclude that, with the exception of a number of "star patients," no implants routinely provide recognizable speech perception.

Somewhere, between the electrochemical and electromechanical data reviewed in the Kim and Khanna chapters, the biochemical principles presented in the Bobbin and associates and Wenthold and Martin chapters, and the coding rules in the Sachs chapter, future attempts at stimulating ears that have no hair cell receptors will be more successful. At present, however, it is safe to say that patients who need to be "put back in touch with the world of sound around them" are pleased to have implants which are at worst lipreading aids, and at best assist in understanding closed set speech messages without visual cues.

The chapters by Kim (chap. 7), Cant and Morest (chap. 11), and Young (chap. 12), are close to each other in this book to encourage the reader to synthesize a global picture of the inner and outer hair cells' subsystems, their projection into the cochlear nuclei, and the extremely complex multicellular nature of the cochlear nuclei. Young injected a solution of horseradish peroxidase into the cell from which he recorded, and which allowed him to visualize the cell later on via the residual opaque precipitate. Young predicts that with such techniques the next few years should bring great progress in the analysis of the function of the cochlear nucleus in hearing. It is a critical way-station in the auditory system because of both its multicellular nature and its critical role in assisting signal processing in noise as well as in processing complex stimuli. The work which suggests that the cochlear nucleus can affect cochlear function in an efferent mode dovetails well with Kim's notions of outer hair cell modulation and control via efferent pathways. Young's chapter outlines various types of units with different response characteristics, such as pausers and choppers.

Young summarized his chapter in an earlier version of his manuscript:

"The cochlear nuclei (CN) contain a number of recognizable distinct subsystems. These subsystems are distinguished by their synaptic and cellular morphology, their connectivity with the other parts of the auditory system, and the properties of their responses to sound. This chapter reviews current knowledge about the response characteristics of single neurons in the CN. A variety of response types has been observed; two schemes for classifying these responses have been developed. In most cases, it is possible to assign specific response types to morphological cell types and to understand certain salient features of the response types from the cellular and synaptic morphology of the cell types. This information is valuable because it allows the generation of a wiring diagram for the CN in which the functional characteristics of the nodes of the diagram are known. Such a diagram is an essential foundation for the study of information processing in the CN."

Cant and Morest attempt to define cell types and subdivisions as they relate to specific synaptic connections with other kinds of neurons in particular locations. It is this approach they hope will provide a structural basis for explaining information processing in the cochlear nucleus and assist scientists in generating functional models. Cant and Morest suggest that it will be necessary to make use of labeling methods of individual cells identified as to type by both light and electron microscopy; they suggest that the approach is tedious and time consuming but feasible. Young's and Ryan's chapters show some of this histochemical type of work and highlight the important interrelationships of structure and function.

The final chapter in this book is a reprise of one of the original themes laid down by Stebbins and associates in the first chapter. In it they discuss laterality and hemispheric differences in various species. In our final chapter we discuss evoked potential asymmetries seen in early, middle, and late responses. The most provocative of our findings shows that left-handed subjects have a 7-ms later Pb wave than do right-handed subjects. If this finding is duplicated by other workers it may allow us to determine when and how laterality develops in humans and other species, whether certain types of "mixed laterality" have physiologic concomitants, and may tell us whether certain right-handed subjects are in fact biological left-handers.

It has been exciting to read these chapters and compile this volume. The authors were invited to write for the highest level of readership; hopefully the book's nature and contents will be inspirational to mature professionals as well as to their beginning students, and will broaden their scope of what might legitimately be called "hearing science." These reports encourage us all to develop professional descendants who ultimately will use what we call here "recent advances" as their "basic principles."

Charles I. Berlin

Acknowledgments

My thanks to the many colleagues who helped to read and contribute to this volume including the diligent and scholarly authors, and Nancie Roark, Cindy Frazier, Vibha Flax and Jack Grove. Linda Hood, Gary Jenison, Harriet Berlin, and my children deserve special thanks for their support and forebearance. Special acknowledgments must go for support from LSU via our Dean Paul Larson, our Chief of Otolaryngology, George D. Lyons, Jr., and grants from NINCDS including NS 07058, NS 11647, and support from the Kresge Foundation, and Kam's Fund. Special support at critical times came from BMDR Program No. 1549, The Eye and Ear Institute of Louisiana, and the Louisiana Lions Eye Foundation.

Chapter 1

Comparative Psychoacoustics: New Directions

William C. Stebbins

Sheryl Coombs

Cynthia Prosen

In this chapter we present recent findings and discuss current issues in the analysis of comparative vertebrate hearing. The chapter is divided into three parts. The first is concerned with the study of biologically significant acoustic stimuli and their perception and localization by animals. The second part examines how different psychophysical approaches help to reveal mechanisms of auditory processing. The relationship, for example, between peripheral auditory structure and auditory acuity is examined. The stress on comparative hearing underscores the significance of adaptation and natural selection on auditory form and function in the course of evolution. The final section elaborates on the search for structure–function relationships by examining the role of the inner ear in hearing. Experiments are described in which ototoxic drugs or intense noise are employed to selectively destroy certain receptive structures while sparing others. Throughout we emphasize the importance of behavior and animal psychophysics in understanding signal processing by the vertebrate auditory system in addition to its ontogeny and phylogeny.

What animals hear and how finely they discriminate the various features of acoustic signals may tell us something about the origins of our own hearing in the course of biological evolution; it also represents the end product of biomechanical and neural processing at the various levels of the auditory system so aptly described elsewhere in this book. It is the functional consequence of the mechanisms that are now being revealed by microscope and microelectrode. Comparative psychoacoustics refers both to a set of procedures for questioning nonhuman animals about the fine details of their sensory acuity (Moody, Stebbins, Johnsson, & Hawkins, 1976a; Stebbins, Brown, & Petersen, 1984; Stebbins, 1970) and to the findings themselves that describe the resolving power and the perceptual capabilities of animals with reference to the many dimensions of acoustic stimulation.

Animal conditioning techniques and their refinement have made it possible to bridge the language gap between animal subject and human experimenter. Under carefully formulated training procedures animals learn to behave differentially to differing conditions of stimulation. They may come to respond when a stimulus is present and refrain from responding in its absence. Psychophysical procedures such as constant stimuli or tracking are then employed to determine statistically that fine line we define as a threshold. More complex training programs are designed to uncover an animal's ability to localize the source of a sound in space (Brown, Beecher, Moody, & Stebbins, 1978), to provide evidence of frequency selectivity as in psychophysical tuning curves (Serafin, Moody, & Stebbins, 1982), or to discriminate between the subtle variants of a biologically relevant signal such as a call that might be uttered by a conspecific (Beecher, Petersen, Zoloth, Moody, & Stebbins, 1979; Petersen, Beecher, Zoloth, Moody, & Stebbins, 1978). It is the results of programs like these that characterize recent developments in comparative psychoacoustics.

The astonishing progress in recent years in auditory physiology, morphology, and human psychoacoustics (see other chapters in this book) has added considerably to our knowledge of the basic mechanisms in normal and impaired hearing and, at the same time, has increased the demand for similar advances in comparative psychoacoustics. As the structural and physiological complexities of the inner ear, for example, are unraveled in experimental animal models, it becomes increasingly urgent to assay, behaviorally, the many dimensions of sensory experience in these same animals. That we can do so is in large measure due to the animal psychophysicist's ability to describe an animal's hearing in all its many and varied facets.

In this chapter we examine three recent developments in comparative psychoacoustics which emphasize the variety of information we can obtain from nonhuman observers. The first underscores an interest in matters of concern to an animal in interaction with its environment. At issue is the biological significance of the sounds to which an animal attends. Are there, for example, perceptual specializations in the auditory system for human speech or for the commmunication sounds of a species? The behavioral evidence from animal subjects suggests that there are. In the second part of the chapter a closer tie is sought between morphological and physiological findings on the one hand, and behavior on the other. When we observe differences in sensory acuity between closely related species, for example, do we also find these differences reflected in variation in peripheral sensory structures and, too, in underlying physiological differences? In the third part of the chapter selective tissue destruction is considered as a means of estimating the behavioral function of that tissue in the normal state. The antibiotic kanamycin destroys basal cochlear outer hair cells while leaving inner hair cells largely intact and presumably functioning normally in the ears of some animals. If threshold sensitivity in that region is impaired but intensity discrimination is unaffected, can we then argue that the outer hair cells play an important role in signal detection near threshold but fail to contribute to the fine resolution of intensity differences?

We are not suggesting that we have final and definitive answers to questions such as these, but we do contend that the methods and findings of comparative psychoacoustics will be a major factor in their eventual resolution. This chapter is illustrative rather than exhaustive and presents a picture of animal psychophysics not as an isolated technique applied to a few "humanlike" animal models, but as part of an integrated approach to the study of auditory processing in all vertebrate species.

THE COMPARATIVE PERCEPTION
OF BIOLOGICAL SIGNALS

The idea that naturally occurring biologically relevant acoustic signals might be processed and even perceived differently than the tones and clicks manufactured in the laboratory was cogently expressed in the proceedings of a workshop edited by Worden and Galambos in 1972. Recent physiological studies of coding and processing at almost every level of the nervous system have offered support for this notion by demonstrating that individual nerve cells are sensitive to certain key features in complex, biologically relevant stimuli (Newman & Wollberg, 1973; Sachs, Woolf, & Sinnott, 1980; Suga, 1978). A hierarchical arrangement has been suggested for the auditory system, with progressively greater abstraction of the acoustic signal between the peripheral receptor and the higher sensory areas of the brain (Bullock, 1977; Sachs et al., 1980). The arrangement is far from simple, however. At least in mammals, and perhaps in birds at higher levels in the nervous system, neuronal responses are labile and dependent on, among other things, selective attention and conditioning history (Manley & Mueller-Preuss, 1978; Miller, Beaton, O'Connor, & Pfingst, 1974).

Although we have learned a great deal about transduction and sensory processing by using tones and clicks as stimuli, it is clear that the nervous system has evolved, at least in part, for the effective reception and processing of information obtained directly from the environment. Such complex information-bearing signals must then be subjected to analysis and treatment at many levels of the nervous system. The resulting behavior of the animal as potential predator, prey, or mate provides it with a selective advantage in its interaction with other animals and with the world around it.

It is behaviors such as these under natural conditions that have occupied the attention of evolutionary biologists and ethologists. New techniques, increased objectivity, and fresh theoretical approaches (e.g., sociobiology; see, for example, Dawkins & Krebs, 1978) have brought forth new findings in the area of animal communication (Green, 1975; Green & Marler, 1979; Peters, 1980; Seyfarth, Cheney, & Marler, 1980). At the communication end of the hearing–communication continuum we are beginning to discover something about the actual function of different biological signals within the natural context of the activities of conspecifics in a social group.

However, there are significant questions about sensory function that cannot be addressed by either physiologists or field behaviorists. Inquiry into the resolution and perception of acoustic signals requires the analytic techniques of animal psychophysics in the laboratory setting. Electrical potentials recorded from the afferent pathway in response to sound can rarely be substituted for behavioral measures of sensory acuity obtained from an intact, trained animal. At the same time perception is not amenable to study in the field because of the lack of control over the acoustic signals and the inability to separate them from their rich and complex environmental context.

It is this separation from context that enables the psychophysicist to chart so precisely the relationship between signal and perception.

The strategy is not without its limitations. The difficulties in treating complex stimuli are immediately obvious; it quickly becomes clear why we used clicks and tones for so many years. Biological signals almost defy accurate measurement (beyond a somewhat qualitative sonographic display). Such stimuli are multidimensional and it is always difficult to determine the specific properties or components of the signals that are driving particular behaviors. The neurophysiologist confronts a similar dilemma in attempting to decide if a particular neuron is a "call detector" or merely sensitive to a particular feature of the call. Comparable problems face the speech scientist who often deals with the component parts of speech signals in an attempt to determine their role in human speech perception. Moreover, under putative natural conditions, visual and/or olfactory stimulation may potentiate or influence in some manner an animal's perception of an acoustic event. There are clearly constraints on the psychophysical approach in the laboratory; it is isolationist and analytic. It is, however, clear that perceptual questions cannot be answered satisfactorily in any other way with the requisite rigor and reliability.

The psychophysical experiment is designed simply to measure capability. Generally the questions are structured so as to secure unequivocal information regarding the resolving power or the discriminative acuity of the sensory system as reflected in the behavior of the intact animal in response to stimulation. Whereas the field biologist may ask, "What does the animal do in its natural surroundings?" the psychophysicist, in removing the animal from those surroundings, wants to know what it can do — that is, what limits must be placed on its ability to perceive environmental events. There is nothing new or startling about these comments, but we too often lose sight of one important distinction between field and laboratory in simple terms of "can" and "does." For example, under natural conditions animals do orient to certain sounds that may represent prey, predator, or mate. Their ability to localize and identify the source may well be one of their most important adaptations. The accuracy with which they do so may be a complex function of acoustic signal structure, environmental conditions, the availability of input from other sensory modalities, and so on. To begin to tease apart the relative influence of these various factors and to assign a specific contribution to the auditory system we must know what that system "can do" in the absence of the participation by other systems and other influences.

The psychophysicist who must deal with biological signals is unquestionably dependent on the observations of the trained field behaviorist, who plays the major role in determining the significance of these signals. Quantitative field research with good instrumental recording and observational techniques provides the laboratory scientist with important information regarding the function of acoustic signals in the social–biological context. With their communicative or other function identified, laboratory research can proceed with an analysis of an animal's ability to resolve such signals, to discriminate between them (the basis of individual or kin recognition, for example), to localize them in space, and so on. Collaboration between field and laboratory is a sine qua non for such research to be carried out effectively.

The motivation behind these experiments is related to a consuming interest in our biological origins. More to the point, it is the evolution of human language, of our ability to speak it and to interpret its acoustic message, and the long history of an evolving relationship between perception and communication that forms the basis of these inquiries.

Experimental questions generally have been of two kinds. In one form of inquiry animals have been examined for their ability to perceive human speech sounds, such as phonemes, categorically. In part, this is an attempt to resolve a theoretical controversy that goes to the very roots of human speech perception. Is the processing of speech signals qualitatively similar to processing of simpler (tonal) stimuli? Put in another way, can the perception of speech be accounted for in the same psychoacoustic framework that has dealt so effectively with simple sinusoids? Or is the whole more than the sum of its parts? Can we agree with Alvin Liberman (1982) that "speech is special"? The argument centers around acoustic versus phonetic levels of processing. If animals, presumably without recourse to phonetic levels of processing, can be shown to perceive speech sounds similarly to man, then, the argument goes, a fairly strong case can be made for a simpler acoustic interpretation of speech perception.

A second, quite different, series of experimental questions is directed at an animal's ability to perceive, under controlled laboratory conditions and in the absence of other cues from the natural context, the sounds of other animals — most often those transmitted vocally by members of its own species. We know that conspecifics share a vocal repertoire at least part of which is species typical. For many vertebrate as well as invertebrate species such signals function as species-isolating mechanisms. Can we find similar specificity, whether ontogenetically or phylogenetically established, in an animal's ability to perceive such signals? The signals would function in identification, recognition, localization, and so on.

It is, of course, well known that animals respond to the sounds of human language. The basis on which they do so is still poorly understood. Discrimination between simple vowel sounds in the laboratory is easily accomplished by cats (Dewson, 1964), monkeys (Dewson, Pribram, & Lynch, 1969), chinchillas (Burdick & Miller, 1975), and dogs (Baru, 1975), and is maintained in spite of changes in speaker (male to female), in sound intensity, in the number of formants present, in duration, and even when the vowels are synthesized (see the review by Miller, 1977). Monkeys have little difficulty in discriminating between phonemes such as /ba/ and /da/, either presented by a speaker or when synthesized (Sinnott, Beecher, Moody, & Stebbins, 1976; Morse & Snowdon, 1975). Using the techniques of animal psychophysics based on either a conditioned avoidance paradigm (see Miller, 1970) or positive reinforcement (Stebbins, 1970), animals have exhibited a considerable degree of perceptual constancy in transferring across stimulus conditions. In general, animals appear to be somewhat less acute than humans in making these discriminations of human speech elements, which may be a reflection of their higher difference thresholds for tonal stimuli (see Fay, 1974; Nelson & Keister, 1978; Stebbins, 1975). But, in fact, are these differences between man and other animals in the discrimination of speech sounds attributable to differences in sensory acuity to simple stimuli, per se, or is man's possession of a special linguistic feature detector or phonetic processor the key factor?

The results of earlier work by Miller, Kuhl, and Burdick and associates (1978) on the chinchilla's perception of speech sounds, and Kuhl and Padden's more recent work on the discrimination of speech sounds by monkeys (Kuhl & Padden, 1982, 1983), would certainly argue against a strict "for humans only" interpretation of speech perception. Clearly, as Kuhl, Miller, and others have shown, many animals are capable of making the fine auditory discriminations required by the elements of speech without much greater difficulty than they exhibit in discriminating between pure tones. The distinction, then, between man and other animals in the perception of speech is more likely quantitative than qualitative. Sensitivity to certain features in complex biologically meaningful signals such as speech and animal communication may be shared between man and other animals, as Miller (1982) has suggested. At the same time the discrimination of variation in feature parameters may be more acute in man. Whether this enhanced acuity can be derived in a straightforward manner from the psychoacoustic data is not yet known. It would be premature to close with an explanation of speech perception based merely on psychoacoustic findings. In fact, research with other animals on the perception of species-typical signals, meager though it is, would indicate that a simple psychoacoustic interpretation of the perception of communicatively relevant sounds may be insufficient to account for the data. The relationship between perception and communication is probably not that simple.

If animals, like humans, exhibit perceptual constancy, as Burdick and Miller (1975) and others have shown, they also discriminate along speech sound continua as humans do and, in fact, categorize these speech sounds in much the same way. Given, for example, a continuum of sounds between /da/ and /ta/, a gradual change in signal structure is accompanied by a discontinuous change in the perception of that signal: A perceptual boundary occurs between /da/ and /ta/ with signals on one side identified as /da/ and those on the other side as /ta/. In addition, discrimination between speech signals that have been identified similarly is poor, but across the boundary between signals that have been identified differently it is very good. Like perceptual constancy, categorical perception has been considered an important hallmark of speech perception and as a species-specific characteristic of man. Kuhl and Miller's chinchillas have provided convincing evidence to the contrary (Kuhl & Miller, 1978). Their animals were trained to discriminate end points of different continua (/ba-pa/, /da-ta/, and /ga-ka/), and then tested for their generalization to intermediate values. The results were consistent with those for English-speaking human listeners; the animals perceived the speech sounds categorically, setting up boundaries near the same locations on the continua as did humans. An example from the /da-ta/ continuum is shown in Figure 1-1. Further, the location depended on the place of articulation – bilabial (/ba-pa/), alveolar (/da-ta/), or velar (/ga-ka/) – in both chinchillas and humans. In a subsequent experiment Kuhl (1981) was able to show that when chinchillas were tested for their discrimination along the entire speech sound continuum (in this instance /da/-/ta/) they were most acute close to the previously determined category boundary.

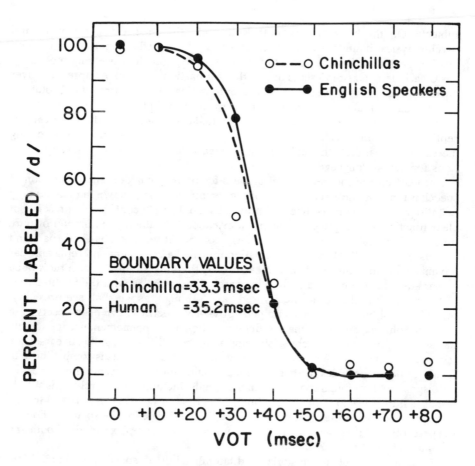

Figure 1-1. Mean percentage of /d/ responses by chinchilla and human subjects to synthetic speech sounds constructed to simulate a continuum ranging from /da/ to /ta/. The animals were trained on the two "endpoint" stimuli (0 and +80 ms VOT) and then tested with stimuli ranging from +10 to +70 ms in a generalization paradigm (feedback always arranged to indicate a correct response) (from Kuhl & Miller, 1978).

Further support for categorical perception of speech sounds in animals has been provided by recent studies on nonhuman primates. For example, Kuhl has trained Japanese monkeys to discriminate between pairs of speech sounds along continua of voice onset time (/ba–pa/, /da–ta/, and /ga–ka/) (Kuhl & Padden, 1982) and, in a second study, place of articulation (/b, d, g/) (Kuhl & Padden, 1983). In both experiments discrimination was enhanced when members of a stimulus pair were from opposite sides of the category boundary established in prior experiments with human subjects. On the basis of their data Kuhl and Miller suggest "a set of 'natural psychophysical boundaries' based on rather simple acoustic properties" to account for the categorical findings rather than the earlier phonetic processing model.

Clearly language represents one of the last bastions of human supremacy over lower animals in the sense that it is thought to indicate a discontinuity in evolution, or at least a quantal jump for man over ancestral forms in the scheme of things. But with evidence that other animals show perceptual constancy for, and categorical perception of, human speech sounds, this view has begun to erode since it is becoming increasingly clear that other animals show at least some of the perceptual specializations for human language.

At least part of the morphological basis for both production and perception of speech is found in the cerebral hemispheric asymmetry long known in man but only just discovered in animals. Recent findings by Pohl (1983) confirm the presence of clear functional perceptual asymmetries in baboons in the discrimination of pure tones and musical chords, but particularly consonant vowels (/ba/ and /pa/) and vowels (/a/ and /i/). Monaural stimulation revealed a consistent and replicable ear advantage in individual animals as measured by their discriminative accuracy. Such an ear advantage implies an underlying cerebral asymmetry with the targeted area of the brain contralateral to the favored ear. Although, as we shall see presently, other forms of both productive and perceptive asymmetries have been observed in animals, Pohl's experiment is the first demonstration of the phenomenon using speech-like stimuli. The results are robust, showing a highly statistically significant ear advantage in all animals. The similarity to findings with human subjects is compelling and, if substantiated, provides further evidence of some form of perceptual readiness or predisposition for human speech in other animals, including ancestral forms. While it makes little sense to imply that animals in man's lineage were preadapted for the perception of signals they had not yet heard, it does argue for the specialization for the perception of those acoustic features common to the complex sounds of both animal and human communication.

If animals are able to categorize and lateralize human speech and, in addition, generalize successfully across wide variations in signal structure (perceptual constancy), how then do they process their own communication sounds or other acoustic signals that assume a greater biological significance to them? Sinnott and her colleagues, having first determined that the normal hearing capabilities of red-winged blackbirds and brown-headed cowbirds were essentially the same, examined these birds for their ability to discriminate features of blackbird and cowbird song (Sinnott, 1980). The songs of the two species are shown in sonograph form in Figure 1-2. When the longer terminal portion of the song was separated from the brief introductory notes the birds were significantly more accurate at identifying their own conspecific song (see Figure 1-3). Whether this form of species-specific perceptual specialization is acquired in the course of normal development or is present at birth is an important unanswered question, but it in no way detracts from the clear and unequivocal evidence for the relationship between the perception of a signal and its biological relevance.

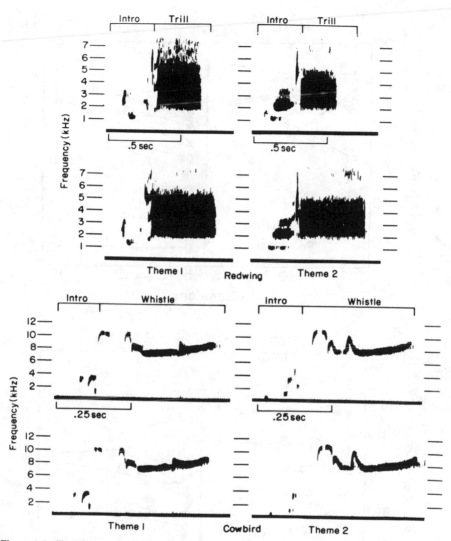

Figure 1-2. (Top) Sonograms of four tokens of red-winged blackbird song themes. (Bottom) Sonograms of four tokens of brown-headed cowbird song themes. Brackets indicate the point where introductory notes were separated from trills during the tests with isolated elements (from Sinnott, 1980).

Our own research on the Japanese monkey (*Macaca fuscata*) (Beecher et al., 1979; Petersen et al., 1978; Stebbins, 1978) is supportive of the work of Sinnott and her colleagues and confirms the notion of species-specific perceptual specialization for species calls. Green's earlier field research (Green, 1975) on the structure and function

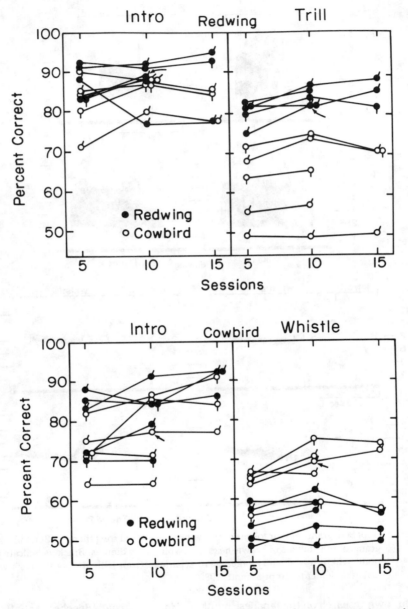

Figure 1-3. The percentage of correct identification scores for red-winged blackbird song elements (top) and brown-headed cowbird song elements (bottom). Males are denoted by a mark at the upper right of circle and females with a mark at bottom center (from Sinnott, 1980).

of the Japanese monkey's communication system made it possible for our laboratory group to examine perceptual specificity in this species. Among his findings Green had pointed to a possible vocal continuum in the Japanese monkey communication system resembling continua for human speech sounds. The "coo" or clear call shown in Figure 1-4 contains a brief but gradual frequency modulation (an increase followed by decrease in frequency) that may occur in any one of several temporal locations in the call. If the pitch shift occurs early in the call (SE or smooth early), as in Figure 1-4, it most often serves as a contact call by a young monkey that has strayed from its nearest kin, or by an older animal that has wandered out of visual contact with the main troop. A pitch shift late in the call (SL or smooth late), on the other hand, functions also as a contact call but is usually given by an estrous female as a form of sexual solicitation early in the courtship.

We asked in the laboratory if these calls had any particular perceptual significance for the Japanese monkey. In the design of the experiment we included as controls animals of the same genus, different species (*M. nemestrina*), as well as those of an entirely different genus, *Cercopithecus*. In the first experiment animals were required to discriminate between a considerable sample of SEs and SLs – with the critical variable being the temporal position of the pitch shift or frequency modulation within the call. The experiment began simply with one example of each call variant, and then, as animals mastered the discrimination (better than 90% correct), additional calls of each type were added. The Japanese monkeys in all instances showed more rapid learning of the discrimination than did the controls, who found each stage of the discrimination extremely difficult. Results from several of the animals are shown in Figure 1-5. To counter a potential objection with regard to greater cognitive abilities for Japanese monkeys, different animals were selected for a new discrimination that was based not on the temporal position of the pitch shift (peak position) but instead on the starting or initial frequency of the calls. Such calls normally vary in fundamental frequency. Animals were now required to discriminate on the basis of starting frequency and to ignore the temporal position of the frequency modulation within the call. The tables were turned. The Japanese monkeys found the discrimination of this (presumably to them) irrelevant dimension extremely difficult and required much longer to learn the discrimination than the subjects of the control species, who had little difficulty in mastering it.

Again, whether the discrimination of this call feature (peak position) by the Japanese monkey is based on experience is not known, but it does seem clear from these data that this is a feature for which the Japanese monkey shows convincing evidence of perceptual specialization.

In the course of these experiments the calls were presented randomly to the right or to the left ear in order to determine whether there was an ear advantage for these species-specific stimuli which might then argue for hemispheric laterality, and thus additionally for perceptual specialization. The five Japanese macaques showed a significant right ear advantage, the three other macaques showed no ear advantage, but the one nonmacaque (a vervet monkey) also showed a significant right ear advantage.

The results on the discrimination and lateralization of animal (nonhuman) commu-

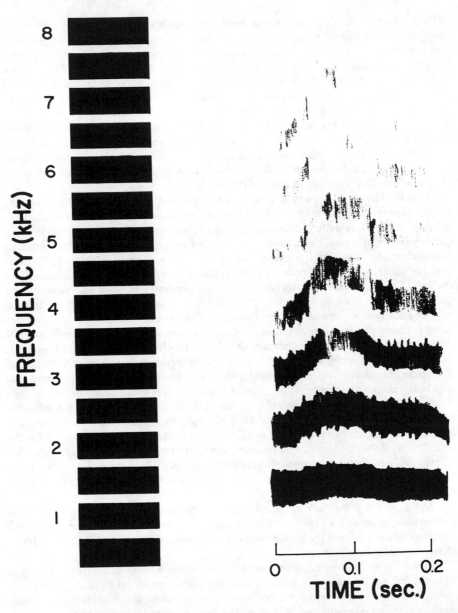

Figure 1-4. Sonograph of a Japanese monkey clear call. From Green, S. 1975). Variation of vocal pattern with social situation in the Japanese monkey (*Macaca fuscata*): A field study. In L. Rosenblum (Ed.), *Primate behavior* (Vol. 4, pp. 1–102). New York, Academic Press. Reprinted with permission.

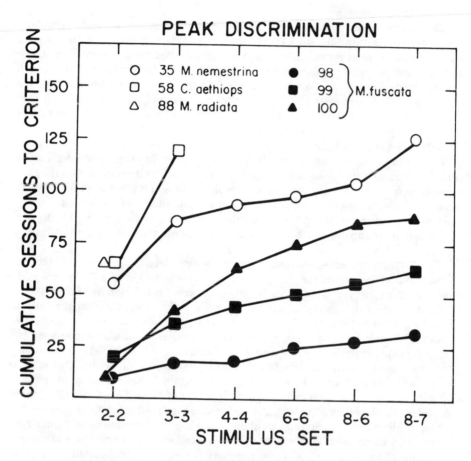

Figure 1-5. Cumulative sessions to criterion for the six animals as a function of the size of the stimulus set. For example, "8-7" means that there were 8 SLs and 7 SEs in the set, "4-4" that there were 4 of each. Thus, the horizontal dimension represents increasing complexity or difficulty of the discrimination. M58 was unable to reach criterion at 3-3, M88 at 2-2; they were switched to another, easier version of the discrimination (not shown) (from Beecher et al., 1979).

nication sounds provides an interesting and supportive parallel to the findings on the discrimination and lateralization of human speech sounds by animals. To offer a theoretical account of the origins of human and animal language on the basis of such preliminary evidence would be premature. However, new directions are indicated, and a rethinking of old theoretical positions, particularly those based so exclusively on the results from human subjects, seems in order.

The perception of acoustic communication – that is, the identification of and the discrimination between species signals, was only one of the roles imposed on the auditory system in the course of evolution. At least in the mammals, and particularly in the primates, it has attained a level of complexity in form and function well beyond what we observe in other animals. The pressures imposed by a terrestrial existence and concomitant social organization were very likely the driving forces behind such developments. Perhaps an even more primitive, important, and ubiquitous function of the auditory system is its role in the accurate location of a sound source. It may mean the difference between eating or being eaten, and it certainly helps to ensure successful reproduction by finding an appropriate mate.

While classical theories of sound localization have been founded on clicks and pure tones as locatable stimuli, we still know very little about the characteristics of complex, naturally occurring stimuli and the ease or difficulty with which they are localized in space. One conventional measure of localization is in terms of the subject's accuracy in identifying the change in location of a sound source from a standard or fixed position in space. Clearly, the smaller the detectable change, measured in degrees of arc around the subject and from the standard position, the greater the localization acuity.

In several experiments in our laboratory by Brown, Beecher, Moody, and Stebbins (1978, 1979), we examined the ability of nonhuman primates to localize several variants of species calls. Our hypothesis, based on an earlier prediction by Marler (1955), was that the clear or contact calls described previously would be more difficult to localize than the more guttural or strident barks or growls that these animals use in both inter- and intragroup encounters. Our hypothesis was also encouraged by earlier evidence from Brown and associates (Brown, Beecher, Moody, & Stebbins, 1980) that signal bandwidth was directly related to localization acuity. Our results on call localization supported the hypothesis. The animals had significantly greater difficulty localizing the clear calls (angular distances of 10–15° were required) than the noisier calls (less than 5° of separation between sound source locations were necessary for localization). The findings from this experiment are presented in Figure 1-6. Further research on the characteristics of the clear call itself uncovered some interesting findings. The extent to which the clear call is frequency modulated appears to determine the accuracy with which it will be localized. The modulation is apparently a way of increasing the bandwidth of the call, thus enhancing its localization. As in the detection and discrimination of communicatively relevant calls, their localization appears to be intimately related to their acoustic structure and, in all likelihood (see the recent review by Brown, 1983), in turn to their social function.

The findings, admittedly few and preliminary, argue against extreme theoretical positions. Both a strict phonetic processor model and an explanation based solely on pure tone psychoacoustics seem limited in their ability to account for the data. A third possibility, which incorporates certain key aspects of the other two, suggests that there may be feature-sensitive neural elements in the auditory systems of man and certain other animals that respond to distinctive properties common to both human speech and animal communication sounds. Frequency modulation (FM) is one such feature that often appears as a distinctive and even defining property of stop consonants in speech, of bird song, of echo-ranging signals in certain bats, of

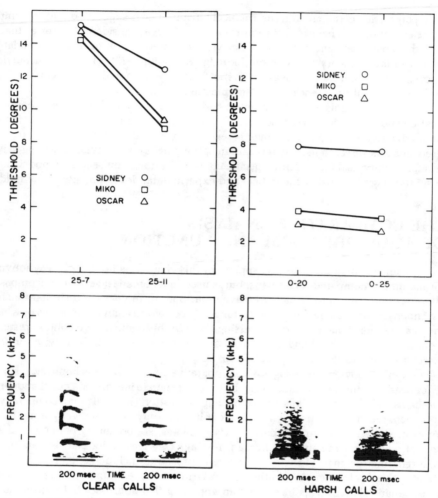

Figure 1-6. Minimum audible angles for two clear calls and two harsh calls (upper panel). The bottom panel presents sonograms corresponding to each vocalization (from Brown et al., 1979).

contact calls in macaque monkeys, and so on. FM detectors have been discovered in electrophysiological experiments with animals (Evans & Whitfield, 1964; Suga, 1973; and others) and hypothesized in psychophysical adaptation experiments with human subjects (Kay & Matthews, 1972; Regan & Tansley, 1979; and others).

The concept of feature sensitivity is certainly not new, but in suggesting a compromise it offers an alternative theoretical approach to the study of the perception of communication sounds than either the phonetic processing model or the psychoacoustic one. The former is highly anthropocentric. Although it pays lip service to physiology by hypothesizing certain neural control mechanisms, it does suggest a quantum jump in the evolution of language that requires a time interval considerably shorter than even the most recent and radical neo-Darwinians would be willing to accommodate in their saltatory theory of evolution (Eldredge & Gould, 1972). The psychoacoustic theory, on the other hand, at least in its most extreme form makes little concession to the perceptual uniqueness of communication sounds.

A concern of animal behaviorists interested in the broader study of animal communication and perception is that theories of human speech perception, whatever their other advantages or limitations, may be exercising undue influence with regard to directions that research in animal communication might take. Human language may be a far-too-atypical form of intraspecific communication to be used as a model and to set the stage for further theoretical and experimental developments in the field.

THE COMPARATIVE ANALYSIS
OF AUDITORY FORM AND FUNCTION

The term comparative, as it is applied in this chapter, is not simply a synonym for mammals "compared" to humans, but is used in its broadest sense to encompass all vertebrate species for which we have data. Both differences and similarities in psychophysical functions from a broad range of species are analyzed in terms of what they can tell us about auditory processing. Within this comparative context results from neurophysiological and anatomical studies have been combined with, or are directly related to, psychophysical findings.

One of the obvious advantages of a comparative approach to psychophysical studies of hearing is that animal models can be used to generate information about auditory mechanisms in humans. While animal modeling is a strong rationale for a comparative approach, it can also be unduly restrictive if it is the only rationale. Why study fish, for example, when mammals, particularly primates, are obviously better suited as animal models for the study of human hearing? One way to look at this question is to redefine the goals of the comparative approach to include general knowledge about species differences in addition to similarities between humans and their close mammalian relatives. It is likely that an approach that addresses both differences and similarities will provide us with critical insight into (1) the evolution of auditory systems and (2) general principles of auditory processing in all vertebrates. These ideas are certainly not new, but have only recently received direct attention in the general study of hearing (Popper & Fay, 1980).

We have just begun to compile a catalogue of hearing capabilities for various vertebrate groups, including fish (Fay & Popper, 1980; Hawkins, 1981), birds (Dooling, 1980; Sachs, Sinnott, & Hienz, 1978) and mammals (Ehret, 1977; Gourevitch, 1980; Stebbins, 1980). The value of cataloging is twofold: (1) it provides a more detailed and generalized view of vertebrate hearing – that is, a context in which human hearing can be better understood, and (2) it allows us to examine similarities and differences in hearing capabilities in relation to their physiological and anatomical correlates.

Correlations between hearing capabilities and differences in peripheral auditory structures often point to the role of structural variation in mechanical processing at the periphery. For example, different frequency ranges of hearing in terrestrial vertebrates appear to be related to different middle ear characteristics (Ehret, 1977; Saunders & Johnstone, 1972) and to basilar membrane dimensions (Manley, 1971). Perhaps one of the clearest demonstrations of a structural correlate to psychophysical findings comes from recent comparative work on the greater horseshoe bat. Psychophysical measures of auditory sensitivity (Long & Schnitzler, 1975) and frequency resolution (Long, 1977, 1980, 1981) show a restricted region of sensitivity around 83 kHz. This sharp tuning is unlike that seen for any other animal and has been related to structural anomalies of the basilar membrane (Bruns, 1980; Neuweiler, 1980). Broader psychophysical sampling from animals, such as the horseshoe bat, which differ from others in peripheral structure, will greatly enhance our understanding of which architectural features of the ear may be important for mechanical filtering at the auditory periphery.

Until recently comparative sampling has been largely incidental to the primary direction of research. Psychoacoustic research on fishes (Coombs & Popper, 1979, 1982), however, has capitalized on the extraordinary diversity among species in both ultrastructural and gross features of the auditory periphery. The focus of this research has been to compare fishes with such differences in the periphery for the express purpose of demonstrating hearing differences. Fish species were chosen on the basis of differences in the relationship between the swimbladder (an air-filled, sound pressure-transducing cavity) and the inner ear, although several additional features of the auditory system differed as well. Results from these studies have clearly demonstrated dramatic differences in both audiograms and psychophysical tuning curves, as shown in Figure 1-7. Furthermore, differences in these psychophysical functions could be "grouped" into two general categories or types of auditory systems – those with and those without specializations for bringing air-filled cavities close to the inner ear.

While differences in hearing sensitivity could be related to differences in the middle-ear analog of these fishes (i.e., the absence or presence of a structural link between the air cavity and the inner ear), other hearing differences are not so easily understood relative to morphology. Thus, while this approach is not capable of isolating specific structural correlates of auditory capabilities, it can identify functional differences that can later be probed with other physiological and anatomical techniques for underlying mechanisms.

Equally important is the potential afforded by this psychophysical approach for the study of the evolution of the auditory system. What is of particular interest here is that taxonomically unrelated species having nonhomologous air-cavity specializations were found to have similar hearing capabilities, whereas species differing in the relationship between swimbladder and ear, even though they were closely related (i.e., members of the same family), were shown to have marked differences in hearing capabilities (Figure 1-7). The tentative suggestion from these results is that air-cavity/inner ear specializations have evolved independently in several different species of fish to perform similar functions (Popper & Coombs, 1980, 1982). Clearly, animal

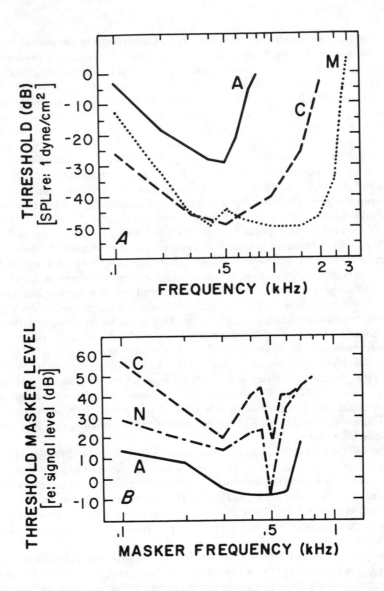

Figure 1-7. Audiograms (A) and psychophysical tuning curves (B) from species of fish differing in the peripheral anatomy of the auditory system. The goldfish, *Carassius auratus* (C), the soldierfish, *Myripristis kuntee* (M) and the clown knifefish, *Notopterus chitala* (N) all have adaptations for linking the swimbladder to the inner ear, whereas the squirrelfish, *Adioryx xantherythrus* (A) does not. Note that *Adioryx* and *Myripristis* are members of the same family, but that other species are from different orders.

psychophysics can play a vital role in determining how or if the actual auditory function of these phylogenetically distant, yet apparently convergent systems, are similar.

Further psychophysical evidence for species differences in auditory processing has come from studies conducted in independent laboratories. Species-specific differences in the temporal modulation transfer function (TMTF) (see below), for example, have recently led to some interesting questions about how animals process temporally modulated information. Not only is the TMTF an elegant example of how a psychophysical approach first applied to the visual system (Cornsweet, 1970) can be adapted for use with the auditory system (Viemeister, 1977), but it is also an efficient way of systematically and quantitatively analyzing auditory capabilities in the temporal domain. Given the paucity of psychophysical techniques for analyzing temporal capabilities relative to techniques being used for spectral analyses, this is indeed a welcome development.

The TMTF is a general description of a system's capacity to detect amplitude fluctuations in various signals. Either a noise carrier or tonal carrier is multiplied by a DC-biased sinusoidal signal, the modulator, to produce an amplitude-modulated (AM) signal. The waveform fine structure of this signal is determined by the waveform of the carrier (F_c), but the waveform envelope undergoes changes in amplitude at the rate of the modulation frequency (F_m), as illustrated in Figure 1-8. The TMTF is a plot of the modulation depth (m) of the AM signal that is just discriminable from the unmodulated carrier as a function of the modulation frequency.

For noise carriers with a flat spectrum, only temporal cues (time-varying changes in amplitude) are available for the AM detection task, because the spectrum of the modulated signal remains flat (Figure 1-8). Noise TMTFs are qualitatively similar for chinchilla (Salvi, Giraudi, Henderson, & Hamernik, 1982a), parakeet (Dooling & Searcy, 1981), and man (Fay, 1980; Viemeister, 1977, 1979), in that they are relatively flat out to a particular modulation frequency, but show signs of rolling off beyond that frequency (see Figure 1-9a). The 3-dB down point from where they begin rolling off (f_0) can be used to determine the minimum integration time constant (where $T = (2f_0)^{-1}$). This value is about 3 ms for humans, mammals, and birds (Dooling & Searcy, 1981; Fay, 1980; Salvi et al., 1982; Viemeister, 1977, 1979), and can be regarded as a measure of temporal resolution comparable to other measures of minimum integration times (Dooling, Zoloth, & Baylis, 1978; Giraudi, Salvi, Henderson, & Hamernik, 1980; Salvi et al., 1982a; Wilkenson & Howse, 1975). The noise function for the goldfish, however, differs qualitatively from that in other vertebrates in that it is essentially flat and shows no signs of rolling off out to 400 Hz (Fay, 1980) (Figure 1-9b). What this means in terms of a minimum integration time for the goldfish is not clear, but it is apparent that the goldfish's ability to detect amplitude changes does not decline at higher modulation frequencies and in fact may be superior to that in other vertebrates at those modulation rates.

For tonal carriers both temporal and spectral cues in the form of side bands (energy bands located at frequencies of $F_c + F_m$ and at $F_c - F_m$) (Figure 1-8) are available for AM detection. The slope of an 800-Hz TMTF for the goldfish increases at a rate of about 3 dB/octave up to modulation frequencies as high as 200 Hz (Fay, 1980)

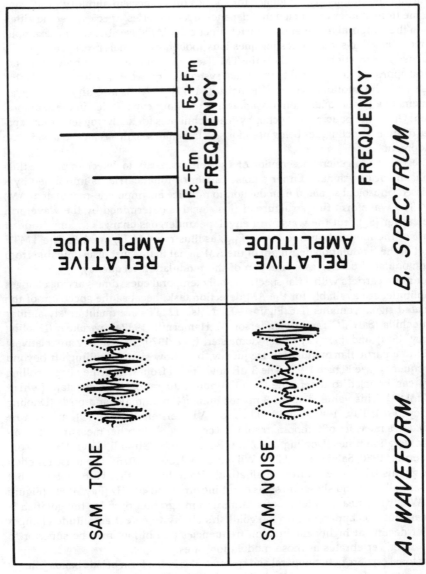

Figure 1-8. (A) Schematic representation of the waveform fine structure (Fc) and envelope (Fm) of a sinusoidally amplitude modulated (SAM) tone and noise. (B) Spectra corresponding to the SAM noise and tone.

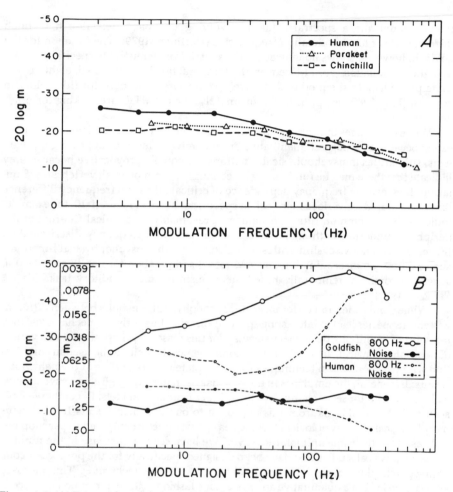

Figure 1-9. (A) Temporal modulation transfer functions obtained with SAM broad band white noise for humans (H) (Viemeister, 1979), parakeet (P) (Dooling & Searcy, 1981) and chinchilla (C) (Salvi et al., 1982). (B) TMTF's obtained with two SAM carriers: an 800-Hz tone (open circles) and white noise that has been low-pass filtered at 800 Hz after modulation (filled circles) for humans (----) and goldfish (——) (from Fay, 1980).

(Figure 1-9b). In contrast, this function in humans decreases rapidly above modulation frequencies of 5 Hz before it reverses and begins increasing again at a modulation frequency around 25 Hz (Fay, 1980). This is particularly interesting since the complex shape of the human function has been interpreted as evidence of a temporal analysis of the modulation envelope at low frequencies (i.e., the detection of a "beat-like" phenomenon) and a spectral solution involving side band detection (i.e., pitch differences) for high modulation frequencies (Hartman, 1979). The function for the goldfish, however, shows no indication of a switch from temporal to spectral analyses at higher modulation rates. Moreover, the temporal fidelity with which eighth nerve units phase lock to the modulation envelope appears to account for this ability in goldfish (Fay, 1980; see p. 312). Unfortunately, tonal TMTFs are lacking for other vertebrates.

While differences in hearing capabilities between vertebrate species may be interesting because they suggest quantitative or qualitative differences in hearing mechanisms, similarities in psychophysical functions are equally provocative because they indicate that there may be fundamental mechanisms common to all vertebrates. Similarities between the frequency dependence of critical ratios and frequency difference limens measured for various mammalian species as shown in Figure 1-10, for example, indicate that a common filter mechanism (presumably mechanical filtering at the periphery) underlies both signal detection in noise and frequency discrimination (Ehret, 1977). Likewise, similarities in the shape of other psychophysical functions, such as duration discrimination and AM rate discrimination for fish (Figure 1-10b), suggest a common, temporally based mechanism for these auditory tasks (Fay & Passow, 1982).

While similarities and differences in psychophysical functions between different vertebrate species lead to interesting speculations about underlying mechanisms, they fall short of identifying these mechanisms. For this reason it is important that a variety of neurophysiological, anatomical, and biomechanical techniques be used in combination with psychophysical techniques for a complete understanding of the behavioral results. In general, the emphasis in the past has been to compare human psychophysical results with those using invasive techniques in animal models. Recently we have seen a shift in emphasis from this approach to one in which results from various morphological and physiological techniques can be directly compared to psychophysical results in the same animal. Moreover, we have seen an increase in the number of psychophysical studies that have been designed specifically for the purpose of comparing psychophysical results to results obtained with other techniques. This approach allows us to look in a quantitative and systematic fashion at the contribution of processing occurring at different levels of the auditory system as measured by a variety of procedures to the processing of the whole intact system as measured psychophysically.

For example, relatively simple comparisons between psychophysical and neural measures of hearing sensitivity can be made at the level of the eighth nerve (Fay, 1978b; Konishi, 1969; Kiang, Watanabe, Thomas, & Clark, 1965) and from various levels of the brain (Dooling & Walsh, 1976; Henderson, Hamernik, Woodford, Sitler, & Salvi, 1973; Jun, Coombs, Fay, Popper, & Saidel, 1982; Long & Schnitzler, 1975; Schnitzler, 1973). In addition, positive correlations can be drawn between psychophysical measures of sensitivity and anatomical measures of innervation density (Burda & Voldrich, 1980; Sachs et al., 1978) and between noise- and drug-induced hearing loss and hair cell damage, as discussed in the final section of this chapter.

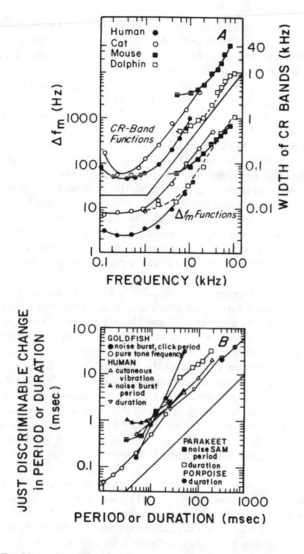

Figure 1-10. (A) Frequency dependence of the width of CR bands and of the frequency difference limen (f_m) for various mammalian species (from Ehret, 1977). (B) A comparison between several vertebrate species drawn by Fay and Passow (1982) for temporal discriminability functions on (1) the just-detectable change in periods between noise bursts for different noise burst repetition rates (noise burst period); (2) the just-detectable difference in silent interval durations delineated by tone burst markers (duration); (3) the just-discriminable change in the period of F_m for a SAM noise (noise SAM period); and (4) pure-tone frequency discrimination and cutaneous vibration rate discrimination.

More recently, comparisons between neural and psychophysical measures of more complex analytical capabilities have emerged. One of these comparisons involves the psychophysical tuning curve (PTC) as a behavioral measure of frequency selectivity of the auditory system (Rodenburg, Brocaar, & Verschuure, 1974; Vogten, 1974; Zwicker, 1974). This curve is generated by a masking technique in which the signal is fixed in frequency and in intensity; the level of the masker is then varied and the threshold of the masked signal is determined. The masker level at signal threshold is then determined for maskers of different frequencies in order to generate a PTC.

The major advantages of the PTC measure of frequency selectivity over older measures, such as the critical band or critical ratio, is that this single function describes the range both of masker frequencies and of intensities that will interfere with the detection of a low-level signal (which presumably stimulates only a small population of neurons) and, as such, describes the shape of an auditory filter in much the same way as does the neural tuning curve (NTC). The qualitative similarity between neural and psychophysical tuning curves for mammals and birds (Figures 1-11a and b) strengthens this supposition and suggests that filtering occurring at the periphery prior to the level of the eighth nerve accounts for most of the tuning revealed psychophysically.

For the goldfish, however, NTCs and PTCs are qualitatively dissimilar in that the PTC is very sharply tuned and irregularly peaked relative to the NTC (Figure 1-11c). PTCs from another species of fish, the clown knifefish, show these same characteristics when obtained with simultaneous masking techniques, but become smoother and broader when generated by forward masking techniques (Figure 1-11d). Although neural tuning curve data are lacking for the knifefish, it has been suggested that the relationship between forward and simultaneously masked PTCs in this species is not unlike the relationship between NTCs and simultaneously masked PTCs for the goldfish (Coombs & Popper, 1982). If this is the case, then forward-masked PTCs and possibly a portion of simultaneously masked PTCs (see the low-frequency portion of the goldfish curves) may reveal a mechanical filtering process at the periphery (i.e., a place-like mechanism) (Coombs & Popper, 1982; Fay, Ahrron, & Orawski, 1978).

The sharp tuning and irregular peaks (i.e., those occurring at masker-probe frequency separations of approximately 100 Hz) apparent in the simultaneously masked curves, however, more likely reveal an additional process. The most plausible explanation for these peaks is that the fish auditory system is employing a temporally based mechanism for detecting "beats" or amplitude fluctuations caused by probe–masker waveform interactions. While the ability to detect beats generated by frequency separations as great as 100 Hz seems unusual in view of human capabilities (Viemeister, 1979), this ability in fish is consistent with results discussed earlier. That is, the goldfish may base its superior ability to detect rapid amplitude modulations (Figure 1-9b) on the ability of eighth nerve units to synchronize their discharge patterns to the modulation envelope (Fay, 1980; see also below for further discussion). Thus PTCs obtained with simultaneous masking techniques may reflect both temporal and mechanical (place) mechanisms for some species of fish, but perhaps not for others (see Figure 1-7b).

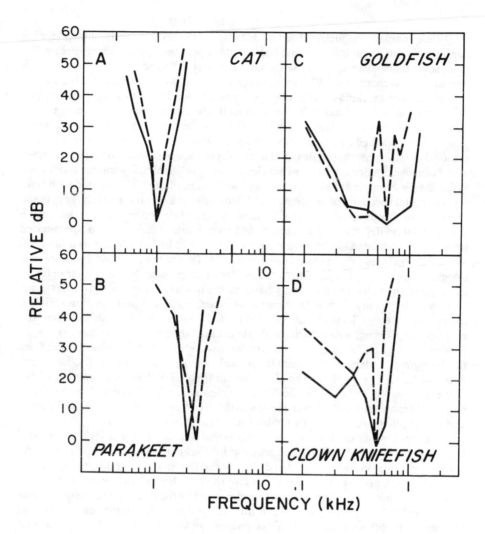

Figure 1-11. A comparsion between neural (———) and psychophysical (----) tuning curves for (A) cat (from Kiang 1965, and Pickles, 1979), (B) bird (from Sachs et al., 1974, for pigeon; Saunders et al., 1978 for parakeet) and (C) goldfish (from Fay, 1978 and Fay et al., 1978b). Tips of neural and psychophysical TC's are normalized to 0 dB. Neural tuning are based on iso-rate criteria; PTC's are based on simultaneous tone-on-tone masking techniques with probe tones set at 10–15 dB SL. (D) Simultaneous (----) and forward-masked (———) PTC's for the clown knifefish (from Coombs & Popper, 1982).

While comparisons such as those made between neural and psychophysical tuning curves yield important information about auditory processing, they nonetheless suffer from several disadvantages. These include stimulus differences in the way in which neural and psychophysical PTCs are typically generated (i.e., PTCs involve a tone-on-tone masking technique, whereas iso-rate responses delineating NTCs are elicited by single tones) and other differences which are a consequence of comparisons between independent laboratories or experiments. One solution to this general problem has been adopted by Fay and his colleagues who have developed an experimental protocol in which psychophysical and neurophysiological experiments are conducted in the same laboratory for the same species under nearly identical stimulus conditions.

A simple example of how this strategy has been used can be illustrated with findings on neural correlates of amplitude modulation detection in the goldfish (Fay, 1980). The basic psychophysical paradigm for measuring AM detection involves decreasing the modulation depth m of a sinusoidal AM signal until it can just be discriminated from an unmodulated signal; m at detection threshold is then plotted as a function of modulation frequency in order to generate a TMTF. For the comparable neurophysiological experiment, Fay measured the ability of single saccular eighth nerve fibers in the goldfish to phase lock their discharge to the modulation envelope of AM signals (presented at the same SL as in the behavioral experiments) as a function of modulation depth. Data were collected in the form of period histograms (the distribution of the number of spikes occurring during a single cycle of the stimulus – in this case, F_m). A measure of phase locking, the synchronization coefficient (R), can be derived from this histogram (Anderson, 1973), and the modulation depth necessary to produce some criterion level of synchronization $(R = .5)$ can then be plotted as a function of F_m to yield a neural TMTF. These results are summarized in Figure 1-12 and show a close correspondence between the best sensitivity of the ensemble of neural curves and the psychophysical TMTFs for both modulated noise and tone.

The conclusion from these experiments is that neural phase locking to the modulation envelope of an AM signal can account for the goldfish's ability to discriminate between modulated and unmodulated signals and that major neural transformations between eighth nerve input to the brain and the final behavioral response need not occur. The validity of this conclusion is strengthened by the fact that these experiments were done by the same investigator, in the same animal, and under nearly identical acoustical conditions with the express purpose of comparing psychophysical and neural results. This approach has been used recently in a number of experiments on the goldfish to demonstrate neural correlates of frequency discrimination (Fay, 1978b), intensity discrimination (Hall, Patricoski, & Fay, 1981), AM rate and noise burst period discrimination (Fay, 1982; Fay & Passow, 1982), and signal detection in noise and temporal summation (Fay & Coombs, 1983).

Clearly, one of the challenges for animal psychoacoustics in the future is to create new and improve existing psychophysical procedures so that the results can be more faithfully interpreted in light of similar neurophysiological experiments. Recent refinements in psychophysical tuning curve paradigms (O'Loughlin & Moore, 1981), for example, are a step in this direction. Ways to tap other neural response properties

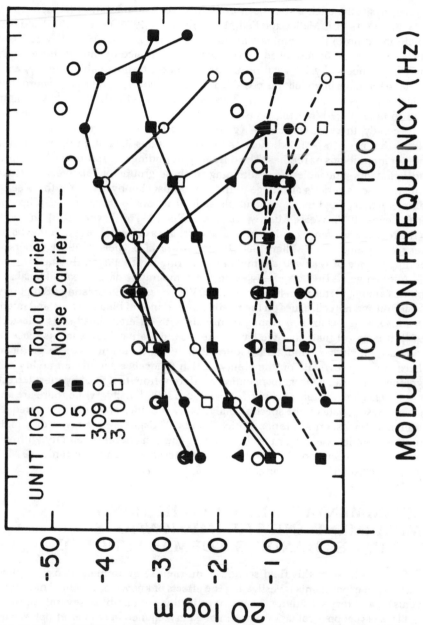

Figure 1-12. Neural TMTFs for noise and an 800-Hz tone for various units (filled symbols) compared to psychophysical TMTFs obtained with the same stimuli (open circles) (see Fay 1980, for further detail).

psychophysically, such as has been done for two-tone inhibition (Houtgast, 1972, 1973; Moore, 1978; O'Malley and Feth, 1979; Shannon, 1976; Vogten, 1978) and neural synchronization to the stimulus waveform (Fay, 1978, 1980, 1982; Fay & Passow, 1982; Zwicker, 1976), also need to be devised and applied to animals for which the comparable neurophysiological results are available or obtainable. Finally, experimental paradigms in which it is possible to simultaneously gather both neurophysiological and psychophysical data in an awake, unanesthetized, and behaving animal need to be explored (Martin, Lonsbury-Martin, & Kimm, 1980) (see also below).

Secondly, there are considerable gaps in our catalogue of vertebrate hearing capabilities that need to be filled, such as the conspicuous lack of any psychophysical data for amphibians or reptiles. The difficulty in finding the appropriate reinforcers and behaviors amenable to conditioning in these groups of relatively intractable animals poses a serious challenge to the animal psychophysicist. Yet the wealth of complementary field biological and physiological data in these groups (Capranica, 1976; Lewis, 1978; Weiss, Mulroy, Turner, & Pike, 1976; Wever, 1978), in addition to the recent emergence of ultrastructural correlates of neural function (Lewis, Leverenz, & Koyama, 1982; Miller, 1980; Turner, Muraski, & Nielsen, 1981), underscores the importance of renewed attempts at gathering psychophysical data.

Another gap is the lack of any extensive comparative data on sound localization abilities among vertebrates (Gourevitch, 1980). Given the interesting predictions by Masterton and his colleagues on the relative importance of binaural time and intensity cues for sound localization among mammals with different head sizes (Masterton, 1974), it is unfortunate that we have so few comparative data, such as those from lateralization studies (Houben & Gourevitch, 1979), to evaluate these predictions. There are very few data on the ability of fish to localize sound – an ability which hypothetically uses a mechanism entirely different from that used by most terrestrial vertebrates (Schuijf, 1981; Schuijf & Buwalda, 1980). Finally, while there are ample psychophysical data on the spectral analytical capabilities of animals (i.e., frequency difference limens, critical ratios, critical bands, PTCs), there are fewer data on temporal capabilities – a further pity considering the behavioral specificity with which many vertebrates respond to the temporal patterns of sound (Capranica & Moffat, 1975; Gerhardt, 1978; Myrberg, Spanier, & Ha, 1978).

EXPERIMENTALLY INDUCED HEARING IMPAIRMENT AND THE IMPLICATIONS FOR UNDERSTANDING NORMAL FUNCTION

The emphasis of this final section is on the use of animals as psychophysical observers in experiments investigating the effects of known or potential ototraumatic events on auditory sensitivity. These investigations often utilize several approaches. That is, a psychophysical task is implemented in conjunction with electrophysiological and histopathological studies to illuminate the effects of the traumatic agent on hearing, to explore the response properties of neurons located in the auditory periphery, and to document the anatomical state of these neurons and their surrounding tissue. Such experiments seek correlations among these measures of auditory system pathology, thereby promoting an understanding of the normal function of a given portion of the auditory system by demonstrating how the entire system (that is, the listener) functions in the absence of that segment. There are obvious clinical correlates to these experiments; in fact, the human pathological condition frequently suggests the laboratory experiment. A systematic exploration of the condition is often possible only with non-human subjects for obvious ethical reasons and reasons of experimental control.

The effects of noise exposure are traditionally evaluated in three ways: surveys of workers exposed to noisy factory environments for long durations, laboratory studies with human subjects, and laboratory studies with animal subjects. The first type of evaluation suffers from a lack of control; that is, the workers may have been exposed to noise outside of the workplace or treated with ototoxic drugs. In the second type of experiment it is ethically permissible to use only brief low-level exposures, capable of producing a temporary threshold shift (TTS), a hearing loss whose relationship to a permanent threshold shift (PTS) is unclear. In laboratory experiments with animals, these problems are eliminated. Thus, animals have been used in experiments investigating the effects of changing several parameters of noise exposure on hearing (Blakeslee, Hynson, Hamernik, & Henderson, 1978; Burdick, 1980, 1982; Burdick, Patterson, Mozo, & Camp, 1978; Hamernik, Henderson, & Salvi, 1980; Henderson, Hamernik, & Hynson, 1979; Henderson, Salvi, & Hamernik, 1982; Nielsen, Elliott, Boisvert, & Hunter-Duvar, 1981; Stebbins, Moody, & Serafin, 1982; and Ward & Turner, 1982).

Yet the basic assumption underlying this research, that animals respond like humans to auditory insults, is questionable. Generally, animal psychophysical experiments use a small number of subjects and, while the noise may be intense, it never extends for the duration of human industrial noise exposures. Further, Saunders and Tilney (1982) suggest that a variety of anatomical variations between species makes it unlikely that all animals have the same susceptibility to noise; thus a given noise band may produce a unique pattern of receptor cell stimulation for each species. Moody, Stebbins, Hawkins, and Johnsson (1978) and Hamernik and associates (1980) concur that animals are best used in noise research in which changes in hearing ability are related to physiological and anatomical changes (see also Stebbins et al., 1982).

Following this mode of investigation, Bohne (1976) began a series of experiments attempting to correlate noise exposure with receptor cell damage using behaviorally trained chinchillas. During exposure to impulse noise, hearing loss in both humans and animals grows for 4–48 hr. and then stabilizes at a level referred to as the asymptotic threshold shift (ATS). The ATS presumably represents the maximum amount of hearing loss which the listener will sustain postexposure. Bohne observed that while the behaviorally trained chinchilla may completely recover from ATS, moderate receptor cell destruction frequently occurrred, suggesting that no noise exposure is truly "safe." Bohne reported that for a given level of noise exposure, longer duration exposures always caused more sensory cell damage than shorter duration exposures, suggesting that sensory cell destruction continues after hearing loss has become asymptotic. Somewhat later, Clark and Bohne (1978) reported that following exposures producing identical ATSs, (1) damage to the high-frequency region of the cochlea increased and, (2) permanent threshold shift (PTS) increased with increasing exposure durations, a finding supported by Henderson and associates (1979), also for the chinchilla. These data indicate that cochlear integrity is best assessed with more than one technique; the extent of the cochlear damage suggested that hearing loss would be moderate, while normal sensitivity indicated that the cochlea was undamaged. Concurring with Clark and Bohne, Moody and co-workers (1978) and Henderson and Hamernik (1982) suggested cochlear damage is probably proportional to exposure duration.

Finally, animal psychophysics has been used to investigate the mechanisms of noise-induced hearing loss. Henderson and Hamernik (1982), using the chinchilla, and Ryan and Bone (1978), using the Mongolian gerbil, reported that the relationship between threshold shift and noise exposure level is not simple. These investigators suggested that the mode of noise-induced cochlear destruction may shift from primarily metabolic to mechanical with increasing level.

Saunders and Tilney (1982) attempted to uncover the anatomical basis of temporary threshold shift (TTS) and the mechanism of recovery from TTS by exposing chicks to noise, behaviorally ascertaining hearing impairment, and then immediately sacrificing the subject and examining the cochlear microstructure. They reported that a loss of stereocilia rigidity may result in TTS by a disruption of the macromolecular structure of the actin filaments contained within the stereocilia. Recovery from TTS may occur following a restoration of the normal order of the actin filaments.

Salvi and co-workers (1978, 1982b) have included electrophysiological measures in investigating noise-induced cochlear destruction. In the 1978 study they exposed chinchillas to a 4.0-kHz octave band noise (OBN), observed an elevation of pure-tone thresholds between 4 and 16 kHz, and then examined the response properties of cochlear nucleus neurons. Neurons with a characteristic frequency greater than 2 kHz had elevated thresholds, broad tuning curves, and a low spontaneous rate, suggesting that a pure-tone hearing loss may be accompanied by other alterations in auditory sensitivity. Indeed, their 1982 study indicates that both neural and psychophysical tuning curves (PTCs) broaden in the presence of an absolute threshold shift, although the latter were narrower than the neural tuning curves, suggesting that PTCs incorporate a contribution from more central locations. Comparing behavioral and neural (eighth nerve) absolute thresholds, Salvi and colleagues (1982b) reported that the former may be lower than the latter, indicating that behavioral thresholds reflect the activity of the most sensitive neural units, a conclusion that is reached in other studies combining neural and behavioral measures of threshold detection (Fay & Coombs, 1983).

Additional animal studies have also examined measures other than pure-tone threshold following noise exposure (Giraudi, Salvi, & Henderson, 1982; Moody, Stebbins, & Serafin, 1982; Syka & Popelav, 1980). The rationale for conducting these experiments is based in part on data from the human literature indicating that while pure-tone thresholds are normal, other measures of auditory sensitivity, such as psychophysical tuning curves (McFadden & Plattsmier, 1982) and lateral suppression

(Mills, 1982), may indicate impairment. These measures may be more sensitive indices of an impaired auditory system than a shift in the pure-tone audiogram.

Just as animals have been used to evaluate the effects of noise on hearing, they also have a long history as subjects in investigations evaluating the effects of drugs on hearing. Again, a variety of drug-related questions have been asked of animal subjects. For example, Hawkins, Stebbins, Johnsson, Moody, & Muraski (1977), having established that few animals have the same sensitivity to dihydrostreptomycin (DHSM) as man, used a positive reinforcement conditioning technique to show that the DHSM-treated *Erythrocebus patas* monkeys' sensitivity is in fact similar to man's. Such species-specific differences emphasize questions about underlying mechanisms – in this case, the biochemical mode of DHSM-induced ototoxicity. Animals have also participated in experiments comparing noise- and drug-induced hearing loss and cochlear pathology (Vertes & Nábêlek, 1977). Finally, animal psychophysics has been used to evaluate the effects of drugs of abuse, such as sedatives or hallucinogens, on auditory perception (Hienz, Lukas, & Brady, 1981).

Experiments abound in which drugs and noise are used to create a particular pattern of cochlear destruction. Many of these studies may aid in understanding normal cochlear function. Clark, Clark, Moody, and Stebbins (1974) exposed chinchillas to a midrange frequency noise band and reported a correlation between the absolute threshold shift and the pattern of cochlear destruction assessed by light microscopy. Although the contribution of the outer hair cells (OHCs) to hearing remains uncertain (Ehret, 1979; Hans, Henderson, & Hamernik, 1975; Henderson, Hamernik, & Sitler, 1974; Ward & Duvall, 1971), recent evidence supports the hypothesis arrived at by Clark and associates that normal hearing is impossible with significant OHC loss (Moody, Beecher, & Stebbins, 1976b; Prosen, Petersen, Moody, & Stebbins, 1978; Ryan & Bone, 1978). The data of Clark and Bohne (1978) suggest that OHCs in the base of the cochlea may function differently than those in the apex. Noting that anatomical changes following noise exposure may be less than predicted based on neural and psychophysical thresholds, Salvi and associates (1982b) suggest that the integrity of the supporting cells may be compromised although the receptor cells appear normal.

Generally the correlation between receptor cell destruction and pure-tone sensitivity changes is quite good. In 1969, Stebbins, Miller, Johnsson, and Hawkins correlated a drug-induced hearing loss with the place and extent of organ of Corti lesions in the kanamycin- or neomycin-treated monkey. Their finding, that destruction of a particular cochlear region was behaviorally manifested in a hearing loss of a restricted frequency range, provided firm behavioral support for the place principle of hearing. Later Eldredge and colleagues (1981), using a variety of noise bands to create specific cochlear lesions, primarily of the OHCs in the chinchilla, observed the resultant changes in hearing at frequencies affected by the receptor cell destruction and correlated the two measures to construct a frequency–position map for the chinchilla cochlea.

Many drug-induced hearing loss studies have attempted to describe the contributions of the individual rows of receptor cells to hearing. Using the aminoglycoside-treated guinea pig, Ylikoski (1974) reported an 18-dB hearing loss associated with destruction of the first row of OHCs, a 38-dB loss with destruction of rows 1 and 2, and a 42-dB loss with OHC but IHC (inner hair cell) retention. Ylikoski also noted that some drugs precipitated a delayed hearing loss such that sensitivity continued to deteriorate long after the termination of drug treatment. A delayed hearing loss was similarly reported by Feitosa, Moody, and Stebbins (1981) in the DHSM-treated patas monkey. Clinically, many humans suffering from tuberculosis and treated with DHSM noted changing auditory sensitivity only long after treatment termination (Glorig, 1951; Shambaugh et al., 1959). An aminoglycoside-induced mechanism of cochlear destruction that accounts for a delayed hearing loss is difficult to formulate.

Kanamycin (KM) has the unusual property of destroying OHCs while leaving the IHCs relatively intact when given to chinchillas and guinea pigs. This fortuitous finding has encouraged many investigators to treat these rodents with KM and then assess various measures of acoustic sensitivity behaviorally and/or electrophysiologically, thus theoretically determining the differential contribution of the OHCs and the IHCs to sensitivity. These studies assume that the remaining IHCs function normally in the presence of OHC destruction. Ryan, Woolf, and Bone (1980) concluded that the IHCs are normal in appearance when examined with the transmission electron microscope if the adjacent supporting cells are undamaged. Anatomical integrity, however, is no guarantee of functional integrity. Further, OHC destruction may alter the cochlear mechanics such that the IHCs are no longer stimulated normally and cannot, therefore, transduce the acoustic signal in a normal fashion. One might conservatively conclude that the following studies assess hearing in the absence of the OHCs rather than differentiating OHC and IHC activity.

Ryan and Dallos (1975) found that chinchilla thresholds were elevated at least 40 dB when OHCs were eliminated but IHCs remained when examined with light microscopy. Prosen, Petersen, Moody, & Stebbins (1978) reported similar results for the guinea pig. Both studies employed a low-pass masker to ensure that responsivity of the remaining IHCs, rather than that of the undamaged apical OHCs, was measured. Dallos and associates (1978) expanded the behavioral and histological data and measured the compound action potential and single auditory nerve fiber thresholds of the KM-treated gerbil and chinchilla. Their results and those of Salvi and colleagues (1982b) suggest that behavioral thresholds are more sensitive than AP or single unit thresholds. Dallos and co-workers (1978) reported that both the AP and the unit thresholds were elevated when originating from cochlear areas where OHCs were eliminated. While a good correspondence existed between behavioral compound action potential and single unit thresholds, the electrophysiological measures generally showed a more drastic threshold shift, especially at the high frequencies.

In experiments investigating measures other than pure-tone thresholds following OHC destruction, Nienhuys and Clark (1978) found no change in frequency discrimination ability in the cat. In a later paper (Nienhuys & Clark, 1979) they reported that the size of the critical band was unaffected by OHC loss alone; only when more than 40% of the IHCs were also destroyed were critical bands enlarged. Ryan, Dallos and McGee (1979) suggested that OHC destruction does not affect PTC sharpness, concluding that the IHCs are capable of transducing fine frequency information. Dallos, Ryan, Harris, McGee, and Özdamer (1977) reported correlative electrophysiological data; the Q_{10}s of single nerve fibers presumably originating from IHC-only cochlear areas were unchanged from the Q_{10}s of fibers found in undamaged cochleas. Finally, Prosen, Moody, Stebbins, & Hawkins (1981) reported that intensity discrimination thresholds were unaffected by OHC destruction. These studies in sum suggest that the IHC-only cochlea may function quite normally in transmitting some suprathreshold information.

The intensity discrimination experiment reported by Prosen and colleagues (1981) is in general illustrative of the approach taken by many of the cited studies. Intensity discrimination ability in the guinea pig was assessed at both a high frequency, 8.0 kHz, where the absolute threshold would shift after KM treatment by approximately 50 dB, and a relatively low frequency, 2.0 kHz, where the absolute threshold would remain unchanged throughout treatment. Difference thresholds were determined at two sound levels, at 20 and 70 dB sensation level (SL), or 20 and 70 dB above the animal's absolute threshold at that test frequency. Following a 50-dB absolute threshold shift at 8 kHz post-KM treatment, what had been 70 dB SL to the untreated guinea pig would now be 20 dB SL. This permitted a comparison of intensity discrimination ability at the same sensation level (20-dB SL) and the same sound pressure level (what was 70 dB SL to the untreated subject) before and after KM treatment, and presumably before and after a restricted OHC loss. After absolute and difference thresholds had stabilized subjects were treated with KM until a 30-dB threshold shift at 8.0 kHz was noted. During treatment subjects were tested daily; following treatment termination thresholds were assessed until they had been stable for at least one month posttreatment. Subjects were then sacrificed and their cochleas removed and prepared for light microscopy in order that receptor cell integrity might be evaluated. The behavioral data were subsequently compared with cytocochleograms to ascertain that the 50-dB absolute threshold shift at 8 kHz was associated with OHC loss and IHC retention, while the unchanged 2-kHz threshold was associated with normal morphology.

As noted earlier, intensity discrimination ability at 8.0 kHz was unchanged following OHC destruction. The extent of the receptor cell destruction is seen in Figure 1-13; only 2% of the OHCs remain in the basal one third of the less-damaged cochlea of this animal, while 97% of the IHCs remain. Before treatment began the 70-dB SL intensity difference limen (IDL) was 3 dB lower than the 20-dB SL IDL. Posttreatment, the IDL remained at the 70-dB SL value; hence, intensity discrimination appeared to improve when assessed at a constant SL before and after drugging, while it was unchanged when measured at a constant SPL throughout this time period, as seen in Figure 1-14.

The results of this experiment concur with intensity discrimination data from hearing-impaired humans. For years it was believed that the hearing impaired could discriminate smaller differences in intensity than normal-hearing listeners; this assumption formed the basis of the Short Increment Sensitivity Index (SISI) test, used clinically to diagnose a hearing loss of cochlear origin. In recent years clinicians have noted that it is the SPL at which the SISI test is conducted, rather than the presence

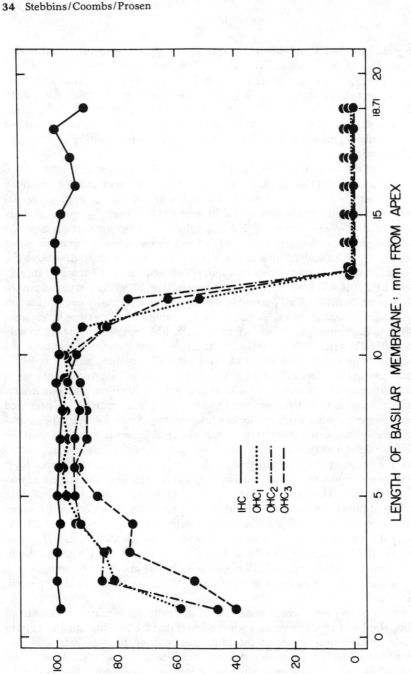

Figure 1-13. Right ear cytocochleogram of a guinea pig treated with kanamycin. Complete outer hair cell destruction and good inner hair cell retention in the base of the cochlea was associated with a 55- to 60-dB absolute hearing loss at 8.0 kHz.

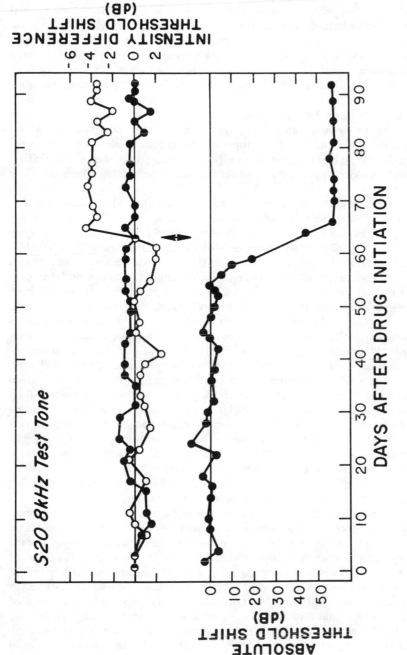

Figure 1-14. Absolute and intensity difference threshold shifts at 8.0 kHz from the subject whose cytocochleogram is portrayed in Figure 1-13. Closed circles in the upper half of the figure represent discrimination data collected at a constant sound pressure level; open circles represent discrimination data collected at a constant sensation level. The arrow indicates the termination of drug treatment.

or absence of cochlear pathology, which determines the size of the IDL. Both normal and hearing-impaired humans detect equally small increments when tested at high SPLs.

We also drew several tentative conclusions about normal cochlear function from this study. OHC presence, needed for normal absolute sensitivity, is not necessary for intensity discrimination nor, as other investigators have concluded, for frequency discrimination, critical bands, or PTCs. Perhaps the moderately compromised cochlea transmits information to higher auditory centers normally if the signals are sufficiently intense to be transduced. Smith and Brachman (1980) reported that single auditory nerve fibers have a dynamic range only slightly smaller than the range over which humans can distinguish different intensities. If the single unit is able to encode intensity information at high SPLs prior to damage, it is perhaps not so remarkable that it continues to do so following a cochlear insult which presumably affects only low SPL encoding.

Finally, there are at least three areas of auditory research to which animal psychophysics may contribute more significantly in the future.

The first of these involves combining standard animal psychophysical techniques and histological preparations with chronic single unit recordings conducted while the subject performs the psychophysical task. This procedure has several advantages over more traditional approaches of obtaining psychophysical data first and then conducting the electrophysiological experiment. First, the same animals are used in both parts of the experiment. Second, since the recording is chronic, effects of anesthesia are absent. Third, the influence of drug- or noise-induced trauma can be evaluated not only behaviorally but also electrophysiologically as the damage occurs. An excellent example of this kind of experiment was performed by Lonsbury-Martin and co-workers (Lonsbury-Martin and Martin, 1981; Lonsbury-Martin, Martin, & Bohne, 1981). Rhesus monkeys with chronic electrodes implanted in the cochlear nucleus and inferior colliculus were trained to respond to pure-tone stimuli in a reaction-time procedure using positive reinforcement. Subjects were then exposed for 6–18 months to intense pure-tone stimuli 3 min. in duration; the brief exposure duration permitted observation of the same neural unit both before and after exposure. The experimental objective was to identify those cellular mechanisms underlying the transition from a temporary to a permanent noise-induced hearing loss. Pfingst and O'Connor (1981) have also combined behavioral and chronic electrophysiological techniques recording from more centrally located auditory neurons in the monkey.

A second area of research which has not been extensively pursued by animal psychophysicists concerns the effects of central auditory nervous system lesions on hearing. We can perhaps attribute this to the vast amount of energy directed toward the auditory periphery; as the periphery becomes better understood, the focus of research may shift. The idea of assessing some aspect of auditory sensitivity before and after destroying part of the central auditory system dates back to 1946 (Raab & Ades, 1946; Rosenzweig, 1946) when two laboratories independently investigated the effects of cortical and midbrain lesions on intensity discrimination in the cat. More recently, Chung and Colavita (1976) trained cats to perform a frequency discrimination and also to report periodicity pitch perception prior to ablation of several cortical areas. Several studies (Cranford & Oberholtzer, 1976; Heffner, 1981; Jenkins & Masterton, 1981; Neff and Casseday, 1977), have examined auditory localization following either unilateral or bilateral central auditory nervous system lesions. Neff suggested (1977) that clinicians and animal researchers collaborate, with animal researchers investigating the effects of known lesions on several indices of auditory integrity and clinicians carefully testing humans with identifiable lesions on a variety of auditory tasks. Potential benefits are twofold; first, the site of a lesion in a newly brain-damaged human would be more easily identified, and second, the normal activity of subareas of the brain would be better understood.

The development of the auditory system and the effects of abnormal early experience on development are areas of inquiry to which animal psychophysics may be applied. Physiological and anatomical data suggest that auditory development is immature at birth (Brugge, 1982; Brugge, Kitzer, & Javel, 1981; Pujol, 1982; Rubel, 1982; Shnerson & Pujol, 1982; Shnerson, Devigne, & Pujol, 1982; Shofner & Feng, 1981) and that the infant auditory system passes through one or more critical periods (Bock & Seifter, 1978; Danto, 1980; Gottlieb, 1981; Saunders & Tilney, 1982). Further, the notion that the development of the neonatal auditory system is affected by the particular acoustic environment that the infant experiences is supported by the electrophysiological and anatomical work of Silverman and colleagues (Silverman, Clopton, & Flamnino, 1975; Clopton and Silverman, 1977; Silverman & Clopton, 1977) and of Webster and Webster (1977). Remarkably few behavioral developmental studies have tested the hypothesis that a critical period exists during which proper, meaningful acoustic stimulation must be received for normal maturation of the central auditory nervous system (Batkin & Ansberry, 1964; Clements & Kelly, 1978; Tees, 1967).

The participants of a conference on otitis media (Ruben, 1979) recently concluded that the temporary fluctuating hearing loss affecting otitis media sufferers may well influence normal development. The experimental data cited above suggest that anatomical and physiological abnormalities accompany auditory deprivation. Well-controlled studies in which the auditory environment of infant animals is restricted, with subsequent behavioral testing of auditory function, might reveal how detrimental abnormal early auditory experience is on adult auditory function. These studies might also elucidate the extent of the plasticity of the developing auditory system.

In this chapter we have attempted to review and to evaluate some of the contributions of comparative psychoacoustics to our understanding of information processing by the auditory system and of auditory perception. The techniques of animal psychophysics (see Stebbins, 1970) make it possible to subject a variety of vertebrate species to exact and detailed questioning regarding their sensory experiences. Under the appropriate training regimens animals become well-qualified psychophysical observers suitable for testing in a wide range of experimental paradigms. We have, for example, examined their perceptual capabilities in the discrimination of human speech sounds as well as the sounds of their own species for what they might reveal about the origins of communication and even language. Then, too, differences in auditory acuity in closely related taxa can be compared with significant morphological and physiological differences in the auditory systems of these animals. Such comparisons are important for what they may tell us about auditory system phylogeny and about general organizing principles of vertebrate auditory systems. In addition, measures of hearing impairment induced in experimental animals by either drugs or intense noise, when accompanied by light and electron microscopic analysis of the inner ear, can disclose important information regarding normal as well as abnormal inner ear function. Finally, several research areas have been identified that could profit from increased attention from comparative psychoacoustics.

REFERENCES

Anderson, D. (1973). Quantitative model for the effects of stimulus frequency upon synchronization of auditory nerve discharges. *Journal of the Acoustical Society of America, 54,* 361-364.

Baru, A.V. (1975). Discrimination of synthesized vowels /a/ and /i/ with varying parameters in dog. In G. Fant & M.A.A. Tatham (Eds.), *Auditory analysis and perception of speech* (pp. 91-101). New York: Academic Press.

Batkin, S., & Ansberry, M. (1964). Effect of auditory deprivation. *Journal of the Acoustical Society of America, 36,* 598.

Beecher, M.D., Petersen, M.R., Zoloth, S.R., Moody, D.B., & Stebbins, W.C. (1979). Macaque perception of conspecific communication sounds. *Brain, Behavior and Evolution, 16,* 443-460.

Blakeslee, E.A., Hynson, K., Hamernik, R.P., & Henderson, D. (1978). Asymptotic threshold shift in chinchillas exposed to impulse noise. *Journal of the Acoustical Society of America, 63,* 876-882.

Bock, G.R., & Seifter, E.J. (1978). Developmental changes of susceptibility to auditory fatigue in young hamsters. *Audiology, 17,* 193-203.

Bohne, B.A. (1976). Safe level for noise exposure? *Annals of Otology, Rhinology and Laryngology, 85,* 711-724.

Brown, C.H. (1983). Auditory localization and primate vocal behavior. In T.C. Snowdon, C.H. Brown, and M.R. Petersen (Eds.), *Primate communication* (pp. 144-164). New York: Cambridge Univ. Press.

Brown, C.H., Beecher, M.D., Moody, D.B., & Stebbins, W.C. (1980). Localization of noise bands by Old World monkeys. *Journal of the Acoustical Society of America, 68,* 127-132.

Brown, C.H., Beecher, M.D., Moody, D.B., & Stebbins, W.C. (1978). Localization of primate calls by Old World monkeys. *Science, 201,* 753-754.

Brown, C.H., Beecher, M.D., Moody, D.B., & Stebbins, W.C. (1979). Locatability of vocal signals in Old World monkeys: Design features for the communication of position. *Journal of Comparative and Physiological Psychology, 93,* 806-819.

Brugge, J.F., Kitzer, L.M., & Javel, E. (1981). Postnatal development of frequency and intensity sensitivity of neurons in the anteroventral cochlear nucleus of kittens. *Hearing Research, 5,* 217-229.

Brugge, J.F. (1982). Functional development within the cochlear nuclei. *Journal of the Acoustical Society of America, 71,* S2.

Bruns, V. (1980). Structural adaptation in the cochlea of the horseshoe bat for the analysis of the long CF-FM echolocating signals. In R.-G. Busnel & J.F. Fish (Eds.), *Animal sonar systems* (pp. 867-869). New York: Plenum.

Bullock, T.H. (Ed.) (1977). *Recognition of complex acoustic signals.* Berlin: Dahlem Konferenzen.

Burda, H., & Voldrich, L. (1980). Correlation between the hair cell density and the auditory threshold in the white rat. *Hearing Research, 3,* 91-93.

Burdick, C.K. (1982). Hearing loss from low-frequency noise. In R.P. Hamernik, D. Henderson, & R. J. Salvi (Eds.) *New perspectives on noise-induced hearing loss* (pp. 321–324). New York: Raven Press.

Burdick, C.K. (1980). Hearing loss in chinchillas exposed to octave bands of noise centered at 31.5 and 250 Hz. *Journal of the Acoustical Society of America, 67,* S58.

Burdick, C.K., & Miller, J.D. (1975). Speech perception by the chinchilla: Discrimination of sustained /a/ and /i/. *Journal of the Acoustical Society of America, 58,* 415–427.

Burdick, C.K., Patterson, J.H., Mozo, B.T., & Camp, R.T., Jr. (1978). Threshold shifts in chinchillas exposed to octave bands of noise centered at 63 and 1000 Hz for 3 days. *Journal of the Acoustical Society of America, 64,* 458–466.

Chung, D.Y., & Colavita, F.B. (1976). Periodicity pitch perception in cortically ablated cats. *Journal of the Acoustical Society of America, 60,* S88.

Clark, W.W., & Bohne, B.A. (1978). Animal model for the 4-kHz tonal dip. *Annals of Otology, Rhinology and Laryngology, Supplement 51.*

Clark, W.W., Clark, C.S., Moody, D.B., & Stebbins, W.C. (1974). Noise-induced hearing loss in the chinchilla, as determined by a positive reinforcement technique. *Journal of the Acoustical Society of America, 56,* 1202–1209.

Clements, M., & Kelly, J.B. (1978). Auditory spatial responses of young guinea pigs *(Cavia porcellus)* during and after ear blocking. *Journal of Comparative Physiology and Psychology, 92,* 34–44.

Clopton, B.M., & Silverman, M.S. (1977). Plasticity of binaural interaction. II. Critical period and changes in midline response. *Journal of Neurophysiology, 40,* 1275–1280.

Coombs, S., & Popper, A.N. (1979). Hearing differences among Hawaiian squirrelfish (family Holocentridae) related to differences in the peripheral auditory system. *Journal of Comparative Physiology, 132A,* 203–207.

Coombs, S., & Popper, A.N. (1982). Comparative frequency selectivity in fishes: Simultaneously and forward-masked psychophysical tuning curves. *Journal of the Acoustical Society of America, 71,* 133–141.

Cornsweet, T.N. (1970). *Visual perception.* New York: Academic Press.

Cranford, J.L., & Oberholtzer, M. (1976). Role of the neocortex in binaural hearing in the cat. II. The "precedence effect" in sound localization. *Brain Research, 111,* 225–239.

Dallos, P., Harris, D., Özdamer, Ö., & Ryan, A. (1978). Behavioral, compound action potential, and single unit thresholds: Relationship in normal and abnormal ears. *Journal of the Acoustical Society of America, 64,* 151–157.

Dallos, P., Ryan, A.F., Harris, D.M., McGee, T., & Özdamer, Ö. (1977). Cochlear frequency selectivity in the presence of hair cell damage. In E.F. Evans & J.P. Wilson (Eds), *Psychophysics and physiology of hearing* (pp. 249–261). New York: Academic Press.

Danto, J. (1980). Effects of noise on infant and adult guinea pigs. *Journal of the Acoustical Society of America, 68,* S98.

Dawkins, R., & Krebs, J.R. (1978). Animal signals: Information or manipulation? In J.R. Krebs & N.B. Davies (Eds.) *Behavioural ecology: An evolutionary approach* (pp. 282–309). Sunderland, MA: Sinauer Associates.

Dewson, J.H. III (1964). Speech sound discrimination by cats. *Science, 144,* 555–556.

Dewson, J.H. III, Pribram, K.H., & Lynch, J.C. (1969). Effects of ablations and temporal cortex upon speech sound discrimination in monkey. *Experimental Neurology, 24,* 579–591.

Dooling, R.J. (1980). Behavior and psychophysics of hearing in birds. In A.N. Popper & R.R. Fay (Eds.), *Comparative studies of hearing in vertebrates* (pp. 261–288). New York: Springer-Verlag.

Dooling, R.J., & Searcy, M.H. (1981). Amplitude modulation thresholds for the parakeet *(Melopsittacus undulatus). Journal of Comparative Physiology, 143,* 383–388.

Dooling, R.J., & Walsh, J.K. (1976). Auditory evoked response correlates of hearing in the parakeet *(Melopsittacus undulatus)*. *Physiological Psychology, 4*, 224–232.

Dooling R.J., Zoloth, S.R., & Baylis, J.R. (1978). Auditory sensitivity, equal loudness, temporal power, and vocalizations in house finch *(Carpodacus mexicanus)*. *Journal of Comparative and Physiological Psychology, 92*, 867–876.

Ehret, G. (1977). Comparative psychoacoustics: Perspectives of peripheral sound analysis in mammals. *Naturwissenschaften, 64*, 461–470.

Ehret, G. (1979). Correlations between cochlear hair cell loss and shifts of masked and absolute behavioral auditory thresholds in the house mouse. *Acta Otolaryngologica, 87*, 28–38.

Eldredge, D.H., Miller, J.D., & Bohne, B.A. (1981). A frequency-position map for the chinchilla cochlea. *Journal of the Acoustical Society of America, 69*, 1091–1095.

Eldredge, N., & Gould, S.J. (1972). Punctuated equilibria: An alternative to phyletic gradualism. In T.J. Schopf (Ed.) *Models in paleobiology* (pp. 82–115). San Francisco: Freeman.

Evans, E.F., & Whitfield, I.C. (1964). Classification of unit responses in the auditory cortex of the unanaesthetized and unrestrained cat. *Journal of Physiology, 171*, 476–493.

Fay, R.R., Ahrron, W., & Orawski, A. (1978). Auditory masking patterns in the goldfish *Carassius auratus:* Psychophysical tuning curves. *Journal of Experimental Biology, 74*, 83–100.

Fay, R.R. (1974). Auditory frequency discrimination in vertebrates. *Journal of the Acoustical Society of America, 56*, 206–209.

Fay, R.R. (1978a). Phase-locking in goldfish saccular nerve fibres accounts for frequency discrimination capacities. *Nature (London), 275*, 320–322.

Fay, R.R. (1978b). The coding of information in single auditory nerve fibers of the goldfish. *Journal of the Acoustical Society of America, 63*, 136–146.

Fay, R.R. (1980). Psychophysics and neurophysiology of temporal factors in hearing by the goldfish: Amplitude modulation detection. *Journal of Neurophysiology, 44*, 312–332.

Fay, R.R. (1982). Neural mechanisms of an auditory temporal discrimination by the goldfish. *Journal of Comparative Physiology, 147*, 201–216.

Fay, R.R., & Coombs, S. (1983). Neural mechanisms in sound detection and temporal summation. *Hearing Research, 10*, 69–92.

Fay, R.R., & Passow, B. (1982). Temporal discrimination in the goldfish. *Journal of the Acoustical Society of America, 72*, 753–760.

Fay, R.R., & Popper, A.N. (1980). Structure and function in teleost auditory systems. In A.N. Popper & R.R. Fay (Eds.), *Comparative studies of hearing in vertebrates* (pp. 3–42). New York: Springer-Verlag.

Feitosa, A.G., Moody, D.B., & Stebbins, W.C., (1981). Loudness recruitment in the dihydro-streptomycin-treated patas monkey. *Journal of the Acoustical Society of America, 70*, S27.

Giraudi, D.M., Salvi, R.J., & Henderson, D. (1982). Gap-detection in hearing-impaired chinchillas. *Association for Research in Otolaryngology, 50* (Abstract).

Giraudi, D., Salvi, R.J., Henderson, D., & Hamernik, D. (1980). Gap detection by the chinchilla. *Journal of the Acoustical Society of America, 68*, 802–806.

Glorig, A., (1951). The effect of dihydrostreptomycin hydrochloride and sulfate on auditory mechanisms. *Annals of Otology, Rhinology and Laryngology, 60*, 327–335.

Gottlieb, G. (1981). Development of species identification in ducklings: VIII. Embryonic vs. postnatal critical period for the maintenance of species-typical perception. *Journal of Comparative and Physiological Psychology, 95*, 540–547.

Gourevitch, G. (1980). Directional hearing in terrestrial mammals. In A.N. Popper & R.R. Fay (Eds.), *Comparative studies of hearing in vertebrates* (pp. 357–372). New York: Springer-Verlag.

Green, S. (1975). Variation of vocal pattern with social situation in the Japanese monkey *(Macaca fuscata)*: A field study. In L. Rosenblum (Ed.), *Primate behavior* (Vol. 4, pp. 1–102). New York: Academic Press.

Green, S., & Marler, P. (1979). The analysis of animal communication. In P. Marler & J.G. Vandenberg (Eds.), *Handbook of behavioral neurobiology, Vol. 3: Social behavior and communication* (pp 73–158). New York: Plenum.

Hall, L., Patricoski, M., & Fay, R.R. (1981). Neurophysiological mechanisms of intensity discrimination in the goldfish. In W.N. Tavolga, A.N. Popper, & R.R. Fay (Eds.), *Hearing and sound communication in fishes* (pp. 179–186). New York: Springer-Verlag.

Hamernik, R.P., Henderson, D., & Salvi, R.J. (1980). Contribution of animal studies to our understanding of impulse noise-induced hearing loss. *Scandinavian Audiology, Supplement 12*, 128–146.

Hans, J., Henderson, D., & Hamernik, R.P. (1975). Effect of impulse noise on the temporal integration function of the chinchilla. *Journal of the Acoustical Society of America, 57*, S41.

Hartman, W. (1979). Detection of amplitude modulation. *Journal of the Acoustical Society of America, 65*, F59.

Hawkins, A.D. (1981). The hearing abilities of fish. In W.N. Tavolga, A.N. Popper, & R.R. Fay (Eds.), *Hearing and Sound Communication in Fishes* (pp. 109–138). New York: Springer-Verlag.

Hawkins, J.E., Jr., Stebbins, W.C., Johnsson, L.-G., Moody, D.B., & Muraski, A. (1977). The patas monkey as a model for dihydrostreptomycin ototoxicity. *Acta Otolaryngologica, 83*, 123–129.

Heffner, H. (1981). Role of the forebrain in sound localization. *Journal of the Acoustical Society of America, 69*, S12.

Henderson, D., & Hamernik, R.P. (1982). Asymptotic threshold shift from impulse noise. In R.P. Hamernik, D. Henderson, & R.J. Salvi (Eds.), *New perspectives on noise-induced hearing loss* (pp. 265–281). New York: Raven Press.

Henderson, D., Hamernik, R.P., & Hynson, K. (1979). Hearing loss from simulated work-week exposure to impulse noise. *Journal of the Acoustical Society of America, 65*, 1231–1237.

Henderson, D., Hamernik, R.P., Woodford, C., Sitler, R.W., & Salvi, R.J. (1973). The evoked response audibility curve of the chinchilla. *Journal of the Acoustical Society of America, 54*, 1099–1101.

Henderson, D., Hamernik, R.P., & Sitler, R. (1974). Audiometric and histological correlates of exposure to 1-msec impulses in the chinchilla. *Journal of the Acoustical Society of America, 56*, 1210–1221.

Henderson, D., Salvi, R.J., & Hamernik, R.P. (1982). Is the equal energy rule applicable to impact noise? *Journal of the Acoustical Society of America, 71*, S50.

Hienz, R.D., Lukas, S.E., & Brady, J.V. (1981). The effects of pentobarbital upon auditory and visual thresholds in the baboon. *Pharmacology, Biochemistry and Behavior, 15*, 799–805.

Jenkins, W.M., & Masterton, R.B. (1981). Effects of unilateral lesions in the central auditory system on sound localization behavior. *Journal of the Acoustical Society of America, 69*, S11.

Jun, S., Coombs, S., Fay, R.R., Popper, A.N., & Saidel, W.N. (1982). Hearing in the jewel cichlid. *Journal of the Acoustical Society of America, Supplement 71*, S49.

Kay, R., & Matthews, D. (1972). On the existence in human auditory pathways of channels selectively tuned to the modulation present in frequency modulated tones. *Journal of Physiology, 225*, 657–677.

Kiang, N., Watanabe, T., Thomas, F.C., & Clark, L.S. (1965). *Discharge patterns of single fibers in the cat's auditory nerve*. Cambridge, MA: MIT Press.

Konishi, M. (1969). Hearing, single-unit analysis, and vocalization in songbirds. *Science, 166*, 1178–1179.

Kuhl, P.K. (1981). Discrimination of speech by nonhuman animals: Basic auditory sensitivities conducive to the perception of speech-sound categories. *Journal of the Acoustical Society of America, 70,* 340-349.

Kuhl, P.K., & Miller, J.D. (1978). Speech perception by the chinchilla: Identification functions for synthetic VOT stimuli. *Journal of the Acoustical Society of America, 63,* 905-917.

Kuhl, P.K., & Padden, D.M. (1983). Enhanced discriminability at the phonetic boundaries for the place feature in macaques. *Journal of the Acoustical Society of America, 73,* 1003-1010.

Kuhl, P.K., & Padden, D.M. (1982). Enhanced discriminability at the phonetic boundaries for the voicing feature in macaques. *Perceptual Psychophysics, 32,* 542-550.

Liberman, A.M. (1982). On finding that speech is special. *American Psychologist, 37,* 148-167.

Long, G. (1980). Further studies of masking in the greater horseshoe bat, *Rhinolophus ferrumequinum.* In R.-G. Busnel & J.F. Fish (Eds.), *Animal sonar systems* (pp. 929-932). New York: Plenum.

Long, G. (1977). Masked auditory thresholds from the bat, *Rhinolophus ferrumequinum. Journal of Comparative Physiology, 116,* 247-255.

Long, G. (1981). Some psychophysical measurements of frequency processing in the greater horseshoe bat. In G. van den Brink & F.A. Bilsen (Eds.), *Psychophysical, physiological and behavioral studies in hearing* (pp. 132-135). Delft: Delft Univ.

Long, G., & Schnitzler, H.-U. (1975). Behavioral audiograms from the bat, *Rhinolophus ferrumequinum. Journal of Comparative Physiology, 100,* 211-219.

Lonsbury-Martin, B.L., & Martin, G.K. (1981). Effects of moderately intense sound on auditory sensitivity in rhesus monkeys: Behavioral and neural observations. *Journal of Neurophysiology, 46,* 563-586.

Lonsbury-Martin, B.L., Martin, G.K., & Bohne, B.A. (1981). Slowly developing hearing loss in rhesus monkeys from repeated exposures to moderate tones. *Association for Research in Otolaryngology, 55* (Abstract).

Manley, G.A. (1971). Some aspects of the evolution of hearing in vertebrates. *Nature (London), 230,* 506-509.

Manley, G.A., & Mueller-Preuss, P. (1978). Response variability in the mammalian auditory cortex: An objection to feature detection? *Federation Proceedings, 37,* 2355-2359.

McFadden, D., & Plattsmier, H.S. (1982). Suprathreshold aftereffects of exposure to intense sound. In R.P. Hamernik, D. Henderson, & R.J. Salvi (Eds.), *New perspectives on noise-induced hearing loss* (pp. 363-373). New York: Raven Press.

Miller, J.D. (1970). Audibility curve of the chinchilla. *Journal of the Acoustical Society of America, 48,* 513-523.

Miller, J.D. (1982). Auditory-perceptual approaches to phonetic perception. *Journal of the Acoustical Society of America, 71,* S112.

Miller, J.D. (1977). Perception of speech sounds in animals: Evidence for speech processing by mammalian auditory mechanisms. In T.H. Bullock (Ed.), *Recognition of complex acoustic signals* (pp. 49-58). Berlin: Dahlem Konferenzen.

Miller, J.M., Beaton, R.D., O'Connor, T., Pfingst, B.E. (1974). Response pattern complexity of auditory cells in the cortex of unanesthetized monkeys. *Brain Research, 69,* 101-113.

Miller, M.R. (1980). The reptilian cochlear duct. In A.N. Popper & R.R. Fay (Eds.), *Comparative studies of hearing in vertebrates* (pp. 169-204). New York: Springer-Verlag.

Mills, J.H. (1982). Effects of noise on auditory sensitivity, psychophysical tuning curves, and suppression. In R.P. Hamernik, D. Henderson, & R.J. Salvi (Eds.), *New perspectives on noise-induced hearing loss* (pp. 249-263). New York: Raven Press.

Moody, D.B., Beecher, M.D., & Stebbins, W.C. (1976a). Behavioral methods in auditory research. In C. Smith and J. Vernon (Eds.), *Handbook of auditory and vestibular research methods* (pp. 439–497). Springfield: Thomas.

Moody, D.B., Stebbins, W.C., & Serafin, J.V. (1982). Psychophysical tuning curves following noise-induced temporary threshold shift in monkey. *Association for Research in Otolaryngology, 54* (Abstract).

Moody, D.B., Stebbins, W.C., Hawkins, J.E., Jr., & Johnsson, L.-G. (1978). Hearing loss and cochlear pathology in the monkey (Macaca) following exposure to high levels of noise. *Archives of Oto-Rhino-Laryngology, 220,* 47–72.

Moody, D.B., Stebbins, W.C., Johnsson, L.-G., & Hawkins, J.E., Jr. (1976b). Noise-induced hearing loss in the monkey. In D. Henderson, R.P. Hamernik, D. Dosanjh, & J.H. Mills (Eds.), *Effects of noise on hearing* (pp. 309–325). New York: Raven Press.

Moore, B.C.J. (1978). Psychophysical tuning curves measured in simultaneous and forward masking. *Journal of the Acoustical Society of America, 63,* 524–532.

Morse, P.A., & Snowdon, C.T. (1975). An investigation of categorical speech discrimination by rhesus monkeys. *Perception and Psychophysics, 17,* 9–16.

Neff, W.D. (1977). The brain and hearing: Auditory discriminations affected by brain lesions. *Annals of Otology, Rhinology and Laryngology, 86,* 500–506.

Neff, W.D., & Casseday, J.H. (1977). Effects of unilateral ablation of auditory cortex on monaural cats' ability to localize sound. *Journal of Neurophysiology, 40,* 44–52.

Nelson, D.A., & Keister, T.E. (1978). Frequency discrimination in the chinchilla. *Journal of the Acoustical Society of America, 64,* 114–126.

Neuweiler, G. (1980). How bats detect flying insects. *Physics Today, 33,* 34–40.

Newman, J.D., & Wollberg, Z. (1973). Multiple coding of species-specific vocalizations in the auditory cortex of squirrel monkeys. *Brain Research, 54,* 287–304.

Nielsen, D.W., Elliot, D.N., Boisvert, P., & Hunter-Duvar, I. (1981). Temporary threshold shift to 8-hour noise exposure in man and monkey. *Journal of the Acoustical Society of America, 69,* S73.

Nienhuys, T.G.W., & Clark, G.M. (1979). Critical bands following the selective destruction of cochlear inner and outer hair cells. *Acta Otolaryngologica, 88,* 350–358.

Nienhuys, T.G.W., & Clark, G.M. (1978). Frequency discrimination following the selective destruction of cochlear inner and outer hair cells. *Science, 199,* 1356–1357.

O'Loughlin, B.J., & Moore, B.C.J. (1981). Improving psychoacoustical tuning curves. *Hearing Research, 5,* 343–346.

Peters, R. (1980). *Mammalian communication: A behavioral analysis of meaning.* Monterey, CA: Brooks/Cole.

Petersen, M.R., Beecher, M.D., Zoloth, S.R., Moody, D.B., & Stebbins, W.C. (1978). Neural lateralization of species-specific vocalizations by Japanese macaques *(Macaca fuscata). Science, 202,* 324–327.

Pfingst, B.E., & O'Connor, T.A. (1981). Characteristics of neurons in auditory cortex of monkeys performing a simple auditory task. *Journal of Neurophysiology, 45,* 16–34.

Pickles, J.O. (1979). Psychophysical frequency resolution in the cat as determined by simultaneous masking and its relation to auditory nerve resolution. *Journal of the Acoustical Society of America, 66,* 1725–1732.

Pohl, P. (1983). Central auditory processing: V. Ear advantages for acoustic stimuli in baboons. *Brain and Language, 20,* 44–53.

Popper, A.N., & Coombs, S. (1980). Auditory mechanisms in teleost fishes. *American Scientist, 68* 429–440.

Popper, A.N., & Coombs, S. (1982). The morphology and evolution of the ear in Actinopterygian fishes. *American Zoology, 22,* 311–328.

Popper, A.N., & Fay, R.R. (1980). *Comparative studies of hearing in vertebrates.* New York: Springer-Verlag.

Prosen, C.A., Moody, D.B., Stebbins, W.C., & Hawkins, J.E., Jr. (1981). Auditory intensity discrimination after selective loss of cochlear outer hair cells. *Science, 212,* 1286–1288.

Prosen, C.A., Petersen, M.R., Moody, D.B., & Stebbins, W.C. (1978). Auditory thresholds and kanamycin-induced hearing loss in the guinea pig assessed by a positive reinforcement procedure. *Journal of the Acoustical Society of America, 63,* 559–566.

Pujol, R. (1982). Synaptogenesis and first coding in the developing cochlea. *Journal of the Acoustical Society of America, 71,* S2.

Raab, D.H., & Ades, H.W. (1946). Cortical and midbrain mediation of a conditioned discrimination of acoustic intensities. *American Journal of Psychology, 59,* 59–83.

Regan, D., & Tansley, B. (1979). Selective adaptation to frequency-modulated tones: Evidence for an information processing channel selectively sensitive to frequency changes. *Journal of the Acoustical Society of America, 65,* 1249–1257.

Rodenburg, M., Brocaar, M.P., & Verschuure, J.V. (1974). Comparison of two masking methods. *Acustica, 31,* 99–106.

Rosenzweig, M. (1946). Discrimination of auditory intensities in the cat. *American Journal of Psychology, 59,* 127–136.

Rubel, E.W. (1982). Structure–function relationships and the role of experience in auditory system ontogeny. *Journal of the Acoustical Society of America, 71,* S3.

Ruben, R.J. (1979). Otitis media and child development. *Annals of Otology, Rhinology and Laryngology, Supplement, 60,* 107–111.

Ryan, A., & Bone, R.C. (1978). Noise-induced threshold shift and cochlear pathology in the Mongolian gerbil. *Journal of the Acoustical Society of America, 63,* 1145–1151.

Ryan, A., & Dallos, P. (1975). Effect of absence of cochlear outer hair cells on behavioral auditory thresholds. *Nature, (London), 253,* 44–46.

Ryan, A., Dallos, P., & McGee, T. (1979). Psychophysical tuning curves and auditory thresholds after hair cell damage in the chinchilla. *Journal of the Acoustical Society of America, 66,* 370–378.

Ryan, A., Woolf, N.K., & Bone, R.C. (1980). Ultrastructural correlates of selective outer hair cell destruction following kanamycin intoxication in the chinchilla. *Hearing Research, 3,* 335–351.

Sachs, M.B., Sinnott, J.M., & Hienz, R.D. (1978). Behavioral and physiological studies of hearing in birds. *Federation Proceedings, 37,* 431–447.

Sachs, M.B., Woolf, N.K., & Sinnott, J.M. (1980). Response properties of neurons in the avian auditory system: Comparison with mammalian homologues and consideration of the neural encoding of complex stimuli. In A.N. Popper & R.R. Fay (Eds.) *Comparative studies of hearing in vertebrates* (pp. 323–353). New York: Springer-Verlag.

Sachs, M.B., Young. E.D., & Lewis, R.H. (1974). Discharge patterns of single fibers in the pigeon auditory nerve. *Brain Research, 70,* 431–447.

Salvi, R.J., Hamernik, R.P., & Henderson, D. (1978). Discharge patterns in the cochlear nucleus of the chinchilla following noise-induced asymptotic threshold shift. *Experimental Brain Research, 32,* 301–320.

Salvi, R.J., Giraudi, D.M., Henderson, D., & Hamernik, R.P. (1982a). Detection of sinusoidally amplitude modulated noise by the chinchilla. *Journal of the Acoustical Society of America, 71,* 424–429.

Salvi, R.J., Perry, J., Hamernik, R.P., & Henderson, D. (1982b). Relationships between cochlear pathologies and auditory and behavioral responses following acoustic trauma. In R.P. Hamernik, D. Henderson, & R. Salvi (Eds.), *New perspectives on noise-induced hearing loss* (pp. 165–188). New York: Raven Press.

Saunders, J.C., & Johnstone, B.M. (1972). A comparative analysis of middle ear function in non-mammalian vertebrates. *Acta Otolaryngologica, 73*, 353–361.

Saunders, J.C., & Tilney, L.G. (1982). Species differences in susceptibility to noise exposure. In R.P. Hamernik, D. Henderson, & R.J. Salvi (Eds.), *New perspectives on noise-induced hearing loss* (pp. 229–248). New York: Raven Press.

Schnitzler, H.-U. (1973). Die Echoortung der Fledermause und ihre hörphysiologischen Grundlagen. *Fortschritte der Zoologie, 21*, 136–189.

Serafin, J.V., Moody, D.B., & Stebbins, W.C. (1982). Frequency selectivity of the monkeys' auditory system: Psychophysical tuning curves. *Journal of the Acoustical Society of America, 71*, 1513–1518.

Seyfarth, R.M., Cheney, D.L., & Marler, P. (1980). Vervet monkey alarm calls: Semantic communication in a free-ranging primate. *Animal Behavior, 28*, 1070–1094.

Shambaugh, G.E., Jr., Derlacki, E.L., Harrison, W.H., House, H., House, W., Hildyard, V., Schuknecht, H., & Shen, J.J. (1959). Dihydrostreptomycin deafness. *Journal of the American Medical Association, 170*, 1657–1660.

Shnerson, A., & Pujol, R. (1982). Age-related changes in the C57BL/6J mouse cochlea. I. Physiological findings. *Developmental Brain Research, 2*, 65–75.

Schnerson, A., Devigne, C., & Pujol, R. (1982). Age-related changes in the C57BL/6J mouse cochlea. II. Ultrastructural findings. *Developmental Brain Research, 2*, 77–88.

Shofner, W.P., & Feng, A.S. (1981). Post-metamorphic development of the frequency selectivities and sensitivities of the peripheral auditory system of the bullfrog, *Rana catesbeiana. Journal of Experimental Biology, 93*, 181–196.

Silverman, M.S., & Clopton, B.M. (1977). Plasticity of binaural interaction. I. Effect of early auditory deprivation. *Journal of Neurophysiology, 40*, 1266–1274.

Silverman, M.S., Clopton. B.M., & Flamnino, F. (1975). Development of single-cell binaural interactions in the inferior colliculus of the rat. *Journal of the Acoustical Society of America, 57*, S54.

Sinnott, J.M. (1980). Species-specific coding in bird song. *Journal of the Acoustical Society of America, 68*, 494–497.

Sinnott, J.M., Beecher, M.D., Moody, D.B., & Stebbins, W.C. (1976). Speech sound discrimination by monkeys and humans. *Journal of the Acoustical Society of America, 60*, 687–695.

Smith, R.L., & Brachman, M.L. (1980). Operating range and maximum response of single auditory nerve fibers. *Brain Research, 184*, 499–505.

Stebbins, W.C. (1970). *Animal psychophysics: The design and conduct of sensory experiments.* New York: Appleton–Century–Crofts.

Stebbins, W.C. (1975). Hearing of the anthropoid primates: A behavioral analysis. In E.L. Eagles (Ed.), *The nervous system: Human communication and its disorders* (Vol. 3, pp. 113–124). New York: Raven Press.

Stebbins, W.C. (1978). Hearing of the primates. In D. Chivers & J. Herbert (Eds.), *Recent advances in primatology* (Vol. 1, pp. 705–720). New York: Academic Press.

Stebbins, W.C. (1980). The evolution of hearing in mammals. In A.N. Popper & R.R. Fay (Eds.), *Comparative studies of hearing in vertebrates* (pp. 421–436). New York: Springer-Verlag.

Stebbins, W.C., Brown, C.H., & Petersen, M.R. (1984). Sensory processes in animals. In I. Darian-Smith, J. Brookhart, & V.B. Mountcastle (Eds.), *Handbook of physiology, sensory processes* (Vol. 1, pp. 123-148). Bethesda, MD: American Physiological Society.

Stebbins, W.C., Miller, J.M., Johnsson, L.-G., & Hawkins, J.E., Jr. (1969). Ototoxic hearing loss and cochlear pathology in the monkey. *Annals of Otology, Rhinology and Laryngology, 78,* 1007-1025.

Stebbins, W.C., Moody, D.B., & Serafin, J.V. (1982). Some principle issues in the analysis of noise effects on hearing in experimental animals. *American Journal of Otolaryngology, 3,* 295-304.

Suga, N. (1973). Feature extraction in the auditory system of bats. In A.R. Moller (Ed.), *Basic mechanisms in hearing* (pp. 675-744). New York: Academic Press.

Suga, N. (1978). Specialization of the auditory system for reception and processing of species-specific sounds. *Federation Proceedings, 37,* 2342-2354.

Syka, J., & Popelav, J. (1980). Hearing threshold shifts from prolonged exposure to noise in guinea pigs. *Hearing Research, 3,* 205-213.

Tees, R.C. (1967). The effects of early auditory restriction in the rat on adult duration discrimination. *Journal of Auditory Research, 7,* 195-207.

Vertes, D., & Nábêlek, I.V. (1977). An audiometric and histologic comparison of noise- and drug-induced cochlear pathology in the chinchilla. In M. Portmann & J.-M. Aran (Eds.), *Inner ear biology* (Vol. 68, pp. 397-403). Bordeaux: Colloques INSERM.

Viemeister, N. (1977). Temporal factors in audition: A system analysis approach. In E. Evans & J. Wilson (Eds.), *Psychophysics and physiology of hearing* (pp. 419-428). London: Academic Press.

Viemeister, N. (1979). Temporal modulation transfer functions based upon modulation thresholds. *Journal of the Acoustical Society of America, 66,* 1364-1380.

Vogten, L.L.M. (1974). Pure-tone masking: A new result from a new method. In E. Zwicker & E. Terhardt (Eds.), *Facts and models in hearing* (pp. 142-155). New York: Springer-Verlag.

Ward, W.D., & Duvall, A.J. (1971). Behavioral and ultrastructural correlates of acoustic trauma. *Annals of Otology, Rhinology and Laryngology, 80,* 881-895.

Ward, W.D., & Turner, C.W. (1982). The total energy concept as a unifying approach to the prediction of noise trauma and its application to exposure criteria. In R.P. Hamernik, D. Henderson, & R.J. Salvi (Eds.), *New perspectives on noise-induced hearing loss* (pp. 423-435). New York: Raven Press.

Webster, D.B., & Webster, M. (1977). Neonatal sound deprivation affects brain stem auditory nuclei. *Archives of Otolaryngology, 103,* 392-396.

Wilkenson, R., & Howse, P.E. (1975). Time resolution of acoustic signals by birds. *Nature (London), 258,* 320-321.

Worden, F.G., & Galambos, R. (1972). Auditory processing of biologically significant sounds: A report based on an NRP work session. *Neurosciences Research Program Bulletin, 10.*

Ylikoski, J. (1974). Correlation between pure-tone audiogram and cochlear pathology in guinea pigs intoxicated with ototoxic antibiotics. *Acta Oto-Laryngologica, Supplement 326,* 5-62.

Zwicker, E. (1976). Psychoacoustic equivalent of period histograms. *Journal of the Acoustical Society of America, 59,* 166-175.

Chapter 2

Developmental Mechanisms of Mammalian Inner Ear Formation[1,2,3]

Thomas R. Van De Water

INTRODUCTION

Formation of the inner ear within the developing embryo is the result of a complex series of tissue interactions occurring over time between the different cell types that compose the local microenvironment which surrounds the developing anlage of the inner ear. To comprehend the series of morphological and cytological changes which result in the formation of the mature membranous and bony labyrinth (see Figure 2-1), it is necessary to understand the developmental mechanisms that provide the inductive influences which effect these changes in cell differentiation and organ geometry. These embryological events are presented as a continuum rather than as unrelated isolated events in the ensuing text, with a stress on mammalian development with reference to both avian and amphibian experiments on inner ear development.

EARLY STAGES

The otic fields are induced at approximately the same time as the neural axis of the embryo by the chorda mesoderm (Yntema, 1950) and are greater in size than the areas of surface ectoderm that actually participate in the formation of the bilateral

[1]This chapter is dedicated to Robert J. Ruben, MD, valued friend and collaborator, to honor the occasion (6/1/83) of his 15th year as department chairman, and to my wife Jeanette, for her understanding and support for all of the late nights and missed weekends that went into its preparation.

[2]Much of the research of this chapter was supported by grants-in-aid to the author from the National Institutes of Health (NSO8365), the March of Dimes, Birth Defects Foundation (I-372), the American Otological Society Research Fund, and the Deafness Research Foundation.

[3]Thanks are given to Cheuk W. Li, PhD, former staff member; Elisabetta Conley, MD, Didier Peron, MD, postdoctoral fellows; Joseph R. McPhee, III, graduate student; Vera Schwartz, MS, and summer students, too numerous to name (eg. Joseph Eviatar and Jeffrey Saver) for their research contributions; to my daughter Ann Marie for her art work of Figures 2-12 and 2-40; Drew Noden, PhD, for Figures 2-21 to 2-23; to Howard Rubin for photographic assistance, and to Susan Montalvo and Janice Cavalcante for their excellent typing of this manuscript.

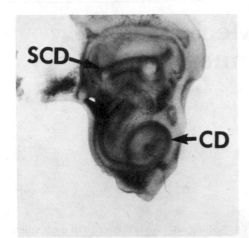

Figure 2-1. A 13-day-old embryonic mouse inner ear that developed for 8 days in organ culture. Two prominent features are a horizontal semicircular duct (SCD) and a coiled cochlear duct (CD). × 32.

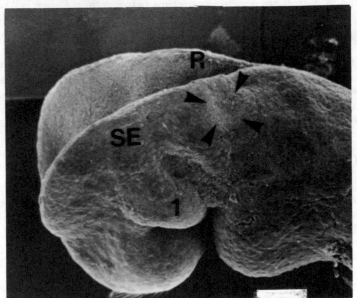

Figure 2-2. *Early stages:* An otic placode (arrowheads) is seen as it forms from the surface ectoderm (SE) just caudal to the first branchial arch (I) and lateral to the fusing edges of the neural tube as it closes to form the rhombencephalon (R) in an 8.5-day-old mouse embryo. Bar = 1 μm.

otic placodes (Harrison, 1945). The otic placodes form from the surface ectoderm (Figures 2-2 and 2-3) in response to inductive cues provided by underlying periaxial mesoderm (Yntema, 1950).

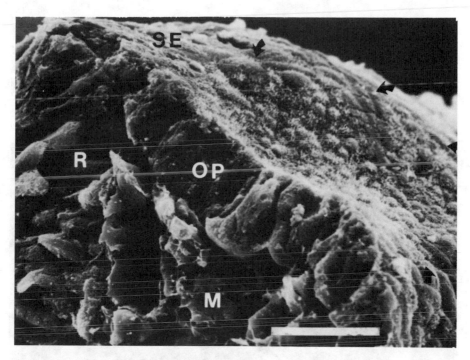

Figure 2-3. *Early stages:* A transverse fracture of an 8.5-day-old mouse embryo at the level of the optic placode (OP) shows its relationships with underlying periaxial mesoderm (M) and adjacent rhombencephalic tissue. The boundaries of this neuroepithelial placode are marked by arrows. Bar = 25 μm.

As the otic placodes invaginate to form otic cups, neuroepithelial cells of this anlage come into close association with neuroepithelial cells of the adjacent rhomb-encephalon (Figures 2-4 and 2-5). Ultrastructural examination of an area of close apposition (Figure 2-6) reveals that the separation between these two apposing neuro-epithelial tissues often consists only of interposed processes of periotic mesenchyme cells. An ultrastructural study (Model, Jarrett, & Bonazzoli, 1981) of the period of inductive interaction between otic anlage and rhomencephalon of an amphibian embryo has demonstrated an area of extensive cellular contacts between these two tissues that have the appearance of focal gap junctions. Similar studies of a comparable period of a developing mammalian inner ear (Van De Water & Conley, 1982) have not demonstrated any areas of cellular contact between closely apposed rhomben-cephalon and otic anlage cells (see also Van De Water, 1980). As the otic cup deepens and begins to separate from the surface ectoderm and form an auditory vesicle, there is an increase in mesenchymal cell processes (Figure 2-7) that form a vellum of cytoplasmic processes which fill the cleft between the otocyst and adjacent brainstem

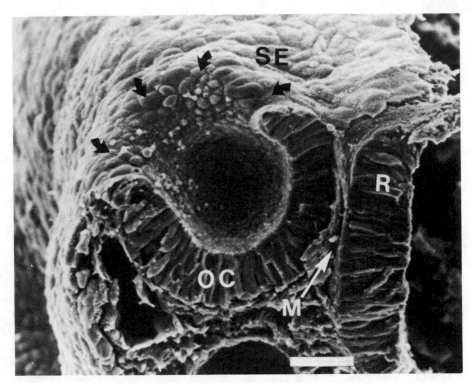

Figure 2-4. *Early stages:* An otic cup (OC) and its relationships to periaxial mesoderm and adjacent rhombencephalon are evident (white arrows) in this scanning electron micrograph of a transverse fractured 9-day-old mouse embryo. Bar = 25 μm.

(rhombencephalon) tissue. At this time, there is also a marked increase in the extracellular matrix material of the cleft between these two neuroepithelial tissues. It is at this stage of inner ear development that the phenomena of the inductive interaction between rhombencephalon and inner ear anlage (otocyst) can first be studied in vitro in the mammal.

NEURAL INFLUENCE

Studies of avian and amphibian embryos have demonstrated that development of their inner ears is dependent upon the inductive influence of rhombencephalon tissue (Chuang, 1959; Detwiler, 1948; Detwiler & Van Dyke, 1950; Harrison, 1924, 1936; Yntema, 1950; and Zwilling, 1941). Waddington (1937) further proposed that other inducing factors in addition to those of the rhombencephalon are active during differentiation of the chick otic ectoderm. One of these factors, he suggested, was the mesoderm adjacent to the otic ectoderm. Yntema (1950), in studying induction

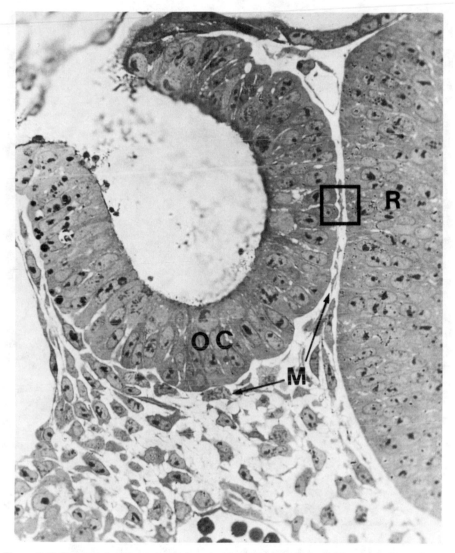

Figure 2-5. *Early stages:* The area of closest apposition between an otic cup and its adjacent rhombencephalon is seen in this 1 μm Epon cross section. Whole mesenchyme cells and their cytoplasmic processes (arrow) invade the cleft between the otic cup and adjacent rhombencephalon. × 500.

of a salamander inner ear, demonstrated that induction of the otic placode is dependent upon mesodermal influences, and that differentiation of the otic vesicle depends on inductive influences of the rhombencephalon (see Figure 2-8).

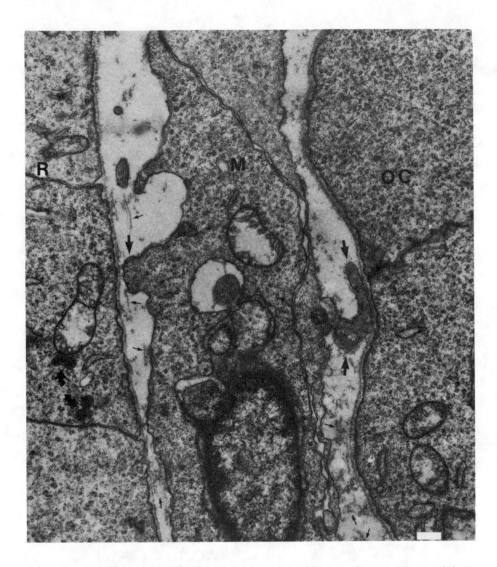

Figure 2-6. *Early stages:* Mesenchyme cells are seen in the cleft between the otic cup and rhombencephalon (area of box in Figure 2-5) with cell processes coming into contact with the basal lamina of both neuroepithelial cell types (large arrows). Extracellular matrix material (small arrows) is present in the cleft and dense core vesicles (large arrows) are present in the basal portions of the neuroepithelial cells of the rhombencephalon. Bar = 1 μm.

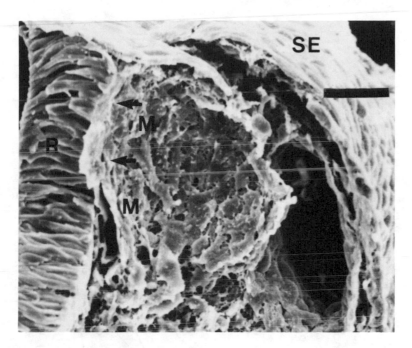

Figure 2-7. *Early stages:* Removal of the otic cup from a transversely fractured 9-day-old mouse
embryo shows the relationship of mesenchyme cells (arrows) to rhombencephalic
and otic tissues at this stage of development. Bar = 25 μm.

In studying the fate map of the mouse otocyst, Li and colleagues (1978a) demonstrated that isolated 10-day-old mouse otocysts fail to differentiate in vitro; while
explants of 11-day-old otocysts differentiated into labyrinths with well-formed sensory
structures.

A preliminary report of the results of a transfilter study by Li, Van De Water,
& Ruben (1978b) suggested that the rhombencephalon exerts an inductive influence
on in vitro differentiation on 10-day-old explants of mouse otocysts.

Further transfilter studies (Van De Water, 1983; Van De Water, Li, Ruben, & Shea,
1980) have shown that 9.5- and 10-day-old otocysts are dependent upon interaction
with rhombencephalic (brainstem) tissue for continued development (see Figure 2-9)
and that 10.5-day-old otocysts are capable of limited vestibular differentiation in the
absence of rhombencephalon, but that development of auditory sensory structures
requires the continuing inductive influence of rhombencephalon (see Table 2-1).

These results, suggesting the continued nature of the inductive influence of the
rhombencephalon upon otic differentiation, were confirmed by a temporal series of
organ culture experiments (see Figure 2-10) in which the spatial relationship between
the otocyst and its adjacent rhombencephalic tissue was kept intact.

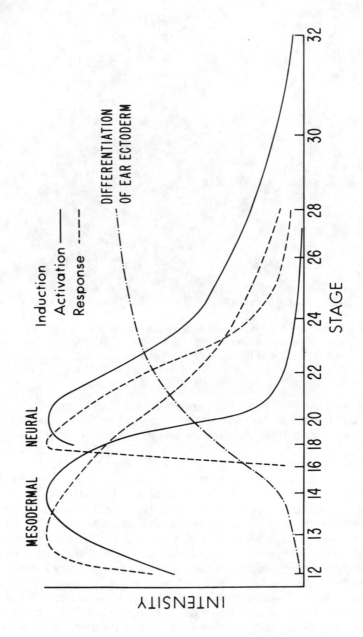

Figure 2-8. *Early stages*: A graphic display of the inductive relationships between ear ectoderm and mesodermal and neural influences based upon results from 1500 amphibian embryo grafts (Yntema, 1950).

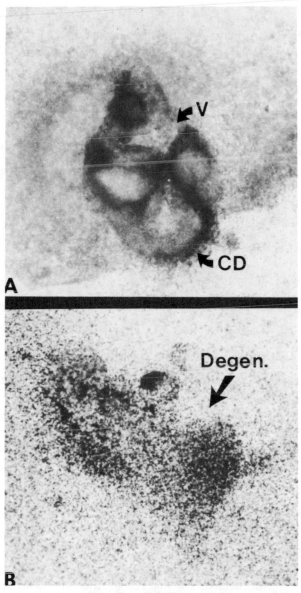

Figure 2-9. *Neural influence:* Transfilter otocyst/rhombencephalon interaction. (A) a 9.5-day-old otocyst interacted with plasma clot-secured rhombencephalic tissue after 10 days of organ culture. Vestibule (V) and cochlear duct compartments have formed. (B) a 9.5-day-old otocyst interacted with only a plasma clot after 10 days in vitro. The otic explant has degenerated (Degen.) × 32.

TABLE 2-1

IN VITRO RESULTS OF OTIC DEVELOPMENT WHEN TRANSFILTER
INTERACTED WITH RHOMBENCEPHALON OR A PLASMA CLOT

	Otocyst/Rhombencephalon			Otocyst/Plasma clot		
	9.5 Day	10 Day	10.5 Day	9.5 Day	10 Day	10.5 Day
Embryonic age						
Cartilaginous capsule	72*	78*	100*	0*	5*	100*
Statoacoustic ganglion	41	67	56	0	5	80
Utriculosaccular space	46	67	56	0	5	100
Maculae: Two	30	33	67	0	5	40
One only	22	33	33	0	5	60
Rudimentary semicircular Ducts with ampulla	51	72	100	0	5	100
Cristae: Three	30	28	67	0	5	40
Two only	19	39	33	0	0	40
One only	5	11	0	0	0	20
Rudimentary cochlear duct	62	67	100	0	5	80
Rudimentary organ of corti	51	67	100	0	5	60
Tectorial membrane	30	44	100	0	5	20
Tissue degeneration	27	22	0	100	95	0
Total No. of specimens	37	18	9	32	21	5

*Percentage = $\dfrac{\text{No. of otic structures observed}}{\text{Total No. of specimens}} \times 100$.

Serial photomicrographs (Figure 2-11) of live 10.5-day inner ear explants that were explanted and grown for 10 days in vitro illustrate the profound effects of the rhombencephalon's continuing inductive influence upon cochlear duct development of a mammalian inner ear.

Both series of organ culture experiments with 9.5-, 10-, and 10.5-day-old mouse embryo otocyst explants demonstrate that rhombencephalic tissue is necessary for continued development of the inner ear in the in vitro system. In the absence of rhombencephalic inductive influence, dysmorphogenesis of the inner ear occurs and cytodifferentiation of otocyst ectoderm into specific sensory structures is impaired. The temporal response of the otocyst to disruption of the inductive influence of brainstem

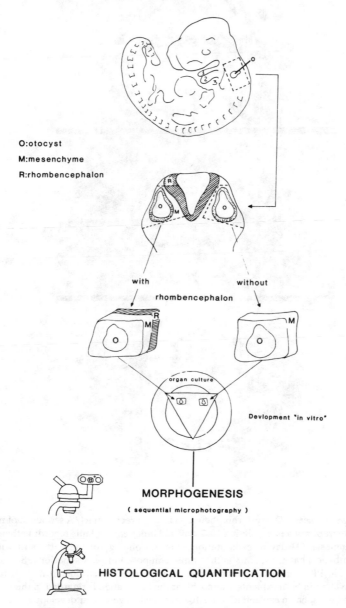

Figure 2-10. *Neural influences:* Design of the otocyst/rhombencephalon direct contact series of experiments.

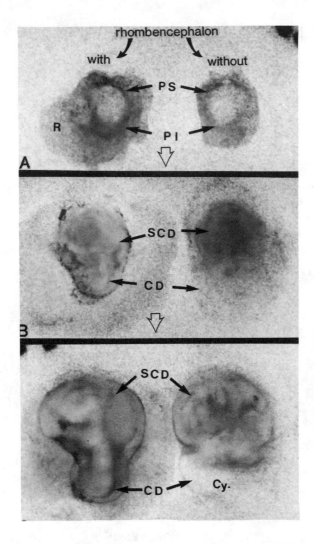

Figure 2-11. *Neural influence:* Otocyst/rhombencephalon – direct contact. A sequence of macrophotographs of a pair of living 10.5-day-old inner ear explants recording their morphogenesis: (A) day of explantation – the morphology of the with- and without-
rhombencephalon explants is the same, composed of pars superior (PS) and pars
inferior (PI) segments; (B) after 6 days in vitro, semicircular duct formation appears
equivalent in both explants, but cochlear duct formation is retarded in the without-
rhombencephalon explant; (C) after 10 days in vitro, vestibular development is similar
in both explants, but dysmorphogenesis of the cochlear duct, cystic outpocket (Cy.),
has occurred in the explant that was explanted without rhombencephalic tissue. × 50.

tissue is graded, with the most severe malformations occurring within the earliest (9.5-day-old) otic explants, while the older (10.5-day-old) inner ear explants confine the expression of dysmorphogenesis and lack of cytodifferentiation to the area of the forming cochlea. The results of this experimental series are presented in diagramatic form in Figure 2-12.

Another series of in vitro experiments transfilter interacted 9.5-day-old otic explants with 10-day-old rhombencephalon. The variable factor in this experiment was the average pore diameter (APD) of the filter membrane channels. Filter channels with an APD of greater than 0.2 μm allow passage of cellular processes and, therefore, contact between interacted tissues; while channels with an APD of less than 0.2 μm preclude cell contact, but allow free exchange of molecules. The results of this study, which utlizes nuclepore filters with an APD of 0.4, 0.2, 0.1, or 0.05 μm and blank filter membranes, demonstrate that cell contact is not required for the passage of the rhombencephalon's inductive message, but that molecular exchange is essential (see Figure 2-13) for this inductive interaction. Inductive interaction between the otocyst and adjacent rhombencephalon is essential for continued development of the inner ear; this brainstem tissue exerts a continuing influence on inner ear development.

EPITHELIOMESENCHYMAL INTERACTIONS

Morphogenesis within an organ system requires the organization of specific cell populations of the forming organ into unique configurations which will ultimately result in the final structure of the organ. What causes and controls the organization of these specific cell populations during the process of morphogenesis? Certain portions of the developmental process are under direct genomic control, but substantial evidence (Bernfield, Cohen, & Banerjee, 1973; Grobstein, 1967, 1968; Hay, 1981; Hay & Meier, 1974; McLoughlin, 1968; Wessells, 1977) suggests that tissue interactions are the primary mechanism for regulating the assembly of specific populations of cells into organs. The development of organs composed of epithelial and mesenchymal components is particularly convenient for study since the interaction involves only two tissues. The interaction occurring between epithelial and mesenchymal tissues appears not to be a series of isolated events, but rather a continuous process. The role of a mammalian otocyst as an inductor tissue in an epitheliomesenchymal tissue interaction was first reported by Grobstein and Holtzer (1955), who demonstrated that a mouse otocyst could act as an inductor of chondrogenesis in somitic mesenchyme in vitro. Benoit (1960, 1964) showed that crude saline extracts of 3- and 4-day-old chick embryo otocysts could induce explants of cephalic mesenchyme to form cartilage, while the cephalic mesenchyme receiving as a control did not undergo chondrogenesis in vitro. Orr and Hafft (1980) have demonstrated that in vitro development of the chick embryo otocyst is dependent upon influences received from its otic mesenchyme. In the following section, experiments defining the role of epitheliomesenchymal tissue interactions in the development of a mammalian embryo inner ear are presented.

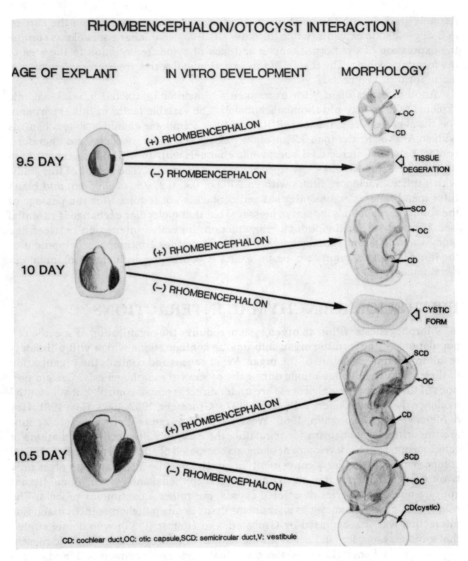

RHOMBENCEPHALON/OTOCYST INTERACTION

AGE OF EXPLANT   IN VITRO DEVELOPMENT   MORPHOLOGY

9.5 DAY

(+) RHOMBENCEPHALON

(−) RHOMBENCEPHALON

V
OC
CD

TISSUE DEGERATION

10 DAY

(+) RHOMBENCEPHALON

(−) RHOMBENCEPHALON

SCD
OC
CD

CYSTIC FORM

10.5 DAY

(+) RHOMBENCEPHALON

(−) RHOMBENCEPHALON

SCD
OC
CD

SCD
OC
CD(cystic)

CD: cochlear duct, OC: otic capsule, SCD: semicircular duct, V: vestibule

Figure 2-12. *Neural influence:* A pictorial summary of the results of the otocyst/rhombencephalon direct series of experiments.

1. Influence of periotic mesenchyme upon otic development. A series of experiments were performed to investigate the nature of the tissue interactions occurring between the otocyst and its surrounding periotic mesenchyme. At the time of explantation, one otocyst was excised in the normal manner with its surrounding periotic

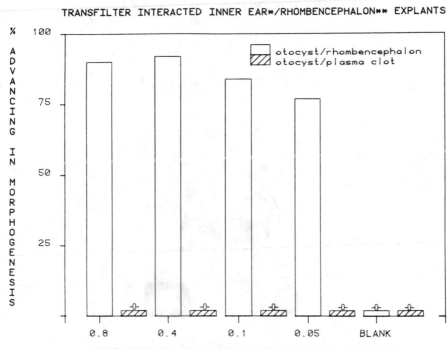

Figure 2-13. *Neural influence:* The results of a series of transfilter-otocyst/rhombencephalon explants in which the average pore diameter of the filter channels was the variable.

mesenchyme (M) intact, while the contralateral otocyst was dissected with as little adhering periotic mesenchyme (m) as possible. Only matched pairs of otocysts derived from the same embryo were employed in this study, to provide exact control for the development stage at the time of surgical manipulation. A schematic drawing depicting the design of this experiment is presented in Figure 2-14. Photomicrographs of all of the specimens were taken, to record gross morphology, at the time of explantation and again at the end of the period of development in vitro. Six gestational ages were studied consisting of explants extirpated from 10.5-, 11-, 11.5-, 12-, 12.5-, and 13-day-old embryos. Embryonic age was determined by somite counts (Rugh, 1968; Theiler, 1972).

The experiment was divided into three groups for each gestational age studied. The first group consisted of explanted otocysts with adequate amounts of adhering periotic mesenchyme (M), while a second group consisted of otocysts that were explanted with minimal amount of adhering periotic mesenchyme (m). The third group

MOUSE   EMBRYO (10.5–13 DAY)

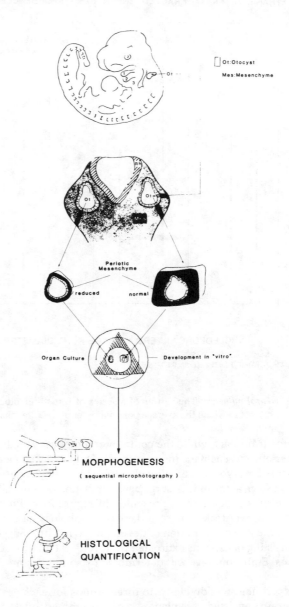

Figure 2-14. *Epitheliomesenchymal interactions:* The design of an experimental series that examined the role of a critical mass of periotic mesenchyme on otic development.

was composed of pairs of otocysts explanted from the same embryo. Otocysts of this third group were cocultured in the same culture dish in proximity to one another, with one otocyst being grown with its mesenchyme intact (M) as in group 1, while the other was a mesenchyme reduced (m) explant as in group 2. Group 3 was included in the study to explore the possibility that there may be some factor from the normal mesenchyme (M) specimens that could be transmitted through the culture medium to the specimens with reduced mesenchyme, thus causing differences in morphogenesis when these reduced mesenchyme specimens were compared to those of group 2 with reduced mesenchyme (m) that were not cocultured with normal mesenchyme specimens.

The morphogenesis observed in the organ-cultured specimens with reduced mesenchyme (m) was comparable in explant groups 2 and 3. The coculturing of (M) and (m) specimens in proximity within the same organ culture dish did not appear to affect the course of morphogenesis of the specimen with reduced mesenchyme (m). A series of macrophotographs recording the morphogenesis of a cocultured pair of 11-day-old inner ear explants with normal (M) and reduced (m) mesenchyme is seen in Figure 2-15. The most striking feature is the size difference, due primarily to the development of a cartilaginous otic capsule in the (M) specimen and the apparent lack of such a capsule in the (m) specimen. Histological analysis of these specimens revealed that the (M) specimens had undergone morphogenesis into areas of vestibule and cochlear duct, whereas the (m) specimens did not undergo any organized pattern of morphogenesis, but formed several small vesicular structures. The photomicrographs in Figures 2-16A and C are cross sections of the (M) and (m) specimens, respectively, whose morphogenesis is recorded in the macrophotographs of Figure 2-15. Histologic analysis of the serial sections of these and other 11-day-old specimens shows that the reduced mesenchyme specimens did not form specific sensory structures, as did the normal mesenchyme explants. Cytodifferentiation of sensory cells occurred within both explants, but was sparse and restricted to a single area of vestibular character in the reduced mesenchyme (m) explant (see Figures 2-16B, D).

Histologic analysis of inner ear morphogenesis and development of sensory structures was performed on serial sections of the 256 inner ear explants which comprised the six gestational ages studied. This analysis, comparing development in the normal (M) and reduced (m) mesenchyme explants, yielded the following observations: (1) 10.5-day reduced mesenchyme explants produced simple flat areas of sensory cells in less than one-half of the cultures and did not form any specific sensory structures; (2) histogenesis of vestibular sensory structures in the reduced mesenchyme explants began in specimens explanted at Day 11 and increased thereafter with age until embryonic Day 12.5, when it attained maximal expression; (3) cytodifferentiation of sensory hair cells of auditory sensory areas first occurred in a few of the reduced mesenchyme explants of Day 11.5 and then increased in frequency of occurrence within these reduced mesenchyme otic explants in direct relationship to their increasing embryonic age. The effects of reduced periotic mesenchymal tissue mass on the development of the embryonic inner ear explants were evident most dramatically in the explants

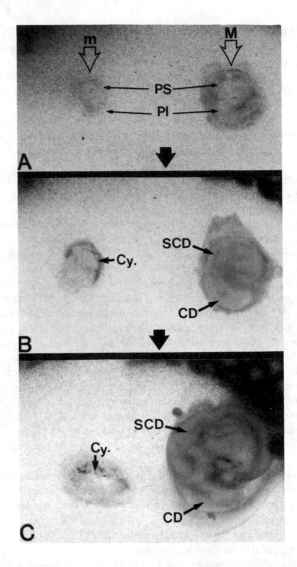

Figure 2-15. *Epitheliomesenchymal interactions:* Sequential macrophotographs of a live pair of 11-day-old otic explants, recording their morphogenesis. (A) day of explantation – the morphology of the otocysts in the normal (M) and reduced (m) mesenchyme explants is similar; (B) after 3 days in vitro, the normal mesenchyme (M) explant has developed into vestibular and cochlear areas, while the reduced mesenchyme (m) explant has expanded its cystic form; (C) after 9 days in vitro, the normal mesenchyme otocyst has formed a labyrinth complete with an otic capsule, while the reduced mesenchyme otocyst has formed a flattened epithelial cyst. × 32.

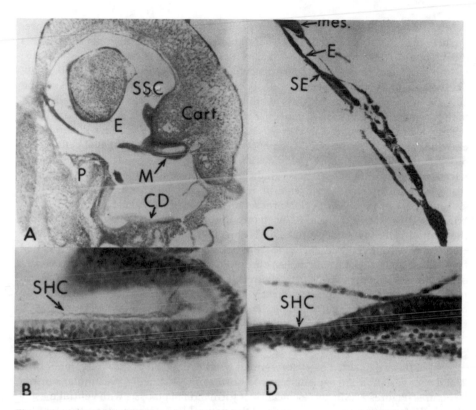

Figure 2-16. *Epitheliomesenchymal interactions:* Histological features of the 11-day-old (M) and (m) inner ear explants (Figure 2-15) that developed for 10 days in vitro: (A) normal mesenchyme (M) explant in cross section. Normal development of vestibular (SSC, M) and cochlear areas is evident with development of endolymphatic (E) and perio-lymphatic (P) spaces. A cartilaginous (Cart.) capsule surrounds this membranous labyrinth. (B) a normal macula of the utriculus of the (M) explant; (C) reduced mesenchyme (m) explant in cross section. Cystic shape is retained with no special-ized areas of sensory epithelial (SE) evident. A reduced endolymphatic space is present, but no perilymphatic spaces or cartilaginous capsule have formed. Only sparse mesenchyme (mes.) is present; (D) the limited area of sensory hair cells (SHC) that differentiated in this (m) explant. The hair cells are vestibular in character (light miscroscopy) but form no specialized sensory structure.

of embryonic Days 10.5 and 11, and decreased thereafter in relationship to the increas-ing embryonic age of the inner ear explants. Thus, some interaction or interactions occurring between the epithelium of the otocyst and its surrounding (periotic) mesen-chyme tissue appear to play a role in the determination and the sequential expression of the developmental program occurring within the epithelial cells of the otocyst.

When this interaction or interactions are prevented or modified, the following consequences are noted in progressively earlier reduced mesenchyme (m) inner ear explants during in vitro development: (1) decreased morphogenesis of labyrinthine form (13- to 10.5-day-old explants); (2) absence of cochlear sensory structures (12.5- to 10.5-day-old explants); (3) lack of formation of specific vestibular sensory structures (11- to 10.5-day-old explants), and (4) loss of ability to differentiate sensory hair cells prior to the formation of any specific inner ear structure (10.5-day-old explants). A graphic portrayal of these results is presented in Figure 2-17. These findings illustrate the essential nature of tissue interactions occurring between the epithelial cells of the otocyst and its surrounding periotic mesenchyme. These tissue interactions are necessary for morphogenesis and cytodifferentiation of the inner ear; disruption of these interactions results in dysmorphogenesis of the labyrinth.

   2. Effect of localized periotic mesenchyme deficiency. Fate map studies (Li, Van De Water, Ruben, & Shea, 1978a) have shown that the cochlear duct forms from the ventral half of the otocyst. Li and McPhee (1979) have studied the effects of the removal of a section of mesenchyme from the ventral portion of otocysts explanted from 11-, 12-, and 13-day-old mouse embryos. Each gestational age group was subdivided into two groups: In the first, controls (CM) underwent no further microsurgical manipulation and were explanted directly to the in vitro system with a normal amount of periotic mesenchyme surrounding the ventral sector of the otocyst (Figure 2-18C); the second, reduced ventral-mesenchyme (VM) group, had adhering periotic mesenchyme dissected away from the ventral portion of the otocyst prior to explantation (Figure 2-18A).

   All of these explanted otocysts were allowed to develop to the equivalent of the 21st day of gestation. All explants showed normal development of vestibular sensory structures (Figures 2-18B, D). Cochlear duct formation of otocysts with ventral mesenchyme (VM) removed was impaired and the ventral half of these otocysts expanded in an unrestrained manner, forming cyst-like extrusions (Figure 2-18B) in place of a normal cochlea. Cochlear ducts of the control specimens (CM) exhibited a normal pattern of morphogenesis in vitro, coiling in a spiral pattern (Figure 18D).

   Additionally, a progressive amount of coiling was observed in specimens of the control groups, corresponding to the embryonic age at the time of explantation to organ culture. Thirteen-day-old otocysts exhibited coiling of the cochlea ranging from one to one-and-a-half turns, while the 11-day-old otocysts produced cochlae in the form of a one-fourth turn hook. The 12-day-old otocysts showed varying degrees of coiling ranging from one-half to one full turn. It is evident that the growth and shape of the cochlea are influenced by the presence of associated periotic mesenchyme. Coiling of the cochlea may be the result of interactions at the epitheliomesenchymal tissue interface occurring between the developing otocyst and its surrounding periotic mesenchyme; another mechanism could be simply the presence of a physical barrier, provided by the cartilage, which differentiates from this surrounding ventral periotic mesenchyme. A combination of both of these factors may be involved in coiling of the cochlea.

   3. Influence of otocyst upon otic capsule formation. The otocyst has been shown to be an essential factor in the formation of its otic capsule and that ablation

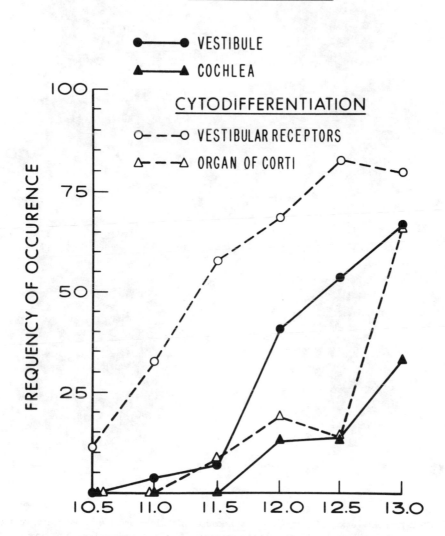

Figure 2-17. *Epitheliomesenchymal interactions:* A graphic presentation of the temporal aspect of the developmental consequences of reduction of mesenchyme volume on in vitro organogenesis of the inner ear.

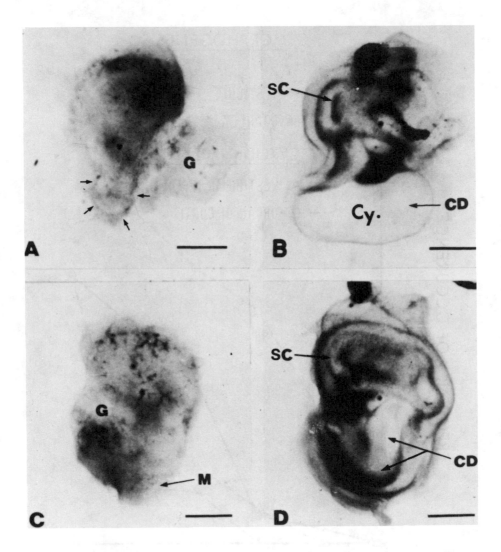

Figure 2-18. *Epitheliomesenchymal interactions:* Localized periotic mesenchyme deficiency (ventral mesenchyme) in 12-day-old otic explants: (A) day of explantation – an otic explant with ventral mesenchyme (VM) removed (arrows); (B) the (VM) explant after 8 days in organ culture. The vestibular labyrinth has developed normally, but the cochlear duct is cystic (Cy.) and has not coiled; (C) day of explantation – otic explant with a normal amount of ventral mesenchyme (CM); (D) the (CM) explant of (C) after 8 days in vitro. Normal otic morphogenesis of both the vestibular and auditory portions of the inner ear are evident. × 32.

of the otocyst during development results in the absence of an otic capsule (Lewis, 1906; Reagan, 1917). The two preceding subsections have demonstrated that the otocyst is dependent upon interaction with its surrounding periotic mesenchyme for normal morphogenesis of a membranous labyrinth. In this subsection, the dependency of the periotic mesenchyme upon the otocyst for its formation into an otic capsule will be presented.

A series of in vitro experiments was performed to investigate the process of inductive interaction between the mouse otocyst and its periotic mesenchyme during otic capsule formation. A chronologic series of otocyst with periotic mesenchyme (Otocyst/Mesenchyme) specimens were extirpated from mouse embryos ranging in age from 10 to 15 days of gestation. A parallel series of isolated periotic mesenchyme (Mesenchyme) specimens were also explanted to in vitro with both series cultured until all specimens attained the equivalent age of 16 days gestation. The specimens were fixed, histologically processed, and stained with toluidine blue stain. Chondrogenesis was rated by the presence of metachromasia and cytologic characteristics of mature chondrocytes. The histogenesis of otic capsule cartilage within 13-day-old explants of isolated periotic mesenchyme after 3 days in vitro is seen in Figure 2-19A. In comparison, 11-day-old isolated periotic mesenchyme explants after 5 days in vitro did not undergo chondrogenesis (Figure 2-19B) and exhibited limited areas of necrosis. A summary histogram depicting the results of histological analysis of all of the mesenchyme with otocyst and isolated mesenchyme explants is presented in Figure 2-20. From these results, it can be concluded that (1) prior to embryonic Day 11.5, the otocyst alone is not a sufficiently strong inductor to control otic capsule formation, and that other factors (i.e., rhombencephal and notochord) are required for otic capsule formation; (2) the otocyst begins to act as an inductor of otic capsule formation on embryonic Day 11.5; (3) determination of the periotic mesenchyme to form a cartilaginous otic capsule is graded and occurs between embryonic Days 11.5 to 13; and (4) by embryonic Day 13, the periotic mesenchyme is sufficiently induced (determined) to be able to undergo chondrogenesis in the absence of the otocyst's inductive influence. The otocyst plays a limited but essential role in organization and induction of its cartilaginous otic capsule.

ORIGIN OF THE STATOACOUSTIC GANGLION

Van De Water and Ruben (1976) reviewed the literature extensively on this subject and concluded that there was strong evidence that the otic anlage makes a major contribution to the formation of its statoacoustic ganglion complex (i.e., Yntema, 1937; 1944) but there was also a growing amount of evidence that neural crest cells participate in some aspect of the formation of this ganglion complex (i.e., Deol, 1967; 1970). New experimental techniques have recently provided more definitive answers to the question of the specific origin of the statoacoustic (eighth nerve) ganglion. Embryonic tissue transplants between quail and chick embryos provide a naturally occurring biological replicating marker (Le Douarin, 1969; 1971) with which to follow the origins

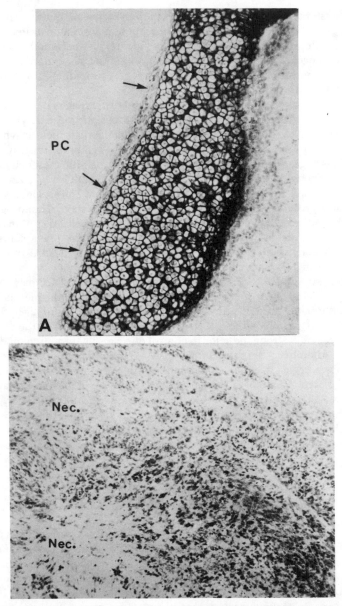

Figure 2-19. *Epitheliomesenchymal interactions:* Isolated periotic mesenchyme explants: (A) a 13-day-old explant after 3 days in vitro has formed a bar of cartilage with a well-defined periochondrium (PC, arrows); (B) an 11-day-old explant after 5 days in vitro has remained as undifferentiated mesenchyme with necrotic foci (Nec.). × 250.

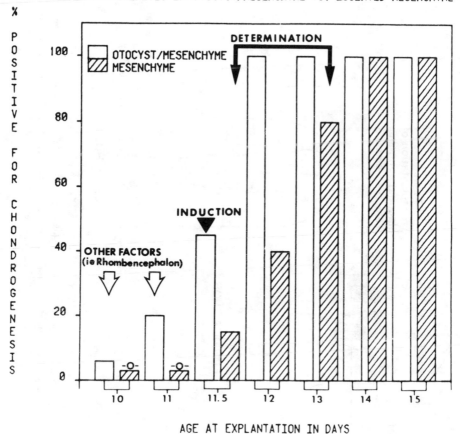

Figure 2-20. *Epitheliomesenchymal interactions:* A summary of the results depicting the in vitro chondrogenic potential of periotic mesenchyme in isolation in comparison to mesenchyme explants with an inductor tissue (otocyst).

of the avian statoacoustic ganglion (Figure 2-21). In a comprehensive study (D'Amico-Martel & Noden, 1983) on placodal and neural crest origins of avian peripheral ganglia these researchers have reported that the acoustic and most, if not all, of the vestibular portion of the eighth cranial nerve ganglion is purely of placodal origin. The neural crest was found to contribute to the formation of all of the eighth cranial nerve ganglion satellite and Schwann sheath cells (Figure 2-22). Further studies by Noden (in press) analyzed chimeric inner ears that were not wholly derived from the placodal transplant. His results (Figure 2-23) show that all of the statoacoustic ganglion neurons have their origin from areas of the otic epithelium that will later form the medial

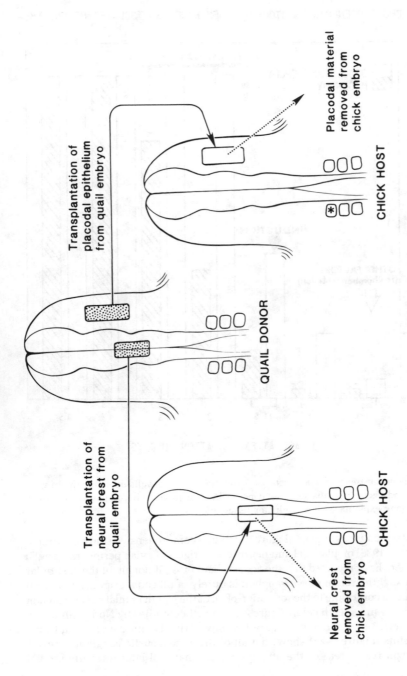

Figure 2-21. *Statoacoustic ganglion:* Schematic drawing of stage 9+ quail and chick embryos showing the method of orthotopic transplantation. Presumptive placodal epithelialium or neural crest is surgically excised from a chick host embryo and replaced with an homologous piece of tissue from a quail donor embryo, somite one.

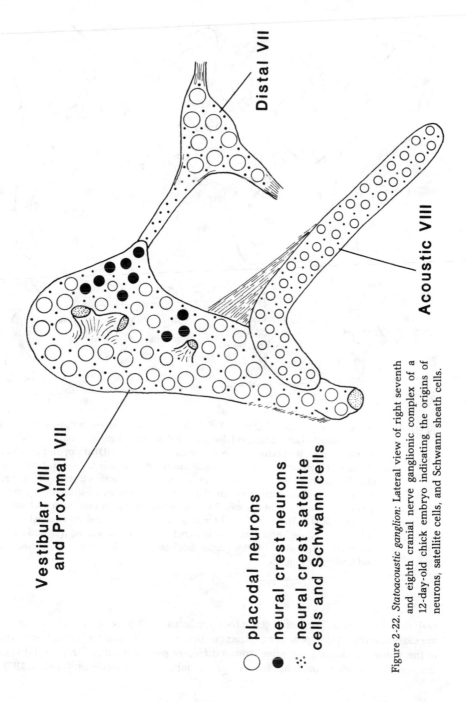

Distal VII

Acoustic VIII

Vestibular VIII
and Proximal VII

○ placodal neurons

● neural crest neurons

∴ neural crest satellite
cells and Schwann cells

Figure 2-22. *Statoacoustic ganglion:* Lateral view of right seventh and eighth cranial nerve ganglionic complex of a 12-day-old chick embryo indicating the origins of neurons, satellite cells, and Schwann sheath cells.

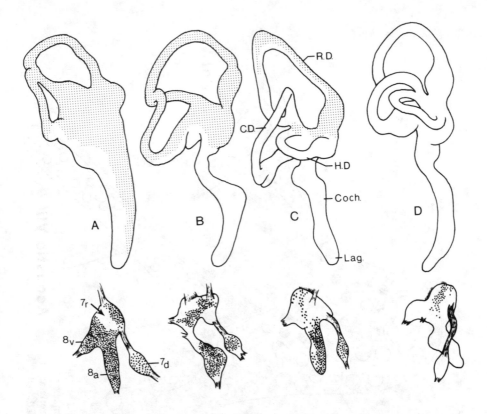

Figure 2-23. *Statoacoustic ganglion:* Figures (A–D) illustrate the different patterns of labeling in reconstructed membranous labyrinths following grafting of small pieces of quail dorsolateral surface ectoderm (A–C) or the neural crest (D) at the mid-myelencephalic level. Strippling indicates quail epithelium. Below are reconstructions of ganglia associated with the seventh and eighth cranial nerves in each of these four hosts. Dots indicate quail neurons. These reconstructions are used to map the origins both of each part of the membranous labyrinth and of vestibular and acoustic neurons. (R.D.), (H.D.), and (C.D.) indicate rostral, horizontal, and caudal semicircular ducts; (Coch.) and (Lag.) are the cochlear duct and lagena; (7p) and (7d) are the proximal (root) and distal (geniculate) ganglia; (8a) and (8v) are the acoustic and vestibular ganglia.

wall of the utriculus. The neurogenic foci producing vestibular and auditory neurons are close together and appear to be either contiguous or overlapping. Thus, the neurons of the statoacoustic ganglion arise from a different part of the membranous labyrinth than that which forms most of their peripheral targets for innervation (Li et al, 1978a).

NEUROTROPHIC INTERACTIONS

Trophic interactions are best defined as interactions between nerves and other cells that initiate or control molecular modification in the other cells and/or the neuron. The earliest observations of a trophic influence were made by Todd (1823) in regenerating amphibian limbs. Farbman (1974) has demonstrated a trophic effect of the gustatory nerve ganglia upon development of taste buds in organ-cultured explants of fetal tongue. The relationship between the statoacoustic ganglion and the developing sensory structures of the labyrinth was an unresolved question. Aspects, pro and con, have perviously been presented by Van De Water and Ruben (1976).

1. Statoacoustic (eighth nerve) ganglion – Sensory receptors. An experiment was designed to answer the question whether or not the neural elements of the statoacoustic ganglion complex exert a trophic effect upon the development of sensory structures within organ-cultured explants of embryonic mouse inner ears. A detailed report of this experiment has been published (Van De Water, 1976). Light micrographs of cross sections of otocyst ventromedial walls from 11, 12, and 13 gestational day specimens are seen in Figure 2-24. These three gestational age groups represent distinct stages of interaction between neural elements of the statoacoustic ganglion complex and the ectodermal cells which compose the otocyst. In 11-day-old otocysts, there are no neural elements penetrating the otocyst; by 12 days of gestation, pioneering nerve fibers penetrate the otocyst wall, and on the 13th day of development, there are fascicles of nerve fibers seen within the epithelial wall of the mouse otocyst. Embryonic otic anlagen with associated periotic mesenchyme and statoacoustic ganglion complexes were excised from CBA/J mouse embryos of 11, 12, and 13 days gestation. These explanted inner ears of each gestational age group were then subdivided into two groups: the first group, A (with statoacoustic ganglion) were explanted to the organ culture system (Van De Water, Heywood, & Ruben, 1973) without further surgical intervention; the second group, B (without statoacoustic ganglion), underwent further microsurgical manipulation, during which their statoacoustic ganglion complexes were dissected away prior to explantation in vitro, and the resultant surgical wound was filled with a section of cephalic mesenchyme. These explants were grown in identical organ culture systems; the A (with ganglion) and B (without ganglion) cultures were grown in separate dishes to control for possible inductive factors that could be transmitted via the culture medium. The explanted inner ears developed in organ culture until the equivalent of embryonic Day 21 was reached for each age group; all cultures were then fixed and histologically processed with a stain for nerve fibers (Bodian's Protargol), in combination with a stain for glycoprotein membranes (Schiff's periodic acid). The resultant histologic specimens were scored (Van De Water & Ruben, 1973) for light microscopic evidence of differentiation of sensory structures and morphogenesis.

The in vitro morphogenesis of the 11-, 12-, and 13-day-old otocysts was similar for both groups A and B. The macrophotographs of Figure 2-25 illustrate this similar pattern of morphogenesis for the explanted 13-day-old otocysts from both groups A and B after 8 days of organ culture. Formations of the organ of Corti in 13-day-old

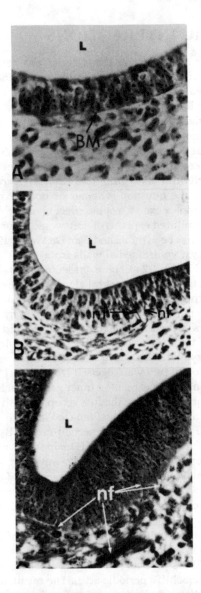

Figure 2-24. *Neurotrophic interactions.* Statoacoustic ganglion–sensory receptors: ventromedial walls of 11- to 13-day-old mouse embryo otocysts stained by Bodian's silver protein method for nerve fibers. (A) an 11-day-old otocyst – no nerve fibers penetrate the basement membrane (BM) of the otocyst; (B) 12-day-old otocyst – pioneering nerve fibers (nf) penetrate otocyst basal lamina; (C) 13-day-old otocyst – fascicles of nerve fibers can be seen penetrating into the otocyst wall.

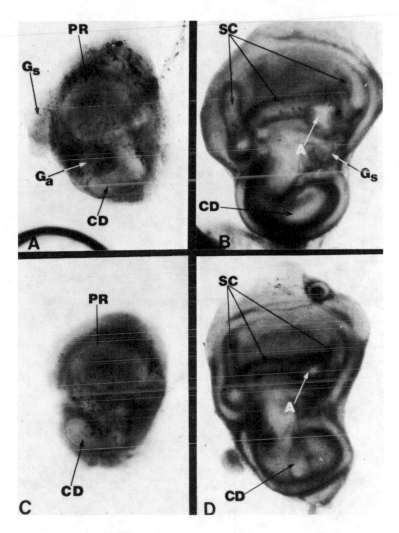

Figure 2-25. *Neurotrophic interactions.* Statoacoustic ganglion–sensory receptors: 13-day-old inner ear explants. (A) and (C), day of explantation; (B) and (D), after 8 days in organ culture. Explants in (A) and (B) have an intact stato- (Gc) acoustic (Ga) ganglion complex. Explants in (C) and (D) have had their statoacoustic ganglion complex excised prior to explantation. × 50.

explants from groups A and B that developed for 8 days in vitro are seen in Figure 2-26. The level of cytodifferentiation in vitro attained by these two groups of specimens is essentially similar in character. The organ of Corti was observed to histologically differentiate in a base-to-apex pattern in the explants in vitro in both group

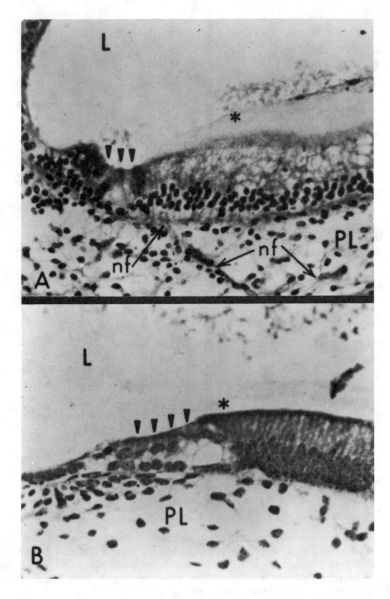

Figure 2-26. *Neurotrophic interactions.* Statoacoustic ganglion–sensory receptors: two 13-day-old inner ear explants, after 8 days in organ culture. (A) with ganglion explant – Corti's organ with nerve fibers originating from the statoacoustic ganglion complex; (B) without ganglion complex explant – Corti's organ that developed without neural elements. Bodian stain, × 500.

A and group B of all gestational ages. In the analysis of the histodifferentiation in vitro of the explanted embryonic inner ears from both groups, the histologic sections were observed with oil immersion objectives for the structure of hair cells. The following histologic qualities were observed: cell morphology, staining characteristics of the nucleus and cytoplasm, morphology of sensory hair tufts, and relationships of sensory membranes to the hair cells. In each gestational age group observed, these characteristics were found to be similar in the specimens from groups A (with statoacoustic ganglion) and B (without statoacoustic ganglion).

The combined results of the histologic quantification of the group A and group B inner ear specimens obtained from 11-, 12-, and 13-day-old embryos are presented in histographic form (Figure 2-27), so that the significant features of the data are easily visualized. Light microscopic observations confirmed that in cultures of group A, statoacoustic ganglion neurons and their nerve fibers were present in association with the developed sensory structures; neither ganglion cell neurons nor their nerve fibers were found to be present in the sensory structures that developed in the organ-cultured specimens of group B. Quantification revealed no consistent trend toward greater occurrence of any sensory structure in any of the groups of explants analyzed.

The presence of such a trend would have signified the probable existence of a trophic effect of the statoacoustic ganglion neural elements on development of the inner ear's sensory structures in the explants of group A when compared to the aganglionic cultured otocysts of group B. Microscopic comparison of the sensory structures and their sensory hair cells revealed no qualitative differences in the histodifferentiation of sensory structures of either group A or group B explants. A base-to-apex pattern of cytodifferentiation of the organ of Corti's sensory structures, which pattern has been reported to occur in vivo, was also respect to whether neural elements were present (A) or absent (B) during development. It was concluded from the above observations that the neuronal elements of the eighth nerve do not exert a trophic influence upon the development of sensory structures of explanted mouse inner ears.

2. Sensory receptors — statoacoustic (eighth nerve) ganglion. The original report (Van De Water, 1976) of the absence of a stimulatory effect of ingrowing neuronal elements of the eighth cranial nerve ganglion upon differentiation of inner ear sensory structures had hypothesized the possible existence of a trophic effect of differentiating inner ear sensory areas upon the ingrowth of nerve fibers from the statoacoustic (eighth nerve) ganglion to these sensory areas. It was suggested that overt cytodifferentiation of presumptive sensory receptor areas is preceded by a wave of chemodifferentiation which would in turn establish fields of chemotaxis that could act to attract the ingrowing neural elements of the eighth nerve ganglion.

An experiment was designed to begin to test the hypothesis that presumptive sensory receptor areas may attract ingrowing neuronal elements of the eighth nerve ganglion by chemotaxis. This study was based upon information obtained from the first set of neurotrophic interaction experiments (Van De Water, 1976) and is reported in detail in a recent publication (Van De Water & Ruben, 1983). Pairs of otocysts were removed from 11-, 12.5-, and 14-day-old embryos; from one otocyst (−), the statoacoustic ganglion was excised while in the other otocyst (+), this ganglion was

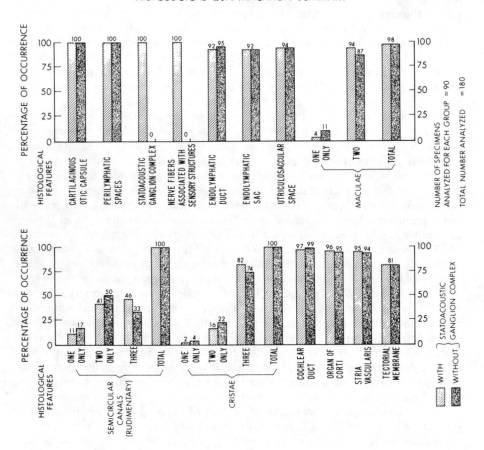

Figure 2-27. *Neurotrophic interactions.* Statoacoustic ganglion–sensory receptors: the confined results of histological quantification of 11-, 12-, and 13-day-old with and without statoacoustic ganglion complex inner ear explants.

left intact. These pairs of otocysts were then explanted into organ culture chambers and cocultured in an orientation so that the statoacoustic ganglion of the intact otocyst (+) was adjacent to the site of ganglion removal of the other (−) otocyst (Figure 2-28). These cocultured inner ear explants developed in vitro to the equivalent of 20 days gestation and were then processed histologically to show both cytodifferentiation of sensory structures and the presence of neuronal elements. Analysis with light microscopic techniques showed that afferent nerve fibers (Figures 2-29A, B) had grown into the areas of developing sensory structures within both otocysts in the 11- and

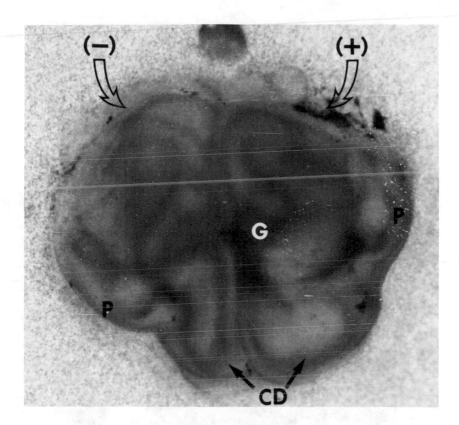

Figure 2-28. *Neurotrophic interactions.* Sensory receptor–statoacoustic ganglion: cocultured 12.5-day-old otic explants after 8 days of organ culture. Right (+) otocyst was explanted with an intact statoacoustic ganglion; left (−) otocyst explanted without its ganglion complex. × 50.

12.5-day-old explants, but not within the 14-day-old explants. These results show that an ingrowth of eighth nerve neurities into (−) aganglionic 11- and 12.5-day-old (−) otocysts had occurred and that these nerve fibers grew preferentially to the sites of differentiating sensory structures which were located close to their source within cocultured (+) otocyst explants.

The results of the 12.5-day-old cocultured explants (Figure 2-30) suggest that those areas of the otocyst committed to forming sensory receptors may, prior to overt cytodifferentiation, undergo a biochemical differentiation and consequently be active in establishing chemoattractant fields that may act to direct the ingrowth of neuronal elements from a nearby source to their target sites.

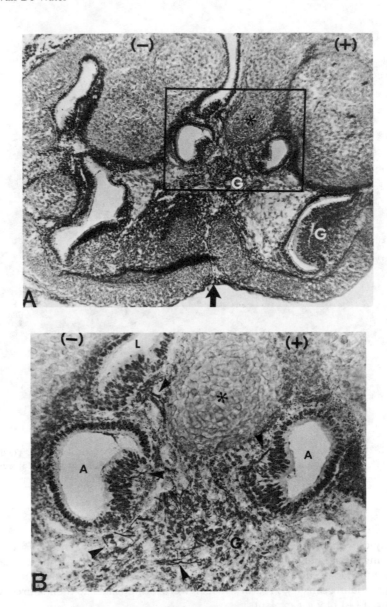

Figure 2-29. *Neurotrophic interactions.* Sensory receptor–statoacoustic ganglion: cocultured 12.5-day-old otic explants after 8 days in vitro. (A) a cross section of the explants of Figure 2-28 showing positional relationships in these explants. The asterisk indicates a common capsular wall and heavy arrow, the site of abutment of cochlear ducts. × 130; (B) the area of the box of (A). Nerve fibers are present in association with the cristae of both (+) and (−) ganglion otic explants. × 310.

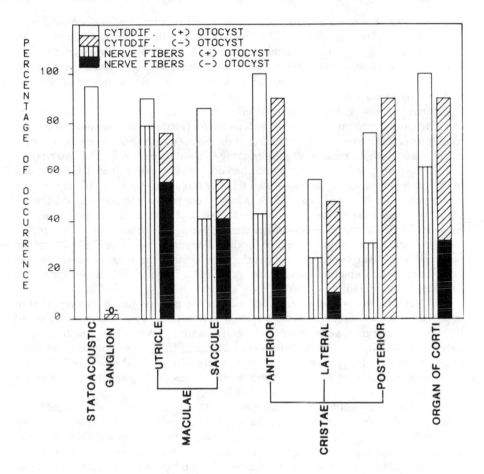

Figure 2-30. *Neurotrophic interactions.* Sensory receptor–statoacoustic ganglion: The results of quantification of cystodifferentiation and presence of nerve fibers in cocultured 12.5-day-old (+) and (−) ganglion inner ear explants.

These results, combined with the observations in the 11- and 14-day-old cocultured inner ear explants, support the hypothesis of a limited period of chemotrophic gradient fields and chemotaxis as a mechanism for the establishment of the pattern of innervation of inner ear sensory receptors by its statoacoustic (eighth nerve) ganglion.

FATE MAPPING

Levy (1906) observed that the cells of the amphibian otic cup developed independent of their environment, and that the fates of these cells were not yet determined. He postulated that any half of the otic cup would develop into a complete labyrinth half the size of a normal ear. Streeter (1914) and Spemann (1918) arrived at a different conclusion and stated that the otic cup was not a harmonic equipotential system, and that these cells were determined by the time of otic cup formation.

Harrison (1924, 1936) demonstrated that at the time of neural fold closure, the otic placode of *Amblystoma punctatum* was no longer isotropic, but was polarized along its anteroposterior axis. This polarization of the placode cells determines the arrangement of labyrinthine sensory structures along this anteroposterior axis. Polarization along the dorsoventral axis of the placode had not yet been determined. Determination of this dorsoventral axis appears at a slightly later stage (early tail bud) of labyrinthine development (Hall, 1939; Kaan, 1926). Kaan (1926) performed surgical ablation of otocysts in *Amblystoma punctatum* and concluded that after the developing inner ear passed the otic cup stage, regeneration was difficult. She demonstrated that reproducible characteristic defects could be produced depending on which portions of the otic cup were ablated and at which developmental stage the surgical operation was performed. Kaan's ablation experiments provided a fate map for the anlage of the developing amphibian inner ear.

1. Normal otocyst. An in vitro fate map of the mouse otocyst was reported in detail by Li and colleagues (1978a). Otocysts of 11 and 12 days gestation were dissected into six anatomic groups of either dorsal/ventral, anterior/posterior, or medial/lateral halves. The dorsal and ventral halves were obtained by an anteroposterior incision midway through the 11- and 12-day-old otocysts; anterior and posterior halves by a dorsoventral incision, and medial and lateral halves by surgical ablation of either the respective lateral or medial wall of the otocyst.

Because of surgical trauma difficulties, the 11-day-old otocyst was not included in the medial/lateral anatomic group. Each anatomic group of otocysts was cultured separately for 10 days. At the end of the experiment, the explants were histologically processed and analyzed with light microscopy. Histological control showed the 11- and 12-day-old mouse otocysts to be composed of undifferentiated ectodermal cells, ranging from pseudostratified columnar to low cuboidal cells. Macrophotographs of dorsal and ventral explants of the 12-day-old mouse otocysts after 10 days of in vitro development illustrate formation of vestibular and cochlear structures from dorsal and ventral halves, respectively (Figure 2-31). The results of this fate-mapping study indicate that by the 11th day of gestation, the mouse otocyst is already a mosaic for the development of otic sensory structures with respect to its dorsoventral and anteroposterior axes. Analysis of the 12-day-old explants reveals that mosaicism of otic sensory structures relative to the mediolateral axis is present by the 12th day of gestation. The fate map of the mouse otocyst is summarized by eight anatomic sectors presented in Figure 2-32. The anterior semicircular duct and its associated crista ampullaris develop from the dorsoanterior portion of the otocyst and its associated crista ampul-

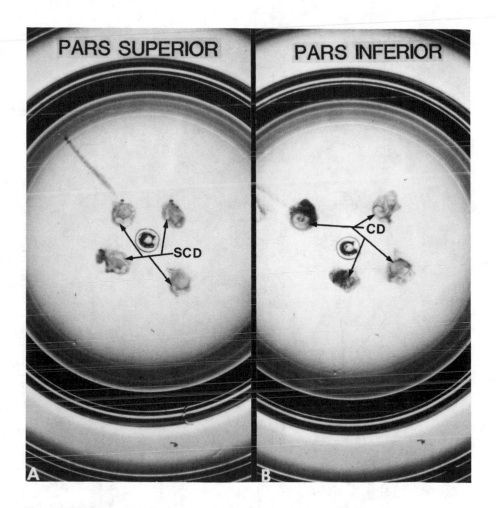

Figure 2-31. *Fate map (normal):* Otic explants (12-day-old) after 10 days in organ culture. (A) Par superior (dorsal halves) formed vestibular structures; (B) pars inferior (ventral halves) formed auditory structures. × 15.

laris from the anterior dorsolateral sector. The posterior duct and its associated crista ampullaris form from the dorsoposterior portion of the otocyst. The utricle derives from the dorsal segment of the middle third of the otocyst and its macula from the anterior portion of this same segment. The saccule and its associated macula develop from the middle third of the anterior wall, ventral to the site of origin of the utricle. The cochlear duct and its sensory epithelium differentiate from the ventral portion of the otocyst.

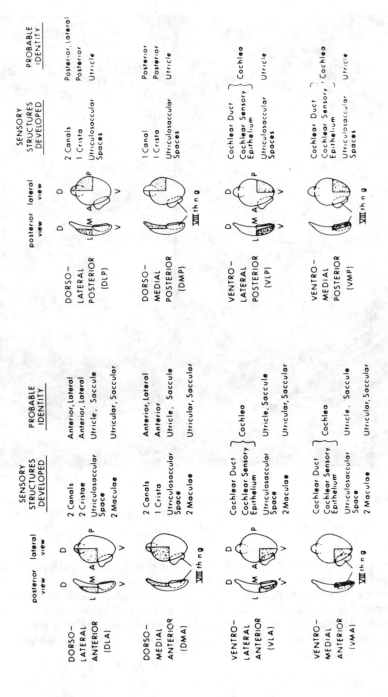

Figure 2-32. *Fate map (normal):* Summary chart of the fates of eight anatomical sectors of mammalian otocyst.

A fate map of the mouse otocyst provides two important pieces of information. First, it shows that cell determination has occurred on or prior to the 11th day of gestation. Ten-day-old otocysts, grown in isolation from rhombencephalon, failed to show gross morphologic differentiation (see Neural induction). Secondly, the fate map of a normal mouse otocyst provides a model for normal structural development of the inner ear that can be used to compare the pathologic morphogenesis of congenitally malformed labyrinths.

2. Abnormal otocyst. Van De Water and Ruben (1974) reported that in vitro explants of homozygotic kreisler otocysts reproduced the phenotypic expression of this congenital malformation as it occurs in vivo (Hertwig, 1944). Li (1979) examined the cell determination of the kreisler mouse and found that the heterozygotic kreisler (+/kr) otocyst (Figure 2-33A) differentiated according to the fate map of a normal mouse otocyst (Li et al, 1978a). In contrast, the homozygotic kreisler (kr/kr) otocyst followed a developmental course that was both variable and different from that of the heterozygotic kreisler otocyst, and which resulted in the formation of malformed labyrinth (Figure 2-33B). However, in spite of this variable pattern of development, the kr/kr otocyst appeared to follow, in a general pattern, the normal outline of dorsoventral pattern of development of otic sensory structures (Table 2-2). Sensory structures, abnormal in size and shape, were often recognizable in histologic preparations of both dorsal and ventral explants of homozygotic kreisler (kr/kr) otocysts. Deformed semicircular ducts and their cristae differentiated in the dorsal halves of explanted kr/kr otocysts, and the middle portions of these kr/kr otocysts developed into utriculosaccular structures. Cystic structures in place of cochlear ducts were derived from the ventral halves of kr/kr otocysts in vitro. The homozygotic kreisler otocyst, although abnormal in its pattern of morphogenesis, did exhibit a dorsoventral polarity of sensory receptor development.

ROLE OF THE ENDOLYMPHATIC DUCT AND SAC ANLAGE

Harrison (1945) suggested that the intactness of the endolymphatic appendage may be an essential factor in the orderly organogenesis of the amphibian inner ear. Bonnevie (1936) and Hertwig (1944), when studying the development of mutant mouse embryos (shaker-short and kreisler mice, respectively) that had congenitally malformed inner ears, noted that both homozygotic genotypes did not develop endolymphatic duct and sac anlage in the early otocystic stage of inner ear development. A report of histological findings in malformed human fetal material (Partsch, 1966) drew the conclusion that the absence of an endolymphatic duct and sac system impaired the regulation of labyrinthine pressure which, in turn, impaired labyrinthine differentiation. Hendricks and Toerien (1973) experimented with endolymphatic duct and sac anlage extirpation in chick embryos in ovo and concluded that an intact endolympatic duct and sac anlage was essential for orderly organogenesis of the chick labyrinth. Van De Water and Ruben (1974) organ-cultured homozygotic and heterozygotic

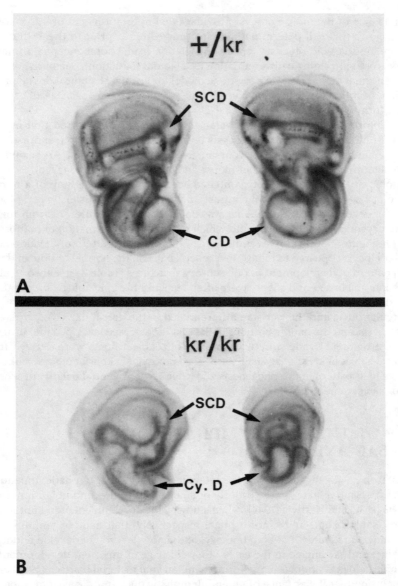

Figure 2-33. *Fate map (normal):* Otocysts (12-day-old) after 8 days in vitro. (A) heterozygotic kreisler (+/kr) otic explants show a normal pattern of inner ear morphogenesis; (B) homozygotic kreisler (kr/kr) otic explants produce congenitally malformed labyrinths with a variable pattern of phenotypic expression, but usually with short blunt semicircular ducts that may end blindly and uncoiled short cystic cochlear ducts (Cy. D). × 40.

TABLE 2-2

FATE MAP OF HOMO- AND HETEROZYGOTIC
12-DAY-OLD KREISLER OTOCYSTS

	Dorsal half of otocyst		Ventral half of otocyst	
	Homozygotic (kr/kr)	Heterozygotic (+/kr)	Homozygotic (kr/kr)	Heterozygotic (+/kr)
OTIC STRUCTURES				
Cartilaginous capsule	87*	100	93	100
Statoacoustic ganglion	7	7	36	63
Perilymphatic space	40	93	14	88
Endolymphatic duct and sac	0	57	0	0
Utriculosaccular space	73	93	36	43
Maculae: Two	13	36	29	43
One only	53	50	29	43
Rudiments of semicircular				
Ducts: Three	13	79	0	0
Two only	40	14	0	0
One only	27	7	0	0
Cristae: Three	13	79	0	0
Two only	40	14	0	0
One only	27	7	0	0
Cochlear duct	0	0	64	100
Cochlear sensory epithelia	0	0	36	94
Tectorial membrane	0	0	29	81
Tectorial membrane	0	0	29	81
Stria vascularis	0	0	0	25
Total No. of specimens	15	14	14	16

*Percentage = No. of otic structures observed × 100.
              Total No. of specimens

kreisler otocysts. They reported that the homozygotic kreisler otocyst in vitro phenotypically reproduced its in vivo pattern of malformation. These homozygotic kreisler explants were observed to lack an endolymphatic appendage at the time of explantation to the organ culture system, relative to otocysts explanted from heterozygotic littermates of a comparable stage of development. This observation suggests that lack of an endolymphatic duct and sac anlage is in some way involved in the production of the cystic malformation of the homozygotic kreisler labyrinth.

1. Ablation experiments. An experiment was designed to observe the effects of removal of the endolymphatic duct and sac anlage upon the organogenesis of a normal mouse's inner ear in vitro. Twelve- and 13-day-old mouse otocysts were excised and each gestational age group of specimens was further divided into two groups. The first group did not undergo further surgical manipulation and was explanted directly into organ culture; the second group underwent further microsurgical dissection which effected the complete removal of the endolymphatic duct and sac anlage at the point at which the anlage joined the dorsomedial aspect of the otocyst's pars superior. No other otocystic ectodermal tissue was excised. A piece of cephalic mesenchyme was placed in the operative site to effect wound closure, and the "without" explants were then placed into organ culture.

All specimens were allowed to develop in vitro to the equivalent of 21 days of gestation. The specimens were then fixed and processed histologically with a conventional hematoxylin and eosin staining technique. The specimens were code-labeled and histologically quantified for development with the aid of a light microscope. Figure 2-34 presents a dark-field photomicrograph of two 13-day-old explants after 8 days of development in vitro, one with an intact and the other without an endolymphatic appendage grown in the same culture dish.

The in vitro morphogenesis of these specimens is similar, with no gross distortion evident in either specimen. A photomicrograph of a histologic cross section of a 13-day-old otic explant "without" endolymphatic duct and sac anlage after 8 days in vitro is shown in Figure 2-35. The histologic features of this organ-cultured specimen were similar to those observed in comparable stages "with" endolymphatic duct and sac anlage specimens. The histologic quantification data obtained from 13-day-old explants are presented in the histogram of Figure 2-36. The 12-day-old explant results were similar to these observations of the 13-day-old specimens.

The resultant histologic quantification of the in vitro embryogenesis of the inner ear explants from either 12- or 13-day-old embryos did not reveal any significant differences in morphogenesis or cytodifferentiation of labyrinthine sensory structures, nor any presence of hydrops of the endolymphatic cavities in any of these organ-cultured specimens. It was concluded that, in the system studied, the absence of the endolymphatic duct and sac anlage did not have a significant effect on the organogenesis of the inner ear, with the exception of the resultant lack of development of an endolymphatic duct and sac. A detailed presentation of these results is contained in a published report (Van De Water, 1977).

2. Cannulation experiments. The role of internal pressure has been shown to be of great importance in the development of the eye (Coloumbre, 1956) and brain (Desmond & Jacobson, 1977). A previous in vitro study (Van De Water, 1977) indicated that removal of the endolymphatic duct and sac anlage does not interfere with development of the inner ear. The role of intralabyrinthine pressure, which may be exerted by the fluid of the endolymphatic space during organogenesis of the inner ear, has

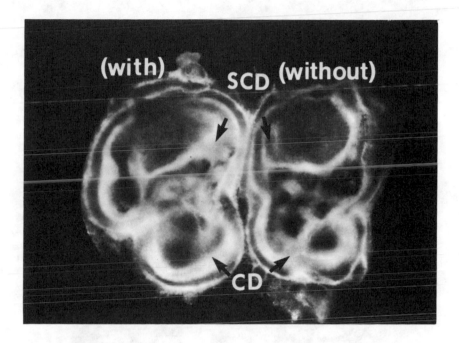

Figure 2-34. *ED&S anlage (ablation):* Dark field macrophotograph of pair of 13-day-old otic
explants after 8 days in vitro. The right otocyst was explanted with an intact endolymphatic duct and sac anlage while this anlage was ablated in the left otocyst
prior to explantation. The in vitro morphogenesis of both these otocysts is of a
normal pattern for both vestibular and auditory structures. × 20.

not been directly studied. The present study is designed to evaluate the role of intro-
labyrinthine fluid pressure on inner ear development.

Inner ear explants excised from 12-, 12.5-, 13-, and 14-day mouse embryos were
the experimental subjects. In the first two groups, the endolymphatic sac anlage was
incised at its distal end and either a hollow glass tube or a solid glass rod of 50μm
diameter was inserted through the endolymphatic duct to the level of entry of this
duct into the utriculosaccular anlage. The explants with the inserted glass tubes with
a patent lumen had permanent communication between the endolymphatic compartment and the culture medium. The second group of explants, with solid glass rods
cannulating the endolymphatic ducts, underwent a surgical procedure identical to
that of the first group but had no communication between the developing endolymphatic spaces and the culture medium. The third group of explants consisted of intact
otocysts with no surgical intervention other than explantation into the organ-culture
system. The morphogenesis of the otocysts was evaluated by daily microscopic examination. A pair of 12.5-day-old inner ear explants that were cannulated with a patent

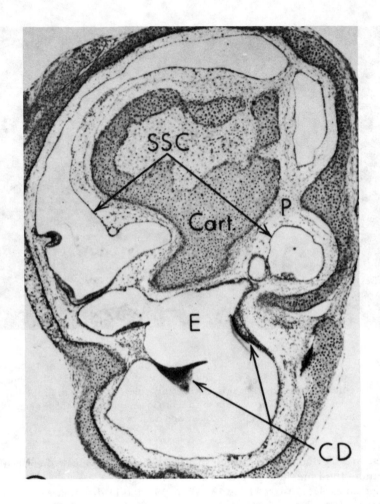

Figure 2-35. *ED&S anlage (ablation):* Otocyst (13-day-old) explanted without an endolymphatic
duct and sac anlage, after 8 days in vitro. This cross section of an explant shows
normal development of all sensory structures, endolymphatic and perilymphatic
spaces, and an otic capsule. × 55.

tube and a solid rod are presented on day of explantation and then after 2 and 9 days
of in vitro development in Figure 2-37. The morphogenesis of labyrinthine form in
both of these specimens is of similar geometry. At an in vitro day equivalent to the
21st day of embryonic development, the inner ear explants were processed histologically with standard paraffin techniques and stained with hematoxylin and eosin.

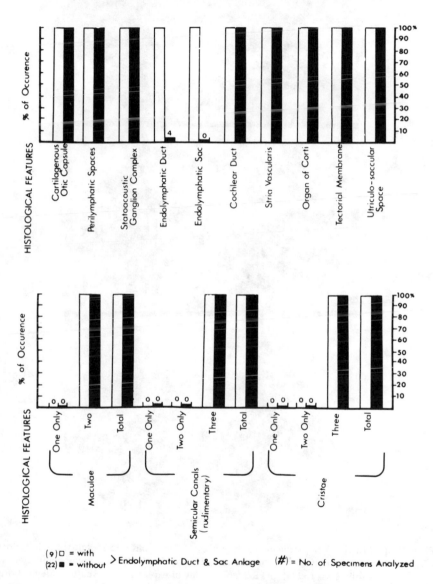

13th - GESTATION DAY SPECIMEN
HISTOLOGICAL QUANTIFICATION SUMMARY

Figure 2-36. *ED&S anlage (ablation):* A summary of the results of histological quantification of 13-day-old with and without endolymphatic duct and sac anlage otic explants.

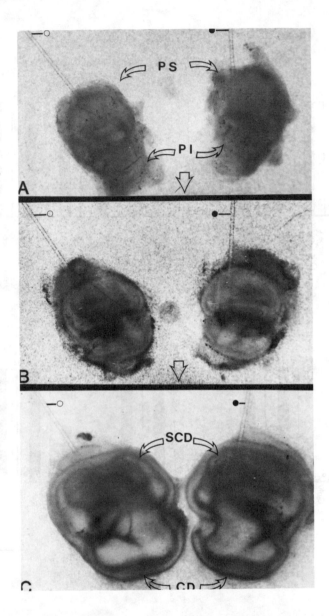

Figure 2-37. *ED&S anlage (cannulation):* A pair of 12.5-day-old otic explants; the left otocyst was cannulated with a glass tube (o) while the right otocyst was cannulated with a solid glass rod (•). (A) Explants of day of explantation; (B) after 2 days of organ culture; (C) after 9 days in vitro. The morphogenesis of these otocysts are similar and follow a normal pattern of otic development. × 50.

No difference in the development of the inner ears was found among the three groups. There was no delay in morphogenesis of labyrinthine geometry in any of the three groups of explants. The development of inner ear neurosensory structures was normal in all of the groups. It is concluded that neither the cannulation of the endolymphatic sac nor intralabyrinthine fluid pressure were influencing the morphogenesis or differentiation of sensory structures of the developing otocyst within the organ-culture environment.

CONGENITAL MALFORMATION

There are more than 50 genetically different strains of deaf mice (Altman & Katz, 1979), of which a number have been histologically studied (Deol, 1980). One of these, the kreisler strain, is of particular interest in that the expression of the malformation in the homozygote (kr/kr) involves the entire bony and membranous labyrinth (Hertwig, 1944). The cell kinetics of the otocyst epithelium of the homozygotic kreisler embryos has been documented (Ruben, 1973) and found to be abnormal compared to otocysts of heterozygotic littermates and a normal inbred strain of mice (CBA-J). The expression of the labyrinthine lesion in the kreisler mouse is pleomorphic (Ruben, 1973). Some ears consist only of a large cyst which can be of significant enough size as to compromise and compress the brainstem (Figure 2-38), while other inner ears may have a near-normal bony labyrinth but be devoid of sensory structures. This variability of genetic expression into a phenotype must be taken into account in studies of the kreisler mouse inner ear.

Organ-culture studies (Van De Water & Ruben, 1974) have shown that inner ear explants from homozygotic (kr/kr) mutant embryos and their heterozygotic (+/kr) littermates will express their genotype in vitro (Figure 2-33), thereby providing a model system with which to investigate the mechanism of congenital malformation of a mammalian inner ear.

Fate map studies (Li, 1979; Table 2-2) show that by the 11th day of gestation determination of the homozygous (kr/kr) otocyst into dorsal and ventral patterns of labyrinthine development is evident.

Deol (1966) has suggested that the site of action of the kreisler gene may be a localized defect in the rhombencephalon that in turn causes faulty induction of the otic anlage, ultimately resulting in a malformed labyrinth. To study the validity of this hypothesis, a series of studies were undertaken to study the consequence of interacting normal (CBA/C57) rhombencephalon with homozygotic kreisler (kr/kr) otocysts and conversely homozygotic kreisler (kr/kr) rhombencephalon with normal (CBA/C57) otocysts. These experiments were performed in vitro by explanting an otocyst, of either a normal or mutant genotype, and allowing it to develop in direct contact with a rhombencephalon explant of either a normal or mutant genotype. The experiments are difficult to perform because of the low fertility of the kreisler strain of mice and, consequently, these experiments must be carried out over a number of years. Additionally, any interpretation of the results must take into account the variability of the phenotypic expression of the kreisler inner ear malformation. This

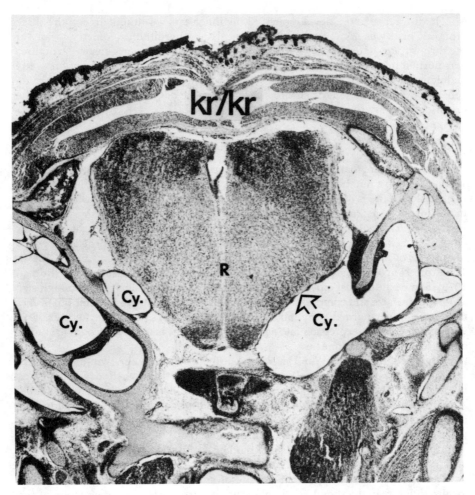

Figure 2-38. *Congenital malformation:* A homozygotic kreisler (kr/kr) fetus at birth showing bilateral cyst formation extruding through an anomolous internal auditory meatus and
compressing the brainstem (rhombencephalon). There were no normal-appearing
labyrinthine structures. × 10.

requires that a large number of studies be done, which further extends the length
of time which is needed for this particular series of experiments. Preliminary findings
show that a homozygotic kreisler (kr/kr) otocyst will develop less abnormally when
interacted with a normal (CBA/C57) rhombencephalon. Additionally, there appears
to be little or no effect on the in vitro pattern of normal (CBA/C57) otocyst
development when interacted with homozygotic kreisler (kr/kr) rhombencephalon

when compared to normal otocysts interacted with normal rhombencephalon. These results do not implicate the rhombencephalon as the primary site of action of the kreisler gene since abnormal rhombencephalon is ineffective in changing the developmental course of a normal otocyst. Deol (1974, 1980) also described a greater distance of separation in the otocyst/rhombencephalon relationship of homozygotic (kr/kr) kreisler embryos. An ultrastructural study of homozygotic (kr/kr) and heterozygotic (+/kr) kreisler embryos has confirmed these observations. The distance separating the rhombencephalic tissue from the otic anlage in homozygotic kreisler embryos (Figure 2-39) can be as much as 100 times the normal separating distance observed in kreisler heterozygotes and normal (CBA/C57) mouse embryos.

The combined findings suggest that the site of gene action in the kreisler mouse may be a very early developmental event (i.e., regional defect in the chorda mesoderm) which then acts as a faulty inductor of both the rhombencephalon and otic fields which in turn affects the normal spaciotemporal pattern of tissue interactions. If a primary inductive event is disrupted or abnormal, then subsequent inductive events (i.e., otocyst/rhombencephalon) are likely to be affected.

These observations are useful in furthering our understanding of genetic disease of the inner ear, as they suggest that some genetic abnormalities may not directly affect the inner ear, but may be the result of abnormalities interfering with the expression of the normal sequence of inductive tissue interactions which direct the formation of the inner ear. This type of mechanism may be operant in a genetic syndrome which is associated with other abnormalities, for example, Waardenburg's disease, Apert's disease, Pendred's disease. This, then, allows the investigator to focus attention on what could be a common mechanism that could result in a heterogeneous phenotype instead of only focusing on the description of abnormalities of the inner ear.

SYNTHESIS OF DEVELOPMENTAL MECHANISMS

Condensations of experimental results which seek to define embryonic mechanisms of vertebrate inner ear development have been presented in this chapter. To synthesize an overall view of the embryogenesis of the inner ear, these data on development are combined with other experimental data relating to inner ear development (Van De Water & Ruben, 1976; Van De Water et al., 1980; Van De Water, 1983). These combined data on development of a tetrapod inner ear have formed the basis for the formulation of a flow chart depicting developmental mechanisms of the inner ear formation (Figure 2-40).

Determination of an otic field in head ectoderm by the inductive action of the chorda mesoderm has been verified in both amphibian (Yntema, 1950; Zwilling, 1941) and avian embryos (Waddington, 1937). Ultrastructural studies in the chick embryo at the stage of otic placode formation (Meier, 1978a, b) suggest that cell contacts between ectoderm cells of the otic field and what were suggested to be migrating neural crest cells are an important event in placodal formation. Earlier studies by Noden (1972) have shown that migrating neural crest cells pass both anterior and posterior

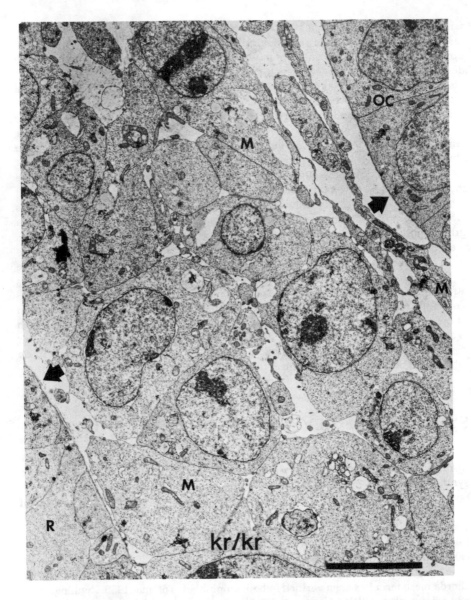

Figure 2-39. *Congenital malformation:* A 9-day-old homozygotic kreisler (kr/kr) embryo at the area of closest apposition between rhombencephalon and otic cup. The separation between these two neuroepithelials is approximately 100 times the normal cleft width in the area of closest apposition in a normal mouse embryo of this developmental stage. Bar = 1 μm.

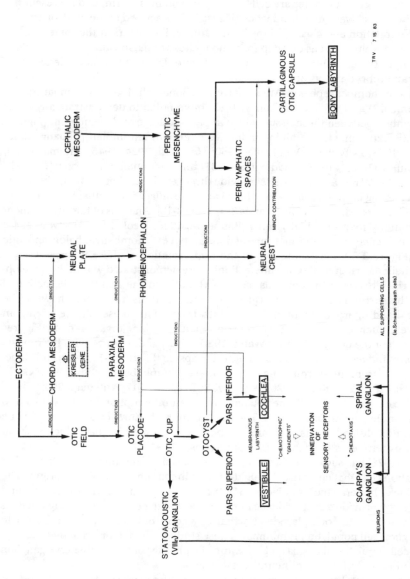

Figure 2-40. *Development mechanisms*: A flow chart depicting the major developmental interactions which influence and control formation of the inner ear and a suggested site of action of the kreisler gene. Heavy lines trace the sequence of changes in otic structures. Light lines indicate the influences which operate at each step or steps.

to the developing otic placode, but not under this ectodermal placode. It may, therefore, be concluded that these cells in close relationship to the ear field are not of neural crest origin, but rather are cells of the paraxial mesoderm, and represent the early mesodermal wave of otic induction (Figure 2-8) described in the work of Yntema (1950). Neuralation and closure of the hindbrain, which occurs at the same stage of embryonic development as otic cup formation, causes this otic anlage to be in close apposition to the adjacent rhombencephalon tissue. Ultrastructural evidence in an amphibian embryo shows areas of focal cell contact between cells of the otic cup and adjacent rhombencephalon (Model, Jarrett, & Bonazzoli, 1981), but similar studies of a mammal (Van De Water & Conley, 1982) have failed to demonstrate any areas of cell contact between these tissues at a comparable stage of development (Figures 2-6, 2-13). Experiments examining inductive events in amphibian (Chuang, 1959; Detwiler, 1948; Detwiler & Van Dyke, 1950; Harrison, 1924, 1945; Yntema, 1950), avian (Muria-Garcia, 1962; Waddington, 1937) and mammalian embryos (Li et al., 1978a; Van De Water & Conley, 1982) provide direct evidence that the inductive interaction occurring between rhombencephalon and otic anlage is essential for the continuation of inner ear development (Figures 2-9, 2-11, 2-12). Analysis of the development of congenitally malformed labyrinths (Bonnevie, 1936; Deol, 1978; Hertwig, 1944) provide evidence that abnormal interactions between rhombencephalon and otic anlage (Figure 2-39) play some role in the malformation of these inner ears.

Epitheliomesenchymal tissue interactions were demonstrated within the developing labyrinth between the epithelial cells of the otic anlage and the mesenchymal cells of the surrounding periotic tissue. These interactions have been shown to be reciprocal and interdependent in nature, with the periotic mesenchyme having an inductive influence on the orderly expression of labyrinthine organogenesis (Figures 2-5 to 2-17) of the otocyst (Van De Water, 1980, 1981), and, in turn, with the otocyst acting as an inducer of the formation of its otic capsule (Figures 2-19, 2-20) and stapedial footplate from the surrounding periotic mesenchyme (Benoit, 1960, 1964; Grobstein & Holtzer, 1955; Kaan, 1926, 1930, 1938; Reagan, 1917; Yntema, 1950). These events are closely timed and interrelated so that an interruption in one will lead to a corresponding deficit in the other. The contribution of neural crest cells to the otic capsule and columella auris in avians has been documented in quail/chick embryo chimera experiments (Noden, 1978a, b; in press).

Deol (1978) has suggested, based upon his analysis of neural crest mutants, that the ganglion cells that comprise the eighth nerve in mammals are of dual origin. The quail/chick chimera studies of Noden (1978a; b; in press) and D'Amico-Martel and Noden (1983) provide direct evidence in the chick that the eighth nerve ganglion cells are derived from the otic placode and that any contribution of the neural crest to this ganglion cell population is minimal. These studies also demonstrate that the supporting cell population (i.e., glia and Schwann sheath cells) of the eighth nerve ganglion is formed entirely by cranial neural crest cells.

In experimental studies of neurotrophic interactions, no support was found for the hypothesis that nerve fibers exert a trophic influence on the development of sensory structures (Van De Water, 1976). Recent investigations of trophic interactions in cocultured otocysts that share a single ganglion have provided support for the hypothesis the areas of differentiating sensory cells provide a trophic effect on ingrowing neurites on the eighth nerve ganglion (Figures 2-28 to 2-30).

The possible site ("?") of gene action of the kreisler mutation (Hertwig, 1944) is placed on the flow chart in Figure 2-40. This proposed site of gene action as a regional defect in the chorda mesoderm is based upon the information obtained from in vitro fate map and otocyst/rhombencephalon experiments, combined with ultrastructural observations of the tissue relationships of the otic area, and could serve to explain the regional defect in the rhombencephalon in combination with abnormal positioning of the otic fields in the kreisler homozygote. Additional measurement of early ultrastructural relationships in early stages of otic development of homozygotic and heterozygotic kreisler embryos will provide definitive data to either confirm or disprove this suggested site of kreisler gene action.

The series of inductive events that are presented in the inner ear development flow chart of Figure 2-40 should not be viewed as isolated events, but rather as a continuum of interrelated tissue interactions, each dependent upon or necessary to some completed or still ongoing inductive interaction that either permits or directs the orderly embryogenesis of the labyrinthine form of the inner ear. A disruption of an inductive tissue interaction cannot, therefore, be viewed in isolation, but as an event that may effect a whole series of inductive interactions that follow the original disruption. Thus, the time in inner ear embryogenesis during which the original insult (i.e., teratogen or mutant gene action) occurs will profoundly influence the localization (i.e., vestibule, cochlea, or both) and severity of its effect upon development of the inner ear.

REFERENCES

Altman, P.L., & Katz, D.D. (1979). *Inbred and genetically defined strains of laboratory animals: Part 1, mouse and rat,* Bethesda; Biological Handbooks III, Federation of American Societies for Experimental Biology.

Benoit, J.A.A. (1960). Etude experimentale des facteurs de l'induction du cartilage otique chez les embryons de poulet et de truite. *Annale des Science Naturelle Zoologique, 12,* 327-385.

Benoit, J.A.A. (1964). Action inductrice de dureé variable sur le mesenchyme otique de l'embryon de poulet en culture in vitro. *Comptes Rendus Academie des Sciences Paris (D), 258,* 334-336.

Bernfield, M.R., Cohen, R.H., & Banerjee, S.D. (1973). Glycosaminoglycans and epithelial organ formation. *American Zoologist, 13,* 1067-1083.

Bonnevie, K. (1936). Abortive differentiation of the ear vesicle following a hereditary brain-anomaly in the short-tailed-waltzing mice. *Genetica, 18,* 105-125.

Chuang, H.H. (1959). Experiments concerning the induction and morphogenesis of the otic vesicle in urodelian amphibian. *Acta Biologica Experimentia Sinica, 6,* 352-363.

Coulombre, A.J. (1956). The role of intraocular pressure in the development of the chick eye 1. control of size. *Journal of Experimental Zoology, 133,* 211-225.

D'Amico-Martel, A., & Noden, D.M. (1983). Contributions of placodal and neural crest cells to avian cranial peripheral ganglia. *American Journal of Anatomy, 166,* 445-468.

Deol, M.S. (1966). Influence of the neural tube on the differentiation of the inner ear in the mammalian embryo. *Nature (London), 209*, 219–220.

Deol, M.S. (1967). The neural crest and the acoustic ganglion. *Journal of Embryology and Experimental Morphology, 17*, 533–541.

Deol, M.S. (1970). The relationship between abnormalities of pigmentation and the inner ear. *Proceedings of the Royal Society of London in Biology, 175*, 201–217.

Deol, M.S. (1978). Deficiencies of the inner ear in the mouse and their origin. In *Mechanisms of the embryogenesis of the organs of vertebrate embryos. Colloques Internationaux CNRS, 266*, 163–171.

Deol, M.S. (1980). Genetic malformations of the inner ear in the mouse and man. In R.J. Gorlin (Ed.), *Morphogenesis and malformation of the ear* (pp. 243–261), *Birth defects, original article series, Vol. XVI, No. 4*. New York: Alan R. Liss.

Desmond, M.E., & Jacobson, A.G. (1977). Embryonic brain enlargement requires cerebrospinal fluid pressure. *Developmental Biology, 57*, 188–198.

Detwiler, S.R. (1948). Further quantitative studies on locomotor capacity of larval Amblystoma following surgical procedures upon the embryonic brain. *Journal of Experimental Zoology, 108*, 45–74.

Detwiler, S.R., & Van Dyke, R.H. (1950). The role of the medulla in the differentiation of the otic vesicle. *Journal of Experimental Zoology, 113*, 197-199.

Farbman, A.I. (1974). Taste bud regeneration in organ culture. *Annals of the New York Academy of Science, 228*, 350–354.

Grobstein, C. (1967). Mechanisms of organogenetic tissue interaction. *National Cancer Institute Monographs, 26*, 279–299.

Grobstein, C. (1968). Developmental significance of interface materials in epitheliomesenchymal interaction. In R. Fleischmajer & R.E. Billingham (Eds.), *Epithelial–Mesenchymal Interaction* (pp. 173–176). Baltimore: Williams & Wilkins.

Grobstein, C., & Holtzer, H. (1955). "In vitro" studies of cartilage induction in mouse somite mesoderm. *Experimental Zoology, 28*, 333–357.

Hall, E.K. (1939). On the duration of the polarization process in the ear primordium of embryos of *Amblystoma punctatum* (Linn.). *Journal of Experimental Zoology, 82*, 173–192.

Harrison, R.G. (1924). Experiments on the development of the internal ear. *Science, 59*, 448–450.

Harrison, R.G. (1936). Relations of symmetry in the developing ear of *Amblystoma punctatum*. *Proceedings of the National Academy of Science, 22*, 238–247.

Harrison, R.G. (1945). Relations of symmetry in the developing embryo. *Transaction's Connecticut Academy of Arts and Sciences, 36*, 277–330.

Hay, E.D., & Meier, S. (1974). Glycosaminoglycan synthesis by embryonic inductors: Neural tube, notochord, and lens. *Journal of Cell Biology, 62*, 889–898.

Hay, E.D. (1981). *Cell biology of extracellular matrix*. New York: Plenum.

Hendricks, D.M., & Toerien, M.J. (1973). Experimental endolymphatic hydrops. *South African Medical Journal, 47*, 2294–2300.

Hertwig, P. (1944). Die Genese der Hirn- und Gehörganmissibildungen bei rontgenmutierten Kreisler-mäusen. *Zeitschrift Menschgeschlecht Verebungs-forschung Konstanthaltung, 18*, 327–354.

Kaan, H.W. (1926). Experiments of the development of the ear of *Amblystoma punctatum. Journal of Experimental Zoology, 46*, 13–61.

Kaan, H.W. (1930). The relation of the developing auditory vesicle to the formation of the cartilage capsule in *Amblystoma punctatum. Journal of Experimental Zoology, 55*, 263–291.

Kaan, H.W. (1938). Further studies on the auditory vesicle and cartilaginous capsule of *Amblystoma punctatum*. *Journal of Experimental Zoology, 78*, 159–183.

Le Douarin, N.M. (1969). Particularities du noyau interphasique chez la caille japonaise *(Coturnix coturnix japonica)*. *Bulletin Biologie France et Belgium, 103*, 435–442.

Le Douarin, N.M. (1971). Caracteristiques ultrastructurales du noyau interphasique chez la caille et chez le poulet et utilisation des cellules de caille comme "marqueurs biologiques" en embryologie experimentale. *Annals Embryologie Morphologie, 4*, 125–135.

Levy, O. (1906). Entwicklungsmechanische Studien am Embryo von *Triton taeniatus*. (1). *Orientierungsversuche. Wilhelm Roux' Archives Entwicklungsmechanische, 20*, 335–379.

Lewis, W.H. (1906). On the origin and differentiation of the otic vesicle in amphibian embryos. *Anatomical Record, 1*, 142–145.

Li, C.W. (1979). Congenital malformation of inner ear: I. An "in vitro" study of cell determination of the homozygotic and heterozygotic kreisler mouse otocysts. *Developmental Neuroscience, 2*, 7–18.

Li, C.W., & McPhee, J. 1979). Influences on the coiling of the cochlea. *Annals of Otology, Rhinology and Laryngology, 88*, 280–287.

Li, C.W., Van De Water, T.R., Ruben, R.J., & Shea, C.A. (1978a). *Rhombencephalic induction on the differentiation of the tenth gestation day mouse otocyst*. (Abstract). Association for Research in Otolaryngology, Midwinter Meeting, Clearwater, Florida, January, 1978.

Li, C.W., Van De Water, T.R., & Ruben, R.J. (1978b). The fate mapping of the eleventh and twelfth day mouse otocyst: An "in vitro" study of the sites of origin of the embryonic inner ear sensory structures. *Journal of Morphology, 157*, 249–268.

McLoughlin, C.B. (1968). Interaction of epidermis with various types of foreign mesenchyme. In R. Fleischmajer & R.E. Billingham (Eds.), *Epithelial–Mesenchymal Interaction* (pp. 244–251). Baltimore: Williams & Wilkins.

Meier, S. (1978a). Development of the embryonic chick otic placode: I. Light microscopic analysis. *Anatomical Record, 191*, 447–458.

Meier, S. (1978b). Development of the embryonic chick otic placode: II. Electron microscopic analysis. *Anatomical Record, 191*, 459–478.

Model, P.G., Jarrett, L.S., & Bonazzoli, R. (1981). Cellular contacts between hindbrain and prospective ear during inductive interaction in the axolotl embryo. *Journal of Embryology and Experimental Morphology, 66*, 27–41.

Muria-Garcia, F. (1962). Experimental contribution to the study of the neural influence in the development of the organ of hearing. *Revista Español Otoneuronatal, 21*, 230–232.

Noden, D.W. (1972). *An autoradiographic analysis of the migration of avian neural crest cells*. PhD dissertation, Washington University, St. Louis, MO.

Noden, D.W. (1978a). The control of avian cephalic neural crest cytodifferentiation. I. Skeletal and connective tissues. *Developmental Biology, 67*, 296–312.

Noden, D.W. (1978b). The control of avian cephalic neural crest cytodifferentiation. II. Neural tissues. *Developmental Biology, 67*, 313–329.

Noden, D.W. (in press). The use of chimeras in analysis of craniofacial development. In Le Douarin, N.M. & McLaren, A., (Eds.), *Chimeras in development*. London: Academic Press.

Orr, M.F., & Hafft, L.P. (1980). The influence of mesenchyme on the development of the embryonic otocyst: An electron microscopic study. *Journal of Cell Biology, 87*, 27a.

Partsch, C.J. (1966). Entwicklungsstörungen des ductus und saccus endolymphaticus als Ursache der Innenohrmissbildung. *Zeitschrift Laryngology Rhinology Otology, 45*, 529–538.

Reagan, J. (1917). The role of the auditory sensory epithelium in the formation of the stapedial plate. *Journal of Experimental Zoology, 23*, 85–105.

Ruben, R.J. (1973). Development and cell kinetics of the kreisler (kr/kr) mouse. *Laryngoscope,* *83,* 1440–1468.

Rugh, R. (1968). *The mouse: Its reproduction and development.* Minneapolis: Burgess.

Saxen, L. (1961). Transfilter neural induction of amphibian ectoderm. *Developmental Biology,* *3,* 14–152.

Spemann, H. (1918). Über die Determination der ersten Organanlagen des Amphibien Embryo, I–VI. *Wilhelm Roux' Archives Entwicklungsmechanische, 43,* 448–555.

Streeter, G.L. (1914). Experimental evidence concerning the determination of posture of the membranous labyrinth in amphibian embryos. *Journal of Experimental Zoology, 16,* 149–176.

Sobkowicz, H.M., Bereman, B., & Rose, J.E. (1975). Organotypic development of the organ of corti in culture. *Neurocytology, 4,* 543–572.

Theiler, K. (1972). *The house mouse: Development and normal stages from fertilization to 4 weeks of age.* Berlin: Springer-Verlag.

Todd, J.R. (1823). On the process of reproduction of the members of the aquatic salamander. *Quarterly Journal of Science Literature and Arts, 16,* 84–96.

Van De Water, T.R. (1976). Effects of removal of the statoacoustic ganglion complex upon the growing otocyst. *Annals of Otology Rhinology, and Laryngology, 85* (Suppl. 33), 1–32.

Van De Water, T.R. (1977). The effect of the removal of the endolymphatic duct and sac anlage upon the organogenesis of the mammalian inner ear in vitro. *Archives of Otolaryngology, 217,* 297–311.

Van De Water, T.R. (1980). The role of epitheliomesenchymal interactions in development of the mammalian inner ear. *Anatomical Record, 196,* 194A.

Van De Water, T.R. (1981). Epitheliomesenchymal tissue interactions effect upon development of the inner ear. *Anatomical Record, 199,* 262A.

Van De Water, T.R. (1983). Embryogenesis of the inner ear: In vitro studies. In R. Romand (Ed.), *Development of Auditory and Vestibular Systems.* New York: Academic Press.

Van De Water, T.R., & Conley, E. (1982). Neural inductive message to the developing mammalian inner ear: Contact mediated versus extracellular matrix interaction. *Anatomical Record, 202,* 195A.

Van De Water, T.R., & Ruben, R.J. (1973). Quantification of the "in vitro" development of the mouse embryo inner ear. *Otology, Rhinology, and Laryngology, 82* (Suppl. 4), 19–21.

Van De Water, T.R., & Ruben, R.J. (1974). Symposium: New data for noise standards (III). Organ culture of the mammalian inner ear: A tool to study inner ear deafness. *Laryngoscope, 86,* 738–749.

Van De Water, T.R., & Ruben, R.J. (1976). Organogenesis of the ear. In R. Hinchcliffe & D. Harrison (Eds.), *Scientific Foundation of Otolaryngology.* (pp. 173–184). London: Heinemann.

Van De Water, T.R., & Ruben, R.J. (1983). A possible embryonic mechanism for the establishment of innervation of inner ear sensory structures. *Otology, 95,* 470–479.

Van De Water, T.R., Heywood, P., & Ruben, R.J. (1973). Development of sensory structures in organ cultures of the twelfth and thirteenth gestation day mouse embryo inner ears. *Annals of Otology, Rhinology, and Laryngology, 82* (Suppl. 4), 1–18.

Van De Water, T.R., Li, C.W., Ruben, R.J., & Shea, C.A. (1980). Ontogenic aspects of mammalian inner ear development. In R.J. Gorlin (Ed.), *Morphogenesis and malformation of the ear.* Birth defects: Original article series, Vol. XVI, No. 4. New York: Alan R. Liss.

Waddington, C.H. (1937). The determination of the auditory placode in the chick. *Journal of Experimental Biology, 14,* 232–239.

Wessells, N.K. (1977). *Tissue interactions and development.* Menlo Park, CA: Benjamin/Cummings.

Yntema, C.L. (1933). Experiments on determination of the ear ectoderm of *Amblystoma punctatum*. *Journal of Experimental Zoology, 65,* 317–357.

Yntema, C.L. (1937). An experimental study of the origin of the cells which constitute the VIIth and VIIIth cranial ganglia and nerves in the embryo of *Amblystoma punctatum*. *Journal of Experimental Zoology, 75,* 75–101.

Yntema, C.L. (1944). Experiments on the origin of the sensory ganglia of the facial nerve in the chick. *Journal of Comparative Neurology, 81,* 147–167.

Yntema, C.L. (1950). An analysis of induction of the ear from foreign ectoderm in the salamander embryo. *Journal of Experimental Zoology, 113,* 211–243.

Zwilling, E. (1941). The determination of the otic vesicle in *Rana pipiens*. *Journal of Experimental Zoology, 86,* 333–342.

Chapter 3

Recent Advances Toward Understanding Auditory System Development[1]

Edwin W Rubel, Donald E. Born,
Jeffrey S. Deitch, and Dianne Durham

When choosing processes for ontogenetic studies (or reviews) it is well to keep in mind that attempts to describe the ontogeny of mature function are only as good as our understanding of the endpoint. Developmental studies are only of value to the extent that currently held concepts are an accurate reflection of the most important principles for mature function. Generally the more fundamental and the more secure our knowledge of the adult structure and function, the greater is the potential for making a lasting contribution by investigating its ontogeny. Thus, we have biased this review toward ontogenetic analyses of those morphological and physiological processes which we best understand and which, arbitrarily, have been judged to be of the most significance. Space limitations required that many important areas be ignored and that the contributions of many investigators be left out.

In choosing processes for ontogenetic study, one must also consider the underlying purposes of these studies. One purpose is to understand the development of audition, per se. Examples of this approach are studies of endocochlear potential development (Bosher & Warren, 1971) or recent studies on the ontogeny of the frequency/place principle (Lippe & Rubel, 1983; Rubel & Ryals, 1983). Another purpose is to utilize unique qualities of the auditory system to approach more general issues of developmental neurobiology (Rubel, 1978). Such studies include the classical demonstration

[1]Support for the empirical investigations from the authors' laboratory was provided by NIH Grants NS 15478 and NS 15395, the Deafness Research Foundation, and The Lions of Virginia Hearing Foundation. Support for the authors was provided by the University of Virginia Neuroscience Program, NIH RCDA 00305 (EWR), NIH training Grant T NSO 719902 (DD), and NIH MSTP 5T 32 GM 07267 (DB). The authors thank Ms. Sharon Davis for expert secretarial and editorial assistance and Dr. O. Steward, Mr. S.R. Young, Dr. Z.D. Smith. Dr. B. Ryals, Dr. W. Lippe, and Dr. T.N. Parks for collection of some of the data presented in this chapter. Ms. Patricia Palmer, Ms. Doris Hannum, and Ms. Margaret Wells provided expert histological assistance.

that afferents influence cell death (Levi-Montalcini, 1949) and the recent study of Jackson and Parks (1982) suggesting ontogenetic elimination of supernumerary inputs in the central nervous system. A third reason for ontogenetic investigations is to understand mature function. This approach is exemplified by the work of Pujol and his colleagues. They have used the fact that differentiation of inner hair cells precedes that of outer hair cells and that synaptogenesis of afferents precedes efferents to contribute to our understanding of the differential contributions of inner and outer hair cells in the encoding of sound (Pujol, Carlier, & Lenoir, 1980). (See later chapters of Khanna and Kim.)

DEVELOPMENT OF CONDUCTIVE ELEMENTS – EXTERNAL EAR AND MIDDLE EAR

Development of the elements that collect, focus, and transmit mechanical motion to the cochlea sets physical limits on the capacities of the maturing inner ear and central processing network. Saunders, Kaltenbach, & Relkin (1983) have recently reviewed the functional development of these elements. The embryology has been considered by Van de Water, Maderson, & Jaskoll (1980b) and Noden (1980), and the maturational pattern found in humans has been described by Anson and Donaldson (1981).

Growth of the ear canal and pinna continues well into the postnatal period. The shape of the pinna and size of the ear canal influence sound reaching the tympanic membrane differentially as a function of frequency (Shaw, 1974). Therefore, as the pinna and ear canal grow we might expect to see major changes in the pattern of spectral sensitivity. In fact, Saunders, Kaltenbach, & Relkin (1983) point out that the relatively small ear canal and pinna would tend to produce resonance at a higher frequency in the neonate than in the adult. On the other hand, because the immature ear canal is more compliant than that of the adult, the maximum gain due to resonance will be considerably less in the neonate. Calculations for adult mice and humans indicate resonant frequencies of 21.2 and 3.4 kHz, respectively (Saunders & Rosowski, 1979), which correspond well with measured values (Djupesland & Zwislocki, 1973; Saunders & Garfinkle, 1982). The predicted value for 11-day-old mice is almost 30 kHz (Saunders et al., 1983) and in newborn humans calculations indicate that peak resonances should be at approximately 4 kHz. The gain due to resonance can be considerable in adults, on the order of 10–20 dB. However, as we will point out later, young animals tend to be less sensitive to high frequencies. Thus, although the resonance of the ear canal is at relatively higher frequencies in neonates, the reduced gain due to greater compliance and high-frequency insensitivity of the immature auditory system probably results in an overall loss of sensitivity in the upper half of their dynamic range.

This slight relative loss at high frequencies along with reduced head size of neonates also has implications for binaural sound localization. Interaural intensity differences are important for frequencies high enough to be reflected by the head, thereby causing a mild pressure gain at the ipsilateral ear and a large pressure loss at the contralateral ear (Shaw, 1974). When the frequency is lowered, sound is diffracted around the head and the pressure at the two ears is approximately equal. In this case, interaural time differences become increasingly important. The smaller head size of neonates means that the maximum interaural intensity differences will occur at higher frequencies, and that neonates must rely more on interaural time differences for sound localization. As the head approaches adult size, progressively lower frequencies produce an interaural intensity difference (Moore & Irvine, 1979a). The conclusion to be drawn is that low-frequency sound localization using binaural cues should be more difficult for the neonate because interaural intensity cues play less of a role. Furthermore, as we shall see later in this chapter, the temporal microstructure of receptor and neural responses remain immature for a long period during functional development. Since these properties are usually thought to be especially important for the processing of interaural time differences, we might expect young mammals to show difficulties with sound localization. While it has been shown that young animals and humans can localize sounds (Clements & Kelly, 1978a, b; Muir, 1984), neither the extent to which binaural cues are used nor the accuracy of localization ability has been examined as a function of development. Developmental investigations of the relative accuracy of sound localization as a function of frequency will be of considerable value.

Functional development of the middle ear has been studied in more detail. Since middle ear structures (tympanic membrane and ossicular chain) provide a 35 to 40dB pressure gain, their development can impose strict boundary conditions on the ontogeny of auditory sensitivity. Saunders and colleagues (1983) provide a detailed and lucid review of this material. Only the most important points will be mentioned here.

Several authors have used tympanometry to measure developmental changes in middle ear admittance. This parameter (the reciprocal of stiffness), is thought to dramatically influence low-frequency sensitivity. Saunders and colleagues (1983) point out that most studies have found a precipitous drop in simple admittance between 40 and 80 days after birth in human neonates (Brooks, 1971; Jerger, Jerger, Mauldin, & Segal, 1974; Keith, 1973, 1975; Stream, Stream, Walker, & Brehingstall, 1978). Recent studies, however, indicate that when the compliance of the immature ear canal is taken into account a different pattern emerges. Himelfarb, Popelka, & Shanon (1979) found an *increase* in admittance during the first three months after birth under some testing conditions. The latter results are in accord with recent ontogenetic studies of admittance changes with age in hamster and chick (Relkin, Saunders, & Konkle, 1979; Saunders et al., 1983). These reports indicate that admittance gradually *increases* over age. There appears to be a good temporal correspondence between the ontogeny of middle ear admittance and low-frequency sensitivity in the hamster (Bock & Seifter, 1978). However, this correspondence breaks down in the chick; admittance gradually increases from hatching until about 70 days of age. Yet, thresholds to frequencies below 2 kHz appear to be at adult levels within the first week or two after hatching (Gray & Rubel, 1984; Kerr, Ostapoff, & Rubel, 1979; Rebillard & Rubel, 1981; Saunders, Coles, & Gates, 1973). Therefore, either other mechanisms must be compensating for the relatively low admittance values found in the neonate, the relationship between admittance and low-frequency sensitivity should be reassessed, or the measurement of sensitivity by electrophysiological and behavioral methods is grossly inaccurate.

Using a capacitive probe, Relkin and Saunders (1980) were able to measure developmental changes in displacement of the tympanic membrane at the tip of the hamster malleus at frequencies up to 35 kHz and over a 60 dB dynamic range. Developmental increases in displacement were shown up to 75 days. Below 10 kHz the development change was flat across frequency. However, above 10 kHz displacement appeared to decrease more dramatically with increasing frequency in the young animals. These findings are interpreted as probably resulting from changes in the effective volume of the middle ear for low frequencies and effective mass of the ossicular chain for high frequencies. They also are in general agreement with developmental trends in sensitivity. There can be little doubt that at the youngest ages middle ear function is one factor limiting hearing sensitivity. On the other hand, the ontogeny of sensitivity can not be "explained" by middle ear changes. Bock and Seifter's (1978) results indicate that hearing sensitivity reaches adult levels *prior* to middle ear function, at least for low frequencies. Second, as pointed out by Relkin and Saunders (1980), the high frequency roll-off in middle ear function in the young animals can not account for ontogenetic changes in sensitivity across frequency. Malleus displacement matures first at the most sensitive frequency of the hamster (approximately 10 kHz) and last at low frequencies. In contrast (see below), most animals' sensitivity matures *first* to *low-middle* frequencies and *last* to *high* frequencies.

While we are beginning to make important advances toward understanding the functional ontogeny of the middle ear, much more work is before us. To understand the development of hearing we must first understand changes in the efficiency and spectral purity of information transfer from the acoustic environment to the inner ear. Future studies which simultaneously measure input–output functions of the middle ear and the cochlea across age will be very important. In addition to measurements of sensitivity as a function of age, we need to know how spectral information in the signal is altered in young animals. Considering the differences that may exist between animals which hear prenatally (such as humans, most ungulates, and precocial birds) and those which begin hearing after birth (such as most rodents and carnivores), our dearth of understanding becomes particularly apparent. In the latter case the conductive mechanism must initially emerge to compensate for the impedance mismatch between air and the fluid-filled cochlea. In animals that hear prenatally, such as humans or precocial birds, however, the conductive elements of the middle ear must play a very different role. As in aquatic organisms, the external and middle ear spaces in utero or in ovo are fluid filled. There is little or no impedance mismatch and the specific gravity of the soft tissues is similar to the amniotic environment. Therefore, in the fetus, the roles of the tympanic membrane and ossicular chain must be very different than after birth; presumably the conduction of sound to the inner ear will follow principles similar to bone conduction. On the other hand, actual studies of the transfer function under these conditions have not been made as yet. We hope that this important gap in our understanding of fetal hearing will soon be corrected.

DIFFERENTIATION OF THE INNER EAR

Reviews of normal inner ear development can be found in Yntema (1950), Van de Water and Ruben (1976), Rubel (1978), and Van de Water et al., (1980b). The tissue interactions important for the determination and early differentiation of inner ear tissues are being intensely investigated in vivo (Ginzberg & Gilula, 1979) and in vitro (Orr, 1968; Sobkowicz, Rose, Scott, & Slapnick, 1982; and Van De Water, Li, Ruben & Shea, 1980a). In this chapter, we provide a brief overview of early stages of differentiation, followed by a discussion of the final stages of differentiation which immediately precede and overlap with the maturation of auditory function.

The inner ear of all vertebrates forms from a placodal thickening on the side of the head, which then invaginates and, in higher vertebrates, splits off from the overlying ectoderm to form the auditory vesicle, or otocyst. This vesicle then evaginates to form three primary ducts – the endolymphatic duct, the utricule, and the saccule. All of the sensory structures of the inner ear, including both the auditory and vestibular end organs as well as their ganglion cells, are derived from this primitive otocyst. In man, otocyst formation and the beginnings of evagination into the three primary ducts occur during the third to sixth weeks of gestation.

The cochlear duct grows as an extension of the sacculus (Figure 3-1). In the human fetus, this occurs quite early; by 10–12 weeks of gestation the cochlea has attained a full 2½ turns. The membranous labryinth then forms within this cartilaginous capsule. The capsule itself is derived from mesenchyme which has surrounded the primitive otocyst. Inductive interactions between the mesenchyme and the ectodermal placode were investigated during the first half of this century in lower vertebrates (see Yntema, 1950) and are currently being explored in mammals, principally using in vitro preparations of the mouse otocyst (see Van de Water et al., 1980a, and chap. 2 of this volume).

During the early period of otocyst formation, the presumptive cochlear ganglion cells bud off from the marginal cells of the lumen of the otic vesicle. While there has been some controversy as to the origin of the cochlear ganglion cells, there is now considerable evidence that in all vertebrates the ganglion cells are derived from the otic placode (see Noden, 1980; Rubel, 1978). The conjecture that this ganglion may be of dual origin (placode and neural crest) has received no support either from direct observation or from experimental studies using chimera preparations (see Noden, 1980).

The pattern of cell proliferation of the sensory and supporting cells of the inner ear and of the ganglion cells has received remarkably little attention. The only thorough investigation known to us is that of Ruben (1967), in which tritiated thymidine was used to label dividing cells at various times of gestation in the mouse. This technique allowed Ruben to determine the "birth dates" of hair cells and supporting cells as a function of position along the cochlear duct. As indicated in Figure 3-2A, the first ganglion cells to go through their final division do so on Day 12 of gestation and contribute primarily to the basal region of the mature cochlea. After Day 12, there are progressively fewer labeled cells in the basal region. Ganglion cells produced

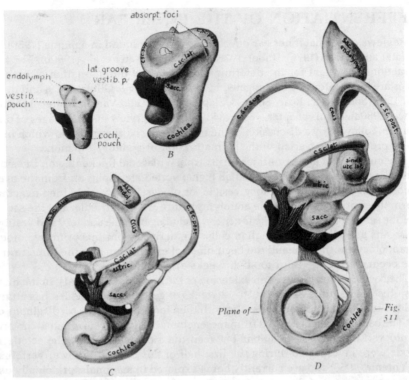

Figure 3-1. Development of the human left membranous labyrinth, shown in lateral views ×
25 at (A) 6.6 mm; (B) 13 mm; (C) 20 mm; and (D) 30 mm stages. Abbreviations:
absorpt. foci, area where absorption is complete; *crus,* crus commune; *c. sc. lat., c.
sc. post., c. sc. sup.,* lateral, posterior, and superior semicircular ducts; *endolymph,*
endolymph duct; *sacc.,* sacculus; *sac. endol.,* endolymph sac; *utric.,* utriculus. (From
Arey, 1966).

at progressively later ages (up to gestation Day 16) contribute to progressively more
apical regions. Most of the cells of the organ of Corti, however, show the reverse
pattern; the cells that undergo terminal mitosis first contribute to the apex of the
mature cochlea, while those that are "born" later contribute to progressively more
basal regions. Cell types showing this apical-to-basal pattern include the inner and
outer hair cells (see Figure 3–2B), pilar cells and several types of supporting cells.
The cellular factors underlying these two distinctly different sequences of cell proliferation are not at all clear and the result needs to be replicated. Ruben (1969) further
suggested that the earliest cells of the organ of Corti are, in fact, produced at the
junction of the cochlear duct and the sacculus. Subsequent to final mitosis they are
"pushed" apically by later proliferating cells. Confirmation of this sequence of events
will be important for understanding the dynamics of cochlear development.

Like neurons, hair cells of the cochlea do not continue to proliferate throughout life; the full complement of hair cells is produced during embryogenesis. In fact, the 4½-month-old human fetus has more hair cells than it will have at birth. Bredberg (1968) has shown that there is a continuous gradual loss of hair cells from the midfetal period until old age. The early loss of hair cells seems to involve outer hair cells to a greater extent than inner hair cells and has now been confirmed in a nonhuman species (Coleman, 1976; Rubel & Ryals, 1982).

Some of the best descriptions of the final stages of inner ear differentiation are those of Retzius (1884). Over the past century his observations (e.g., Figure 3-3) have been confirmed and elaborated using modern methods and in a variety of animals. Wada (1923) provided a detailed description of the changes in the rat cochlea that can be seen at the light microscopic level. The major events in a variety of species is summarized by Pujol and Hilding (1973) and much of the literature is summarized by Rubel (1978). More recent studies (Carlier & Pujol, 1978; Lenoir, Schnerson, & Pujol, 1980; Pujol, Carlier, & Devigne, 1978; Pujol, Carlier, & Lenoir, 1980; Schnerson & Pujol, 1982) on a variety of mammals at both light and electron microscopic levels confirm the earlier observations and add important details. Some generalizations are possible, including the following: (1) hair cells can be distinguished quite early; (2) nerve fibers initially make contact with supporting cells as well as hair cells; (3) inner hair cells tend to differentiate prior to outer hair cells; (4) the establishment of efferent connections from the central nervous system occurs later than connections between the hair cell and ganglion cell dendritic processes; and (5) hair cells lose their kinocilium prior to onset of function.

A major point to emphasize, however, is that during the final stages of differentiation there are many concomitant major structural and ultrastructural changes which seem to be occurring throughout the cochlear duct (see Wada, 1923). Each of these changes has, by one or more authors, been held responsible for the onset of cochlear function. It now appears that no single event triggers the onset of function. Instead, as first suggested by Wada, the events leading up to the onset of function include the simultaneous and apparently synchronous maturation of many mechanical and neural properties. Some of the important mechanical events are (1) thinning of the basilar membrane; (2) degeneration of the psuedostratified epithelium of the inner spiral sulcus to form a single layer of cuboidal cells; (3) maturation of the pilar cells; (4) freeing of the inferior margin of the tectorial membrane from the organ of Corti; and, (5) development of tissue spaces of the tunnel of Corti and around the outer hair cells.

Neural events which seem to occur at approximately the same time include (1) differentiation of the hair cells; (2) establishment of mature cilia structure and orientation; and (3) the maturation of synaptic connections at the base of the hair cells.

The final stages of maturation do not occur simultaneously throughout the length of the cochlea. As indicated in the original studies of Retzius, there is a clear gradient of differentiation extending in both directions from the midbasal region. The evidence for such a gradient during the final stages of maturation is, in our opinion, overwhelming. Whether examining the general morphology or electron microscopy in species

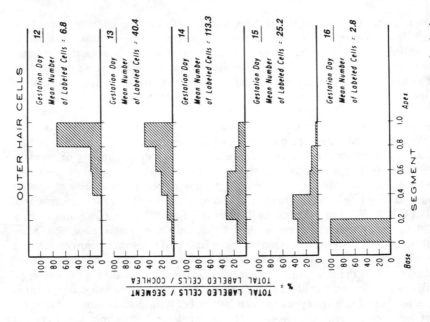

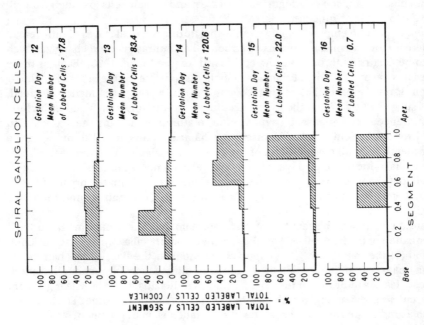

Figure 3-2. Position of labeled (A) outer hair cells or (B) spiral ganglion cells within the mature mouse cochlea. Gestation day is the day of injection of the tritiated thymidine. From Ruben, R. (1967). Development of terminal mitoses. *Acta Otolaryngologica*, Suppl. *220*, 21–44. Reprinted with permission.

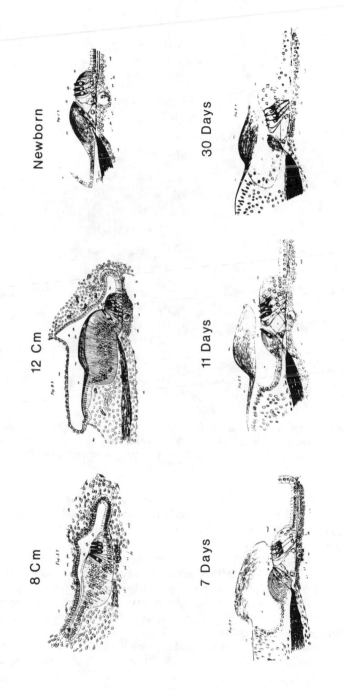

Figure 3-3. Successive stages of organ of Corti differentiation in the cat. (From Retzius, 1884).

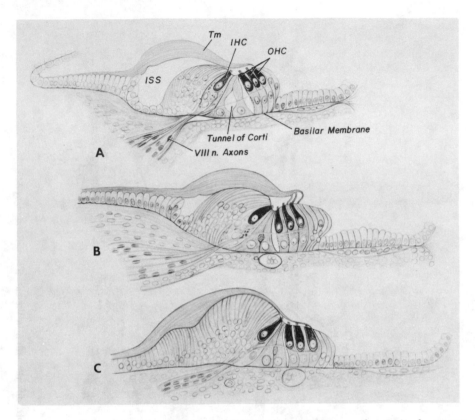

Figure 3-4. Organ of Corti in newborn rabbit. Note successive stages of maturity from apex (bottom) to middle turn (middle) to base (top). IHC, inner hair cells; ISS, inner spiral sulcus; OHC, outer hair cells; TM, tectorial membrane. (Redrawn from Retzius, 1884).

ranging from the chick to man (e.g., Änggard, 1965; Bast & Anson, 1949; Bredberg, 1968; Fermin & Cohen, 1983; Hirokawa, 1978; Pujol & Marty, 1970; Rebillard & Pujol, 1984; Retzius, 1884; Wada, 1923) differentiation occurs first in the midbasal region and spreads in both directions, with the apex maturing last. Figure 3-4 shows the relative maturity of the rabbit organ of Corti at birth in the basal (top), middle (center), and apical (bottom) turns. Interestingly, early stages of inner ear development, including cell proliferation and differentiation, may not conform to this gradient (Cotanche & Sulik, 1983; Ruben, 1967). Thus, the age of the cells, per se, does not seem to be the primary regulative factor.

A pattern of differentiation similar to that found in the cochlea has been identified at more central locations. Romand and Romand (1982) demonstrated this gradient in the myelination of kitten spiral ganglion cells. In the hamster, Schweitzer and Cant (in press) have shown a similar gradient in axons entering the dorsal cochlear nucleus. Axons enter the basal projection region (high-frequency) prior to those entering the apical (low-frequency) region. In the chick a corresponding spatiotemporal gradient has been identified for a variety of morphological and physiological indices of maturation in the brain stem auditory nuclei. These include cell death and neuron lamina formation in n. laminaris (Rubel, Smith, & Miller, 1976), the onset of postsynaptic responses in n. magnocellularis (Jackson, Hackett, & Rubel, 1982), the absorption of immature dendritic processes in n. magnocellularis (Young & Rubel, unpublished observations), and dendritic maturity in n. laminaris (Smith, 1981). Figure 3-5 demonstrates the gradient in the alterations in dendritic processes during development in n. magnocellularis. Jhaveri and Morest (1982) showed these changes as occurring between embryonic Days 11 and 17 in the chick. By embryonic Day 17 all the magnocellularis neurons are "bald," similar to the neuron shown in Figure 3-5C. However, at embryonic Day 14 there is a clear gradient within the nucleus. In the posterolateral region, which receives its projections from the apical end of the cochlea, the cells continue to have long sinuous processes. In the middle region, the processes are shorter and in the anteromedial region, which receives its projection from the basal end of the cochlea, they are gone. Thus, at one age all stages of dendritic maturation can be seen along a spatial axis in n. magnocellularis that corresponds to the pattern of projections from the cochlea.

Functional implications of the midbasal to apical developmental gradient will be discussed below (see Development of the Place Principle). Here it is important to note that although this developmental pattern seems to be pervasive in cochlear ontogeny, essentially nothing is known about how it arises, what factors regulate it, or why it occurs. The fact that it occurs centrally as well as peripherally suggests that cochlear differentiation is guiding the central expression. However, Parks (personal communication) has discovered that at least one variable, elimination of dendrites in n. magnocellularis (Figure 3-5), is independent of peripheral influence in that systematic loss of dendrites occurs following ipsilateral otocyst removal. Developmental studies aimed at further understanding of the factors that influence this remarkable gradient are of considerable interest in that they may provide some clues regarding the mechanisms whereby the orderly projection between the cochlea and the brain is established.

The relationships between stereocilia structure and the tuning properties of the mature cochlea are only beginning to be appreciated (Tilney, DeRosier, & Mulroy, 1980; Tilney, Egelman, DeRosier, & Saunders, 1983; Tilney & Saunders, 1983; see also chapters in this volume by Khanna and by Kim). At present there is little information on the development of these structures. Cotanche and Sulik (1983) reported that in the chick, stereocilia orientation emerges gradually at about the time function begins. The stereocilia and kinocilium in a 5- and a 7-month-old human fetus also have been briefly described (Fujimoto, Yamamoto, Hayabuchi, & Yoshizuka, 1981). In view of the gradient during the final stages of differentiation and recent findings that the frequency organization of the cochlea may shift during ontogeny (see below), it is of obvious importance to examine the developmental relationship between cilia structure and frequency selectivity at anatomically and physiologically defined positions along the cochlea.

In conclusion, we may ask what events trigger the onset and maturation of cochlear function. At present it appears that function emerges because of a precisely regulated synchrony of maturational processes, some of which sculpt the mechanical and chemical properties of the receptor; others allow appropriate energy to be transduced, while still others transmit information to the brain. These events seem to emerge together within a single region along the receptor surface, but there is an orderly progression beginning in the midbasal region. At present, neither the mechanisms responsible for the synchrony nor those for the progression from the basal part of the cochlea are understood. The commonality of such gradients across sensory systems (Easter, 1983) suggests that they are fundamental for the ontogeny of a spatial representation of our physical environment.

DEVELOPMENT OF THE PLACE PRINCIPLE

Most animals do not simultaneously begin hearing all frequencies which are included in their adult dynamic range. Table 3-1 summarizes most of the data available on the frequency range to which animals of a variety of species initially respond and the adult dynamic range of each species. Both behavioral and physiological data were used to construct this table. The important point to note is that in each species initial responses are elicited by low or mid low frequencies for that species. As development proceeds, responsiveness to both lower and higher frequencies increases. Responsiveness to the highest frequencies develops last (see reviews by Gottlieb, 1971, and Rubel, 1978). This sequence seems to be remarkably universal across both avian and mammalian species. Other measures of functional ontogeny also show this developmental sequence. For example, adultlike thresholds develop first for relatively low frequencies and later for high frequencies (Gray & Rubel, 1984; Moore & Irvine, 1979b), "phase-locking" seems to mature first for low frequency units and only later for high frequency units (Brugge, Javel, & Kitzes, 1978), and the most sensitive frequency for a given species seems to shift toward progressively higher frequencies during development (e.g., Saunders, Coles, & Gates, 1973; Rebillard & Rubel, 1981, Ehret & Romand, 1981).

The most fundamental principle of auditory science, from the work of von Békésy (1960), is the place principle. Simply stated, there is a progression of positions along the basilar membrane which are most sensitive to (i.e., tuned to) successively higher frequencies. This relationship is thought to be due to the mechanical properties of basilar membrane motion and the characteristics of the stereocilia (see chaps. 6 & 7). In all birds and mammals, the cochlea is organized such that apical positions are most sensitive to low frequencies and progressively more basal regions are selectively responsive to progressively higher frequencies.

Knowledge of the place principle and of the information on responsiveness as a function of frequency presented above suggests that the apical or midapical region

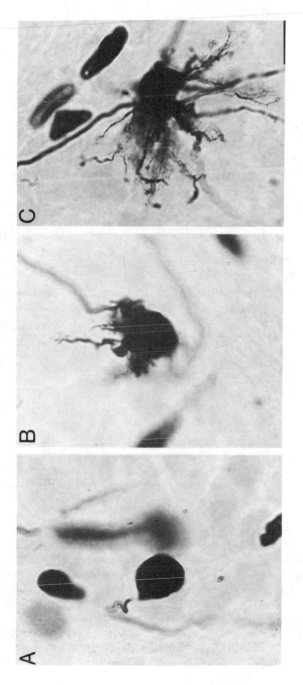

Figure 3-5. Photomicrographs of HRP-filled cells from a 14-day-old chick embryo to demonstrate "gradient" of dendritic morphology in n. magnocellularis. Cells are characteristic of those found in the (A) anteromedial, (B) middle, and (C) caudolateral regions of the nucleus. Calibration bar = 20 μm.

TABLE 3-1

INITIAL FREQUENCY RANGES

Species	Adult frequency range (kHz)*	Initial frequency range (kHz)
Human	.03–20	0.5–1.0 (Hr, Physiol., Beh)
Cat	.06–75	0.5–2.0 (Physiol.) 0.3–0.75 (Beh)
Dog	.04–50	0.5–0.75 (Beh)
Mink	0.1–70	0.5–0.75 (Beh)
Rabbit	.06–50	0.5–3 (Physiol.) 0.3–0.75 (Beh)
Rat	0.3–76	0.2–2 (Physiol.)
Mouse *(Mus)*	1–84	0.6–2 (CM) 1–3 (Beh)
Bat *(Myotis)*	10 –120	7–12 (Physiol.)
Chicken	0.1–7	0.1–0.8 (Physiol., Beh)
Duck	0.1–8	0.1–0.5 (CN)

*Approximate range of audiogram at 70 db (SPL); compiled with the help of Henry Hefner and William Stebbins.

of the cochlea is the first to mature (since in the adult this region is most sensitive to low frequencies), and that maturation of the cochlea then spreads primarily toward the base. Paradoxically, as noted in the previous section, just the opposite result is consistently found; cochlear differentiation occurs first in the basal or midbasal region. Differentiation then spreads in both directions and the *last* part of the cochlea to undergo differentiation is the apex.

There appear to be three ways to resolve this paradox. First, morphological differentiation of the cochlea and brain stem may precede development of function; that is, these two developmental processes, structural and functional differentiation, do not overlap in time. Studies on the chick auditory system rule out this "explanation." The onset of physiological responses to sound (Saunders et al., 1973), the final stages of cochlea differentiation (Fermin & Cohen, 1983; Hirokawa, 1978), cell death and lamination in the brain stem auditory nuclei (Rubel et al., 1976), and the development of functional connections between the periphery and the brain stem auditory nuclei (Jackson et al., 1982), all seem to occur simultaneously. Behavioral responses follow within a day or two (Jackson & Rubel, 1978).

A second resolution of this paradox could be derived from developmental changes in the middle ear transfer function. The suggestion was made that the neonatal middle ear acted as a low-pass filter; high-frequency stimuli, which normally best activate the basal region of the cochlea, were excluded and only low-frequency components impinged upon the cochlea (Saunders et al., 1973). Saunders and his colleagues (1983) have conducted an elegant series of studies examining the development of middle ear admittance and compliance in both mammals and birds. Their findings do not support the above interpretation. Whereas there is an obvious improvement in middle ear transmission during the early stages of hearing, it appears to be relatively flat across frequency. In addition, indirect data from our laboratory strongly suggest that the middle ear transfer properties cannot account for the paradoxical relationship noted above. We exposed 20-day-old chick embryos or 10-day-old posthatch chicks to white noise (125 dB SPL) for 12 hr. If the young animals' middle ear acts as a low-pass filter and the cochleae of the two age groups were working similarly, then cochlear damage should be weighted toward the apex in the embryonic chicks as compared to the posthatch subjects. However, as seen in Figure 3-6, the opposite result occurred. Although the embryos sustained less overall damage than the hatchlings, damage was also limited to the basal half of the cochlea. This result is totally inconsistent with the hypothesis that middle ear high-frequency transmission deficits are responsible for the structure–function paradox noted above. The data presented in Figure 3-6, however, are entirely consistent with the hypothesis described below.

On the basis of the developmental characteristics of the avian brain stem, we suggested a third resolution of this paradox. We hypothesized that the values of the place code along the cochlea were changing during development (Rubel et al., 1976; Rubel, 1978). This hypothesis has recently been tested in the chick (Lippe & Rubel, 1983; Rubel & Ryals, 1983). The model and its implications are shown schematically in Figure 3-7. The upper diagram in each part schematically shows the cochlea, from base to apex, and the relative positions of traveling waves produced by several different tone frequencies. In the adult (right-hand diagram) low frequencies cause a relatively broadly tuned traveling wave which peaks near the apex. Progressively higher frequencies cause more sharply tuned traveling waves which peak at progressively more basal locations (see von Békésy, 1960). Also shown in this diagram is the orderly representation of input from the cochlea to the central nervous system, which produces neurons selectively tuned to the indicated frequencies (in kilohertz). This relationship in the central nervous system is generally referred to as tonotopic organization.

Our hypothesis and its predictions are shown in sequence from left to right (embryo – adult) across these diagrams. We proposed that during the early stages of hearing the base, or midbasal region of the cochlea, and thereby the basal representation areas of the central nervous system, are most sensitive to relatively low frequencies. With maturation of both mechanical and neural processes, the values of the place code shift toward the apex. Restating this hypothesis, low frequencies first cause a maximal response in the basal or midbasal region of the cochlea, and as the organism matures progressively more apical regions become most responsive to low frequencies.

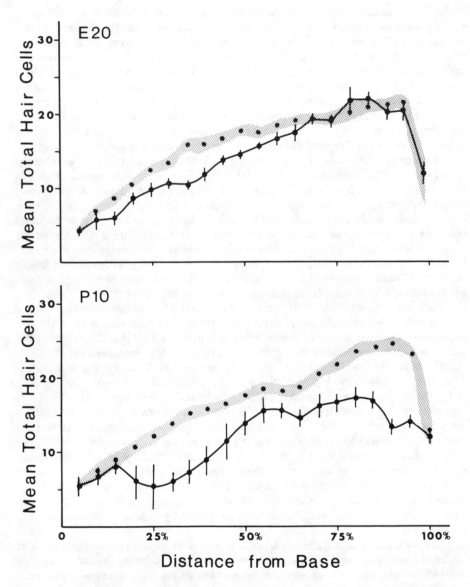

Figure 3-6. Mean total hair cell counts in chicks exposed at embryonic Day 20 (E20, top) or posthatch Day 10 (P10, bottom) to white noise at 125 dB for 12 hr (connected filled circles). In each graph, values within stippling indicate hair cell counts for age-matched controls. Stippling or error bars indicate ±*SEM* (*N* = 5 at E20, *N* = 4 at P10). (From Ryals, 1981).

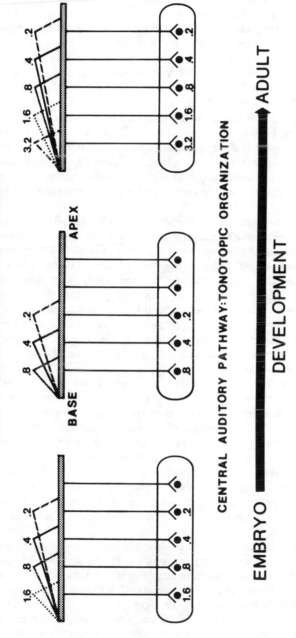

Figure 3-7. Model of inner ear functional development. The sequence of development is shown from left to right. The basilar papilla (cochlea) is depicted at the top of each section and the positions of the traveling waves produced by pure tones of several frequencies (in kilohertz) are indicated. A region of the central auditory pathways which is tonotopically organized is shown connected to each basilar membrane. The numbers here indicate the "best frequency" (in kilohertz) of neurons at each location. At the beginning of auditory function (left diagrams) the basal half of the cochlea is responsive to relatively low frequencies and the central nervous system areas receiving projections from the base respond to low frequencies. With maturation (middle and right sections), the apex of the cochlea begins responding to low frequencies and the base becomes progressively more sensitive to high frequencies. The cochlear shift is accompanied by a shift in neuronal best frequencies.

High frequencies, on the other hand, are initially ineffective because of the mechanical or neural properties of the cochlea. As the basal region matures, it become selectively tuned to progressively higher frequencies. This hypothesis allows two surprising predictions, one regarding the cochlea and the other about central tonotopic organization.

The first prediction, that the frequency organization of the cochlea shifts, is indicated by the upper portions of Figure 3-7. Frequency organization can be demonstrated by examining the area of cochlear damage produced by exposure to high-intensity pure tones. The avian cochlea (basilar papilla) is flat and uncoiled, making it amenable to dissection, reproducible orientation and sectioning, and counting of the number of hair cells at regular intervals along its length (Rubel & Ryals, 1982; Figure 3-8A). We tested the prediction by exposing chickens of different ages to high-intensity pure tones. If the hypothesis were correct, we would expect to observe a systematic ontogenetic shift in the position of hair cell damage. That is, low or mid-range frequencies should produce maximum damage at progressively more apical locations as the animal matures.

The results of our experiments are shown in Figures 3-8, 3-9, and 3-10. In 10-day-old chickens, high-intensity pure tones produce discrete, reliable regions of hair cell loss at characteristic locations along the length of the cochlea (Figure 3-9A). When these same tones are used with animals at two other ages, just before hatching (embryonic Day 20) and 30 days posthatch, the *position* of maximum damage shifted systematically. Figure 3-9B demonstrates this change for animals exposed to 1500 Hz pure tones at different ages. The position of peak hair cell loss shifted toward the apex with increasing age at the time of damage. Figure 3-10 summarizes the data for all frequencies tested with the three age groups; with each frequency, the region of damage shifted toward the apex as a function of increasing age. These results confirmed the first prediction of our hypothesis.

The second prediction of the model indicated in Figure 3-7 has also been tested (Lippe & Rubel, 1983). If the transduction properties of the cochlea are changing during development and the orderly topography of projections from the cochlea to the central nervous system is remaining stable, then in each auditory center of the brain the position at which neurons are responsive to a particular frequency will shift during development. Stated differently, the neurons at any given location within an auditory area of the central nervous system should respond to successively higher frequencies during development. This prediction, indicated at the bottom of Figure 3-7, was tested by electrophysiologically "mapping" the relationship between the location of neurons and the frequency to which they were most sensitive in 17-day-old chick embryos and 2- to 3-week-old hatchlings.

Two areas of the chick brain were examined. Nucleus magnocellularis receives direct projections from the cochlea and, in turn, sends axons bilaterally to nucleus laminaris. Both nuclei have a similar tonotopic organization (Parks & Rubel, 1975; Rubel & Parks, 1975; Young & Rubel, 1983). As summarized in Figure 3-11, the embryonic neurons responded best to frequencies 1–1½ octaves below those that would be predicted by the relationship in adult animals between neuronal position and best frequency. Since neither the total number of neurons nor their relative positions in

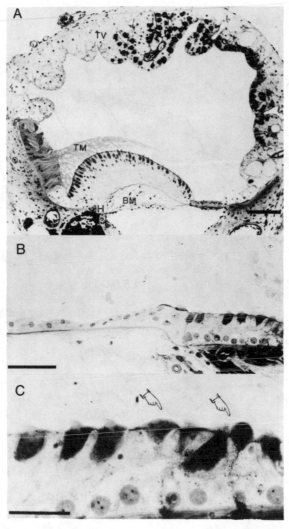

Figure 3-8. Photomicrographs of transverse sections through the basilar papilla (cochlea) in the chick. (A) Normal 40-day-old chicken. Tall hair cells predominate the width of the basilar membrane. BM, basilar membrane; H, habenula; TM, tectorial membrane; TV, tegmentum vasculosum. Bar indicates 100 μm. (B) The basilar membrane of an animal exposed to a 125dB, 1.5kHz pure tone for 4 hr to show the appearance of damaged hair cells. In this section many short hair cells are lost and remaining tall hair cells appear distorted. Bar indicates 50 μm. (C) Higher magnification photomicrograph of damaged hair cells from same animal as in (B). Pointers indicate abnormal cells that did not meet criteria for counting. Bar indicates 20 μm. From Rubel, E.W., & Ryals, B.M. (1982). Patterns of hair cell loss in chick basilar papilla after intense auditory stimulation: Exposure duration and survival time. *Acta Otolaryngologica, 93*, 31–41. Reprinted with permission.

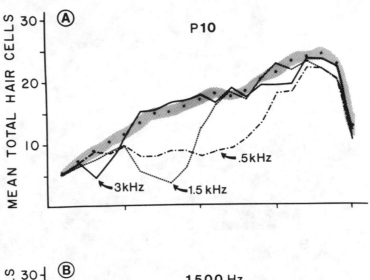

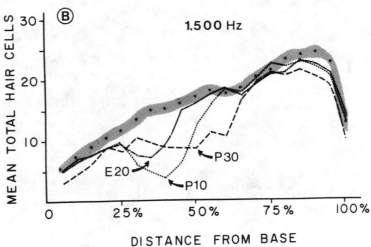

Figure 3-9. Total number of hair cells as a function of position along the chick basilar papilla (cochlea) from base to apex. The mean ±*SEM* for normal animals is shown by the dots and shading. Standard errors for the experimental groups are omitted for clarity but were comparable to those for normal animals. (A) Mean number of hair cells of chicks exposed on postnatal Day 10 to 500, 1500, or 3000-Hz high-intensity pure tones. (B) Mean number of hair cells from chicks exposed to 1500-Hz tone on embryonic Day 20 (E20), postnatal Day 10 (P10), or postnatal Day 30 (P30). Arrows indicate positions of maximum damage. (From Rubel & Ryals, 1983).

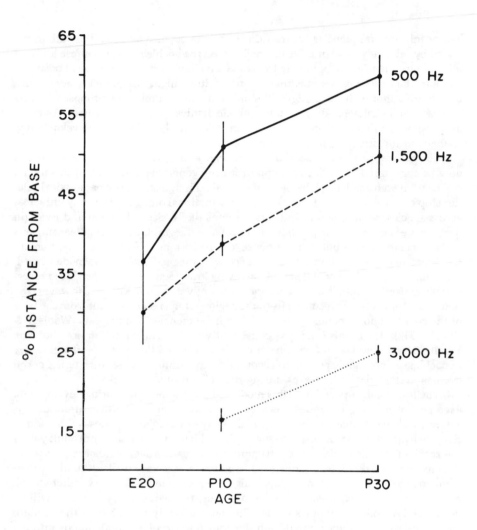

Figure 3-10. Position of maximum hair cell loss following exposure to high-intensity pure tones at 500, 1500, and 3000 Hz as a function of age. The ordinate represents the percentile position along the cochlea, from base to apex, at which maximum hair cell loss occurred. Means ±*SEM* are shown for each group. (From Rubel & Ryals, 1983).

these nuclei change after embryonic Day 7 (Rubel, Smith, & Miller, 1976) these data also support the prediction that the neurons at any given position in the nucleus respond to successively higher frequencies as the animals mature.

Taken together, these two experiments strongly support the model of cochlear development presented above. This model suggests that early in development, only

low or mid-low frequencies are transduced by the cochlea and that they are transduced by relatively basal or midbasal regions. As the cochlea matures, these low and
mid-low frequencies are optimally transduced by successively more apical positions
while the basal regions become tuned to increasingly higher frequencies. Space does
not permit a thorough discussion of the mechanisms that might be proposed for this
process. In all likelihood, they include both mechanical and neural changes. An exciting possibility is that the changing tuning properties are also reflected in developmental
changes in the structure of stereocilia. (See Preface.)

The generality of this process across species and its functional implications can
now be considered. Four lines of support for the general applicability of this model
can be derived from data available on mammals. First, because the paradoxical relationship between cochlear development and functional ontogeny is nearly universal
across species, some general explanation seems likely. Second, Woolf and Ryan (in
press) have shown that the position of neurons in the gerbil dorsal cochlear nucleus
which increase glucose uptake in response to a 3-kHz tone shifts during development;
the direction of the shift is in correspondence with the prediction of this model. Third,
Pujol and Marty (1968) noted that only relatively low-frequency tones produced recognizable evoked potentials in the cerebral cortex of very young kittens. However, the
potentials could only be recorded from the region which receives input from the base
of the cochlea and responds to relatively high frequencies in adult cats (Woolsey &
Walzl, 1942). Again, this finding is consistent with the interpretation noted above.
Finally, Harris and Dallos (1983) have recently reported that the cut-off frequency
of cochlear microphonic potentials recorded from within the basal turn of the gerbil
cochlea systematically increases during the third postnatal week.

The functional implication of this model is that at some point during development
each part of the cochlea, and thereby each tonotopic region of the central nervous
system, will be maximally responsive to relatively low-frequency tones. With maturation, each area will be responsive to successively higher frequencies until adult values
are reached. In this context it is intriguing to evaluate what sounds are present in
the environment of young organisms. Acoustically, it is very difficult to block low-
frequency tones and very easy to block high-frequency tones. Thus, whether an animal lives in a burrow, in an egg, or in a uterus, the acoustic environment will be
dominated by low-frequency sounds. The data currently available on the in utero
sound environment indicate that both the transmission of external sounds into the
uterus and internally generated sounds strongly favor low frequencies, and high-
frequency sounds are markedly attenuated (Bench, 1968; Vince, Armitage, Baldwin,
Toner, & Moore, 1982; Walker, Grimwade, & Wood, 1971, Figure 3-12). The match
between low-frequency dominated sound environments and the sequence of hearing
development we have identified may be coincidental. On the other hand, it is tempting
to speculate that it may represent an example of natural selection for a pattern of
sensory system development which makes use of the stimuli reliably available in
the environment of the developing organism. In the following section we will examine
evidence that the development of hearing and of the auditory areas of the brain is
influenced by cochlear input, particularly the amount or pattern of activity in the

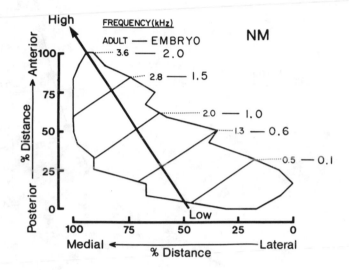

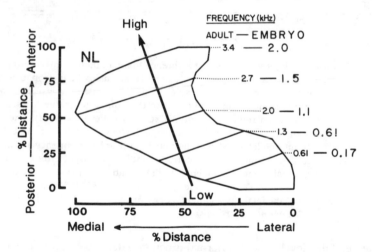

Figure 3-11. Two-dimensional reconstructions of the magnocellular (NM; top) and laminar (NL; bottom) nuclei in the chick brain stem comparing the tonotopic organization in hatchlings and embryos. The nuclei are divided into four equal sectors along the frequency axis (long arrows). The best-frequency ranges (kilohertz) observed in the different sectors in hatchlings and embryos are indicated to the right. Orientation of the frequency axes from posterolateral (low frequencies) to anteromedial (high frequencies) is predicted by multiple linear regression equations (see Rubel & Parks, 1975) that quantitatively describe the tonotopic organization in hatchling chicks.

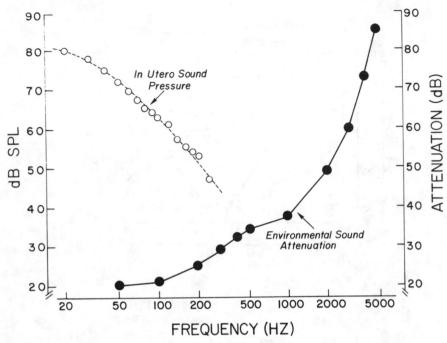

Figure 3-12. Graphs showing two factors that influence the mammalian intrauterine acoustic environment, the sound level from fetal and maternal behavior (open circles) and the attenuation of sound from outside the mother (closed circles). The data ("corrected for impedence of microphone") for the human fetus due to each of these sources have been replotted from Walker and colleagues (1971). These results emphasize the low-frequency domination of the fetal environment. Ambient sound levels (left line and left axes) are relatively intense at low frequency and attenuated with increasing frequency. Attenuation (right line and right ordinate) of low-frequency external sounds is moderate but attenuation increases markedly above 2 kHz. From Walker, D., Grimwade, J., & Wood, C. (1971). Intrauterine noise: A component of the fetal environment. *American Journal of Obstetrics and Gynecology,* *109,* 91–95. *Reprinted by permission.*

eighth nerve. If the development of normal function is dependent on external stimulation, then the developmental pattern we have proposed will provide a mechanism to ensure that each neuronal region, in turn, receives adequate stimulation from the environment.

EXTRINSIC INFLUENCES ON AUDITORY SYSTEM ONTOGENY

Modification of the inputs to central nervous system neurons is known to exert a profound effect on both their development and maintenance (for reviews, see

Cowan, 1970; Globus, 1975; Guillery, 1974; and Smith, 1977). Since environmental influences usually are mediated through the peripheral auditory receptors, we first examine the extent to which they are susceptible to extrinsic ototoxic agents and events with reference to the developing system. The effects of changes in afferent input on developing and mature auditory system neurons are then examined. Experiments designed to examine such effects can be divided into two classes. One approach has been to utilize the auditory system as a "model system" with which to examine how the integrity and activity of afferent axons influence the regulation of morphology and connectivity of neurons. Alternatively, it is of great interest simply to determine whether "normal" input is necessary for normal auditory structure and function. The experiments described below will be examined in light of these different goals.

The Periphery

A number of environmental events may exert a significant ototoxic effect on the auditory periphery (see Chapters 1, 2 and 4). Some pathological influences, such as high-intensity noise or aminoglycoside antibiotics, are known to directly damage hair cells and thus result in a presumed loss of normal eighth nerve activity (Fee, 1980; Hawkins, Johnsson, & Aran, 1969; Johns, Ryals, Guerry, Wenzel, & Rubel, 1980; Rubel & Ryals, 1982; Ryals & Rubel, 1982). Other auditory impairments, such as recurrent otitis media or trauma, may also alter the activity reaching central nervous system (CNS) structures, although in these cases the changes in afferent activity are less well defined. Nevertheless, such alterations may have severe consequences for normal CNS development when they occur in young animals. The extent to which the infant is differentially susceptible to ototoxic agents is of immediate clinical importance, as well as of interest for understanding how the auditory system matures.

Saunders and Bock (1978) summarized the literature on the differential susceptibility to aminoglycosides and noise exposure in young animals. Studies by Pujol, Saunders, and others have now shown that exposure of young animals to drugs or to noise at levels which would not produce damage in adults can cause severe hearing loss and histological damage to the cochlea (e.g., see Bock & Saunders, 1977; Carlier & Pujol, 1980; Lenoir, Bock, & Pujol, 1979; Lenoir & Pujol, 1980; Price, 1976). Pujol and his co-workers have gone on to show that the period of increased susceptibility corresponds to the final stages of anatomical and functional development of the cochlea. They suggest that during this period the cochlea is hypersensitive because of the lack of normal efferent input, but this hypothesis has yet to be validated. Much more work needs to be done to determine the biological mechanisms underlying the differential susceptibility of young animals. In addition, we need to determine if and when hypersensitivity occurs in human infants and if it occurs during other periods of life. For example, are similar processes occurring during aging (Henry, Chole, McGinn, & Frush, 1981) and/or during periods of heightened stress? A fruitful approach toward understanding differential susceptibility may be provided by examining age-related differences in temporary threshold shift (Bock & Seifter, 1978).

The Central Nervous System

The changes in the auditory periphery described above or other changes that are produced experimentally can be used to study the effects of altered afferent input on the central auditory structures. Experimental manipulations range from completely eliminating input by destruction or removal of the entire inner ear and ganglion cells to producing subtle changes in the pattern of input by altering the acoustic environment. If the goal of such manipulations is to determine simply if normal input is necessary for normal structure and function then it is sufficient to know that the manipulation has produced some change. The results of such experiments do not allow mechanistic interpretations, but simply document the existence of a relationship between a particular peripheral change and its importance to normal ontogeny. On the other hand, if the goal of the experiment is to provide a mechanistic interpretation, as when the auditory system is used as a "model" to examine general principles of nervous system ontogeny, then it is essential to examine precisely how each manipulation influences the integrity and activity of the presynaptic neurons.

Examples of the first goal of documenting a relationship between peripheral input and normal neural and behavioral development include studies of the effects of conductive hearing deficits on cell size (Conlee & Parks, 1981; Webster & Webster, 1979), dendritic symmetry in the medial superior olive or nucleus laminaris (Feng & Rogowski, 1980; Gray, Smith, & Rubel, 1982) or the otogeny of behavior (Gottlieb, 1976; Kerr, Ostapoff, & Rubel, 1979). To determine the mechanisms whereby peripheral manipulations affect central neurons we must first document the effects of the manipulations on activity and integrity of both the presynaptic and the postsynaptic elements under investigation. For example, through a series of studies on mammals and birds the changes in eighth nerve activity and integrity have been investigated following cochlea destruction (Koerber, Pfeiffer, Warr, & Kiang, 1966; Lippe, Steward, & Rubel, 1980). For example, Lippe and colleagues (1980) described changes in 2-deoxy-glucose uptake in brain stem auditory areas at various intervals following the lesion.

Cochlea removal. The destruction or removal of the auditory receptor influences the development and maintenance of central nervous system auditory nuclei. In a classic neuroembryological study, Levi-Montalcini (1949) showed that otocyst removal did not noticeably affect the development of cells in the avian cochlear nuclei (n. magnocellularis and n. angularis) until after 11 days of incubation, about the time of normal innervation of these cells by the eighth nerve (Jackson et al., 1982; Jhaveri & Morest, 1982). In a series of experiments we have repeated and expanded on this early work to examine how the integrity of the cochlea influences the development and maintenance of neurons of nucleus magnocellularis and nucleus laminaris of the chick brain auditory system. A schematic representation of this system is shown in Figure 3-13.

In the chick it is possible to take out the cochlea with or without the ganglion cells at various ages, ranging from embryonic Day 2 (by removing the otocyst) to adulthood (by removing the mature cochlea). We have examined the effects of otocyst

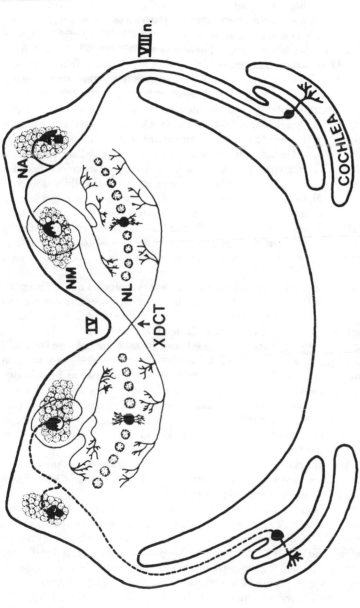

Figure 3-13. Schematic diagram to show the organization of the chick brain stem auditory nuclei. The basilar papilla (cochlea) is innervated by the peripheral processes of eighth nerve ganglion cells. Central processes (eighth nerve) bifurcate and synapse in second-order n. magnocellularis (NM) and n. angularis (NA). Axons from NM bifurcate and project bilaterally to third-order neurons in n. laminaris (NL). NL neurons are arranged in a monolayer sheet and possess dendrites spatially segregated into domains dorsal and ventral to the cell body. The projection from NM is also segregated such that axons from ipsilateral NM terminate on dorsal NL dendrites and cell bodies and axons from the contralateral NM terminate on ventral NL dendrites and somata. Both NM and NL are tonotopically organized. IV, fourth ventricle; XDCT, crossed dorsal cochlear tract.

and of cochlea removal using a number of measures. Parks (1979) confirmed and extended the work of Levi-Montalcini. He measured changes in neuron number and cross-sectional area at several embryonic and one posthatch time point after unilateral otocyst removal in 2- to 3-day-old embryos. There was no evidence of an effect until embryonic Day 11. After this time absence of the inner ear resulted in a decreased neuron number and size (Figure 3-14). The end result was a 30% reduction in neuron number and a 25% decrease in soma size in n. magnocellularis in late embryos and posthatch chickens. These results should be interpreted in light of our knowledge of the development of functional connectivity in the chick auditory system. Acoustically driven responses can first be recorded from the medulla at 11–12 days of incubation (Saunders et al., 1973) and behavioral responses can be evoked by Day 14 (Jackson & Rubel, 1978). Using an in vitro preparation of the brain stem Jackson and colleagues (1982) examined the ontogeny of postsynaptic responses in n. magnocellularis to electrical stimulation of the eighth nerve. They found that postsynaptic responses could not be evoked until after embryonic Day 11, which coincides with the age at which otocyst removal first affects survival and differentiation of brain stem auditory neurons. These results imply that the age at which cell survival and morphology become dependent on presynaptic influences corresponds to the onset of physiological connectivity.

Other experiments examining the effects of an intact receptor on neuron number and morphology indicate that the presence of an intact receptor exerts a profound influence on the brain stem auditory nuclei until well after normal functional maturation (Born & Rubel, submitted for publication; Jackson & Rubel, 1976; Rubel et al., 1981). Cochlea removal in newly hatched chickens and 6-week-old chickens resulted in loss of 20–40% of the neurons in n. magnocellularis and a 15–25% reduction in size of the remaining neurons (Figure 3-15). Neuron loss was evident by one day after the removal of the cochlea. We also observed that 1–2 days after cochlea removal some n. magnocellularis neurons were unstained by Nissl dyes and were thus presumably RNA deficient. These "ghost" neurons were visible due to the presence of membranes and stained nuclei. These observations could account for the rapid loss of neurons that were counted.

Strikingly different effects were found in adult chickens. Removal of the cochlea from 66-week-old chickens produced little or no neuron loss (less than 10%) (Figure 3-16) and caused no significant reduction in soma size.

In summary, the effects of deafferentation on the integrity and size of neurons in n. magnocellularis were similar for embryos and posthatch chickens up to 6 weeks of age but were very different for adult animals (66-week-old chickens). Although these results implicate the age of the animals as one determinant of cellular change due to deafferentation, the fact that there were major differences in the responses of chickens 6 weeks of age and those 66 weeks old is surprising. The auditory system of the chick is considered essentially mature at hatching and certainly adultlike by one month in every way measured (Gray & Rubel, 1981, 1984; Jackson & Rubel, 1978; Rubel & Rosenthal, 1975; Rubel & Ryals, 1983; Saunders et al., 1973; Smith, 1981). This would predict that the major difference would occur either in embryos or

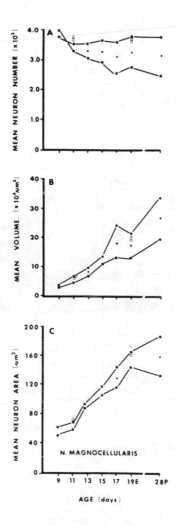

Figure 3-14. The effects of otocyst ablation on the development of n. magnocellularis. On the abscissae are the ages (in days of incubation), which correspond to the Hamburger–Hamilton (1951) stage determined for each embryo. On the ordinates are (A) mean neuron number, (B) mean total nuclear volume, and (C) mean neuronal cross-sectional area. Filled points represent means from three animals at each age, except for the 28-day posthatch group, which is from two animals. Filled circles and squares represent, respectively, the mean values on the normal (unoperated) and operated sides of experimental animals; open circles and squares represent, respectively, mean values from the left and right sides of normal control animals. Stars between the operated and normal curves indicate a statistically significant difference at that age. (From Parks, 1979).

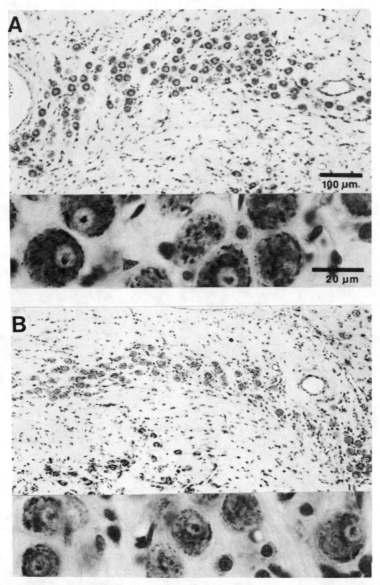

Figure 3-15. Low- and high-power photomicrographs of 10-µm paraffin sections stained with thionin through n. magnocellularis of the chick showing (A) normal (contralateral) and (B) deafferented (ipsilateral) neurons approximately 1 month following cochlea removal performed at 2 weeks posthatch. Note cell loss and cell shrinkage on the deafferented side of the brain.

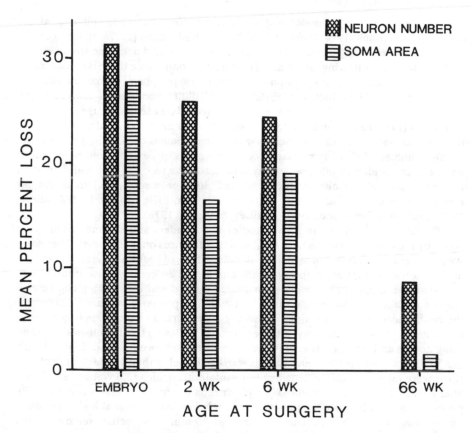

Figure 3-16. Changes in the number and cross-sectional area of neurons in n. magnocellularis
of the chick as a function of age at the time of cochlea removal. The percentage
loss was calculated by comparing the neuron area or number on the operated to
that on the unoperated side of the brain for each animal. Means for four to five
posthatch chickens in each group are shown. Means for embryos are from Parks
(1979).

between hatching and 6 weeks posthatch, during the period of functional development. Since this was not found, other factors must play an important role in controlling
the importance of afferents to these central nervous system neurons. An interesting
possibility is that the hormonal state of the animal is the determining factor.

Although there are not complete data for any single species, it appears that the
results of peripheral receptor destruction will follow a similar pattern in mammals
as in aves. Powell and Erulkar (1962) examined the effects of cochlea destruction
on the cochlear nucleus of cats. While neuron loss was not determined, there was
clearly a significant effect on cell morphology. In other studies of the effects of cochlea

destruction in "mature" animals there is clearly an effect, but again cell loss has not been reported (Kane, 1974; Webster & Webster, 1978). Trune (1982a, b) has recently reported marked changes in neuron number, soma area, and dendritic size in mouse cochlear nucleus following neonatal cochlea destruction. Since there is considerable information available on the development of the mouse peripheral and central auditory system (Ehret, 1976; Webster & Webster, 1980; Willott, 1983) further analysis of the effects of cochlea destruction at a variety of ages would be useful. Nordeen, Killackey, and Kitzes (1983) have found that there is an increased input to the inferior colliculus from the contralateral cochlear nucleus which accompanies cell loss in the ipsilateral cochlear nucleus following neonatal cochlear lesions in newborn but not in adult gerbils. Many studies on other sensory systems also have reported that deafferentation in young animals results in profound cell loss or atrophy, whereas similar manipulations in adults have much less effect (Cowan, 1970; Globus, 1975; Guillery, 1973; Peduzzi & Crossland, 1983; Woolsey & Wann, 1976).

The ultimate goal of the above studies is to understand the molecular basis whereby presynaptic neurons have long-lasting influences on their targets. Therefore, we have begun examining some of the metabolic effects of cochlea removal on neurons of the brain stem auditory pathways in the chick. The 2-deoxy-glucose studies mentioned above (Lippe et al., 1980) demonstrated a rapid and long-lasting decrease in glucose metabolism following cochlea removal. The presence of "ghost" neurons in the deafferented n. magnocellularis also suggested that a change was occurring in the protein synthetic machinery of these neurons. We tested this hypothesis by examining uptake and incorporation of [³H]leucine by n. magnocellularis neurons at various intervals after cochlea removal (Steward & Rubel, submitted for publication). Birds were injected with [³H]leucine after unilateral cochlea removal and sacrificed after 20 min. In subsequent autoradiographic preparations, silver grains over the cytoplasm of neurons indicate the presence of labeled amino acids that had been taken up and incorporated into proteins. As early as 30 min after cochlea removal, most n. magnocellularis neurons ipsilateral to cochlea removal showed a large reduction in the number of silver grains as compared to the opposite side of the brain from the same animal (Figure 3-17). Grain counts revealed a 50% difference between the average number of silver grains over neurons on the two sides of the brain. Between 3 and 24 hr, two populations emerged on the operated side; one group of cells had virtually no silver grains overlying the cytoplasm (see pointer in Figure 3-17). The remaining cells showed a consistent, statistically significant, 10–15% reduction in silver grain density as compared to neurons in the contralateral n. magnocellularis. As with the previously described morphological data, these changes were seen only in hatchlings; in 66-week-old chickens the two sides of the brain were identical. Other investigators have reported changes in protein synthesis following deafferentation in other systems (Fass, Diggs, & Steward, 1983; Fass & Steward, 1981; Meyer & Edwards, 1982) but in no case were the changes as rapid or as dramatic as those described here.

Another assay of the general metabolic state of a neuron is reflected in the levels of metabolic intermediates. As an index of "steady state" carbohydrate metabolism,

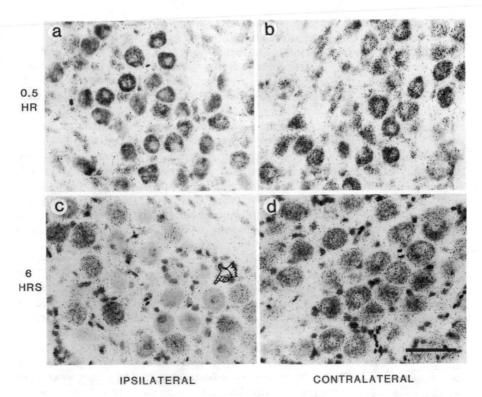

IPSILATERAL   CONTRALATERAL

Figure 3-17. Photomicrographs of 10-μm paraffin sections through n. magnocellularis (NM) prepared for emulsion autoradiography from chicks sustaining unilateral cochlea removal on posthatch Day 10. [³H]Leucine was injected 30 min (top) or 6 hr (bottom) after cochlea removal. Left panels show neurons in NM contralateral to surgery (control); right panels show neurons ipsilateral to surgery. Pointer indicates a group of cells with virtually no label. Bar indicates 50 μm.

we also have examined levels of the mitochondrial enzyme succinate dehydrogenase (SDH) in the brain stem auditory nuclei following cochlea removal (Durham & Rubel, submitted for publication). Using a histochemical stain to demonstrate SDH (Killackey & Belford, 1979; Nachlas, Tsou, deSouza, Cheng, & Seligman, 1957) reaction product is concentrated in the cytoplasm of n. magnocellularis neurons and the dorsal and ventral neuropil regions of n. laminaris. In these experiments the cochlea removal was again unilateral, allowing quantitative intra-animal comparison of "affected" and "control" regions of the two nuclei. Following cochlea removal, we observed a rapid biphasic change in SDH levels in n. magnocellularis. On the side ipsilateral to cochlea removal, from 8 to 60 hr following surgery SDH reaction product *increased*, followed by a decrease that persisted up to 35 days after surgery (Figure 3-18, top).

In n. laminaris, only a decrease in density was observed, confined to the neuropil regions receiving afferent input from the deafferented n. magnocellularis (Figure 3-18, bottom). The change in n. laminaris was first observed 3 days after surgery and also persisted until at least 35 days postoperatively. As with the other data presented above, strikingly different results were obtained with cochlea removal in 66-week-old birds. None of the changes in SDH levels were observed; control and affected regions were identical (Figure 3-18).

Similar changes in metabolic intermediates have been described in other sensory systems following deafferentation or deprivation (Dietrich, Durham, Lowry, & Woolsey, 1981, 1982; Wong-Riley, Merzenich, & Leake, 1978; Wong-Riley & Welt, 1980). Many of the changes observed are phenomenological, although some attempts have been made to elucidate the underlying mechanisms (Kasamatsu & Pettigrew, 1979; Kasamatsu, Pettigrew, & Ary, 1979; Wong-Riley & Riley, 1983). It is likely that this mechanism involves a number of interrelated changes; thus a thorough examination of as many biochemical markers as possible in a well-described pathway like the chick auditory system will be most likely to yield the underlying pattern of biological processes.

Partial deafferentation. Another approach toward understanding the role of afferent integrity on postsynaptic neurons in the auditory system is to examine the time course and specificity of the changes in neuronal morphology during normal development and following elimination of input to a portion of the neuron. The organization of dendrites in n. laminaris provides an ideal model for examining these questions. The dendrites of n. laminaris neurons are divided into distinct dorsal and ventral domains which are symmetrical in size and number (Smith & Rubel, 1979). The dorsal dendrites receive their major excitatory input from the ipsilateral n. magnocellularis while the ventral dendrites are innervated by axons from the contralateral n. magnocellularis, via the crossed dorsal cochlear tract. The development of n. laminaris dendrites has been described by Smith (1981). When first examined in Golgi-stained sections at embryonic Days 8-9, the cells of n. laminaris are uniformly covered with filopodial processes. Starting at approximately embryonic Day 9-10 there is a spatiotemporal gradient of dendrite proliferation from the rostromedial to the caudolateral poles of the nucleus, followed by a wave of process elimination in the same direction, occurring around the same time as the lamina formation and normal cell death (Rubel et al., 1976). These morphological changes will result, in the 25-day-old hatchling, in a systematic 13-fold gradient of dendritic size from the rostromedial to the caudolateral poles of the nucleus, along with a systematic decrease in the number of primary dendrites along the same spatial orientation. This organization matches the tonotopic organization of the nucleus such that, anteromedially, the cells with numerous very short dendrites are excited by high-frequency tones to either ear, whereas cells located posterolaterally have few long highly branched dendrites and are binaurally activated by low-frequency sounds.

This dendritic organization is first detectable at embryonic Day 14, at the time when n. laminaris neurons become driven by cochlear nerve activity (Jackson et al., 1982). From around embryonic Day 15 to posthatch Day 25, the gradient in dendritic

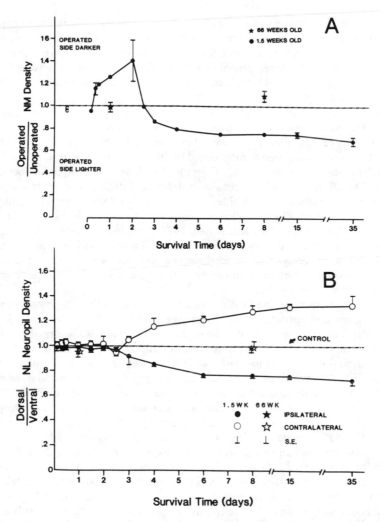

Figure 3-18. Graphs showing changes in density of SDH reaction product in n. magnocellularis (NM) (A) or n. laminaris (NL) (B) as a function of time after unilateral cochlea removal on posthatch Day 10 (circles) or at 66 weeks (stars). In (A), the mean density of 20 NM neurons on each side of the brain was calculated in each bird. Ratios of mean density on the operated (affected) to that on the unoperated (control) sides of the brain were calculated for each bird and the averages for two to five birds plotted ±SEM as a function of survival time. The C indicates average ratio for control birds, and the dotted line the value at which the operated equals the control value. In (B) the mean ratio of density in dorsal to that in ventral NL neuropil is plotted ±SEM for the side ipsilateral (filled symbols) and contralateral (open symbols) to cochlea removal. Dotted line equals control value.

size attains its adult characteristics, and the size symmetry between the dorsal and ventral dendrites of the n. laminaris neurons evolves from a correlation of approximately 0.50 to 0.75 (Gray et al., 1982; Smith & Rubel, 1979). Therefore, the temporal correlation between the development of auditory function (synaptic activity) and the ontogenetic "sculpturing" of dendritic organization again suggests a causal relationship between these events.

The correlation between the development of the dendritic organization and tonotopy within the nucleus prompted us to consider a role for afferent activity in maintaining the receptive surface of the n. laminaris neurons. The atrophy of dendrites after deafferentation has been demonstrated in many neural systems (Caceres & Steward, 1983; Matthews & Powell, 1962; Valverde, 1968). Severing the cross dorsal cochlear tract (XDCT in Figure 3-13) results in deafferentation of the ventral dendrites of n. laminaris neurons on both sides of the brain, while leaving the input to the dorsal dendrites intact. Electron microscopic observations of n. laminaris 4 days after such an operation (Benes, Parks, & Rubel, 1977) revealed a severe loss of dendritic profiles on the ventral side of the nucleus while the dorsal dendrites appeared healthy and of normal size. Along with the dendritic changes, they also observed a disruption of the cytoplasm localized predominantly to the ventral side of the n. laminaris cell bodies.

Recently, we examined the time course and specificity of the atrophy of the ventral dendrites using a quantitative Golgi technique (Deitch & Rubel, in press; Rubel & Smith, 1981). The severity of the atrophy of the ventral dendrites was readily apparent by 2 days after sectioning their afferents and striking by 8 days (Figure 3-19). We then measured the lengths of the dorsal and ventral dentrites at various survival times from 1 hour to 16 days after the operation. On the ventral (deafferented) side there was an immediate and continuous loss of dendrites throughout the nucleus, whereas on the dorsal side there were no changes at any survival interval. The atrophy of the ventral dendrites was quite dramatic, reaching a 20% loss in only 2 hr, and at least a 60% loss by 16 days following deafferentation (Figure 3-20).

Several conclusions can be drawn from this experiment. For one, the morphology of n. laminaris dendrites is dependent on innervation by the n. magnocellularis afferents. In addition, this regulatory action is localized to the postsynaptic surface only; the dorsal dendrites, whose innervation remains intact, were unaffected by the insult to the opposite side of the cell. Finally, any speculation on the nature of this afferent regulation is constrained by the rapidity with which the observed dendritic changes occur. The functional change most likely to occur with the immediacy of the ventral dendrite reaction is the interruption of activity in the presynaptic axons. Indeed, electrophysiological recordings from the ventral neuropil of n. laminaris during and after the operation reveal a sudden and precipitous cessation of the normally high levels of spontaneous and driven activity impinging on the ventral dendrites (Rubel & Deitch, unpublished observations). The activity levels in the dorsal neuropil were unchanged.

Environmental influences. There have now been a number of studies showing that monaural or binaural occlusion influences cell structure, neuronal function, and hearing in aves and mammals. Webster and Webster (1977, 1979) were early contribu-

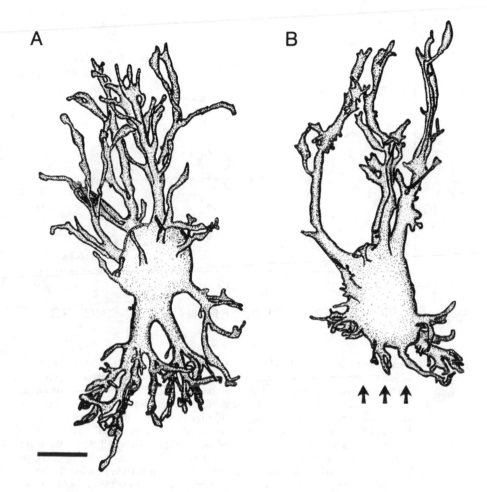

Figure 3-19. Camera lucida drawings of Golgi-impregnated n. laminaris (NL) neurons in the normal chick (A), and 8 days after deafferenting the ventral dendrites (B). Neurons are from similar regions in NL. The ventral dendrites have nearly completely atrophied, whereas the dorsal dendrites are unaffected. Bar = 10 μm.

tors to this area, showing that ear occlusion and quiet rearing resulted in significant reductions of cell size, as defined by Nissl stain, in many areas of the cochlear nucleus and superior olivary complex of mice. Conductive hearing deficits in adult animals did not produce reliable differences. Anatomical changes produced by presumed conductive hearing losses during development have also been shown in the rat and the chick (Coleman & O'Connor, 1979; Conlee & Parks, 1981, 1983; Feng & Rogowski,

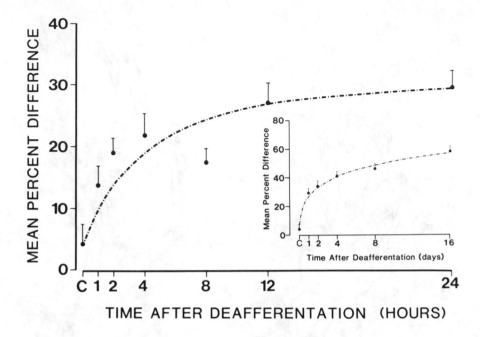

Figure 3-20. Mean percent loss (±SEM) in length of the ventral dendrites of n. laminaris neurons at various survival times after deafferentation. The dendrites are normally symmetrical (zero percent difference), and deafferentation does not change the dorsal dendritic length. Thus, for each cell the dorsal dendritic length was used as a predictor of the ventral dendritic length of that cell prior to deafferentation. The difference between the predicted length (dorsal dendrites) and the observed length (ventral dendrites) is expressed as a percentage of the predicted length. All cells of the same survival time after crossed dorsal cochlear tract transection were averaged to give a mean percent difference between normal and deafferented dendritic lengths. Large graph demonstrates the time course of dendritic atrophy over the first 48 hr. Inset shows the time course over 16 days (from Deitch & Rubel, 1984).

1980; Gray et al., 1982; Smith, Gray, & Rubel, 1983). One serious shortcoming in all of these studies is that the normalcy of inner ear function has not been verified at the end of the deprivation period. Clinically, the existence of normal bone conduction thresholds is required to rule out combined conductive and sensorineural components. At least these same criteria should be applied to experimental investigations.

Another consideration in interpreting the results of "deprivation" studies is the necessity to "calibrate" the deprivation paradigm used. A recent series of studies in our laboratory has sought to determine morphological and behavioral consequences of auditory deprivation on chick brain stem auditory nuclei (Kerr et al., 1979; Gray et al., 1982; Smith et al., 1983). As shown in Figure 3-21, a silicone ear plug produced

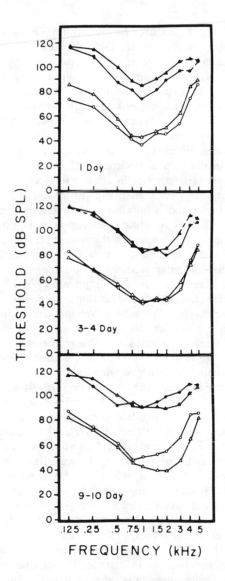

Figure 3-21. Audiographs of brain stem evoked potential thresholds (dB, re: 20N/m²) for 1, 3-4, and 9-10 day hatchling chicks. Points are mean thresholds at each frequency for all ears tested. Triangles refer to acute treatment groups and circles to chronic treatment groups. Open symbols refer to stimulus runs without ear plugs and closed points to stimulus runs with ear plugs for both treatment groups. Dotted lines connect frequencies at which one or more chicks failed to achieve a threshold response at the highest sound level presented in the plugged condition.

a 40 dB conductive loss, as measured by eighth nerve evoked potentials, that was consistent across frequency (Kerr et al., 1979). However, when the morphology of neurons in the second-order n. laminaris was examined after a similar deprivation, a surprising result was obtained (Figure 3-22). Changes in dendrite length varied with frequency, such that dendritic size in low-frequency regions increased while dendritic size decreased in high-frequency regions. One interpretation of these results is that superimposed on the flat conductive hearing loss were alterations in bone conduction and/or neuronal activity resulting from internally generated sound. Thus, it is important to know what changes are occurring in the sound environment of the organism as well as in the "neural environment" in the central nervous system.

What do these studies tell us about the relationship between the acoustic environment, neuronal activity, and development of neurons in the auditory system? Laying aside the caveats mentioned above, they imply that cellular morphology can be altered by chronically abnormal activity. Little more can be concluded at this time. Only a few studies have sought to determine if the abnormal conditions were disrupting the normal developmental trend or producing an abnormal condition following normal ontogeny (Gottlieb, 1976; Solomon & Lessac, 1968). In some cases abnormal development has been found (Gray et al., 1982) or implicated (Feng & Rogowski, 1980). In others it appears that the effects of altered hearing are superimposed on normal development (Conlee & Parks, 1981; Webster & Webster, 1980). In addition, it is not at all clear that a conductive hearing loss will cause a simple reduction in the ongoing activity in the eighth nerve, much less in cochlear nuclei and other auditory nuclei in the brain. The change in dendritic sizes noted above (Smith et al., 1983) is an example of this phenomenon. Finally, we don't know when in development activity from the ear can begin to influence the central nervous system. Webster and Webster (1980) and Brugge and O'Connor (in press) indicate that major anatomical and physiological processes are "independent of environmental events." It is important to consider that activity along eighth nerve fibers, whether influenced by sound in the external environment or not, is part of the "environment" of the cells in the cochlear nuclei. Thus, in order to understand how activity from the ear influences development of central auditory system structures, we need to know when a functional synaptic network is established, what the ontogenetic activity pattern is in the eighth nerve, and how sound influences that activity pattern throughout ontogeny.

Behavioral studies on animals subjected to altered acoustic environments (Gottlieb, 1975, 1976; Kerr et al., 1979; Tees, 1967), examinations of language development in children suffering chronic conductive hearing loss, and observations of clinicians all concur that normal function can be disrupted by an abnormal acoustic environment. Yet, to date there are only scattered results indicating altered physiological function following deprivation or altered stimulation (Clopton & Silverman, 1977, 1978; Sanes & Constantine-Paton, 1982; Silverman & Clopton, 1977). Over the next few years it is certain that considerable effort will be expended in this area and a "battery" of changes will be demonstrated. A theoretical structure with which to interpret such changes, in relation to the environment of the developing organism and to its behavioral abilities, is of paramount importance.

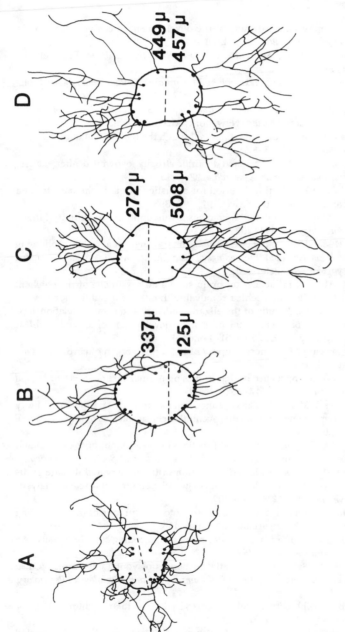

Figure 3-22. Camera lucida tracings of n. laminaris (NL) neurons from monaurally deprived chickens. All neurons are shown as if on the side of the brain contralateral to the deprived ear; therefore the "deprived" dendrite is the ventral dendrite. Numbers next to each neuron indicate the total lengths of the dorsal dendrites and the total length of the ventral dendrites. (A) Neuron with disoriented dendrites. Because some dendrites are both dorsal and ventral, the separate lengths could not be objectively determined. Such neurons were not considered in the quantitative analysis. (B) Neuron from anterior part of NL; deprived (ventral) dendrite is shorter than the nondeprived dendrite. (C) Neuron from the posterolateral third of NL showing the opposite effect as that shown in (B); the deprived (ventral) dendrite is longer than the nondeprived (dorsal) dendrite. (D) Normal-appearing NL neuron from the middle region of the nucleus; note that the lengths of the dorsal and the ventral dendrites are similar. [From Smith et al., 1983].

REFERENCES

Änggard, L. (1965). An electrophysiological study of the development of cochlear function in the rabbit. *Acta Otolaryngologica, 203*, (Suppl.), 1–64.

Anson, B.J., & Donaldson, J.A. (1981). *Surgical anatomy of the temporal bone.* Philadelphia: Saunders.

Arey, L.B. (1966). *Developmental anatomy. A textbook and laboratory manual of embryology.* Philadelphia: Saunders.

Bast, T.H., & Anson, B.J. (1949). *The temporal bone and the ear.* Springfield, IL: Thomas.

Békésy, G. von (1960). *Experiments in hearing.* New York: McGraw–Hill.

Bench, J. (1968). Sound transmission to the human fetus through the maternal abdominal wall. *Journal of Genetic Psychology, 113*, 85–87.

Benes, F.M., Parks, T.N., & Rubel, E.W (1977). Rapid dendritic atrophy following deafferentation: An EM morphometric analysis. *Brain Research, 122*, 1–13.

Bock, G.R., & Saunders, J.C. (1977). A critical period for acoustic trauma in the hamster and its relation to cochlear development. *Science, 197*, 396–398.

Bock, G.R., & Seifter, E.J. (1978). Developmental changes of susceptibility to auditory fatigue in young hamsters. *Audiology, 17*, 193–203.

Born, D.E., & Rubel, E.W (1983). Differential effects of age on transneuronal cell loss following cochlea removal in chickens (Abstract). *Proceedings of the Midwinter Meeting of the Association of Research in Otolaryngology*, St. Petersburg, FL.

Born D.E., & Rubel, E.W. Afferent influences on brain stem auditory nuclei of the chicken: Neuron number and size following cochlea removal. Submitted for publication.

Bosher, S.K., & Warren, R.L. (1971). A study of the electrochemistry and osmotic relationships of the cochlear fluids in the neonatal rat at the time of the development of the endocochlear potential. *Journal of Physiology 6, 212*, 739–61 (London).

Bredberg, G. (1968). Cellular pattern and nerve supply of the human organ of corti. *Acta Otolaryngologica, 236* (Suppl.), 1–135.

Brooks, D. (1971). Electroacoustic impedance bridge studies on normal ears of children. *Journal of Speech and Hearing Research, 14*, 247–253.

Brugge, J.F., Javel, E., & Kitzes, L.M. (1978). Signs of functional maturation of peripheral auditory system in discharge patterns of neurons in anteroventral cochlear nucleus of kittens. *Journal of Neurophysiology, 41*, 1557–1579.

Brugge, J.F., & O'Connor, T.A. (in press). Postnatal functional development of the dorsal and posteroventral cochlear nuclei of the cat. *Journal of the Acoustical Society of America.*

Caceres, A., & Steward, O. (1983). Dendritic reorganization in the denervated dentate gyrus of the rat following entorhinal cortical lesions: A Golgi and electron microscopic analysis. *Journal of Comparative Neurology, 214*, 387–403.

Carlier, E., & Pujol, R. (1980). Supra-normal sensitivity to ototoxic antibiotic of the developing rat cochlea. *Archives of Otorhinolaryngology, 226*, 129–133.

Carlier, E., & Pujol, R. (1978). Role of inner and outer hair cells in coding sound intensity: An ontogenetic approach. *Brain Research, 147*, 174–176.

Clements, M., & Kelly, J.B. (1978a). Auditory spatial responses of young guinea pigs *(Cavia procellus)* during and after ear blocking. *Journal of Comparative and Physiological Psychology, 92*, 34–44.

Clements, M., & Kelly, J.B. (1978b). Directional responses by kittens to an auditory stimulus. *Developmental Psychobiology, 11*, 505–511.

Clopton, B.M., & Silverman, M.S. (1977). Plasticity of binaural interaction: II. Critical period and changes in midline response. *Journal of Neurophysiology, 40*, 1275–1280.

Clopton, B.M., & Silverman, M.S. (1978). Changes in latency and duration of neural responding following developmental auditory deprivation. *Experimental Brain Research, 32*, 39–47.

Coleman, J.W. (1976). Hair cell loss as a function of age in the normal cochlea of the guinea pig. *Acta Otolaryngologica, 82*, 33–40.

Coleman, J.R., & O'Connor, P. (1979). Effects of monaural and binaural sound deprivation on cell development in the anteroventral cochlear nucleus of rats. *Experimental Neurology, 64*, 553–566.

Conlee, J.W., & Parks, T.N. (1981). Age- and position-dependent effects of monaural acoustic deprivation in nucleus magnocellularis of the chicken. *Journal of Comparative Neurology, 202*, 373–384.

Conlee, J.W., & Parks, T.N. (1983). Late appearance and deprivation-sensitive growth of permanent dendrites in the avian cochlear nucleus (nuc. magnocellularis). *Journal of Comparative Neurology, 217*, 216–226.

Cotanche, D.A., & Sulik, K.K. (1983). Morphogenesis of the avian basilar papilla with special emphasis on the differentiation of stereociliary bundles (Abstract). *Proceedings of the Midwinter Meeting of the Association for Research in Otolaryngology.*

Cowan, W.M. (1970). Anterograde and retrograde transneuronal degeneration in the central and peripheral nervous system. In W.J.H. Nauta & S.O.E. Ebbesson (Eds.), *Contemporary research methods in neuroanatomy* (pp. 217–251). New York: Springer-Verlag.

Deitch, J.S., & Rubel, E.W (1982). Time course of changes in dendritic morphology in n. laminaris following deafferentation (Abstract). *Society for Neuroscience Abstracts, 8*, 756.

Deitch, J.S., & Rubel, E.W (in press). Afferent influences on brain stem auditory nuclei of the chicken: Time course and specificity of dendritic atrophy following deafferentation. *Journal of Comparative Neurology.*

Dietrich, W.D., Durham, D., Lowry, O.H., & Woolsey, T.A. (1981). Quantitative histochemical effects of whisker damage on single identified cortical barrels in the adult mouse. *Journal of Neuroscience, 1*, 929–935.

Dietrich, W.D., Durham, D., Lowry, O.H., & Woolsey, T.A. (1982). "Increased" sensory stimulation leads to changes in energy-related enzymes in the brain. *Journal of Neuroscience, 2*, 1608–1613.

Djupesland, G., & Zwislocki, J.J. (1973). Sound pressure distribution in the outer ear. *Acta Otolaryngologica, 75*, 350–352.

Durham, D., & Rubel, E.W. Afferent influences on brain stem auditory nuclei of the chicken: Changes in succinate dehydrogenase activity following cochlea removal. Submitted for publication.

Easter, S.S. (1983). Postnatal neurogenesis and changing connections. *Trends in NeuroSciences, 6*, 53–56.

Ehret, G. (1976). Development of absolute auditory thresholds in the house mouse (*Mus musculus*). *Journal of the American Audiology Society, 1*, 173–184.

Ehret, G., & Romand, R. (1981). Postnatal development of absolute auditory thresholds in kittens. *Journal of Comparative and Physiological Psychology, 95*, 304–311.

Fass, B., Diggs, J., & Steward, O. (1982). Histochemical evidence for increases of RNA in the denervated neuropil of the dentate gyrus during reinnervation. *Society for Neuroscience abstracts, 8*, 304.

Fass, B., & Steward, O. (1981). Increases of protein-precursor incorporation in the denervated neuropil of rat dentate gyrus during sprouting (Abstract). *Anatomical Record, 199*, 80A–81A.

Fee, W.E., Jr. (1980). Aminoglycoside ototoxicity in the human. *Laryngoscope 90, Suppl. 24*, 1–19.

Feng, A.S., & Rogowski, B.A. (1980). Effects of monaural and binaural occlusion on the morphology of neurons in the medial superior olivary nucleus of the rat. *Brain Research, 189,* 530–534.

Fermin, C.F., & Cohen, G.M. (1983). Developmental gradients in the embryonic chick's basilar papilla (Abstract). *Proceedings of the Midwinter Meeting of the Association for Research in Otolaryngology,* St. Petersburg, FL.

Fujimoto, S., Yamamoto, K., Hayabuchi, I., & Yoshizuka, M. (1981). Scanning and transmission electron microscope studies on the organ of corti and stria vascularis in human fetal cochlear ducts. *Archivum Histologicum Japonicum, 44,* 223–235.

Ginzberg, R.D., & Gilula, N.B. (1979). Modulation of cell junctions during differentiation of the chicken otocyst sensory epithelium. *Developmental Biology, 68,* 110–129.

Globus, A. (1975). Brain morphology as a function of presynaptic morphology and activity. In A.H. Riesen (Ed.), *The developmental neuropsychology of sensory deprivation* (pp. 9–91). New York: Academic Press.

Gottlieb, G. (1971). Ontogenesis of sensory function in birds and mammals. In E. Tobach, L.A. Aronson, and E. Shaw (Eds.), *The biopsychology of development* (pp. 67–128). New York: Academic Press.

Gottlieb, G. (1975). Development of species identification in ducklings: I. Nature of perceptual deficit caused by embryonic auditory deprivation. *Journal of Comparative and Physiological Psychology, 89,* 387–399.

Gottlieb, G. (1976). The roles of experience in development of behavior and the nervous system. In G. Gottlieb (Ed.), *Studies on the development of behavior and the nervous system: Neural and behavioral specificity* (Vol. 3, pp. 25–54). New York: Academic Press.

Gray, L., & Rubel, E.W (1981). Development of responsiveness to suprathreshold acoustic stimulation in chickens. *Journal of Comparative and Physiological Psychology, 95,* 188–198.

Gray, L., & Rubel, E.W (1984). Development of auditory thresholds and frequency difference limens in chickens. In G. Gottlieb & N.A. Krasnegor (Eds.), *Measurement of audition and vision during the first year of life: A methodological overview.* Norwood, NJ: Ablex.

Gray, L., Smith, Z.D.J., & Rubel, E.W (1982). Developmental and experiential changes in dendritic symmetry. *Brain Research, 244,* 360–364.

Guillery, R.W. (1973). Quantitative studies of transneuronal atrophy in the dorsal lateral geniculate nucleus of cats and kittens. *Journal of Comparative Neurology, 149,* 423–437.

Guillery, R.W. (1974). On structural changes that can be produced experimentally in the mammalian visual pathways. In R. Bellairs & E.G. Gray (Eds.), *Essays on the nervous system* (pp. 299–326). Oxford: Claredon.

Hamburger, V., & Hamilton, H.L. (1951). A series of normal stages in the development of the chick embryo. *Journal of Morphology, 88,* 49–92.

Harris, D.M., & Dallos, P. (1983). CM measurements of the place/frequency code in developing gerbils (Abstract). *Proceedings of the Midwinter Meeting of the Association for Research in Otolaryngology,* St. Petersburg, FL.

Hawkins, J.E., Jr., Johnsson, L.-G., & Aran, J.-M. (1969). Comparative tests of gentamicin ototoxicity. *Journal of Infectious Diseases, 119,* 417–426.

Henry, K.R., Chole, R.A., McGinn, M.D., & Frush, D.P. (1981). Increased ototoxicity in both young and old mice. *Archives of Otolaryngology, 107,* 92–95.

Himelfarb, M.Z., Popelka, G.R., & Shanon, E. (1979). Tympanometry in normal neonates. *Journal of Speech and Hearing Research, 22,* 179–191.

Hirokawa, N. (1978). The ultrastructure of the basilar papilla of the chick. *Journal of Comparative Neurology, 181,* 361–374.

Jackson, H., Hackett, J.T., & Rubel, E.W (1982). Organization and development of brain stem auditory nuclei in the chick: Ontogeny of postsynaptic responses. *Journal of Comparative Neurology, 210,* 80-86.

Jackson, H., & Parks, T.N., (1982). Functional synapse elimination in the developing avian cochlear nucleus with simultaneous reduction in cochlear-nerve axon branching. *Journal of Neuroscience, 2,* 1736-1743.

Jackson, J.R.H., & Rubel, E.W (1976). Rapid transneuronal degeneration following cochlea removal in chickens (Abstract). *Anatomical Record, 184,* 434-435.

Jackson, H., & Rubel, E.W (1978). Ontogeny of behavioral responsiveness to sound in the chick embryo as indicated by electrical recordings of motility. *Journal of Comparative and Physiological Psychology, 92,* 682-696.

Jerger, S., Jerger, J., Mauldin, L., & Segal, P. (1974). Studies in impedance audiometry. II. Children less than six years old. *Archives of Otolaryngology, 99,* 1-9.

Jhaveri, S., & Morest, D.K. (1982). Sequential alterations of neuronal architecture in nucleus magnocellularis of the developing chicken: A Golgi study. Neuroscience, 7, 837-853.

Johns, M.E., Ryals, B.M., Guerry, T.L., Wenzel, R.P., & Rubel, E.W (1980). Effects of aminoglycoside antibiotics on hair cells of the chick basal papilla (Abstract). *Proceedings of the 1980 Mid-Winter Meeting of the Association for Research in Otolaryngology,* January, 1980.

Kane, E.C. (1974). Patterns of degeneration in the caudal cochlear nucleus of the cat after cochlear ablation. *Anatomical Record, 179,* 67-92.

Kasamatsu, T., & Pettigrew, J.D. (1979). Preservation of binocularity after monocular deprivation in the striate cortex of kittens treated with 6-hydroxydopamine. *Journal of Comparative Neurology, 185,* 139-162.

Kasamatsu, T., Pettigrew, J.D., & Ary, M. (1979). Restoration of visual cortical plasticity by local microperfusion of norepinephrine. *Journal of Comparative Neurology, 185,* 163-182.

Keith, R.W. (1973). Impedance audiometry with neonates. *Archives of Otolaryngology, 97,* 465-467.

Keith, R.W. (1975). Middle ear function in neonates. *Archives of Otolaryngology, 101,* 376-379.

Kerr, L.M., Ostapoff, E.M., & Rubel, E.W (1979). Influence of acoustic experience on the ontogeny of frequency generalization gradients in the chicken. *Journal of Experimental Psychology: Animal Behavior Processes, 5,* 97-115.

Killackey, H.P., & Belford, G.R. (1979). The formation of afferent patterns in the somatosensory cortex of the neonatal rat. *Journal of Comparative Neurology, 183,* 285-304.

Koerber, K.C., & Pfeiffer, R.R., Warr, W.B., & Kiang, N.Y.S. (1966). Spontaneous spike discharges from single units in the cochlear nucleus after destruction of the cochlea. *Experimental Neurology, 16,* 119-130.

Lenoir, M., Bock, G.R., & Pujol, R. (1979. Supra-normal susceptibility to acoustic trauma in the rat pup cochlea. *Journal of Physiology (Paris), 75,* , 521-524.

Lenoir, M., & Pujol, R. (1980). Sensitive period to acoustic trauma in the rat pup cochlea: Histological findings. *Acta Otolaryngologica, 89,* 317-322.

Lenoir, M., Shnerson, A., & Pujol, R. (1980). Cochlear receptor development in the rat with emphasis on synaptogenesis. *Anatomical Embryology, 160,* 253-262.

Levi-Montalcini, R. (1949). The development of the acousticovestibular centers in the chick embryo in the absence of the afferent root fibers and of descending fiber tracts. *Journal of Comparative Neurology, 91,* 209-241.

Lippe, W.R., & Rubel, E.W (1983). Development of the place principle: Tonotopic organization. *Science, 219,* 514-516.

Lippe, W.R., Steward, O., & Rubel, E.W (1980). The effect of unilateral basilar papilla removal upon nuclei laminaris and magnocellularis of the chick examined with [^{3}H]2-deoxy-D-glucose autoradiography. *Brain Research, 196,* 43-58.

Matthews, M.R., & Powell, T.P.S. (1962). Some observations on transneuronal cell degeneration in the olfactory bulb of the rabbit. *Journal of Anatomy, 96*, 89–102.

Meyer, M.R., & Edwards, J.S. (1982). Metabolic changes in deafferented central neurons of an insect, *Acheta domesticus*. I. Effects upon amino acid uptake and incorporation. *Journal of Neuroscience, 2*, 1651–1659.

Moore, D.R., & Irvine, D.R.F. (1979a). A developmental study of the sound pressure transformation by the head of the cat. *Acta Otolaryngologica, 87*, 434–440.

Moore, D.R., & Irvine, D.R.F. (1979b). The development of some peripheral and central auditory responses in the neonatal cat. *Brain Research, 163*, 49–59.

Muir, D. (1984). Infant's orientation to the location of sound sources. In G. Gottlieb & N.A. Krasnegor (Eds.), *Measurement of audition and vision during the first year of life: A methodological overview.* Norwood, NJ: Ablex.

Nachlas, M.M., Tsou, K.-C., deSouza, E., Cheng, S.-S., & Seligman, A.M. (1957). Cytochemical demonstration of succinic dehydrogenase by the use of a new p-nitrophenyl substituted ditetrazole. *Journal of Histochemistry and Cytochemistry, 5*, 420–436.

Noden, D.M. (1980). The migration and cytodifferentiation of cranial neural crest cells. In R.M. Pratt & R.L. Christensen (Eds.), *Current research trends in prenatal craniofacial development* (pp. 3–25). New York: Elsevier.

Nordeen, K.W., Killackey, H.P., & Kitzes, L.M. (1983). Reorganization of ascending projections to the inferior colliculus following unilateral cochlear ablations in the neonatal gerbil, *Meriones unguiculatus. Journal of Comparative Neurology, 214*, 144–153.

Orr, M.F. (1968). Histogenesis of sensory epithelium in reaggregates of dissociated embryonic chick otocysts. *Developmental Biology, 17*, 39–54.

Parks, T.N. (1979). Afferent influences on the development of brain stem auditory nuclei of the chicken: Otocyst ablation. *Journal of Comparative Neurology, 183*, 665–678.

Parks, T.N., & Rubel, E.W (1975). Organization and development of brain stem auditory nuclei of the chicken: Organization of projections from n. magnocellularis to n. laminaris. *Journal of Comparative Neurology, 164*, 435–448.

Peduzzi, J.D., & Crossland, W.J. (1983). Anterograde transneuronal degeneration in the ectomammilary nucleus and ventral lateral geniculate nucleus of the chick. *Journal of Comparative Neurology, 213*, 287–300.

Powell, T.P.S., & Erulkar, S.D. (1962). Transneuronal cell degeneration in the auditory relay nuclei of the cat. *Journal of Anatomy, 96*, 249–268.

Price, G.R. (1976). Age as a factor in susceptibility to hearing loss: Young versus adult ears. *Journal of the Acoustical Society of America, 60*, 886–892.

Pujol, R., Carlier, E., & Devigne, C. (1978). Different patterns of cochlear innervation during the development of the kitten. *Journal of Comparative Neurology, 177*, 529–536.

Pujol, R., Carlier, E., & Lenoir, M. (1980). Ontogenetic approach to inner and outer hair cell function. *Hearing Research, 2*, 423–430.

Pujol, R., & Hilding, D. (1973). Anatomy and physiology of the onset of auditory function. *Acta Otolaryngologica, 76*, 1–10.

Pujol, R., & Marty, R. (1968). Structural and physiological relationships of the maturing auditory system. In L. Jilek & S. Trojan (Eds.), *Ontogenesis of the brain* (pp. 337–385). Prague: Charles Univ. Press.

Pujol, R., & Marty, R. (1970). Postnatal maturation of the cochlea of the cat. *Journal of Comparative Neurology, 139*, 115–125.

Rebillard, M., & Pujol, R. (1984). Innervation of the chicken basilar papilla during its development. *Acta Otolaryngologica, 96*, 379–388.

Rebillard, G., & Rubel, E.W (1981). Electrophysiological study of the maturation of auditory responses from the inner ear of the chick. *Brain Research, 229*, 15-23.

Relkin, E.M., & Saunders, J.C. (1980). Displacement of the malleus in neonatal golden hamsters. *Acta Otolaryngologica, 90*, 6-15.

Relkin, E.M., Saunders, J.C., & Konkle, D.F. (1979). The development of middle-ear admittance in the hamster. *Journal of the Acoustical Society of America, 66*, 133-139.

Retzius, G. (1884). *Das Gehörorgan der Wirbelthiere. II. Das Gehörorgan der Reptilien, der Vögel und Säugethiere.* Stockholm: Samson & Wallin.

Romand, R., & Romand, M.-R. (1982). Myelination kinetics of spiral ganglion cells in kittens. *Journal of Comparative Neurology, 204*, 1-5.

Rubel, E.W (1978). Ontogeny of structure and function in the vertebrate auditory system. In M. Jacobson (Ed.), *Handbook of sensory physiology. Vol. IX. Development of sensory systems* (pp. 135-237). New York: Springer-Verlag.

Rubel, E.W, & Parks, T.N. (1975). Organization and development of brain stem auditory nuclei of the chicken: Tonotopic organization of nucleus magnocellularis and nucleus laminaris. *Journal of Comparative Neurology, 164*, 435-448.

Rubel, E.W, & Rosenthal, M.H. (1975). The ontogeny of auditory frequency generalization in the chicken. *Journal of Experimental Psychology: Animal Behavior Processes, 1*, 287-297.

Rubel, E.W, & Ryals, B.M. (1982). Patterns of hair cell loss in chick basilar papilla after intense auditory stimulation: Exposure duration and survival time. *Acta Otolaryngologica, 93*, 31-41.

Rubel, E.W, & Ryals, B.M. (1983). Development of the place principle: Acoustic trauma. *Science, 219*, 512-514.

Rubel, E.W, & Smith, Z.D.J. (1981). Afferent maintenance of dendritic organization in n. laminaris of the chick (Abstract). *Anatomical Record, 199*, 219A.

Rubel, E.W, Smith, Z.D.J., & Miller, L.C. (1976). Organization and development of brain stem auditory nuclei of the chicken: Ontogeny of n. magnocellularis and n. laminaris. *Journal of Comparative Neurology, 166*, 469-490.

Rubel, E.W, Smith, Z.D.J., & Steward, O. (1981). Sprouting in the avian brain stem auditory pathway: Dependence on dendritic integrity. *Journal of Comparative Neurology, 202*, 397-414.

Ruben, R.J. (1967). Development of the inner ear of the mouse: A radioautographic study of terminal mitoses. *Acta Otolaryngologica 220*, (Suppl.), 1-44.

Ruben, R.J. (1969). The synthesis of DNA and RNA in the developing inner ear. *Laryngoscope, 79*, 1546-1556.

Ryals, B.M. (1981). *Ontogenetic effects of acoustic trauma in chick basilar papilla. Doctoral dissertation presented to the graduate faculty of The University of Virginia.*

Ryals, B.M., & Rubel, E.W (1982). Patterns of hair cell loss in chick basilar papilla after intense auditory stimulation: Frequency organization. *Acta Otolaryngologica, 93*, 205-210.

Sanes, D.H., & Constantine-Paton, M. (1982). The role of temporal activity during auditory maturation (Abstract). *Society for Neuroscience Abstracts, 8*, p. 669.

Saunders, J.C., & Bock, G.R. (1978). Influences of early auditory trauma on auditory development. In G. Gottlieb (Ed.), *Studies on the development of behavior and the nervous system, Vol. 4: Early influences* (pp. 249-287). New York: Academic Press.

Saunders, J.C., Coles, R.B., & Gates, G.R. (1973). The development of auditory evoked responses on the cochlea and cochlear nuclei of the chick. *Brain Research, 63*, 59-74.

Saunders, J.C., & Garfinkle, T. (1983). Peripheral physiology II. In J.F. Willott (Ed.), *Auditory psychobiology of the mouse.* Springfield, IL: Thomas.

Saunders, J.C., Kaltenbach, J.A., & Relkin, E.M. (1983). The structural and functional development of the outer and middle ear. In R. Romand & R. Marty (Eds.), *Development of auditory and vestibular systems.* New York: Academic Press.

Saunders, J.C., & Rosowski, J.J. (1979). Assessment of hearing in animals. In W.F. Rintelmann (Ed.), *Hearing Assessment* (pp. 487–529). Baltimore: University Park Press.

Schweitzer, L., & Cant, N.B. (in press). Development of the cochlear innervation of the dorsal cochlear nucleus of the hamster. *Journal of Comparative Neurology.*

Shaw, E.A.G. (1974). The external ear. In W.D. Keidel & W.D. Neff (Eds.), *Handbook of sensory physiology, auditory system* (Vol. 1, pp. 455–490). New York: Springer-Verlag.

Shnerson, A., & Pujol, R. (1982). Age-related changes in the C57Bl/6J mouse cochlea. I. Physiological findings. *Developmental Brain Research, 2,* 65–75.

Silverman, M.S., & Clopton, B.M. (1977). Plasticity of binaural interaction. I. Effect of early auditory deprivation. *Journal of Neurophysiology, 40,* 1266–1174.

Smith, D.E. (1977). The effect of deafferentation on the development of brain and spinal nuclei. *Progress in Neurobiology, 8,* 349–367.

Smith, Z.D.J. (1981). Organization and development of brain stem auditory nuclei of the chicken: Dendritic development of n. laminaris. *Journal of Comparative Neurology, 203,* 309–333.

Smith, Z.D.J., Gray, L., & Rubel, E.W (1983). Afferent influences on brain stem auditory nuclei of the chicken: N. laminaris dendritic length following monaural acoustic deprivation. *Journal of Comparative Neurology, 220,* 199–205.

Smith, Z.D.J., & Rubel, E.W (1979). Organization and development of brain stem auditory nuclei of the chicken: Dendritic gradients in nucleus laminaris. *Journal of Comparative Neurology, 186,* 213–240.

Sobkowicz, H.M., Rose, J.E., Scott, G.E., & Slapnick, S.M. (1982). Ribbon synapses in the developing intact and cultured organ of Corti in the mouse. *Journal of Neuroscience, 2,* 942–957.

Solomon, R.L., & Lessac, M.S. (1968). A control group design for experimental studies of developmental processes. *Psychological Bulletin, 70,* 145–209.

Steward, O., & Rubel, E.W. Afferent influences on brain stem auditory nuclei of the chicken: Cessation of protein synthesis as an antecedent to age-dependent transneuronal degeneration. Submitted for publication.

Stream, R.W., Stream, K.S., Walker, J.R., & Brehingstall, G. (1978). Emerging characteristics of the acoustic reflex in infants. *Transactions of the American Academy of Ophthalmology and Otolaryngology, 86,* 628–636.

Tees, R.C. (1967). Effects of early auditory restriction in the rat on adult pattern discrimination. *Journal of Comparative Physiological Psychology, 63,* 389–392.

Tilney, L.G., DeRosier, D.J., & Mulroy, M.J. (1980). The organization of actin filaments in the stereocilia of cochlear hair cells. *Journal of Cell Biology, 86,* 244–259.

Tilney, L.G., Egelman, E.H., DeRosier, D.J., & Saunders, J.C. (1983). Actin filaments, stereocilia, and hair cells of the bird cochlea. II. Packing of actin filaments in the stereocilia and in the cuticular plate and what happens to the organization when the stereocilia are bent. *Journal of Cell Biology, 96,* 822–834.

Tilney, L.G., & Saunders, J.C. (1983). Actin filaments, stereocilia, and hair cells of the bird cochlea. 1. Length, number, width, and distribution of stereocilia of each hair cell are related to the position of the hair cell on the cochlea. *Journal of Cell Biology, 96,* 807–821.

Trune, D.R. (1982a). Influence of neonatal cochlear removal on the development of mouse cochlear nucleus: I. Number, size, and density of its neurons. *Journal of Comparative Neurology, 209,* 409–424.

Trune, D.R. (1982b). Influence of neonatal cochlear removal on the development of mouse cochlear nucleus: II. Dendritic morphology of its neurons. *Journal of Comparative Neurology, 209,* 425–434.

Valverde, F. (1968). Structural changes in the area striata of the mouse after enucleation. *Experimental Brain Research, 5,* 274–292.

Van de Water, T.R., Li, C.W., Ruben, R.J., & Shea, C.A. (1980a). Ontogenetic aspects of mammalian inner ear development. In R.J. Gorlin (Ed.), *Morphogenesis and malformation of the ear* (pp. 5–45). New York: Liss.

Van de Water, T.R., Maderson, P.F.A., & Jaskoll, T.F. (1980b). The morphogenesis of the middle and external ear. In R.J. Gorlin (Ed.), *Morphogenesis and malformation of the ear* (pp. 147–180). New York: Liss.

Van de Water, T.R., & Ruben, R.J. (1976). Organogenesis of the ear. In R. Hinchcliffe & D. Harrison (Eds.), *Scientific foundation of otolaryngology* (pp. 173–184). London: Heineman.

Vince, M.A., Armitage, S.E., Baldwin, B.A., Toner, J., & Moore, B.C.J. (1982). The sound environment of the foetal sheep. *Behaviour, 81,* 296–315.

Wada, T. (1923). Anatomical and physiological studies on the growth of the inner ear of the albino rat. *American Anatomical Memoranda, 10,* 1–74.

Walker, D., Grimwade, J., & Wood, C. (1971). Intrauterine noise: A component of the fetal environment. *American Journal of Obstetrics and Gynecology, 109,* 91–95.

Webster, D.B., Webster, M. (1977). Neonatal sound deprivation affects brainstem auditory nuclei. *Archives of Otolaryngology, 103,* 392–396.

Webster, D.B., & Webster, M. (1978). Long-term effects of cochlear nerve destruction on the cochlear nuclei (Abstract). *Anatomical Record, 190,* 578–579.

Webster, D.B., & Webster, M. (1979). Effects of neonatal conductive hearing loss on brainstem auditory nuclei. *Annals of Otology, Rhinology and Laryngology, 88,* 684–688.

Webster, D.B., & Webster, M. (1980). Mouse brainstem auditory nuclei development. *Annals of Otology, Rhinology and Laryngology, 89* (Suppl. 68), 254–256.

Willott, J.F. (1983). *Auditory psychobiology of the mouse.* Springfield, IL: Thomas.

Wong-Riley, M.T.T., Merzenich, M.M., & Leake, P.A. (1978). Changes in endogenous enzymatic reactivity to DAB inducted by neuronal inactivity. *Brain Research, 141,* 185–192.

Wong-Riley, M., & Riley, D.A. (1983). The effect of impulse blockage on cytochrome oxidase activity in the cat visual system. *Brain Research, 261,* 185–193.

Wong-Riley, M.T.T.., & Welt, C. (1980). Histochemical changes in cytochrome oxidase of cortical barrels after vibrissal removal in neonatal and adult mice. *Proceedings of the National Academy of Science. 77,* 2333–2337.

Woolf, N.K., & Ryan, A.F. (in press). Functional ontogeny of neural discharge patterns in the ventral cochlear nucleus of the mongolian gerbil. *Experimental Brain Research.*

Woolsey, T.A., & Wann, J.R. (1976). Areal changes in mouse cortical barrels following vibrissal damage at different postnatal ages. *Journal of Comparative Neurology, 170,* 53–66.

Woolsey, C.N., & Walzl, E.M. (1942). Topical projection of nerve fibers from local regions of the cochlea in the cerebral cortex of the cat. *Bulletin of Johns Hopkins Hospital, 71,* 315–344.

Yntema, C.L. (1950). An analysis of induction of the ear from foreign ectoderm in the salamander embryo. *Journal of Experimental Zoology, 113,* 211–244.

Young, S.R., & Rubel, E.W (1983). Frequency-specific projections of individual neurons in chick brain stem auditory nuclei. *Journal of Neuroscience, 3,* 1373–1378.

Chapter 4

Neurotransmitters of the Cochlea and Lateral Line Organ[1]

Richard P. Bobbin
Sanford C. Bledsoe, Jr.[2]
Gary L. Jenison

INTRODUCTION

This chapter outlines some of the recent developments in the biochemistry and pharmacology of the mammalian cochlea and the amphibian lateral line organ. By convention these sensory structures have been categorized among acousticolateralis systems, or what some prefer to call octavolateralis systems. We restrict our focus to the processes of neurotransmission which intimately involve the hair cells in these systems. In particular, we review currently relevant information available on the identity of the afferent neurotransmitters produced by the hair cells of both the cochlea and the lateral line and the efferent neurotransmitters produced by the terminals of olivocochlear bundle fibers and those of lateral line efferents.

In general, a great deal of the evidence available on the peripheral efferent transmitters of acousticolateralis systems indicates that they are cholinergic (see reviews by Guth, Norris, & Bobbin, 1976; Guth, Sewell, & Tachibana, 1981; Klinke, 1981). Primary afferent nerve fibers of these sensory organs, on the other hand, are typically responsive to a variety of amino acid analogs. This is not to say that the identities of the endogenous ligands have been determined conclusively. On the contrary, a number of the criteria established for such identification still need to be met in all cases. Our discussion begins with a subjective review of those criteria. We then review the data which has been forwarded in support of the candidacy of various substances

[1]Kresge Hearing Research Laboratory of the South Department of Otorhinolaryngology and Biocommunication, Louisiana State University Medical Center, 1100 Florida Avenue, Building 124, New Orleans, Louisiana, 70119. Thanks to Madeline Bobbin and Cindy Frazier for their aid in the preparation of this manuscript. Research was supported by NIH Grants NS-11647, NS-07058, and NS-16080. Laboratory facilities were provided in part through grants from the Kresge Foundation and the Louisiana Lions Eye Foundation.

[2]Kresge Hearing Research Institute, University of Michigan Medical School, Ann Arbor, Michigan, 48109.

as either afferent or efferent neurotransmitters. Bear in mind that the resolution of the vast majority of physiological techniques that have provided these data is not high enough to distinguish outer from inner hair cell mechanisms in the cochlea nor between those of differently oriented hair cells in the lateral line organ. Therefore, we have refrained from addressing any distinctions which potentially exist either between the transmitters such subpopulations produce or between those to which they are responsive.

NEUROTRANSMITTER CRITERIA

Several criteria have been established by convention which must be satisfied in order to verify that a chemical is actually the endogenous neurotransmitter acting at any particular synapse (see discussions by McLennan, 1963; Siegel, Albers, Agranoff, & Katzman, 1981; Werman, 1966). Among these are the following:

1. Identical action: The chemical in question (the candidate), when applied to the synapse, should elicit a postsynaptic response which mimics the response normally elicited by natural stimulation of the presynaptic element.

2. Pharmacological identity: Other substances that influence the natural postsynaptic response when applied to the synapse should also have the same influence on the postsynaptic response elicited by the candidate.

3. Presynaptic location: The candidate must be documented to exist in the presynaptic terminal under normal physiological conditions.

4. Synthetic enzymes: Enzymes responsible for the biosynthesis of the candidate must be present in the presynaptic element of the synapse.

5. Stimulus-induced release: Stimulation of the presynaptic element should result in the release of the candidate and this release should be calcium dependent.

6. Inactivation mechanism: A mechanism must be demonstrated which can either remove the candidate from the synaptic cleft or inactivate its physiological influence on the postsynaptic element.

The logic behind the development of these criteria is based on an ability to monitor the unique functional characteristics of the endogenous transmitter in an unperturbed environment. In those few cases where all of the criteria have been met, nondestructive techniques for gaining access to the synapse in question have been available, as well as the technology to monitor the electrical events occurring across both the pre- and postsynaptic membranes. The pharmacological agents necessary to probe the relevant enzyme systems or transmitter receptors have also been available. In addition, those transmitters which have been positively identified have generally been those substances which are relatively localized to the synaptic sites under investigation. The same has been true of the enzyme systems involved in their synthesis and inactivation. Unfortunately, all of these have not been available to a very large proportion of the investigations intended to identify the transmitters of various synapses. In such cases, the candidacy of a putative transmitter may be supportable on the basis of one or two criteria, but the remaining criteria cannot be satisfied for the lack of adequate technology or specific biochemical probes. This has led to an opinion that some of these criteria are too stringent and need to be modified to take into account less direct evidence. Nevertheless, the criteria outlined do serve as a useful framework for a discussion of the relative merits of different transmitter candidates of acousticolateralis systems.

THE CANDIDATES

To date, most researchers have followed the idea described by Werman (1966) that "At some point a guess as to the nature of the transmitter must be made and the criteria can then be used to challenge the guess." Many chemical "guesses" have been made which can be evaluated in terms of the criteria just discussed. The prominent guesses which have been forwarded regarding the afferent and efferent synapses of acousticolateralis systems include acetylcholine, γ-aminobutyrate (GABA), the excitatory amino acids (glutamate and aspartate), methionine-enkephalin, and two as yet unidentified ligands termed "a GABA-like substance" and "the auditory nerve activating substance" (ANAS).

Acetylcholine as the Afferent Transmitter of the Cochlea

Vinnikov (1974) originally proposed that the afferent transmitter of the cochlea is acetylcholine (ACh). On the contrary, most investigators contend that the evidence supporting the candidacy of ACh as the afferent transmitter is very weak and have discounted the possibility as remote (see discussion by Guth et al., 1976).

Acetylcholine as the Efferent Transmitter of the Cochlea

The most persuasive evidence supporting an efferent role for ACh is the fact that atropine, D-tubocurarine, other anticholinergic agents, and α-bungarotoxin block the effects of efferent stimulation when applied intracochlearly, but do not affect any of the potentials associated with afferent transmission (Bobbin & Konishi, 1974; Fex, 1968a; Fex & Adams, 1978; Konishi, 1972). On the other hand, some of these agents have the potential of acting nonspecifically and, consequently, influencing ion-gating mechanisms of membranes directly (Ascher, Lowy, & Rang, 1979). Another complication in the issue of this candidacy is the observation that the physiological effects of evoking efferent nerve activity can be blocked by strychnine, a glycine antagonist (as discussed by Desmedt, 1975, and Fex, 1974). One mechanism which has been forwarded to explain this action of strychnine is that it inhibits the release of ACh from efferent terminals (Guth et al., 1976).

One of the two enzymes prominently involved in the regulation of ACh is acetyl-cholinesterase. This enzyme inactivates ACh by cleaving it into acetate and choline before it can diffuse beyond the confines of the synaptic cleft. Churchill, Schuknecht, & Doran (1956) and Schuknecht, Churchill, & Doran (1959) demonstrated that when the efferents of the olivocochlear bundle are sectioned and allowed to degenerate, cholinesterase activity declines to an undetectable level. This localization of cholin-esterase exclusively to efferent terminals indicated that the enzymatic inactivation of ACh takes place presynaptically rather than postsynaptically on the surface of the hair cells or the afferent terminals. Potentiation of cochlear efferents has also been demonstrated by the use of anticholinesterases (Klinke, 1981), demonstrating that this enzyme is involved in terminating the action of the efferent transmitter.

Choline acetyltransferase is a synthetic enzyme for ACh which has also been found to be associated solely with olivocochlear nerve endings. Jasser and Guth (1973) demonstrated that choline acetyltransferase activity in the cochlea falls below detect-able levels after the olivocochlear bundle has been sectioned and allowed to degen-erate. Thus the remaining cochlear structures, including the hair cells, appear incapable of synthesizing ACh. This assertion has been confirmed and extended by Fex, Altschuler, Parakkal, & Eckenstein (1982a), who have localized choline acetyl-transferase to the efferent terminals under both inner and outer hair cells using an immunofluorescence technique. Since synthesis of acetylcholine is generally thought to occur only in the neurons which use it as a transmitter, these findings imply that only the efferent fibers of the cochlea use acetylcholine as a transmitter.

Another approach which has been taken regarding the candidacy of ACh as the efferent transmitter is the analysis of perilymph constituents under various stimulus conditions. Both Fex (1968b) and Norris and Guth (1974) have reported the detection of ACh-like activity within perilymph after electrical stimulation of the efferent system. In addition, Norris and Guth (1974) have shown that this ACh-like activity is not altered by exposing the cochlea to sound. It remains to be determined, however, whether or not this change in ACh-like activity is calcium dependent. Nevertheless, these results are entirely consistent with the premise that ACh is released by the efferent terminals.

The "identical activity" criterion for ACh as the efferent transmitter has also been approached by examining its influence on evoked afferent activity. Intracochlear perfusions of ACh in combination with eserine (an acetylcholinesterase inhibitor) produce an increase in the amplitude of the cochlear microphonic (CM) evoked by low frequencies and a concurrent reduction in the amplitude of the auditory nerve compound action potential (AP) (Bobbin & Konishi, 1971). Both of these effects mimic the influence of efferent stimulation and both are blocked by curare (Bobbin & Konishi, 1974). Robertson and Johnstone (1978) and Comis and Leng (1979) have each demon-strated that the decrease in AP reflects the suppression of the firing rates of afferent fibers. One interesting element of these studies was that the effects of efferent stimulation on afferent activity were not sustained but progressively diminished with longer periods of stimulation (Konishi & Slepian, 1971). This presumably reflects either a gradual depletion of transmitter or a desensitization of the efferent neurotransmitter receptor. The receptor desensitization hypothesis has been supported on the basis of the lack of a sustained effect on AP and CM during the continuous perfusion of ACh (Bobbin & Konishi, 1971). Both Robertson and Johnstone (1978) and Comis and Leng (1979), on the other hand, have reported that such a chronic suppressive influence of ACh does exist at the level of individual afferent fibers, implying that the depletion theory cannot be discounted. Thus the question of whether or not the temporal characteristics of ACh-induced alterations in afferent activity are identical to those induced by efferent stimulation remains unresolved.

Acetylcholine as the Afferent Transmitter of the Lateral Line Organ

We are not aware of any evidence directly supporting the candidacy of ACh as the afferent transmitter of the lateral line.

Acetylcholine as the Efferent Transmitter of the Lateral Line Organ

Russell first suggested that the transmitter of the efferent innervation of the *Xenopus laevis* lateral line organ is acetylcholine. He showed that tetanic stimulation of these fibers suppressed spontaneous firing of the afferent units (Russell, 1968, 1971). This effect was related to synaptic transmission by the demonstration of its dependence on extracellular calcium. Efferent fiber-evoked suppression of afferent activity did not take place when preparations were exposed to high extracellular concentrations of magnesium, a competitive antagonist of the calcium necesssary for transmitter release (Russell, 1971). Russell (1968, 1971) also pointed out that curare and atropine both antagonize the effects of efferent stimulation. Cholinesterase activity has also been documented in the lateral line organ, as has the potentiation of efferent stimulation with the anticholinesterase, physostigmine (Russell, 1971). Finally, suppression of spontaneous afferent activity has been achieved with the application of both ACh and ACh-like compounds, and this drug-induced suppression has also been shown to be counteracted by prior treatment with curare or atropine (Russell, 1971). In summary, persuasive evidence has been collected in support of the candidacy of ACh as the efferent transmitter of the lateral line organ on the basis of its identical action, pharmacological identity, and the presence of inactivating enzymes.

One interesting characteristic of the lateral line's response to ACh has surfaced, during our studies involving concurrent application of ACh and other compounds, which tends to complicate a simple concept of efferent transmission. We have discovered that a transient increase in afferent activity occurs prior to the sustained suppression produced by ACh in combination with the anticholinesterase, eserine.

The same biphasic effect is seen when carbachol, a cholinergic agonist resistant to degradation by acetylcholinesterase, is applied by itself. In addition, the transient increase in activity can be detected as a result of concentrations of carbachol lower than those necessary to evoke suppression of spontaneous activity. This transient increase in afferent activity was not reported by Russell as such, although modest increases in unit activity are reflected in some of his data (see Russell, 1971; Figure 1). We have found that the excitatory period induced by carbachol is more apparent in some preparations than in others. In addition, we have found that the entire excitation–inhibition effect induced by carbachol or ACh–eserine can be blocked by atropine without any apparent effect on spontaneous activity (Winbery & Bobbin, 1983), on activity evoked by natural stimulation (Bobbin et al., 1983), or on either the excitation induced by glutamate or the inhibition induced by GABA (Bobbin, Bledsoe, Jenison, Winbery, & Caesar, 1983).

The above observations do not lend themselves to any immediate interpretation of which discrete mechanisms are being regulated by ACh receptors. We do not believe, however, that they can be accounted for by assuming that ACh is an excitatory efferent neurotransmitter with suppression being simply the result of an overstimulation of its postsynaptic target. What seems more likely is that exogenously applied ACh may be acting on more than one receptor, engaging inhibitory mechanisms in one case while potentially initiating excitatory mechanisms in another. Another possibility under consideration is that one of those two mechanisms is under the regulation of an intermediate, which is dependent on the presence of ACh. For example, Fex and Altschuler (1981) have demonstrated the presence of a substance with enkephalin-like immunoreactivity within efferent fibers of the cochlea which presumably coexists with ACh. Though speculative, the same condition may also exist in the lateral line. If so, the activation of ACh receptors may involve both the initiation of mechanisms responsible for the initial transient excitation of afferent activity and the release of an enkephalin, which could in turn regulate the mechanisms responsible for the suppression which follows.

γ-Aminobutyrate as the Afferent Transmitter of the Cochlea

The first suggestion that GABA might be the primary afferent transmitter came from the work of Flock and Lam (1974) who demonstrated the synthesis of GABA from glutamate in several hair cell preparations. These investigators did not, however, include the cochlea in their studies. Tachibana and Kuriyama (1974), on the other hand, were unable to detect the presence of GABA in either inner or outer hair cells of the guinea pig cochlea. Fex and Wenthold (1976) found that, while the synthesis of GABA from glutamate could be detected in the cochlea, this synthesis was of a slow rate. Glutamic acid decarboxylase synthesizes GABA from glutamate. Furthermore, Desmedt and Monaco (1962) and Bobbin and Guth (1970) have shown that thiosemicarbazide, an inhibitor of glutamic acid decarboxylase, has no influence on the compound action potential of the auditory nerve (AP). More recently, Fex and colleagues (1982b) have demonstrated the presence of aspartate aminotransferase (AAT), which degrades GABA, in the spiral ganglion cells and the efferent nerve fibers associated with outer hair cells of the cochlea, but not within the hair cells. Bobbin and Guth (1970) and Bobbin and Gondra (1973) have reported, however, that amino-oxyacetic acid (AOAA), an inhibitor of aspartate aminotransferase, reduces AP but also concurrently reduces CM and the endocochlear potential (EP) generated by the stria vascularis. This last observation does not refute the existence of AAT but introduces the question of whether AAT is restricted to the innervation of the cochlea.

GABA applied both iontophoretically (Tanaka & Katsuki, 1966) and intracochlearly (Bobbin & Guth, 1970; Bobbin & Thompson, 1978; Klinke & Oertel, 1977b) exerts no detectable effect on cochlear potentials. Baclofen, a GABA receptor agonist[3] considered by some to be specific for one class of presynaptic GABA receptors, also apparently has no influence on cochlear potentials (Martin, 1982). Several laboratories (Bobbin & Guth, 1970; Desmedt & Monaco, 1961, 1962; Klinke & Oertel, 1977b) have found that picrotoxin, a GABA antagonist, does not alter guinea pig afferent cochlear potentials. However, bicuculline methiodide, another GABA antagonist, has been found to suppress the guinea pig AP but only at unusually high concentrations (Bobbin & Thompson, 1978; Klinke & Oertel, 1977b). The above observations do not lend themselves to a strong argument in support of GABA as an afferent transmitter.

Studies designed to satisfy the "release" criterion suggest that the candidacy of GABA cannot be ruled out entirely. Initial investigations into the potential for sound-induced release of afferent transmitter did not reveal a significant change in the concentration of GABA within the guinea pig cochlea (Melamed, Norris, Bryant, & Guth, 1982). More recently, Drescher, Drescher, and Medina (1983) demonstrated the presence of a GABA-like compound in guinea pig perilymph and, furthermore, showed that this compound increases in concentration during exposure to noise. The term "GABA-like" was used because the chromatographic analysis of this substance is indistinguishable from that of GABA. Using slightly different chromatographic techniques, we have also detected a primary amine within guinea pig perilymph that we have tentatively identified as taurine, though it frequently cannot be distinguished from GABA. The concentration of this amino acid, among others, increases as a result of perfusing the cochlea with artificial perilymph containing high concentrations of potassium salts (Jenison & Bobbin, 1983b), and the elevation is reduced by low calcium–high magnesium. Though the results of the last two studies are comparable, important methodological differences in the studies producing them must be considered before any conclusions can be made. In our study the cochlear aqueduct was blocked prior to sampling perilymph in order to ensure that all constituents originated from the cochlea rather than from inflowing cerebrospinal fluid. The study by Drescher and colleagues (1983), however, did not include an aqueduct blockade. On the other hand, the high-potassium stimulus we employed may have caused some cytolysis in addition to depolarizing hair cells and inducing the release of their transmitter. This criticism may not apply to the study by Drescher and colleagues if the noise level employed was not excessive. Beyond this, the calcium dependence of

---

[3]A substance which activates a receptor.

stimulus-induced changes in the concentration of the GABA-like substance reported by Drescher and co-workers has yet to be demonstrated. In the case of both studies, however, the origin of these GABA-like substances has not been conclusively determined; yet, both indicate that GABA or a GABA-like substance such as taurine may serve some physiologic role in the cochlea.

γ-Aminobutyrate as the Efferent Transmitter of the Cochlea

The GABA antagonists, picrotoxin and bicuculline, both reduce the influence of efferent stimulation on the cochlea (Klinke & Oertel, 1977b) and GABA uptake has been localized predominantly among the terminals of efferent fibers (Gulley, Fex, & Wenthold, 1979; Schwartz & Ryan, 1983). Aminooxyacetic acid (AOAA) does have rather complex effects on efferent stimulation (Bobbin et al., 1981b), and aspartate aminotransferase, the enzyme that AOAA inhibits, has been demonstrated to exist in efferent nerve fibers associated with the outer hair cells (Fex et al., 1982b). On the other hand, thiosemicarbazide, a glutamic acid decarboxylase inhibitor, does not reduce the effects of efferent stimulation on the evoked activity of the cochlea (Bobbin & Guth, 1970; Desmedt & Monaco, 1962), and, as previously discussed, GABA does not produce any significant alterations in AP or CM when applied intracochlearly except at unusually high concentrations. In addition, stimulus-dependent changes in the concentration of GABA-like substances discussed above (Drescher et al., 1983; Jenison & Bobbin, 1983b) suggest a potential involvement of GABA in synaptic mechanisms, but the methods described do not allow a delineation of which synapses, if any, are involved. In short, evidence does exist which suggests a role for GABA in the efferent system of the cochlea, although the majority of this evidence does not persuasively support its candidacy as the efferent transmitter per se.

γ-Aminobutyrate as the Afferent Transmitter of the Lateral Line Organ

We are unaware of any evidence directly supporting the candidacy of GABA as the afferent transmitter of this sensory system.

γ-Aminobutyrate as the Efferent Transmitter of the Lateral Line Organ

We have discovered GABA to be very potent in suppressing spontaneous activity in the lateral line organ of *Xenopus laevis* (Bledsoe, Chihal, Bobbin, & Morgan, 1983; Chihal, Bledsoe, Bobbin, & Morgan, 1980). This observation is in disagreement with the finding reported by Russell (1976) that GABA did not influence this sensory system. It also illustrates another of the physiological distinctions between the lateral line organ and the mammalian cochlea which, as discussed above, is not responsive to GABA. Preliminary results from our laboratories indicate that bicuculline, a GABA antagonist, does block the inhibition induced by GABA, but does not affect either the activity evoked by natural stimulation or the increase in spontaneous activity induced by L-glutamate or carbachol (Bobbin et al., 1983). Also, baclofen, a GABA agonist effective on some GABA receptors, failed to alter either spontaneous activity or the activity evoked by natural stimulation. These data indicate that GABA acts on receptors separate from those activated by L-glutamate, carbachol, or the endogenous afferent transmitter. Furthermore, it appears that the receptors sensitive to GABA are of a subclass termed GABA-A receptors, in which baclofen is inactive and bicuculline blocks GABA, rather than of the subclass termed GABA-B receptors, which are characteristically insensitive to bicuculline but are sensitive to baclofen (Bowery, Hill, & Hudson, 1983). Our observations do, therefore, support the likelihood that GABA plays some role in efferent transmission. In consideration of the strong support which currently exists for the candidacy of acetylcholine as the efferent transmitter, we suspect that GABA's role is adjunct to that of acetylcholine, possibly as a cotransmitter (Bledsoe et al., 1983). This does not preclude, however, the possibility that GABA is also involved in transmission mechanisms of the lateral line's innervation which are synaptically independent of efferent transmission (Bledsoe et al., 1983).

Excitatory Amino Acids as the Afferent Transmitter of the Cochlea

Support for the candidacy of excitatory amino acids as the afferent transmitter initially stemmed from screening studies intended to determine the relative influence of various putative neurotransmitters on the AP (Bobbin & Thompson, 1978; Klinke & Oertel, 1977a). Of the amino acids introduced into the scala tympani in these studies (including GABA, L-alanine, β-alanine, taurine, and glycine), L-glutamate and L-aspartate were found to most significantly reduce AP without influencing CM. The explanation forwarded to account for the reductions induced by L-glutamate and L-aspartate was that these excitatory amino acids were not inhibitory, but that they were excitatory and increased the discharge rate of afferent units. Both Bobbin (1979) and Comis and Leng (1979) later confirmed this explanation by demonstrating that L-glutamate and L-aspartate both increase the activity of individual afferent fibers and, furthermore, that as a result of this increase, consequent sound-evoked increases in discharge rates were smaller than normal.

Differences in the relative sensitivity of various central nervous system synaptic preparations to a number of more currently available amino acid agonists and antagonists has led to a tentative classification of amino acid receptors on the basis of their preferential susceptibility to one of three agonists: N-methyl-D-aspartate (NMDA), quisqualate, or kainate (McLennan & Lodge, 1979; Watkins, 1978, 1981; Watkins & Evans, 1981). We have found that kainate introduced into the perilymph of the guinea pig cochlea causes both a reduction in the amplitude of AP and an excitation of auditory single units without affecting CM (Bledsoe et al., 1981b). Quisqualate produces comparable effects on AP and CM, but NMDA has virtually no effect on either potential (Jenison & Bobbin, 1983a). On the basis of AP, we have calculated that quisqualate is approximately two orders of magnitude more potent than L-glutamate and approximately fourfold more potent than kainate, but that both NMDA and D-glutamate (another amino acid agonist with a specificity comparable to NMDA) are nearly one order of magnitude less potent than L-glutamate (Jenison & Bobbin, 1983a). These observations argue against the presence of NMDA-preferring receptors and for the presence of quisqualate- and/or kainate-preferring receptors.

Several compounds have been shown to antagonize the activation of amino acid receptors in various vertebrate central nervous system preparations (Biscoe, Evans, Francis, Martin, & Watkins, 1977; Davies, Evans, Francis, & Watkins, 1979a, 1979b; Evans, Francis, Hunt, Oakes, & Watkins, 1979; Martin & Adams, 1979); however, only two studies to date have examined the effects of any of these substances in the cochlea. Fex and Martin (1980) have demonstrated that D-, L-α-aminoadipate has no effect on the AP or CM of the cat. We have found that ($\pm$)-2-amino-5-phosphono-valerate, D-α-aminoadipate, γ-D-glutamylglycine, L($+$)-2-amino-4-phosphono-butyrate, and D-α-aminosuberate were essentially inactive (Bobbin et al., 1981a). cis-2,3-Piperidine dicarboxylate (PDA) caused a moderate reduction in AP (33%) but had no effect on the CM. In addition, glutamate diethyl ester (GDEE) abolished the AP (86%) and caused a reduction in CM (60%) and EP (15%). PDA and GDEE have been proposed to block quisqualate and glutamate receptors more readily than NMDA receptors, and the inactive antagonists to act preferentially on NMDA receptors. These observations concur with those of Fex and Martin (1980) and support their original conclusion that an NMDA-preferring receptor is not involved in hair cell auditory nerve transmission. These data also support our current hypothesis that afferent neurotransmission may involve the activation of quisqualate-preferring receptors.

Several attempts have been made to examine the candidacy of various amino acids as the afferent transmitter on the basis of the stimulus-induced release criterion by demonstrating an increase in the concentration of such candidates in perilymph. Sewell, Norris, Tachibana, and Guth (1978) reported preliminary evidence that the concentrations of glutamate and aspartate in natural perilymph did not change in response to stimulation with sound and concluded that these data were inconsistent with the hypothesis that the afferent transmitter was either of these two amino acids. Medina and Drescher (1981) measured the concentrations of 14 amino acids and ammonia in natural perilymph but reported no significant difference between the constituents of fluids taken from guinea pigs maintained in silence and those retrieved after exposure to noise. The constituents examined included the presumptive amino acid neurotransmitters taurine, aspartate, glutamate, and glycine. Melamed, Norris, Bryant, and Guth (1982) perfused the cochlea with artificial perilymph and measured the concentrations of glutamate, aspartate, and nine other amino acids including GABA (which Medina and Drescher did not measure) and reported that exposure to sound did not produce any alteration in amino acid concentrations. Bledsoe and colleagues (1981a) reported preliminary results of an increase in the concentration of glutamate in the artificial perilmyph used to perfuse cochleae during periods of exposure to sound. Drescher and co-workers (1983), measuring up to 81 different primary amines in natural perilymph under conditions of sound and silence, reported increases in a GABA-like component, aspartate, methionine-enkephalin, and two unknown derivatives labeled "A" and "B". They concluded that the GABA-like substance may mediate excitatory receptoneuronal transmission since its concentration was the most highly correlated with the different levels of noise used, and that aspartate may have been conveyed from the cochlear nucleus by the influx of cerebrospinal fluid through the patent cochlear aqueduct. Finally, in an extension of our priliminary studies (Jenison & Bobbin, 1983b) we have chromatographically detected two primary amines which were significantly elevated as a result of perfusing cochleae with artificial perilymph containing high concentrations of potassium salts (HIGH K+) with the elevation being reduced by low calcium–high magnesium. We have tentatively identified these primary amines as glutamate and taurine.

We have no a priori basis upon which to predict which, if any, of the methodological differences which distinguish these studies might produce differences in the detection of any of the substances mentioned above. Perfusion techniques are known to enhance amino acid release in central nervous system preparations (Collins, Anson, & Probett, 1981; Cotman & Hamberger, 1978; Cox & Bradford, 1978) and are likely to reduce background values. Also, occlusion of the cochlear aqueduct must also stand out as a stabilizing influence as it prevents large quantities of cerebrospinal fluid from entering the sampling site and, consequently, eliminates one potential source of contamination (Carlborg, Densert, & Densert, 1982). Additional methodological differences include the stimulus used to evoke release. We (Jenison & Bobbin, 1983b) have used HIGH K+ which, in addition to depolarizing more than hair cells, probably induces some cellular edema and potentially some cytolysis which might result in the production of holes into the scala media (Bohne, 1976). Thus the glutamate shown to be in scala media endolymph (Thalmann, Comegys, & DeMott, 1981; Thalmann, Comegys, & Thalmann, 1982) could be another source of contamination. However, the calcium dependency, coupled with the fact that values derived from the final control perfusion following the perfusion of HIGH K+ approximate those derived from control perfusions conducted at the beginnings of these experiments, suggests that the concentration increases are not due to holes in the reticular lamina or some other irreversible event. It is again important to point out that few of these studies have yet to satisfy the calcium-dependence requirements of the stimulus-induced release criterion.

Glutamate and aspartate have been shown to be present in the organ of Corti (Godfrey, Carter, Sosamma, & Matschinsky, 1976; Thalmann, 1975). Ryan and Schwartz (1984) found a preferential uptake of glutamine by cochlear hair cells. Eybalin, Calas, and Pujol (1981) and Eybalin and Pujol (1983) studied the transport of radioactive L-glutamine and L-glutamate in the cochlea and observed both an uptake of glutamine into inner hair cells and an uptake of glutamate into glial cells. They concluded that these data suggested a metabolic link between glutamine and glutamate which is consistent with the premise that glutamate is the neurotransmitter produced by inner hair cells. These data, taken with those discussed earlier in this section, do lend weight to the candidacy of a limited number of amino acids as auditory neurotransmitters and indicate that glutamate and aspartate must be considered.

Excitatory Amino Acids as the Efferent Transmitter of the Cochlea

The only study of which we are aware which directly addresses the influence of excitatory amino acid analogs on the efferent system is one by Bledsoe and colleagues (1981b), who reported that intracochlear perfusion of kainate has no effect on the slow potentials evoked by efferent stimulation (COCP). Drescher and co-workers (1983) acknowledge the possibility that any one of the elevated primary amines they reported could actually originate from efferent terminals. This same consideration must also apply, possibly to a greater extent, to the amino acids discussed by Jenison and Bobbin (1983b).

Excitatory Amino Acids as the Afferent Transmitter of the Lateral Line Organ

Glutamate and aspartate were among the first substances shown to induce an increase in the firing rate of afferent fibers of the lateral line organ of *Xenopus laevis* (Bledsoe et al., 1983; Bobbin et al., 1981c; Bobbin & Morgan, 1980; Katsuki, 1973; Russell, 1976; Zimmerman, 1979). These responses are not sustained and, in this respect, are different from those which glutamate and aspartate have been reported to induce in other neuronal systems. Rather, they include a rapid trailing suppression of spontaneous activity suggestive of a depolarization blockade. Recently, though, such biphasic responses have been reported to occur in central nervous system preparations (Martin & Adams, 1979; Peet, Malik, & Curtis, 1983). Bledsoe and colleagues (1983) have demonstrated that the responses of the lateral line to quisqualate and kainate are similar to the responses these agonists induce in the cochlea. Unlike the cochlea, however, the lateral line is quite responsive to NMDA, indicating that one distinction between the two acousticolateralis organs is that the amino acid receptors within the lateral line organ include those of the NMDA-preferring subtype. One other distinction between the two acousticolateralis systems that Bledsoe and colleagues (1983) discovered was that the lateral line afferents respond equally well to both the D- and L-isomers of glutamate. As previously discussed, D-glutamate is thought to be specific for the NMDA-subtype of amino acid receptors. These investigators also found lateral line afferents to be responsive to homocysteate. L-Homocysteate, a glutamate analog with sulfonyl substitutions of the carbonyl groups, was determined to be approximately one order of magnitude more potent than either L-glutamate or D-homocysteate.

Support for the classification of the afferent transmitter receptor as NMDA preferring stems from antagonist studies employing D-α-aminoadipate (DAA). Bledsoe and Bobbin (1982a, b) found that DAA reversibly antagonizes the elevation of afferent unit activity of the *Xenopus laevis* lateral line organ induced by NMDA and by natural stimulus of fluid motion. The magnitude of the antagonism by DAA is dose dependent. DAA was also found to antagonize the excitation induced by L-glutamate and L-aspartate; however, the potency of DAA in this regard was found to be less than that related to NMDA antagonism. In contrast to these effects, DAA had no influence on the excitation induced by kainate. Since the concentrations of DAA necessary to block stimulus-evoked afferent activity was also effective in blocking the response to NMDA, it appears that all of these substances, NMDA, DAA, and the endogenous neurotransmitter, act on the same receptors. Furthermore, the fact that kainate-induced excitation was not blocked by DAA suggests that kainate acts on a separate class of endogenous receptors and that the receptor for the endogenous ligand is probably more appropriately classified as NMDA preferring than kainate preferring.

The candidacy of excitatory amino acids as neurotransmitters of the afferent system based on the stimulus-induced criterion has been directly addressed, to our knowledge, by only one study. Bledsoe, Bobbin, Thalmann, and Thalmann (1980) examined the release of aspartate, glutamate, and glycine from skin preparations of *Xenopus laevis*. Enzymatic assays specific for these amino acids were conducted on samples of Ringer solution which had bathed the serosal surfaces of these preparations after subjecting the outer (cupular) surfaces to pulsating water. Values derived from preparations containing lateral line organs (stitch skins) were compared to those derived from preparations without lateral line organs (nonstitch skins). No stimulus-dependent differences in glycine were noted, but samples from stitch skins were found to contain significantly higher concentrations of both glutamate and aspartate than samples taken from nonstitch skins. Samples taken after subsequent stimulation of stitch skins also contained comparable amounts of glutamate, but the amount of aspartate decreased. The reason for the temporal differences in the release of glutamate and aspartate is not yet clear; however, the fact that the stimulus-induced release of both excitatory amino acids and not glycine was correlated with the presence of lateral line organs suggests a role for these amino acids in afferent transmission. Legitimate candidacy on the basis of release, however, must again await the demonstration of a calcium dependence.

Excitatory Amino Acids as the Efferent Neurotransmitter of the Lateral Line Organ

We are not aware of any evidence supporting the candidacy of any excitatory amino acid as the efferent neurotransmitter of the lateral line organ.

Monoamines as Transmitter Candidates of Acousticolateralis Systems

Monoamines do not occur in the organ of Corti, but appear to be restricted to structures in the modiolar, habenular, and lateral wall regions of the cochlea (Eybalin et al., 1983; Rarey, Ross, & Smith, 1981). Rarey and colleagues (1981, 1982) identified norepinephrine in these structures using high performance liquid chromatography (HPLC) and electrochemical detection but did not detect epinephrine, dopamine, or serotonin. Furthermore, epinephrine, norepinephrine, octopamine, dopamine, histamine, and serotonin applied intracochlearly produced no effect on cochlear potentials (Bobbin & Thompson, 1978; Comis & Leng, 1979; Klinke & Evans, 1977; Klinke & Oertel, 1977c; Tanaka & Katsuki, 1966). The reduction in AP demonstrated in response to phenotolamine, an antagonist of epinephrine at alpha adrenergic receptors, and to methysergide, a serotonin antagonist, have been attributed to an effect on the stria vascularis since CM and EP are also reduced (Bobbin & Thompson, 1978; Klinke & Evans, 1977; Thalmann, 1975). On the other hand, it remains to be demonstrated whether or not the response of AP to antagonists targeted for beta adrenergic receptors is due to a direct action on the nerve fibers (Wiederhold, 1980; Wiederhold & Savaki, 1979).

Osborne and Thornhill (1972) and Monaghan (1975) presented data which indicated that synaptic bars of lateral line hair cells are electron dense and behave pharmacologically like catecholamine-bearing synaptic vesicles in that they may be rendered electron lucent by the catecholamine-depleting drugs, reserpine and guanethidine. On the other hand, epinephrine, norepinephrine, 6-hydroxydopamine, and dopamine have been shown not to influence the spontaneous activity of lateral line afferents, and the excitatory effects produced by dopa and 6-hydroxydopa can be attributed to their acting on glutamate receptors (Bledsoe et al., 1983; Chihal et al., 1980). Thus, the possibility that any of these monoamines act as neurotransmitters in these two acousticolateralis systems must be considered very remote at this time.

Prostaglandins as Transmitter Candidates in the Cochlea

Bobbin and Thompson (1978) reported a reduction in the AP with the prostaglandins PGF2 and PGE2. In addition, salicylates cause a reduction in the AP but not the CM in guinea pigs (Bobbin & Thompson, 1978; Thalmann, 1975). Salicylates have been shown to inhibit prostaglandin synthesis. Thus, one explanation for the influence of salicylates on AP might be that they block prostaglandin synthesis in the cochlea. By themselves, however, the effects of PGF2 and PGE2 on AP do not adequately support the candidacy of prostaglandins as transmitter candidates in the cochlea.

Polypeptides as Neurotransmitter Candidates in the Cochlea

Lim, Mogi, O'Dorisio, & Cataland (1981) demonstrated vasoactive intestinal peptide in perilymph. Fex and Altschuler (1981) demonstrated an enkephalin-like immunoreactivity in the efferent olivocochlear neurons of the cochlea, but not in the spiral ganglion cells, the auditory nerve fibers, or the hair cells of the organ of Corti. Hoffman, Altschuler, & Fex (1983) identified two methionine-enkephalin fractions in cochleae from guinea pigs using high performance liquid chromatographic separation and subsequent radioimmunoassay. Drescher and colleagues (1983) detected a methionine-enkephalin-like component in perilymph and found it elevated in response to noise. These last investigators have suggested that the enkephalin they detected may have been released from the efferents. Fex and Altschuler (1981) have speculated that enkephalins may share a role with acetylcholine in efferent transmission. In regard to these data, the candidacy of these polypeptides as cochlear transmitters, cotransmitters, or modulators seems promising though somewhat tentative at this time.

Auditory Nerve Activating Substance as the Afferent Neurotransmitter of the Cochlea

In an innovative study, Sewell and colleagues (1978) collected the perilymph of guinea pigs and frogs during exposure to sound and monitored the influence of this perilymph, when applied to the frog amphibian papilla, on the discharge rate of individual auditory nerve fibers. These investigators found that perilymph collected during exposure to sound induced a relative increase in the discharge rates of individual auditory units as compared to the influence of perilymph collected during periods of silence. They hypothesize that this was evidence for the existence of what they called the auditory nerve activating substance (ANAS) in perilymph and that ANAS is the afferent transmitter. In addition, they compared glutamate and aspartate levels in perilymph collected during sound and silence, as did both Medina and Drescher (1981) and Melamed and co-workers (1982) during subsequent studies, and, like them, reported the lack of any apparent difference. As a consequence, all of these investigators concluded that ANAS could not be either glutamate or aspartate. As previously discussed, Drescher and colleagues (1983) later chromatographically assayed guinea pig perilymph collected under conditions similar to those employed by Sewell and co-workers (1978) and found several primary amines which are apparently released into perilymph as a result of exposure to sound. The positive correlation between the intensity level of the stimuli employed and the concentration of a GABA-like substance led these investigators to suggest that this substance may be the endogenous afferent neurotransmitter. The actual chemical relationship between this GABA-like substance and ANAS has yet to be determined. The discovery of ANAS is undoubtedly an important step towards the elucidation of the biochemistry of the cochlea. It is important to point out, however, that the same qualifications regarding the potential for artifactual release from tissues other than the hair cells, discussed above in reference to the stimulus-induced release of amino acids, also apply here.

CONCLUSIONS

In this review we have separated the information available on the cochlea and the lateral line organ in order to discourage the generalization that all receptoneuronal neurotransmission mechanisms within these two acousticolateralis systems are biochemically or pharmacologically indistinguishable. One of the most pronounced indications that distinctions do exist is that N-methyl-D-aspartate (NMDA) and D-

α-aminoadipate (DAA) have such differential effects on the activity of these two sensory organs. Beyond this, the inhibition induced by GABA in the lateral line organ and the organ's biphasic response to acetylcholine are in sharp contrast with the lack of a GABA-induced response in the cochlea and the purely inhibitory influence of acetylcholine on evoked cochlear activity. These distinctions indicate that it is not appropriate to assume that the receptors mediating synaptic transmission within these two systems are the same.

In regard to afferent neurotransmission in the lateral line organ, we feel the endogenous ligand is most likely an excitatory amino acid. Our interpretation of our data is that DAA blocks the effects of an excitatory amino acid transmitter on the postsynaptic receptors of afferent nerve terminals and that this receptor is of the NMDA-preferring variety. The stimulus-induced release of glutamate and aspartate from lateral line preparations is consistent with this premise, but candidacy on the basis of this criteria must await the demonstration of a calcium dependence. On the contrary, the candidacies of acetylcholine and GABA seem insupportable in light of the fact that neither atropine nor bicuculline have any influence on spontaneous or stimulus-induced afferent activity.

The data presently available on the lateral line efferent neurotransmitter indicate that acetylcholine is the most likely candidate. It should be kept in mind, however, that the suppressive influence of GABA on spontaneous activity and the blockade of GABA by bicuculline each suggest as least an adjunct role for GABA. Cotransmitters and modulators of transmission have been proposed in other synaptic preparations, and it may be that GABA serves in one of these capacities, though, as we have already mentioned, this is no more than speculation on our part at this time.

The potential for a functional interrelationship between GABA and acetylcholine also seems to exist within mechanisms of efferent neurotransmission in the cochlea. This interrelationship may be reflected in the influence of GABA antagonists, the localization of aspartate aminotransferase in efferent fibers, and the correlation of elevated concentrations of GABA-like substances with exposure to different stimuli. In the absence of any demonstrable influence of exogenously applied GABA, however, the above observations do not persuasively support the candidacy of GABA as the efferent transmitter. The presence of methionine-enkephalin in efferent fibers and natural perilymph also suggests the possibility that this peptide is additionally or alternatively involved in a comparable interactive relationship with acetylcholine; however, corroborative pharmacological evidence has not yet been reported. On the other hand, considerable experimental support presently exists in favor of the candidacy of acetylcholine and, lacking any correspondingly convincing evidence to the contrary, we feel that the endogenous efferent ligand can be identified as such.

In regard to afferent neurotransmission in the cochlea, our current hypothesis is that the endogenous ligand is an excitatory amino acid. This assertion was initially based on observations that glutamate and aspartate, like sound, elevate the discharge rates of single afferent cochlear units. To our knowledge, no comparable demonstrations using any of the other candidates proposed have been reported except for ANAS, and the chemical identity of this endogenous substance is presently unknown. The influence of excitatory amino acid agonists on cochlear potentials and, to a lesser extent, the effects of excitatory amino acid antagonists, are consistent with this hypothesis. Given the qualifications discussed in preceding sections, the data generated by our studies on potassium-induced changes in perilymph primary amines are also consistent with this hypothesis. This is not to say, by any means, that proposals regarding the candidacy of ANAS and GABA-like amines are not without significant merit. A great deal of additional information will have to be gathered in order to make a positive identification of the cochlea's afferent neurotransmitter, and it is unlikely that this identification will be possible without more specifically defining the physiological role of ANAS and the GABA-like amines in afferent transmission.

REFERENCES

Ascher, P., Lowy, W.A., & Rang, H.P. (1979). Studies on the mechanism of action of acetylcholine antagonists of rat parasympathetic ganglion cells. *Journal of Physiology (London), 295*, 139–170.

Biscoe, T.J., Evans, R.H., Francis, A.A., Martin, M.R., & Watkins, J.C. (1977). D-α-Aminoadipate as a selective antagonist of amino acid-induced and synaptic excitation of mammalian spinal neurons. *Nature (London), 270*, 22–29.

Bledsoe, S.C., Jr., & Bobbin, R.P. (1982a). Effects of antagonists of excitatory amino acids on the activity of afferent fibers in the *Xenopus laevis* lateral line. *Association for Research in Otolaryngology Abstracts*, St. Petersburg Beach, FL, January 18–21, 1982, p. 88.

Bledsoe, S.C., Jr., & Bobbin, R.P. (1982b). Effects of D, L-aminoadipate on excitation of afferent fibers in the lateral line of *Xenopus laevis*. *Neuroscience Letters, 32*, 315–320.

Bledsoe, S.C., Jr., Bobbin, R.P., & Chihal, D.M. (1981a). Technique for studying sound-induced release of endogenous amino acids from the guinea pig cochlea. *Association for Research in Otolaryngology Abstracts*, St. Petersburg Beach, FL, January 19–21, 1981, p. 24.

Bledsoe, S.C., Jr., Bobbin, R.P., & Chihal, D.M. (1981b). Kainic acid: An evaluation of its action on cochlear potentials. *Hearing Research, 4*, 109–120.

Bledsoe, S.C., Jr., Chihal, D.M., Bobbin, R.P., & Morgan, D.N. (1983). Comparative actions of glutamate and related substances on the lateral line of *Xenopus laevis*. *Comparative Biochemistry and Physiology, 75C*, 119–206.

Bledsoe, S.C., Jr., Bobbin, R.P., Thalmann, R., & Thalmann, I. (1980). Stimulus-induced release of endogenous amino acids from the *Xenopus laevis* lateral-line organ. *Experimental Brain Research, 40*, 97–101.

Bobbin, R.P. (1979). Glutamate and aspartate mimic the afferent transmitter in the cochlea. *Experimental Brain Research, 34*, 389–393.

Bobbin, R.P., Bledsoe, S.C., Jr., & Chihal, D.M. (1981a). Effects of various excitatory amino acid antagonists on guinea pig cochlear potentials. *Association for Research in Otolaryngology Abstracts*, St. Petersburg Beach, FL, January 19–21, 1981, p. 27.

Bobbin, R.P., Bledsoe, S.C., Jr., & Chihal, D.M. (1981b). Effect of asphyxia and aminooxyacetic acid on the slow potential evoked by crossed olivocochlear bundle stimulation. *Hearing Research, 5*, 265–269.

Bobbin, R.P., Bledsoe, S.C., Jr., Chihal, D.M., & Morgan, D.N. (1981c). Comparative actions of glutamate and related substances on the *Xenopus laevis* lateral line. *Comparative Biochemistry and Physiology, 69C*, 145–147.

Bobbin, R.P., Bledsoe, S., Jr., Jenison, G.L., Winbery, S., & Caesar, G. (1983). Actions of atropine and bicuculline on the activity of afferent fibers in the *Xenopus laevis* lateral line. *Society for Neuroscience Abstracts, 9*, 739.

Bobbin, R.P., & Gondra, M. (1973). Effect of intravenous aminooxyacetic acid on guinea pig cochlear potentials. *Neuropharmacology, 12*, 1005–1007.

Bobbin, R.P., & Guth, P.S. (1970). Evidence that gamma-aminobutyric acid is not the inhibitory transmitter at the crossed olivo-cochlear nerve–hair cell junction. *Neuropharmacology, 9*, 567–574.

Bobbin, R.P., & Konishi, T. (1974). Action of cholinergic and anticholinergic drugs at the crossed olivocochlear bundle-hair cell junction. *Acta Otolaryngology, 77*, 56–65.

Bobbin, R.P., & Konishi, T. (1971). Acetylcholine mimics crossed olivocochlear bundle stimulation. *Nature New Biology, 231*, 222–223.

Bobbin, R.P., & Morgan, D.N. (1980). Glutamate mimics the afferent transmitter in the Xenopus laevis lateral line. In R.J. Gorlin (Ed.), *Morphogenesis and malformation of the ear* (Vol. XVI). New York: Alan R. Liss for the March of Dimes Birth Defects Foundation.

Bobbin, R.P., & Thompson, M.H. (1978). Effects of putative transmitters on afferent cochlear transmission. *Annals of Otology, Rhinology and Laryngology, 87*, 185–190.

Bowery, N.G., Hill, D.R., & Hudson, A.L. (1983). Characteristics of GABA receptor binding sites on rat whole brain synaptic membranes. *British Journal of Pharmacology, 78*, 191–206.

Carlborg, B., Densert, B., & Densert, O. (1982). Functional patency of the cochlear aqueduct. *Annals of Otology, Rhinology and Laryngology, 91*, 209–215.

Chihal, D.M., Bledsoe, S.C., Bobbin, R.P., & Morgan, D.N. (1980). The glutamate receptor site in the lateral line of *Xenopus laevis*: Structure activity relationships (SAR). *Association for Research in Otolaryngology Abstracts*, St. Petersburg Beach, FL, January 21–23, 1980, p. 7.

Churchill, J.A., Schuknecht, H.F., & Doran, R. (1956). Acetylcholinesterase activity in the cochlea. *Laryngoscope, 66*, 1–15.

Collins, G.G.S., Anson, J., & Probett, G.A. (1981). Patterns of endogenous amino acid release from slices of rat and guinea-pig olfactory cortex. *Brain Research, 204*, 103–120.

Comis, S.D., & Leng, G. (1979). Action of putative neurotransmitters in the guinea pig cochlea. *Experimental Brain Research, 36*, 119–128.

Cotman, C.W., & Hamberger, A. (1978). Glutamate as a neurotransmitter: Properties of release, inactivation and biosynthesis. In F. Fonnum (Ed.), *Amino acids as chemical transmitters*. New York: Plenum.

Cox, D.W.G., & Bradford, H.F. (1978). Uptake and release of excitatory amino acid transmitters. In E.G. McGeer et al. (Eds.), *Kainic acid as a tool in neurobiology*. New York: Raven Press.

Davies, J., Evans, R.H., Francis, A.A., & Watkins, J.C. (1979a). Excitatory amino acid receptors and synaptic excitation in the mammalian central nervous system. *Journal de Physiologie (Paris), 75*, 641–645.

Davies, J., Evans, R.H., Francis, A.A., & Watkins, J.C. (1979b). Excitatory amino acids: Receptor differentiation by selective antagonists and role in synaptic excitation. In J. Simon (Ed.), *Advances in pharmacology and therapeutics, Vol. 2: Neurotransmitters*. New York: Pergamon.

Desmedt, J.E. (1975). Physiological studies of the efferent recurrent auditory system. In W.D. Keidel & W.D. Neff (Eds.), *Handbook of sensory physiology, Vol. V/2; Auditory system*. New York: Springer-Verlag.

Desmedt, J.E., & Monaco, P. (1961). Mode of action of the efferent olivocochlear bundle on the inner ear. *Nature (London), 193,* 1263–1265.

Desmedt, J.E., & Monaco, P. (1962). The pharmacology of a centrifugal inhibitory pathway in the cat's acoustic system. *Proceedings of the First International Pharmacological Meeting, 8,* 183–188.

Drescher, M.J., Drescher, D.G., & Medina, J.E. (1983). Effect of sound stimulation at several levels on concentrations of primary amines, including neurotransmitter candidates, in perilymph of the guinea pig inner ear. *Journal of Neurochemistry, 41,* 309–320.

Evans, R.H., Francis, A.A., Hunt, K., Oakes, D.J., & Watkins, J.C. (1979). Antagonism of excitatory amino acid-induced responses and of synaptic excitation in the isolated spinal cord of the frog. *British Journal of Pharmacology, 67,* 591–603.

Eybalin, M., Calas, A., & Pujol, R. (1981). *Cochlear neurotransmitters: Morphological approach.* XVIII Workshop on Inner Ear Biology, La Grande Motte, September, 1981.

Eybalin, M., Calas, A., & Pujol, R. (1983). Radioautographic study of the sympathetic fibers in the cochlea. *Acta Otolaryngologica, 96,* 69–74.

Eybalin, M., & Pujol, R. (1983). A radioautographic study of (^{3}H)L-glutamate and (^{3}H)L-glutamine uptake in the guinea-pig cochlea. *Neuroscience, 9,* 863–871.

Fex, J. (1968a). Efferent inhibition in the cochlea by the olivocochlear bundle. In A.V.S. de Reuck & J. Knight (Eds.), *Ciba foundation symposium on hearing mechanisms in verterbrates.* London: Churchill.

Fex, J. (1968b). Discussion. In A.V.S. de Reuck & J. Knight (Eds.), *Ciba foundation symposium on hearing mechanisms in verterbrates.* London: Churchill.

Fex, J. (1974). Neural excitatory processes of the inner ear. In W.D. Keidel & W.D. Neff (Eds.) *Handbook of sensory physiology, Vol. V/1: Auditory system.* New York: Springer-Verlag.

Fex, J., & Adams, J.C. (1978). α-Bungarotoxin blocks reversibly cholinergic inhibition in the cochlea. *Brain Research, 159,* 440–444.

Fex, J., & Altschuler, R.A. (1981). Enkephalin-like immunoreactivity of olivocochlear nerve fibers in cochlea of guinea pig and cat. *Proceedings of the National Academy of Sciences, USA, 78,* 1255–1259.

Fex, J., Altschuler, R.A., Parakkal, M.H., & Eckenstein, F., (1982a). Immunocytochemical localization of choline acetyltransferase-like immunoreactivity in olivocochlear fibers in the guinea pig cochlea. *Society for Neuroscience Abstracts, 8,* 41.

Fex, J., Altschuler, R.A., Wenthold, R.J., & Parakkal, M.H. (1982b). Aspartate aminotransferase immunoreactivity in cochlea of guinea pig. *Hearing Research, 7,* 149–160.

Fex, J., & Martin, M.R. (1980). Lack of effect of DL-α-aminoadipate, an excitatory amino acid antagonist, on cat auditory nerve responses to sound. *Neuropharmacology, 19,* 809–811.

Fex, J., & Wenthold, R. (1976). Choline acetyltransferase, glutamate decarboxylase, and tyrosine hydroxylase in the cochlea and cochlear nucleus of the guinea pig. *Brain Research, 109,* 575-585.

Flock, A., & Lam, D.M.K. (1974). Neurotransmitter synthesis in inner ear and lateral-line sense organs. *Nature (London), 249,* 142–144.

Godfrey, D.A., Carter, J.A., Sosamma, J.B., & Matschinsky, F.M. (1976). Levels of putative transmitter amino acids in the guinea pig cochlea. *Journal of Histochemistry and Cytochemistry, 24,* 468–472.

Gulley, R.L., Fex, J., & Wenthold, R.J. (1979). Uptake of putative neurotransmitters in the organ of Corti. *Acta Otolaryngologica, 88,* 177–182.

Guth, P.S., Norris, C.H., & Bobbin, R.P. (1976). The pharmacology of transmission in the peripheral auditory system. *Pharmacological Reviews, 28,* 95–125.

Guth, P., Sewell, W.F., & Tachibana, M. (1981). The pharmacology of the cochlear afferents and cochlear nucleus. In R.D. Brown & E.A. Daigneault (Eds.), *The pharmacology of hearing.* New York: Wiley.

Hoffman, D.W., Altschuler, R.A., & Fex, J. (1983). High-performance liquid chromatographic identification of enkephalin-like peptides in the cochlea. *Hearing Research, 9,* 71–78.

Jasser, A., & Guth, P.S. (1973). The synthesis of acetylcholine by the olivocochlear bundle. *Journal of Neurochemistry, 20,* 45–54.

Jenison, G.L., & Bobbin, R.P. (1983a). Effects of quisqualate on guinea pig cochlear potentials. *Association for Research in Otolaryngology Abstracts,* St. Petersburg Beach, FL, January 23–27, 1983.

Jenison, G.L., & Bobbin, R.P. (1983b). Potassium-induced changes in the levels of endogenous amino acids of guinea pig perilymph. *Society for Neuroscience Abstracts, 9,* 41.

Katsuki, Y. (1973). The ionic receptive mechanism in acoustico-lateralis system. In A.R. Moller & P. Boston (Eds.), *Basic mechanisms in hearing.* New York: Academic Press.

Klinke, R. (1981). Neurotransmitters in the cochlea and the cochlear nucleus. *Acta Otolaryngologica, 91,* 541–554.

Klinke, R., & Evans, E.F. (1977). Evidence that catecholamines are not the afferent transmitter in the cochlea. *Experimental Brain Research, 28,* 315–324.

Klinke, R., & Oertel, W. (1977a). Amino acids – Putative afferent transmitter in the cochlea? *Experimental Brain Research, 30,* 145–148.

Klinke, R., & Oertel, W. (1977b). Evidence that GABA is not the afferent transmitter in the cochlea. *Experimental Brain Research, 28,* 311–314.

Klinke, R., & Oertel, W. (1977c). Evidence that 5-HT is not the afferent transmitter in the cochlea. *Experimental Brain Research, 30,* 141–143.

Konishi, T. (1972). Action of tubocurarine and atropine on the crossed olivocochlear bundle. *Acta Otolaryngologica, 74,* 252–264.

Konishi, T., & Slepian, J.Z. (1971). Effects of the electrical stimulation of the crossed olivocochlear bundle on cochlear potentials recorded with intracochlear electrodes in guinea pigs. *Journal of the Acoustical Society of America, 49,* 1762–1769.

Lim, D.J., Mogi, G., O'Dorisio, T.M., & Cataland, S. (1981). Vasoactive intestinal peptide in perilymph. *Association for Research in Otolaryngology Abstracts,* St. Petersburg Beach, FL, January 19–21, 1981, p. 25.

Martin, M.R. (1982). Baclofen and the brain stem auditory evoked potential. *Experimental Neurology, 76(3);* 675–680.

Martin, M.R., & Adams, J.C. (1979). Effects of DL-α-aminoadipate on synaptically and chemically evoked excitation of anteroventral cochlear nucleus neurons of the cat. *Neuroscience, 4,* 1097–1105.

McLennan, H., & Lodge, D. (1979). The antagonism of amino acid-induced excitation of spinal neurones in the cat. *Brain Research, 169,* 83–90.

McLennan, J. (1963). *Synaptic transmission.* Philadelphia: Saunders.

Medina, J.E., & Drescher, D.G. (1981). The amino acid content of perilymph and cerebrospinal fluid from guinea pigs and the effect of noise on the amino acid composition of perilymph. *Neuroscience, 6,* 505–509.

Melamed, B., Norris, C., Bryant, G., & Guth, P. (1982). Amino acid contents of guinea pig perilymph collected under conditions of quiet or sound stimulation. *Hearing Research, 7,* 13–18.

Monaghan, P. (1975). Ultrastructural and pharmacological studies on the afferent synapses of the lateral-line sensory cells of the African clawed toad, *Xenopus laevis. Cell and Tissue Research, 163,* 239–247.

Norris, C.H., & Guth, P.S. (1974). The release of acetylcholine by the crossed olivocochlear bundle. *Acta Otolaryngologica, 77,* 318–326.

Peet, M.J., Malik, R., & Curtis, D.R. (1983). Post excitatory depression of neuronal firing by acidic amino acids and acetylcholine in the cat spinal cord. *Brain Research, 263,* 162–166.

Rarey, K.E., Ross, M.D., & Smith, C.B. (1982). Distribution and significance of norepinephrine in the lateral cochlear wall of pigmented and albino rats. *Hearing Research, 6,* 15–23.

Rarey, K.E., Ross, M.D., & Smith, C.B. (1981). Quantitative evidence for cochlear, nonneuronal norepinephrine. *Hearing Research, 5,* 101–108.

Robertson, D., & Johnstone, B.M. (1978). Efferent transmitter substance in the mammalian cochlea: Single neuron support for acetylcholine. *Hearing Research, 1,* 31–34.

Russell, I.J. (1976). Amphibian lateral line receptors. In R. Llinas & W. Precht (Eds.), *Frog neurobiology, a handbook.* New York: Springer-Verlag.

Russell, I.J. (1968). Influence of efferent fibres on a receptor. *Nature (London), 219,* 177–178.

Russell, I.J. (1971). The pharmacology of efferent synapses in the lateral line system of Xenopus laevis. *Journal of Experimental Biology, 54,* 643–658.

Ryan, A.F., & Schwartz, I.R. (1984). Preferential glutamine uptake by cochlear hair cells: Implications for the afferent cochlear transmitter. *Brain Research, 290,* 376–379.

Schuknecht, H.F., Churchill, J.A., & Doran, R. (1959). The localization of acetylcholinesterase in the cochlea. *Archives of Otolaryngology, 69,* 549–559.

Schwartz, I.R., & Ryan, A.F. (1983). Differential labeling of sensory cell and neural populations in the organ of Corti following amino acid incubations. *Hearing Research, 9,* 185–200.

Sewell, W., Norris, C.H., Tachibana, M., & Guth, P.S. (1978). Detection of an auditory nerve-activating substance. *Science, 202,* 910–912.

Siegel, G.J., Albers, R.W., Agranoff, B.W., & Katzman, R.K. (1981). *Basic neurochemistry.* Boston: Little, Brown & Co.

Tachibana, M., & Kuriyama, K. (1974). Gamma-aminobutyric acid in the lower auditory pathway of the guinea pig. *Brain Research, 69,* 370–374.

Tanaka, Y., & Katsuki, Y. (1966). Pharmacological investigations of cochlear responses and of olivocochlear inhibition. *Journal of Neurophysiology, 29,* 94–108.

Thalmann, R. (1975). Biochemical studies of the auditory system. In D. Tower (Ed.), *The nervous system, Vol. 3: Human communication and its disorders.* New York: Raven Press.

Thalmann, R., Comegys, T.H., DeMott, J.E., & Thalmann, I. (1981). Steep gradients of amino acids between cochlear endolymph and perilymph. *Laryngoscope, 91,* 1785–1791.

Thalmann, R., Comegys, T.H., & Thalmann, I. (1982). Amino acid profiles in inner ear fluids and cerebrospinal fluid. *Laryngoscope, 92,* 321–328.

Vinnikov, Y.A. (1974). *Sensory reception, cytology, molecular mechanisms, and evolution.* Heidelberg: Springer-Verlag.

Watkins, J.C. (1978). Excitatory amino acid. In E.G. McGear et al. (Eds.), *Kainic acid as a tool in neurobiology.* New York: Raven Press.

Watkins, J.C. (1981). Pharmacology of excitatory amino acid receptors. In P.J. Roberts, J. Storm-Mathisen, & G.A.R. Johnston (Eds.), *Glutamate: Transmitter in the central nervous system.* New York: Wiley.

Watkins, J.C., & Evans, R.H. (1981). Excitatory amino acid transmitters. In R. George, R. Okun, & A.K. Cho (Eds.), *Annual review of pharmacology and toxicology*. Palo Alto: Annual Reviews.

Werman, R. (1966). A review: Criteria for identification of a central nervous system transmitter. *Comparative Biochemistry and Physiology, 18*, 745–766.

Winbery, S.L., & Bobbin, R.P. (1983). Actions of acetylcholine and carbachol on the spontaneous activity of afferent fibers in the *Xenopus laevis* lateral line. *Association for Research in Otolaryngology Abstracts*, St. Petersburg Beach, FL, January 23–27, 1983, p. 47.

Zimmerman, D. McG. (1979). Onset of neural function in the lateral line. *Nature (London), 282*, 82–84.

Chapter 5

Anatomical Measures of Physiological Parameters in the Cochlea[1]

Allen F. Ryan

INTRODUCTION

Traditionally, there has been a clear distinction between the study of auditory physiology and that of auditory anatomy. However, the past decade has seen the development of a variety of anatomical techniques with which it is possible to assess physiological state or even physiological function. These anatomical measures have provided a valuable supplement to physiological data obtained with more conventional methodologies, such as electrophysiology or psychophysics. They have also extended our understanding of functional processes in new directions, by allowing very close linkage between functional characteristics and anatomical structures.

Several of these techniques have been adapted for use in the central auditory system. Their application in the cochlea has not occurred as rapidly, in part due to the technical problems of obtaining access to inner ear tissues through the bony cochlear capsule. However, there are many questions regarding inner ear function which have been difficult to answer utilizing standard electrophysiological or psychophysical measures. Some of the most interesting unresolved problems include identification of the neurotransmitter at the hair cell/afferent nerve fiber synapse; elucidation of the spatial pattern of activation of cochlear hair cells and neurons during acoustic stimulation; and more precise delineation of cochlear innervation patterns, including

[1]The research upon which this chapter is based was done in collaboration with several individuals. The amino acid studies were performed with Dr. Ilsa Schwartz of University of California at Los Angeles. The 2-DG investigations were the result of collaboration with Dr. Frank R. Sharp and Dr. Nigel K. Woolf of University of California at San Diego. EDXA studies were performed with Dr. Robert C. Bone of the Scripps Clinic and Research Foundation, La Jolla, California. The work of these investigators has been drawn upon quite heavily. They have also reviewed this manuscript and supplied invaluable critical comments. Their contributions are gratefully acknowledged. The research was supported by grants NS14945, NS14503, and NS09823 from the NIH/NINCDS, by the Research Service of the Veterans Administration, and by the Duaei Hearing Research Fund. Dr. Ryan is the recipient of Research Career Development Award NS00176, from the NIH/NINCDS.

the efferent innervation of the two populations of hair cells and the afferent projection of outer hair cell-associated afferent neurons, to name a few.

The development of anatomical measures of auditory physiological function presents challenging technical difficulties. However, their successful application also promises to provide new evidence that will address these unanswered questions. This chapter describes the methods by which three of these techniques have been applied to the cochlea: autoradiographic demonstration of amino acid uptake, 2-deoxy-D-glucose autoradiography to indicate functional activation, and electron microprobe analysis of ion distribution.

COCHLEAR UPTAKE OF AMINO ACIDS

Autoradiographic demonstration of preferential amino acid uptake has been employed in neural tissue to provide information regarding putative neurotransmitters. The presence of specific uptake systems, while by no means providing conclusive evidence, is suggestive of a transmitter function (Iverson & Schon, 1973). An additional use for this methodology is in identifying biochemically distinct neural subpopulations. For example, differential amino acid uptake has been used to distinguish different populations of cholinergic neurons (Mesulam & Dichter, 1981). The significance of high-affinity amino acid uptake in the latter case is not clear. However, it is possible that the amino acids, or derivatives, serve as cotransmitters in neurons which rely upon another substance as the primary neurotransmitter, as has been suggested by Krnjevic (1981). Previous attempts to identify preferential amino acid uptake in the cochlea did not provide evidence for such uptake in hair cells, although preferential amino acid uptake by the cochlear efferents, especially of GABA, was observed (Gulley, Fex, Wenthold, & Wenthold, 1970; Richrath, Kraus, & Fromme, 1974).

To more fully explore amino acid uptake in the cochlea, the inner ears of gerbils were perfused in vivo with artificial perilymph containing micromolar concentrations of one of eight ^{3}H-labeled amino acids. Glutamic and aspartic acid are generally regarded as the amino acids most likely to act at the hair cell/eighth nerve fiber synapse, although the evidence for either is far from convincing (Klinke, 1981). Both the L- and the D-forms of aspartic acid are readily available as radiolabeled reagents. Both were employed since L-aspartic acid is rapidly metabolized in some systems, and uptake of D-aspartic acid can more closely reflect high-affinity transport in such cases. Glycine, alanine, and taurine have also been suggested as neurotransmitters in the cochlea (Klinke & Oertel, 1977), although there is little or no evidence to support such a role for any of the three. Gamma-amino butyric acid (GABA) uptake by cochlear efferents has been described by other investigators (Gulley et al., 1970; Richrath et al., 1974). Uptake of the GABA analog muscimol has been shown to be more specific to neural populations than to glial cells in the retina (Pourcho, 1981). Cochleae were incubated with the labeled amino acids for 20 min. Longer incubations were also employed for taurine. Following incubation, cochleae were briefly perfused with artificial perilymph to remove unbound label, then perfused with a mixed aldehyde fixative. The inner ears were then removed from the bulla, widely opened, osmicated, uranyl acetate block-stained, and embedded in Spurr resin. The embedded cochleae were bisected along the modiolus with a 100-μm jeweler's saw, decalcified in 5% trichloroacetic acid for 10 days, reembedded, and sectioned for light and electron microscopic autoradiography. A more detailed discussion of methodology is available in previous publications (Ryan & Schwartz, 1983; Schwartz & Ryan, 1983).

Organ of Corti

No dramatic preferential uptake into hair cells was noted with any of the amino acids investigated. This result agrees with the findings of previous investigators (Gulley et al., 1970; Richrath et al., 1974). However, two- to threefold higher levels of glycine and alanine uptake were observed in the inner hair cells when compared to the outer hair cells. Preferential uptake was clearly apparent in the cochlear efferents. However, in contrast to the results of previous studies (Gulley et al., 1970; Richrath et al., 1974), two distinctly different patterns of uptake were noted with different amino acids. A high level of aspartic acid uptake, especially D-aspartic acid uptake, as illustrated in Figure 5-1, was observed in nerve fibers and efferent endings terminated upon the inner hair cells. The majority of the efferent endings terminated upon the inner hair cell afferents, while a smaller number terminated directly upon the inner hair cells themselves. No labeling was observed in the efferents under the outer hair cells. As shown in Figure 5-2, preferential uptake of GABA was observed in efferent endings under the outer hair cells, in tunnel-crossing fibers, and in fibers, as well as in some efferent endings under the inner hair cells.

These data suggest that there are two populations of cochlear efferents which are distinguished by amino acid uptake pattern. One population innervates the inner hair cell afferents exclusively and, to a much lesser extent, the inner hair cells themselves. The other population innervates both the outer hair cells and the inner hair cell afferents. It is likely that the two populations distinguished by their preferential amino acid uptake characteristics correspond to the two populations of efferents identified by Warr and Guinan (1979) as originating in separate neural populations in the brainstem. Warr and Guinan, based upon light microscopic analysis of their data, concluded that each efferent population innervates a separate hair cell type. Efferents that originate from neurons medial to the medial superior olivary nucleus innervate the outer hair cells, while efferents originating from neurons near the lateral superior olivary nucleus innervate the inner hair cells. However, the electron microscopic autoradiographs obtained with GABA suggest that the population that supplies the outer hair cells also supplies efferent innervation to the region of the inner hair cells.

The significance of these uptake patterns is not clear. There is strong evidence that the cochlear efferents are cholinergic (Klinke, 1981). Thus it is unlikely that either of the preferential uptake systems demonstrated in efferent nerve fibers and endings relate to the primary neurotransmitter of these two efferent populations. Differences in the metabolic requirements of the two populations of efferents may explain their differential amino acid uptake. However, the possibility that an amino acid might

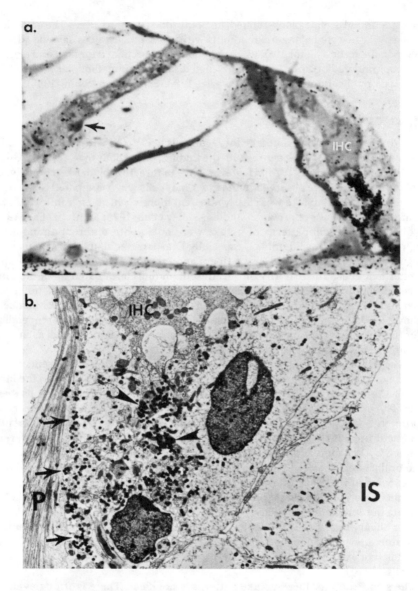

Figure 5-1. (a) Light micrograph illustrating labeling in the region underneath the inner hair cell (IHC) following in vivo incubation with D-[^{3}H]aspartic acid. Note the absence of labeling in the tunnel-crossing fibers and in the ending (arrow) beneath the outer hair cell. (b) Electron micrograph showing the labeling of both fibers (arrows) and efferent endings (arrowheads) underneath an inner hair cell (IHC). (IS) = inner sulcus. (P) = pillar cell. Figure 5-1b was adapted from Schwartz and Ryan (1983).

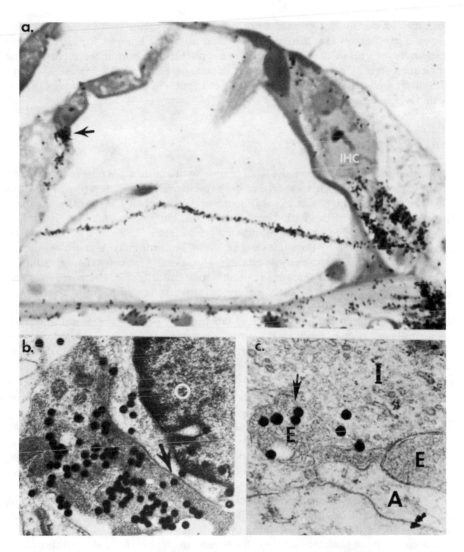

Figure 5-2. (a) Light micrograph illustrating labeling in a tunnel-crossing fiber, in an ending underneath an outer hair cell (arrow), and in the region underneath an inner hair cell (IHC), following in vivo incubation with [3H]GABA. (b) Electron micrograph showing labeling of an efferent terminal adjacent to an outer hair cell (O), with some grains also being present over the hair cell cytoplasm, adjacent to the subsynaptic cistern (arrow). (c) Electron micrograph showing the labeling of an efferent ending (arrow, E), while an adjacent efferent terminal (E) and an afferent dendrite (A) are unlabeled, in the region underneath an inner hair cell (I). Figures 5-2b, c were adapted from Schwartz and Ryan (1983).

serve as a cotransmitter or modulator of efferent synaptic activity, as has been proposed in other systems (Krnjevic, 1981), should not be ignored. This is especially true when the recent demonstration of enkephalin-like immunoreactivity in the cochlear efferents (Fex & Altschuler, 1981, Hoffman, Altschuler, & Fex, 1981) is considered. The pharmacology of the cochlear efferents may be more complex than is currently appreciated.

Spiral ganglion

Within the spiral ganglion, the level of uptake of amino acids observed in neural somas was rather low. This was true of both the heavily myelinated Type I neurons and the more lightly myelinated Type II neurons. An exception was the case of taurine. Preferential uptake of this amino acid was noted, but as illustrated in Figure 5-3, it was restricted to the Type II spiral ganglion neurons.

Uptake of taurine by the somas of the Type II neuron may have no relation to the neurotransmitter released by its endings. However, it indicates that this subpopulation of spiral ganglion neurons is not only anatomically, but also biochemically, distinct from Type I neurons. There is some controversy regarding the central projection of the Type II spiral ganglion neuron, as distinct from that of the Type I neuron (Spoendlin, 1979). Preferential uptake of taurine may prove to be useful in tracing the central projection of the Type II neuron, since amino acids incorporated into proteins within neural somas are often anterogradely transported (Kane, 1977).

DEOXYGLUCOSE UPTAKE IN THE AUDITORY SYSTEM

The 2-deoxy-D-glucose (2-DG) autoradiographic method has been used to map functional activity at many locations in the central nervous system. In sensory systems, this technique has demonstrated functional activity in number of central pathways, including the central auditory system (see Ryan, Woolf, & Sharp, 1982c for a review).

The 2-DG technique is based upon the incorporation of this glucose analog into tissue via the same mechanisms by which glucose itself is transported into cells. The great majority of 2-DG is converted into 2-deoxy-D-glucose-6-phosphate. At this point, the tracer cannot proceed along the glucolytic pathway and is trapped with a half-life of about 24 hr. Some of the 2-DG remains free in the tissue, while a small fraction is converted into glycogen.

2-DG injected as an intravascular pulse is rapidly removed from the circulation, so that within 45–60 min. only a few percent of the tracer remain in circulation. Uptake into tissue depends upon serum concentration of the tracer, serum concentration of glucose, with which 2-DG competes for transport, and the level of metabolic activity of the tissue in question. The net effect is that tissues with high levels of metabolism incorporate higher levels of 2-DG than do tissues with lower metabolic rates. In brain, metabolism is almost entirely glycolytic and activation of

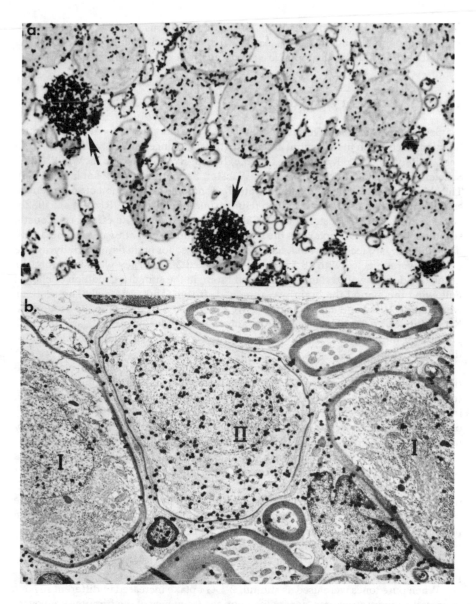

Figure 5-3. (a) Light micrograph illustrating the labeling of a small proportion of spiral ganglion neurons (arrows) following in vivo incubation with [³H]taurine. (b) Electron micrograph demonstrating that the selectively labeled neurons are Type II spiral ganglion cells (II) with their characteristic paucity of myelin and rough endoplasmic reticulum. Figure 5-3b was adapted from Ryan and Schwartz (1983).

neural pathways frequently results in dramatic elevations in 2-DG uptake in the associated neural structures. This can be demonstrated visually if the 2-DG is radiolabeled and autoradiographs are prepared from brain tissue sections.

Central Auditory System

Several investigators have shown that the 2-DG technique can be used to identify functional activation in the central auditory pathway (Hungerbuhler, Saunders, Greenberg, & Reivich, 1981; Ryan et al., 1982b,c; Sharp, Ryan, Goodwin, & Woolf, 1981; Scheich, Bonke, Bonke, & Langer, 1979; Webster, Serviere, Batini, & Laplante, 1978). The ability of the technique to demonstrate the tonotopic organization of some central activity nuclei has also been described (Hungerbuhler et al., 1981; Ryan et al., 1982b; Scheich et al., 1979; Webster et al., 1978). We have explored the effects of acoustic stimulation upon 2-DG uptake in the gerbil central auditory pathway in some detail, using the standard techniques that have been developed for brain tissue. Briefly, awake animals were injected with 16.7 μCi of ^{14}C-labeled 2-DG. They were kept for 1 hr inside of a double-walled sound-attentuated room, in the stimulus condition of choice. Following this period the brain was removed, frozen, and sectioned. The sections were rapidly dried and autoradiographs were generated by exposing the sections to X-ray film for 7 days. The density of the autoradiographic image of a brain structure provided a measure of 2-DG uptake during the 1-hr period following injection of the tracer.

Most central auditory structures showed increases in 2-DG uptake during stimulation with an acoustic stimulus. With increasing stimulus intensity, uptake increased regularly up to about 85 dB SPL, as illustrated in Figure 5-4. Relatively little additional increase was observed between 85 and 105 dB SPL. Figure 5-4 also illustrates one of the differences observed in the evoked metabolic response of different auditory nuclei. By far the greatest degree of stimulus-associated 2-DG uptake was observed in the inferior colliculus. In contrast, the smallest amount of uptake observed in a central auditory structure during stimulation occurred in the medial geniculate nucleus and auditory cortex. In the medial nucleus of the trapezoid body, no change in 2-DG uptake occurred in response to acoustic stimulation. The reasons for the high degree of metabolic response in the inferior colliculus, and the absence of response in the medial nucleus of the trapezoid body, are not clear. The relatively modest response observed in the medial geniculate and auditory cortex, on the other hand, may relate to the greater sensitivity of these structures to such variables as attention and physiologic state.

When pure tones were used as stimuli, 2-DG uptake increased in different regions of central auditory structures, depending upon the frequency of the stimulus employed. This is illustrated in the autoradiographs of Figure 5-5, which show the patterns of 2-DG uptake observed in the cochlear nuclear complex following stimulation with wide band noise or one of three pure tones. In each of the three divisions of the complex, a pure tone produced a focal region of elevated 2-DG uptake in the tonotopic-

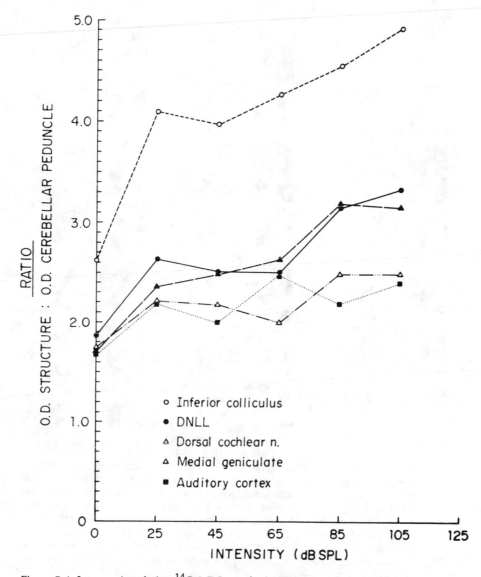

Figure 5-4. Increase in relative ^{14}C-2-DG uptake in various central auditory structures as a
function of wide band noise intensity. Note that the inferior colliculus shows a much
greater metabolic response to stimulation than the typical auditory structure, illustrated by the response of the dorsal cochlear nucleus and the dorsal nucleus of the
lateral lemniscus (DNLL). In contrast, the 2-DG response of the medial geniculate
nucleus and auditory cortex are markedly less pronounced than those of the brainstem and midbrain auditory nuclei. From Sharp et al. (1981).

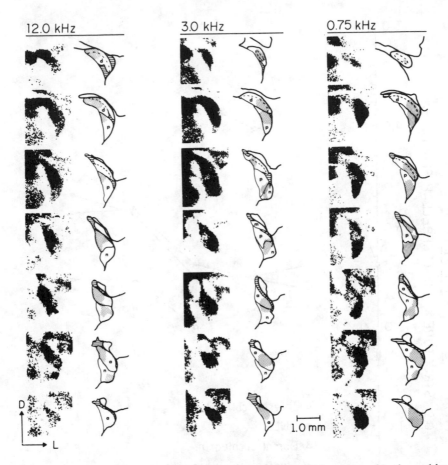

Figure 5-5. Autoradiographs illustrating the patterns of 2-DG uptake observed in the cochlear nuclear complex during exposure to one of three pure tone frequencies, 0.75, 3.0, or 12.0 kHz. In the camera lucida drawings, hatching represents granule cell areas while stippling indicates regions in which 2-DG uptake is high relative to adjacent tissue. Note that localized regions of elevated 2-DG uptake occur not only in the cochlear nuclei, but also in the eighth nerve. Caption: (d) = dorsal cochlear nucleus, (m) = molecular layer of the DCN, (p) = posterior ventral cochlear nucleus, (a) = anterior ventral cochlear nucleus, (n) = eighth nerve. From Ryan and associates (1982c).

ally appropriate area. These regions of locally elevated 2-DG uptake were relatively simple in the cochlear nucleus, as shown in Figure 5-6. In this figure the patterns of 2-DG uptake produced by each of the pure tones have been semiquantitated by measuring optical densities through the autoradiographic image of the structure on a microdensitometer.

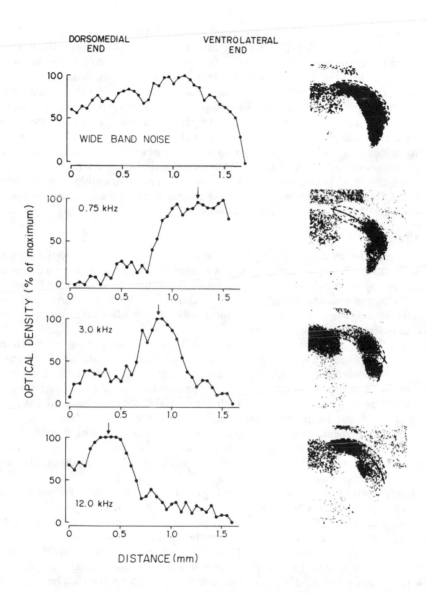

Figure 5-6. Variation in 2-DG uptake, expressed as optical density of the autoradiographic image, along the major axis of the dorsal cochlear nucleus, during stimulation with wide band noise or one of three pure tones. The arrow indicates the location of the center of each band of elevated 2-DG uptake in the pure tone functions. The solid lines in the autoradiographs show the location of optical density measurements. From Ryan and associates (1982c).

In the inferior colliculus, the 2-DG response to pure tones was not as simple. As illustrated in Figure 5-7, 2-DG uptake in the central nucleus of the colliculus did not occur uniformly even with broad band stimulation. Rather, it occurred in a series of 3-4 bands oriented dorsomedially to ventrolaterally. The response to pure tones was also in accordance with this banding pattern. As shown by the densitometry functions, each pure tone activated a tonotopically appropriate portion of the colliculus, but only up to the "ceiling" represented by the wide band noise response. There is thus a metabolic pattern of response in the colliculus which is rigidly defined and within which other responses tend to occur. The basis for this pattern is not at all clear. Neither the cytoarchitecture nor the functional characteristics of neurons in the colliculus have been shown to display any pattern comparable to the banding in the 2-DG response. The pattern is not of binaural origin, since it occurs unchanged in one colliculus of monauralized animals.

Cochlea

As illustrated by the preceding data, the 2-DG technique can be applied readily in the central auditory pathway. It provides a useful tool with which to map the spatial pattern of activity produced by a given stimulus condition. Of course, the technique is limited to single-stimulus conditions of long duration. Within these limits, however, spatial mapping using the 2-DG technique can be accomplished far more easily than it can in electrophysiological experiments.

If the 2-DG autoradiographic technique could be used in the cochlea, it could allow the mapping of activity in various cochlear cell populations as elicited by acoustic stimulation. However, application of this methodology in the cochlea presents several difficulties not present in brain. The primary problems result from the highly water-soluble nature of 2-DG. Once cells containing the tracer are compromised, the 2-DG diffuses freely from its in vivo position. In brain, this problem is solved by freezing, frozen-sectioning, and rapid drying of sections. In the cochlea, with a bony capsule and large fluid spaces adjacent to all of the relevant tissues, this technique is not applicable. Frozen sections would be difficult to obtain, and upon drying the large fluid pools would lead to tracer diffusion.

The following protocol was developed to avoid these difficulties. Following injection of 2-DG (16.7 μCi/100 g of ^{14}C-2-DG), and a 1-hr incubation period in silence or acoustic stimulation, animals were sacrificed and the inner ears rapidly dissected from the temporal bones without breaching the round and oval windows. The intact cochleae were then frozen in Freon 12 slush, cooled to $-159°C$ in liquid nitrogen, lyophilized ($-40°C$, 0.01 Torr, 72 hr), vapor-fixing over 4% osmium tetroxide followed by acrolein, and embedded in Spurr resin using only organic solvents. The embedded cochleae were cut in half along the modiolus using a bone-cutting lathe, and exposed on LKB Ultrafilm. All embedding fluids were counted to ensure that no loss of tracer occurred at any step of the procedure.

This technique was used to assess the effects of acoustic stimulation upon the uptake of deoxyglucose in inner ear tissues. The results of this investigation are presented in Figure 5-8. The figure shows typical autoradiographs prepared from cochleae

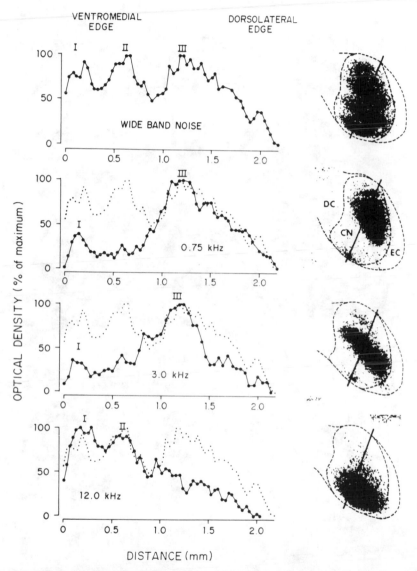

Figure 5-7. Variation in 2-DG incorporation along the ventromedial to dorsolateral axis of the inferior colliculus during stimulation with wide band noise or a pure tone. The dotted line in each pure tone function represents the response to wide band noise. Note the agreement between the maximum optical density in each pure tone condition and the tonotopically appropriate portion of the response to noise. (DC) = dorsal cortex, (CN) = central nucleus, (EC) = external cortex. From Ryan and colleagues (1982c).

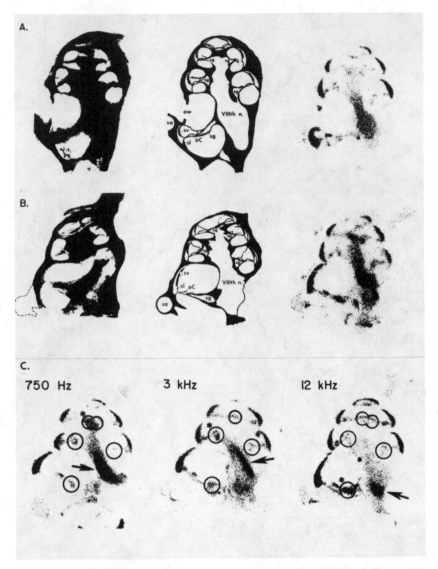

Figure 5-8. Typical autoradiographs obtained from cochleae maintained in silence (A), wide band noise (B), or one of three pure tones (C) for 1 hr following injection of ^{14}C-2-DG. The light micrographs in (A) and (B) show the corresponding plastic sections, which were approximately 200 μm in thickness. The camera lucida drawings show the structures at the surface of each section which was exposed to the film. Caption: (sv) = stria vascularis, (sl) = spiral ligament, (oC) = organ of Corti, (sg) = spiral ganglion, (sa) = stapedial artery, (ow) = oval window. From Ryan et al. (1982a).

which were kept in silence or were exposed to one of four stimulus conditions: wide band noise or one of three pure tones, at an intensity of 85 dB SPL.

The major feature of the 2-DG uptake pattern observed in silence was the very high level of uptake observed in the lateral wall structures, both spiral ligament and stria vascularis, when compared to the remaining cochlear tissues. No marked difference in uptake could be discerned between the ligament and the stria. During exposure to wide band noise at an intensity of 85 dB SPL, 2-DG uptake in the spiral ganglion and the eighth nerve increased dramatically, when compared to lateral wall uptake. Little or no change was observed in the organ of Corti. During exposure to pure tones, localized regions of relatively high 2-DG uptake were observed in tonotopically appropriate areas of the cochlea, just as they were in the brain. With a 0.75-kHz tone, uptake was greatest in the spiral ganglion of the apical turn, and in a band of the eighth nerve along the lateral edge. During exposure to a 3.0-kHz tone, uptake was greatest in the lower middle turn spiral ganglion and in a band of the eighth nerve along its medial edge. With a 12.0-kHz tone, uptake was greatest in the lower basal turn ganglion, and in a small region of the eighth nerve close to the cochlear base. In no case was a localized increase comparable to that seen in the spiral ganglion or the eighth nerve observed in the organ of Corti or the lateral wall structures.

The effects of 85 dB SPL wide band noise on 2-DG uptake were examined quantitatively by obtaining serial serum samples throughout the 1-hr. 2-DG incubation period. Specific activity curves for 2-DG were determined for three noise-exposed and three control subjects using the techniques of Sokoloff and colleagues (1977). This allowed a quantitative comparison of tissue concentrations of 2-DG, obtained by microdensitometry from cochlear autoradiographs, across all subjects. The results of this analysis are illustrated in Figure 5-9, which compares 2-DG uptake in various tissues of the first cochlear turn, in silence versus 85 dB SPL wide band noise. It is apparent from the figure that noise exposure had little effect upon 2-DG uptake in the spiral ligament. Some increase in uptake was observed in the stria vascularis during noise, although the increase was not statistically significant. In the organ of Corti a modest increase in uptake occurred, while in the spiral ganglion and eighth nerve wide band noise produced dramatic increases.

When the pattern of 2-DG uptake in the cochlea was examined across several intensities of wide band noise, it was found that a relative increase in uptake in the ganglion and nerve occurred gradually between 0 and 65 dB SPL, with a very sharp increase at 85 dB SPL. Little additional increase in relative uptake occurred between 85 and 105 dB SPL, as illustrated in Figure 5-10.

To define the pattern of cochlear 2-DG uptake with greater precision, a method for the use of ^{3}H-labeled 2-DG was developed. Essentially the same procedures employed for the ^{14}C-labeled tracer were used. However, a dose of 1.67 mCi/100 gm body weight was employed to compensate for the weaker beta-emissions produced by tritium decay. After bisection of the plastic-embedded cochlea, individual turns were separated, the bony capsule was removed, and 3- to 5-μm sections were cut with glass knives. The sections were flattened on glass slides with xylene or anhydrous glycerol, covered with nearly dry emulsion by the dry-loop technique, and exposed

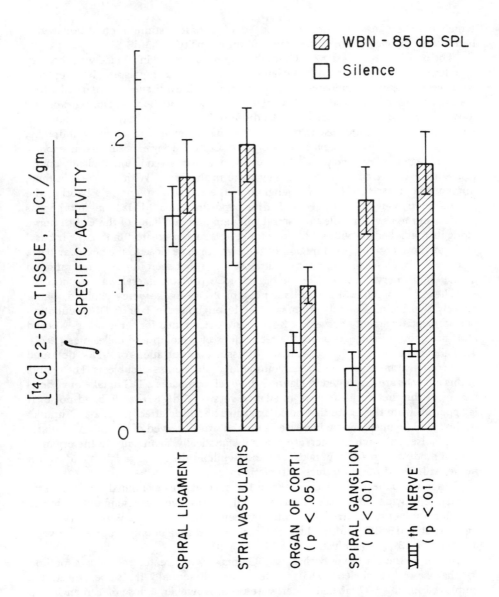

Figure 5-9. Mean 2-DG levels in cochlear tissues of the lower basal turn from inner ears in
silence and in 85 dB SPL wide band noise. Tissue levels have been normalized for
each subject by the integral of the plasma specific activity curve. Each mean represents six cochleae; vertical bars show one standard deviation about each mean. From
Ryan and associates (1982a).

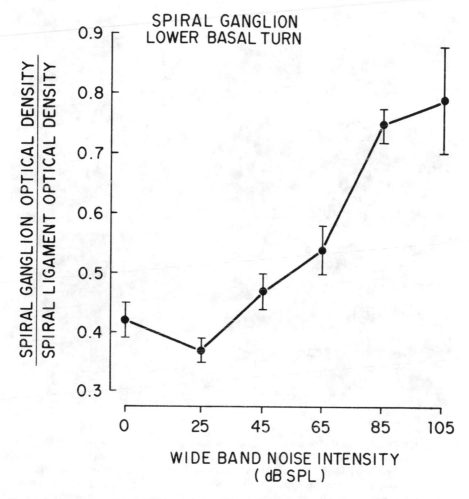

Figure 5-10. Relative 2-DG levels in the spiral ganglion of the lower basal cochlear turn as a function of wide band noise intensity. Tissue levels of 2-DG have been normalized by dividing the optical density obtained from each spiral ganglion image by that of the adjacent spiral ligament. Vertical bars represent one standard error above and below each mean.

for 125 days. Sections from the lower basal turn of noise-exposed cochleae (85 dB SPL wide band noise) were compared with those from cochleae kept in silence.

The results are illustrated in Figure 5-11. Resolution of tracer was achieved at the cellular and subcellular levels. In silence, the greatest numbers of grains were observed over the stria vascularis and spiral ligament, with far fewer grains over other tissues, in agreement with the ^{14}C results. In cochleae exposed to noise, the

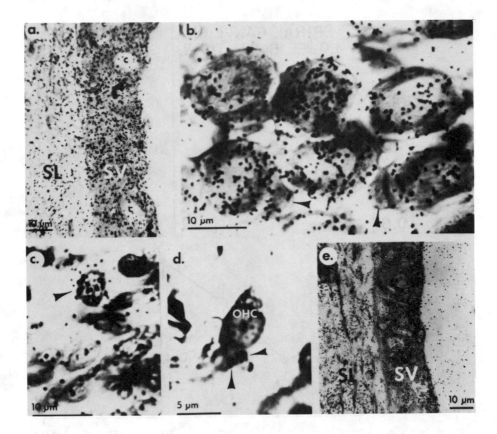

Figure 5-11. Dry-loop autoradiographs of cochlear tissues following injection with ³H-2-DG and exposure to 85 dB SPL wide band noise. (a) Stria vascularis (SV) and spiral ligament (SL). (b) Spiral ganglion neurons and satellite cells (arrowheads). (c) Nerve fibers in the osseus spiral ganglion. Note the fiber with particularly high uptake (arrowhead). (d) Dense accumulations of grains (arrowheads) over the synaptic region under the outer hair cells. (e) Autoradiograph of a section which was dipped in emulsion rather than dry-looped, showing the loss of localized label due to diffusion of the 2-DG. From Ryan and Sharp (1982).

number of grains over spiral ganglion cells and eighth nerve fibers increased, as had been observed with ¹⁴C. However, the increased resolution of the ³H-2-DG technique permitted new observations.

In the lateral wall structures, in contrast to the uniform grain density observed with ¹⁴C, it was apparent that 2-DG uptake was higher in the stria vascularis than in the spiral ligament, especially during exposure to noise. Uptake into the three cell types of the stria (marginal, intermediate, and basal cells) was appropriately equivalent.

During noise exposure, 2-DG uptake increased significantly in all of the cell types of the stria vascularis, but not in the spiral ligament. In the organ of Corti, increased uptake was observed in inner hair cells, but not in supporting cells or outer hair cells. However, increased uptake was apparent in the region of the nerve endings underneath the outer hair cells. Uptake of 2-DG increased in spiral ganglion cells and in eighth nerve fibers in the modiolus, as had been observed with [14]C. However, with ^{3}H-2-DG it was apparent that wide variations in uptake occurred from one individual spiral ganglion cell to the next. Also, increased uptake in individual afferent dendrites within the osseous spiral lamina was observed.

These 2-DG autoradiographic data differ in some respects from those of Canlon and Schacht (1981; Schacht & Canlon, 1981), who utilized a dissection and scintillation counting technique in the mouse cochlea. While they observed increases in 2-DG uptake during noise exposure, they also reported equal levels of uptake in the lateral wall tissues, the organ of Corti, and the eighth nerve, within every stimulus condition. That is, uptake was uniformly low in all three tissues in silence, and increased equally in all three during noise exposure. This is in marked contrast to the different levels of uptake in various cochlear tissues which we observed, and the limitation of stimulus-induced increases in uptake to specific tissues. This difference may reflect the different methodology and species employed in their experiments.

In summary, acoustic stimulation increases the incorporation of 2-DG into cochlear tissues. The 2-DG autoradiographic data indicate that stimulation elicits a metabolic response from some cochlear tissues while leaving others unaffected. The 2-DG technique thus provides a means of mapping sound-evoked activation of inner ear neural tissues, inner hair cells, and stria vascularis. The use of ^{3}H-2-DG permits such mapping at the level of the individual cell.

ENERGY DISPERSIVE X-RAY ANALYSIS OF COCHLEAR ION DISTRIBUTION

The distribution of ions within the complex fluid spaces of the cochlea plays a critical role in cochlear function. The unique extracellular ionic composition of endolymph is a prerequisite of the transduction process. The movement of ions across cell membranes can be presumed to be the mechanism by which the generator potentials of the inner ear arise. The measurement of ion content in the major cochlear fluid spaces has been accomplished with conventional techniques such as micropipet sampling and flame spectrophotometry, or ion-sensitive electrodes. However, it has not been possible to identify the distribution of ions within smaller fluid compartments such as the subtectorial space, or within cochlear tissues themselves.

The development of X-ray microanalysis as a means of identifying element content has allowed the definition of ion distribution in biological samples with extremely high resolution, at the cellular and even subcellular levels (Marshall, 1975; Tousimis, 1969). This technique is based upon the emission of X rays by a sample which is irradiated by an electron beam. Both the energy and the wavelength of the emitted X rays are determined by the atomic number of the atoms in the sample; a sample will emit a characteristic X-ray spectrum which reflects its element content. The most commonly employed spectrometers utilize the differential energy of X rays to identify the element content of samples, hence the term energy dispersive X-ray analysis (EDXA). EDXA spectrometers are usually coupled to an electron microscope, which provides an electron beam and which permits visualization of the sample to be analyzed.

The EDXA technique has several technical limitations that must be considered in the design and interpretation of experiments. First, because fresh biological material cannot be placed in an electron microscope, the in vivo distribution of elements must be preserved while the sample is made compatible with microscopy. This is usually accomplished by cryogenic freezing, with analysis either in a frozen state on a cryogenic microscope stage or in a freeze-dried state at ambient temperature. Second, an electron beam can penetrate biological samples at a depth of up to 100 μm. To obtain a spectrum from a given biological sample, it is necessary to isolate the material from underlying sources of contamination such as an adjacent tissue or fluid. This is accomplished by sectioning, or by microdissection of freeze-dried material. Third, EDXA data are obtained in counts per second of X-ray emission. The volume from which counts are obtained must be very carefully defined if the absolute levels of elements are to be determined. However, the relative levels of various elements are easily calculated, and are often sufficient to answer an experimental question. Fourth, the level of X-ray emission from different elements is not the same. For example, elements lighter than lithium cannot be detected at all, while the level of emission from sodium atoms is only about 24% of that from an equal number of chlorine atoms. These differences can be derived from theory and measured by the use of standards, and are easily correctable. Other, though less major, technical considerations must also be addressed, as discussed elsewhere (Bone & Ryan, 1980, 1982; Ryan, Wickham, & Bone, 1979, 1980).

The electron microprobe has been employed in the cochlea by several investigators. In an early study Ross (1975) reported that the underside of the freeze-dried tectorial membrane contained appreciable quantities of sodium, thus suggesting that the subtectorial fluid is not ionically related to endolymph. Subsequently Flock (1977) examined the ion content of fluid residue in the inner sulcus of intact cochleae which had been frozen, freeze-fractured, and freeze-dried. He found the residue to be rich in potassium, and concluded that the subtectorial fluid was endolymph. Hunter-Duvar, Landolt, and Cameron (1981) and Burgio (1982) studied frozen-hydrated cochleae as bulk specimens and concluded that the ionic composition of inner sulcus fluid was similar to endolymph, while that of the fluid in the organ of Corti spaces was similar to perilymph. Anniko and his associates (Anniko & Nordemar, 1980; Anniko & Wroblewski, 1980, 1981) have characterized the ionic content of the major cochlear fluids in adult and developing animals, using freeze-dried frozen sections to avoid the difficulties inherent in bulk specimens. These previous studies have focused upon the cochlear fluids and upon the ionic composition of fluids in the vicinity of the tectorial membrane. Little or no work has been done concerning the ionic composition of cochlear tissues.

In our studies of ion distribution in the cochlea, we have utilized an EDXA unit in conjunction with a scanning electron microscope. Cochleae were cryogenically frozen intact and freeze-dried. Samples of cochlear fluids and tissues were obtained by microdissection techniques based upon those of Thalmann, Comegys, and Arenberg (1972). EDXA spectra have been obtained from isolated perilymph and endolymph residues, individual outer hair cells, stria vascularis, spiral ligament, otoconia, and the tectorial membrane under a variety of experimental conditions.

Cochlear fluid spaces

A typical EDXA spectrum obtained from perilymph residue is illustrated in Figure 5-12. Freeze-dried perilymph residue consists of dense crystals suspended in a tenuous matrix, as one would expect from an electrolyte solution with low protein content. The principal peaks observed in the perilymph spectrum reflect emission in the chlorine and sodium windows. The level of sodium emission was about 25% of that of chlorine, a level which with the correction for differential emission indicates that the majority of the sample consisted of approximately equal levels of chlorine and sodium. Much smaller peaks were presented in the potassium and calcium windows. This composition is consistent with the known ionic composition of perilymph (Bosher & Warren, 1968), and agrees with the EDXA data of other investigators (Anniko & Wroblewski, 1980, 1981, Burgio, 1982; Hunter-Duvar et al., 1981).

An EDXA spectrum from endolymph residue obtained from the utricle, with an otoconial spectrum as well, are illustrated in Figure 5-13. The endolymph spectrum was dominated by emission in the chlorine and potassium windows, with approximately equal levels of each. No other element contributed a distinct peak to the spectrum, including sodium. Since chlorine emits slightly more X rays than potassium, this indicates that the fluid residue consisted of about 20% more potassium than chlorine. Since no peak was observed for sodium, the level of this ion in utricular endolymph is less than 1 mEq/L, the limit of detectability of this element on an energy dispersive X-ray spectrometer. The EDXA spectrum of endolymph is consistent with the known ionic composition of this fluid (154 mEq potassium, 125 mEq chlorine, < 1 mEq sodium, reference 7). The data were similar to the findings of other investigators with the EDXA technique (Anniko & Nordemar, 1980; Anniko & Wroblewski, 1980, 1981; Burgio, 1982; Hungerbuhler et al., 1981). The otoconial spectrum reflected only its calcium content, since the carbon and oxygen atoms of the carbonate radical emit X rays too weak to be detected.

Figure 5-14 shows EDXA spectra obtained from fluid residue crystals on the underside of the tectorial membrane. This figure illustrates two points. First, it is clear from a comparison of these spectra with the spectrum in Figure 5-13 that the fluid underlying the tectorial membrane was identical in its relative ionic composition to endolymph. We have consistently failed to find any evidence of sodium in this

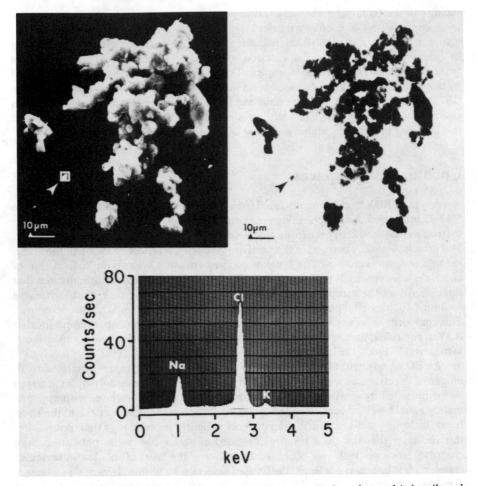

Figure 5-12. A scanning electron micrograph and EDXA spectrum from freeze-dried perilymph residue. The spectrum was obtained from the small crystal indicated by the arrowhead. The spectrum reflects approximately equal levels of sodium and chlorine, although the sodium peak is smaller due to this element's characteristically low X-ray emission rate, with potassium consisting of less than 1% of the total electrolyte content. A small peak in the calcium window, though not present in this example, is often observed in perilymph residue spectra. From Ryan and associates (1980).

fluid, as reported by Ross (1975). Second, the relative ionic composition of endolymph in the cochlea was identical to that in the utricle.

The EDXA data on cochlear fluids illustrate that the major and minor fluid compartments of the cochlea maintain their integrity during freezing and freeze-drying.

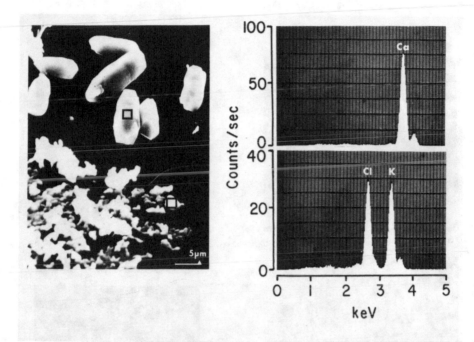

Figure 5-13. Otoconia and endolymph residue from the utricle, with associated EDXA spectra. The spectrum of the otoconium shows only the large α peak, and the smaller β peak, of calcium, since the carbon and oxygen of the carbonate radical emit X-rays too weak to be detected by EDXA. The endolymph spectrum indicates chlorine and potassium almost exclusively, with the latter predominating. (If the two were present in equal amounts, potassium emission would be only about 85% of chlorine emission, due to inherent differences in emission characteristics.) From Ryan and associates (1980).

Also, in the dry state the difficulties of obtaining uncontaminated samples of cochlear fluids are greatly reduced. In fact, obtaining pure samples of endolymph and peri-lymph residue by microdissection is relatively easy, and contaminated samples are rarely encountered if reasonable care is used in the sampling procedure.

Cochlear tissues

EDXA spectra were obtained from those tissues which can be isolated from adja-cent material. This can be accomplished with relative ease in the case of outer hair cells, stria vascularis, and the spiral ligament.

A typical EDXA spectrum from an individual outer hair cell is illustrated in Figure 5-15. The spectrum shows a content high in sodium, chlorine, and potassium. Signifi-cant levels of phosphorus and sulfur are also present. The spectrum is similar to that of many other tissues, such as muscle cells (Wroblewski, Roomans, Jansson, &

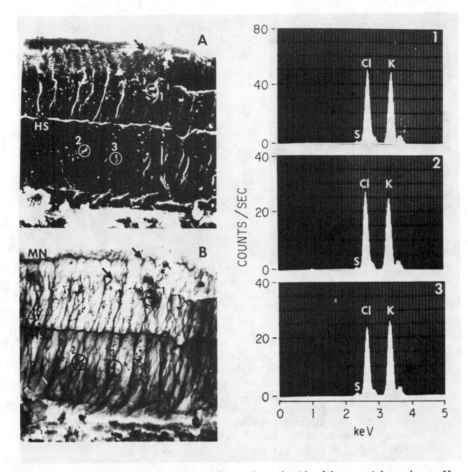

Figure 5-14. EDXA spectra from fluid residue on the underside of the tectorial membrane. Hensen's stripe (HS) and the marginal net (MN) are visible. Stereocilia from other hair cells (arrows) are difficult to distinguish from crystals of fluid residue in the secondary image. In the backscattered image, which reflects primarily specimen density, the sterocilia produce only faint ghosts, while the much denser fluid residue crystals produce an intense image. EDXA spectra (1–3) were obtained from the indicated crystals. In all cases, they share the ionic composition of endolymph residue (Figure 5-13). From Bone and Ryan (1982).

Edstrom, 1978), with the exception of elevated sodium and chlorine. The explanation for this may reside in the fluid which bathes much of the surface of the outer hair cells in vivo. Discrete crystals of fluid residue, such as those observed in the perilymphatic and endolymphatic spaces, were not found in the organ of Corti spaces. It has been suggested that "cortilymph" is similar to perilymph in ionic composition,

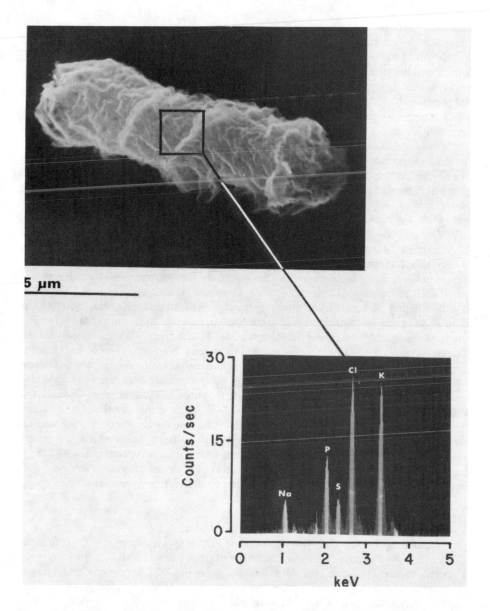

Figure 5-15. EDXA spectrum from the isolated fragment of an outer hair cell. The spectrum is dominated by chlorine and potassium, with lesser amounts of sodium, phosphorus, and sulfur. Perilymph substitution experiments suggest that the sodium and some of the chlorine in the spectrum are of extracellular origin, and represent "corti-lymph" dried on the surfaces of the cells.

although much higher in protein. Fluids with relatively high protein content do not precipitate as crystals during freeze-drying, but form an amorphous material. The high levels of sodium and chlorine in outer hair cell spectra may thus represent Corti-lymph residue precipitated on the outer surface of the hair cell. When the cochlea was perfused with artificial perilymph in which cobaltous chloride was substituted for sodium chloride, the sodium peak in the outer hair cell spectrum disappeared, while the potassium peak was unaffected. This also suggests that the sodium in outer hair cell spectra is extracellular in origin.

A typical EDXA spectrum obtained from the stria vascularis is shown in Figure 5-16. The spectrum shows high levels of phosphorus and potassium, with lower levels of chlorine, sulfur, and sodium. The spectrum characteristic of this tissue is unusual in the high level of phosphorus. Given the high rate of oxidative metabolism characteristic of this tissue (Ryan et al., 1982a; Thalmann et al., 1970) this may reflect inorganic phosphate associated with oxidative phosphorylation. Since there is very little extracellular space in the stria vascularis, the sodium in the strial spectrum is less likely to be of extracellular origin than is that in the outer hair cell spectrum. Strial sodium is also independent of the sodium in the perilymphatic compartment, since substitution of perilymphatic sodium did not change the strial spectrum, even though it eliminated sodium from spiral ligament spectra. Orsulakova, Morgenstern, and Kaufmann (1983), utilizing the LAMMA technique, recently reported that the potassium/sodium ratio of stria increases dramatically from the lateral edge to the luminal surface of the stria vascularis. To confirm this observation, EDXA spectra were obtained across a dry-sectioned stria sample, from the base adjacent to spiral ligament to the scala media surface. As illustrated in Figure 5-17, while the potassium content of the tissue was relatively constant across the tissue, the sodium content decreased substantially toward the scala media surface. This suggests that the changing ratios of Orsulakova and colleagues (1983) reflect lower levels of sodium in the marginal cells of stria vascularis than in the intermediate and basal cells. It has been suggested that the unique ionic composition of endolymph, and the resting potential of scala media, are generated by a Na/K ion transport system located in the stria vascularis. These EDXA data suggest that such a pump may be located at the intermediate cell/marginal cell border, with sodium directed into the intermediate cell compartment.

Effects of noise exposure

The effects of noise exposure on cochlear EDXA spectra were also investigated. Chinchillas were exposed to noise at intensities from 95 to 120 dB SPL for 1 hr. prior to sacrifice and preparation for EDXA. No changes in the EDXA spectra of endolymph, perilymph, and stria vascularis from the appropriate cochlear region were noted at any intensity. Outer hair cells could be reliably obtained only up to an exposure intensity of 105 dB SPL. At higher intensities, the cells were fragile and could only occasionally be recovered intact. After exposure to 105 dB SPL, however, EDXA spectra of outer hair cells were virtually identical to those from control subjects, as illustrated in Figure 5-18. A few outer hair cells were recovered from subjects following 110

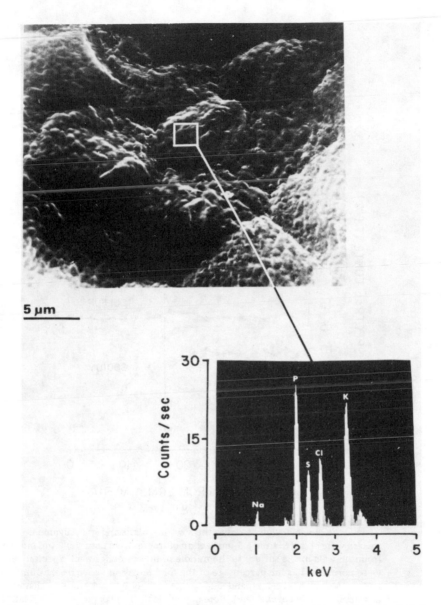

Figure 5-16. EDXA spectrum obtained from isolated stria vascularis. Note the high level of phosphorus and the appreciable sodium content. Although the measurement is obtained from the scala media surface of the stria, the electron beam penetrates to the back of the sample, and the spectrum represents the entire epithelium. From Bone and Ryan (1982).

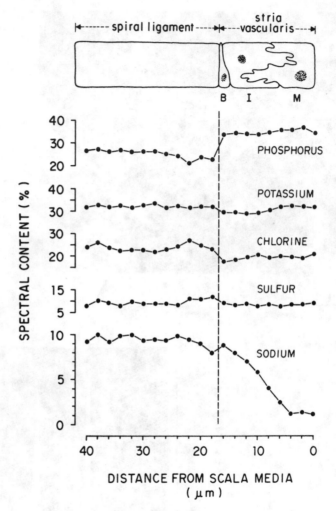

Figure 5-17. Variation in element content across the stria vascularis and spiral ligament. EDXA spectra were obtained from a 5-μm section of freeze-dried tissue, at 2-μm intervals, from the scala media surface to the middle of the spiral ligament. Spectral values were normalized as the percentage of the total emission above background. The scale for sodium has been expanded to compensate for its weak emission characteristics (about 24% that of chlorine). Note that while the level of potassium is relatively constant across both tissues, the percentage of sodium is much lower in the marginal cells of stria than it is in the intermediate or basal cells. The level of chlorine in the stria is also lower than that in the spiral ligament. These differences reflect the differing ionic content of these cell and tissue types. They also suggest that the site of active sodium transport in stria is at the marginal/intermediate cell border.

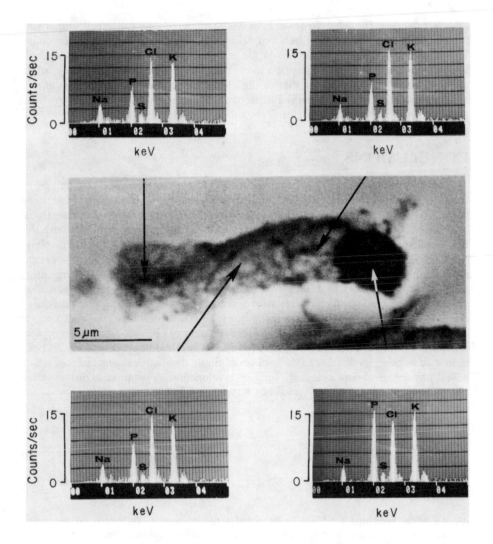

Figure 5-18. EDXA spectra obtained from an isolated outer hair cell which has been exposed for 1 hr. to 105 dB SPL noise. The scanning electron micrograph is a backscattered image which displays internal details such as the cell nucleus. Note that the spectra from the cytoplasmic region of the cell are identical to those of the normal outer hair cell in Figure 5-15. Thus there was no effect of noise exposure upon the element content of the cell. The spectrum from the nucleus shows higher phosphorus, which is typical of cell nuclei.

dB SPL exposure. Though insufficient cells were recovered for a statistical comparison, their spectra also appeared to be identical to those from normal outer hair cells.

In summary, the electron microprobe offers a new technique for the analysis of ion and other element composition in cochlear fluids and tissues. The resolution of this technique is essentially that of the electron microscope, and it thus allows a far closer correlation between ion content and anatomical location than has been possible with other methodologies.

CONCLUSIONS

Anatomical measures of physiologic function represent a methodology in its infancy, yet they have already provided information which could not have been obtained with conventional functional measures. Relationships between functional characteristics and anatomical structure can often be obtained more readily with this methodology than with other techniques. For example, it is possible to characterize the tonotopic organization of the entire auditory pathway of a species in a few experiments utilizing the 2-DG technique. This characterization would require a large number of electrophysiological studies over a much greater period of time. The precision with which physiological characteristics and anatomical location can be correlated can also be much greater with these techniques. Thus the question of the ionic content of the fluid underneath the tectorial membrane could not be resolved by micropipet techniques. Only with the development of EDXA methodology have the ions been identified as being identical with those of endolymph. As anatomical techniques which assess physiological parameters are further developed, they promise to provide even more insights into function in auditory structures.

REFERENCES

Anniko, M., & Nordemar, H. (1980). Embryogenesis of the inner ear. IV. Post-natal maturation of the stria vascularis in correlation with the elemental composition of endolymph. *Archives of Oto-Rhino-Laryngology, 229,* 281–288.

Anniko, M., & Wroblewski, R. (1980). Elemental composition of the mature inner ear. *Acta Otolaryngologica, 90,* 425–430.

Anniko, M., & Wroblewski, R. (1981). Elemental composition of the developing inner ear. *Annals of Otology, Rhinology and Laryngology, 90,* 25–32.

Bone, R.C., & Ryan, A.F. (1980). Cochlear ion shifts during progressive hypoxia. *Laryngoscope, 90,* 1169–1190.

Bone, R.C., & Ryan, A.F. (1982). Intracochlear microprobe analysis. *Laryngoscope, 92,* 385–389.

Bosher, S.K., & Warren, R.L. (1968). Observations on the electro-chemistry of the cochlear endolymph of the rat. *Proceedings of the Royal Society of London, 171,* 227–247.

Burgio, P.A. (1982). *Relation of tectorial membrane to Corti's organ, and nature of Cortilymph and infratectorial fluid: A scanning electron microscopic and X-ray microanalysis study.* Doctoral dissertation, University of Michigan.

Canlon, B., & Schacht, J. (1981). The effect of noise on deoxyglucose uptake into inner ear tissues of the mouse. *Archives of Oto-Rhino-Laryngology, 230,* 171–176.

Fex, J., & Altschuler, R.A. (1981). Enkephalin-like immunoreactivity of olivocochlear fibers in cochlea of guinea pig and cat. *Proceedings of the National Academy of Science, USA, 78,.* 1255–1259.

Flock, A. (1977). Electron probe determination of relative ion distribution in the inner ear. *Acta Otolaryngologica, 83,* 239–244.

Gulley, R.L., Fex, R.L., Wenthold, J., & Wenthold, R.J. (1970). Uptake of putative neurotransmitters in the organ of Corti. *Acta Otolaryngologica, 88,* 177–182.

Hoffman, D.W., Altschuler, R.A., & Fex, J. (1981). Enkephalinergic mechanisms in the cochlea. *Society for Neuroscience Abstacts, 7,* 95.

Hungerbuhler, J.P., Saunders, J.C., Greenberg, J., & Reivich, M. (1981). Functional neuroanatomy of the auditory cortex studied with (2-^{14}C) deoxyglucose. *Experimental Neurology, 71,* 104–121.

Hunter-Duvar, I., Landolt, I., & Cameron, R. (1981). X-ray microanalysis of fluid spaces in the frozen cochlea. *Archives of Oto-Rhino-Laryngology, 230,* 245–249.

Iverson, L.L., & Schon, F. (1973). The use of the autoradiographic techniques for the identification and mapping of transmitter-specific neurons in CNS. In A. Mandell (Ed.), *New concepts in transmitter regulation.* New York: Plenum.

Kane, E.S. (1977). Autoradiographic evidence of primary projections to the caudal cochlear nucleus in cats. *American Journal of Anatomy, 73,* 641–652.

Klinke, R. (1981). Neurotransmitters in the cochlea and the cochlear nucleus. *Acta Otolaryngologica, 91,* 541–554.

Klinke, R., & Oertel, W. (1977). Amino acids – putative afferent transmitter in the cochlea? *Experimental Brain Research, 30,* 145–148.

Krnjevic, K. (1981). Acetyl choline as modulator of amino-acid mediated synaptic transmission. In J.B. Lombardini & A.D. Kenney (Eds.), *The role of peptides and amino acids as neurotransmitters.* New York: Liss.

Marshall, A.T. (1975). Electron probe X-ray microanalysis. In M.A. Hoynt (Ed.), *Principles and techniques of scanning electron microscopy,* Vol. 4. New York: Reinhold.

Mesulam, M.-M., & Dichter, M. (1981). Concurrent acetylcholinesterase staining and γ-aminobutyric acid uptake of cortical neurons in culture. *Journal of Histochemistry and Cytochemistry, 29,* 306–308.

Pourcho, R.G. (1981). Autoradiographic localization of (^{3}H)muscimol in the cat retina. *Brain Research, 215,* 187–199.

Orsulakova, A., Morgenstern, K., & Kaufmann, R. (1983). The LAMMA technique in the studies of the inner ear. *Scanning Electron Microscopy,* 108–114.

Richrath, W., Kraus, H., & Fromme, H.D. (1974). Lokalisation von ^{3}H-γ-Amino- buttersaüre in der Cochlea. *Archives of Otorhinolaryngology, 208,* 283–293.

Ross, M.D. (1975). The tectorial membrane of the rat. *American Journal of Anatomy, 239,* 449–482.

Ryan, A.F., Goodwin, P., Woolf, N.K., & Sharp, F.R. (1982a). Auditory stimulation alters the pattern of 2-deoxyglucose uptake in the inner ear. *Brain Research, 234,* 213–225.

Ryan, A.F., Woolf, N.K., & Sharp, F.R. (1982b). Functional ontogeny in the central auditory pathway of the mongolian gerbil: A deoxyglucose study. *Experimental Brain Research, 47,* 428–436.

Ryan, A.F., Woolf, N.K., & Sharp, F.R. (1982c). Tonotopic organization in the central auditory pathway of the mongolian gerbil: A 2-deoxyglucose study. *Journal of Comparative Neurology,* 207, 369–380.

Ryan, A.F., & Schwartz, I.R. (1983). A biochemically distinct subpopulation of neurons in the spiral ganglion identified by preferential amino acid uptake. *Hearing Research,* 9, 173–184.

Ryan, A.F., & Sharp, F.R. (1982). Localization of (^{3}H) 2-deoxyglucose at the cellular level freeze-dried tissue and dry-looped emulsion. *Brain Research,* 252, 177–180.

Ryan, A.F., Wickham, M.G., & Bone, R.C. (1979). Element content of intracochlear fluids, outer hair cells and stria vascularis determined by energy dispersive X-ray analysis. *Otolaryngology,* 87, 659–665.

Ryan, A.F., Wickham, M.G., & Bone, R.C. (1980). Studies of ion distribution in the inner ear: Scanning electron microscopy and X-ray microanalysis of freeze-dried cochlear specimens. *Hearing Research,* 2, 1–20.

Ryan, A.F., & Woolf, N.K. (1983). Energy dispersive X-ray analysis of inner ear fluids and tissues during the ontogeny of cochlear function. *Scanning Electron Microscopy,* 201–207.

Schacht, J., & Canlon, B. (1981). The effect of noise exposure on deoxyglucose uptake in the inner ear of the mouse. *Neuroscience Abstracts,* 7, 535 (Abstract).

Schwartz, I.R., & Ryan, A.F. (1983). Differential labeling of sensory cell and neural populations in the organ of Corti following amino acid incubations. *Hearing Research,* 9, 185–200.

Scheich, H., Bonke, B.A., Bonke, H., & Langner, G. (1979). Functional organization of some auditory nuclei in the guinea fowl demonstrated by the 2-deoxyglucose technique. *Cell and Tissue Research,* 204, 17–27.

Sharp, F.R., Ryan, A.F., Goodwin, P., Woolf, N.K. (1981). Increasing intensities of wide-band noise increase ^{14}C-2-deoxyglucose uptake in gerbil central auditory structures. *Brain Research,* 230, 87–96.

Sokoloff, L., Reivich, M., Kennedy, C., DesRosiers, M.H., Patlak, C.S., Pettigrew, K.D., Kakaurda, O., & Shinohara, M. (1977). The deoxyglucose method for the measurement of local cerebral glucose utilization: Theory, procedure, and normal values in the conscious and anesthetized albino rat. *Journal of Neurochemistry,* 28, 13–36.

Spoendlin, H. (1979). Neural connections of the outer haircell system. *Acta Otolaryngologica,* 87, 381–387.

Thalmann, R., Comegys, T.H., & Arenberg, I.K. (1972). Evaluation of microdissected, unfixed, freeze-dried tissue for ultramicrochemical study. *Scanning Electron Microscopy,* 281–288.

Thalmann, I., Matschinsky, F.M., & Thalmann, R. (1970). Quantitative study of selected enzymes involved in energy metabolism of the cochlear duct. *Annals of Otology, Rhinology and Laryngology,* 79, 12–29.

Tousimis, A.J. (1969). A combined scanning electron microscopy and electron probe microanalysis of biological soft tissues. *Scanning Electron Microscopy,* 217–230.

Warr, W.B., & Guinan, J.J., Jr. (1979). Efferent innervation of the organ of Corti: Two separate systems. *Brain Research,* 173, 152–155.

Webster, W.R., Serviere, J., Batini, C., & Laplante, S. (1978). Autoradiographic demonstration with 2-(^{14}C)deoxyglucose of frequency selectivity in the auditory system of cats under conditions of functional activity. *Neuroscience Letters,* 10, 43–48.

Wroblewski, R., Roomans, G.M., Jansson, E., & Edstrom, L. (1978). Electron probe X-ray microanalysis of human muscle biopsies. *Histochemistry,* 55, 281–292.

Chapter 6

Inner Ear Function Based on the Mechanical Tuning of the Hair Cells[1]

Shyam M. Khanna

INTRODUCTION

Our understanding of the mechanical function of the inner ear has been steadily increasing. The recent discovery of the sharply turned basilar membrane frequency response in cat (Khanna & Leonard, 1980b; 1981a, 1982a,b) and confirmation of a similar sharply tuned response in the guinea pig cochlea (Sellick, Patuzzi, & Johnstone, 1982) forces us to reevaluate some of our basic concepts of the way the inner ear functions. An analysis and interpretation of these responses indicates that these sharply tuned responses originate in the mechanical tuning of the individual hair cell stereocilia (Khanna, 1983a).

This chapter reviews some of the current concepts of the inner ear mechanics and reinterprets them in light of the recent observations. It must be emphasized that the knowledge of the inner ear function is still quite incomplete and in many aspects lacking altogether. There are many reasons for this situation: (a) The physical dimensions of the cochlea are small; those of the hair cells and cilia even smaller; (b) The vibration amplitudes of the inner ear structures are extremely small; their measurement stretches present-day technology to its limits; (c) The organ of Corti, enclosed in a hard bony shell, is quite inaccessible. Attempts to gain access by opening the cochlea produce trauma and change its mechanical responses; (d) All measuring techniques at present produce some trauma and introduce artifacts in the measurements. In view of the above difficulties, it is not surprising that progress in this area has been slow.

SOME SOURCES OF TRAUMA IN OPENING THE COCHLEA

All basilar membrane measurement techniques at present require surgical opening of the cochlea. Access to the basilar membrane is gained by (a) enlarging the round

[1]Many thanks to M.C. Liberman, J.C. Saunders, L.G. Tilney, T.F. Weiss, and E.G. Wever for allowing me to use information from their papers and books still in press. This work was supported by NIH Grants 5K04 NS 00292 and 2R01 NS 03654.

window opening with a sharpened pick and knife (Johnstone, Taylor, & Boyle, 1970), picking and paring the bone of scala tympani of the first turn (Wilson & Johnstone, 1975), thinning the temporal bone with a dental burr (Rhode, 1971), drilling a hole through the petrous bone apical to the round window (Khanna & Leonard, 1981a), cauterizing and removing the round window membrane (Khanna & Leonard, 1982a), and shaving the first turn with a sharp scalpel (Sellick et al., 1982). The surgical procedures invariably produce some damage to the cochlea. The damage can be seen in the loss of round window cochlear microphonics (CM) response (Khanna & Leonard, 1981b), in the loss of N_1 response measured at the round window (LePage & Johnstone, 1980; Sellick et al., 1982; Wilson & Johnstone, 1975), and in the histological evaluation of the cochlea (Leonard & Khanna, 1984). The loss generally increases with time after opening the cochlea.

The extreme vulnerability of the cochlea to damage was not appreciated until recently. The damage is produced in a variety of ways: (a) Drilling of the bony wall of the cochlea produces trauma by mechanical vibration of the organ of Corti, by exposing the ear to the acoustical noise of the drill, and by the heating of the cochlea due to the frictional heat produced by drilling (Khanna & Leonard, 1981b; Leonard & Khanna, 1984). (b) Even the process of opening the bulla with forceps can produce loss in the cochlear action potential response above 16 kHz. The loss is apparently caused by the mechanical trauma produced by the fracturing of the bulla bone (Brown, Smith, & Nuttall, 1983a). The basal turns of the cochlea seem to be much more susceptible to trauma than the apical ones and the damage due to chipping the cochlear bone should be even more traumatic than that for the bulla bone because the cochlear bone surrounds the organ of Corti. (c) The cooling of the cochlea also produces a loss of high-frequency response. The temperature of the basal turn of the cochlea may be lowered due to heat loss when the middle ear is surgically exposed. Cochlear action potential (CAP) thresholds are elevated at frequencies above 16 kHz and their latencies are increased. The CAP threshold and latency increases are dependent on the degree of cooling and are reversible. Increases up to 38 dB were observed at 40 kHz (Brown et al., 1983b). (d) Cauterizing done to prevent bleeding from blood vessels in the round window membrane produces damage in the high-frequency region of the cochlea (Khanna & Leonard, 1981a, 1982a). Trauma is produced by the heat of the cautery and by the flow of electric current due to the tip potential. (e) In addition to the damage introduced in the process of opening the cochlea, the opened cochlea itself results in additional damage, which accumulates with time.

In an intact cochlea slow pressure changes associated with the flow of perilymph in scala vestibuli are equalized through the helicotrema, so that the pressure is of the same magnitude in the scala vestibuli and scala tympani. As a consequence, these low-frequency pressure changes are not sensed by the organ of Corti. This situation changes when a hole is made in the scala tympani. The pressure in the scala tympani now remains at an atmospheric level while the pressure in the scala vestibuli fluctuates. This pressure differential or the one between scala media and scala tympani acts as a traumatizing stimuli to the cochlea and produces damage to the hair cells. The resulting displacements of the basilar membrane due to the pressure differential and due to the damaging process are often so large that they can be easily seen with a low power [10 × magnification] microscope. The estimated equivalent sound pressure needed to produce such large displacements must exceed 140 dB SPL. The damage can be observed histologically at the apical end where the cochlear partition is more sensitive to low-frequency stimulation (Leonard & Khanna, 1984). Thus, from the moment a hole is made in one of the scala, the entire cochlea is subjected to this course of trauma. In addition, the very large amplitude of the basilar membrane deflection at low frequencies may mask or alter the response measured at the basal end with the high-frequency signals.

TRAUMA AND ARTIFACT DUE TO MEASUREMENT TECHNIQUES

Trauma and artifact may also be introduced by the measuring techniques themselves. Basilar membrane measurements have been made in the past using four basic measurement techniques: (a) Mössbauer method; (b) capacitive probe; (c) interferometry; and (d) speckle interferometry.

Mössbauer Method

A highly radioactive source approximately 70 μm^2 in area is placed on the basilar membrane. The source emits γ rays. An absorber and detector sensitive to γ rays are arranged so that the γ rays penetrating the absorber are detected. When the source vibrates, the emitted γ rays are frequency modulated due to Doppler shift and undergo varying absorption. These absorption–time functions are utilized to obtain magnitude and phase of the unknown vibration velocity. The details of the method and its application to basilar membrane measurements are described by a number of investigators (Gunderson et al., 1978; Helfenstein, 1973; Hillman, 1964; Johnstone & Boyle, 1967; Johnstone et al., 1970; Johnstone & Yates, 1974; Peake & Ling, 1980; Rhode, 1971, 1973, 1974; 1977, 1978, 1980; Rhode & Robles, 1974; Robles, Rhode, & Geisler, 1976; Sellick et al., 1982; Yates & Johnstone, 1979).

The following considerations are important when interpreting the measurements from Mössbauer experiments: (i) The source may not be vibrating with the underlying basilar membrane. (ii) The source may be mechanically loading the vibrating system and altering its response. These two considerations also apply to the interferometric methods, in which a mirror is placed on the basilar membrane (Khanna & Leonard, 1981b, 1982a). (iii) The radioactivity of the source may damage the hair cells in its vicinity, thus altering the local mechanical response of the system. The dose rate from a typical source used in Rhode's Mössbauer experiments, at a distance of 10μm from the foil, has been calculated to be approximately 100 Gy per hour (Kliauga & Khanna, 1983). This high-radiation dose is injurious to the delicate sensory cells. A thirty times stronger radioactive source has been utilized by Sellick and colleagues (1982) in their experiments. They find that the observed basilar membrane vibration amplitude for a given sound pressure decreases progressively. The thresholds of the click evoked action potentials recorded at the round window also increase with time, a result that reflects increasing damage to the cochlea. During the course of an experiment losses up to 50 dB were encountered. Since large change in the sensitivity occur mainly in the sharply tuned tip region and increase progressively with time, the shape of the frequency response curve would depend very much on the order of frequencies at which the measurements are made. If the measurements are made first at the center frequency (when the vibration sensitivity is highest) and later at other frequencies (when the sensitivity has decreased), the sharpness of tuning will be enhanced due to this experimental artifact.

An important point is that the observed decrease in vibration sensitivity in the tip region is most probably produced by damage to the hair cells by the strongly radioactive source.

Capacitive Probe

The method is based upon the measurement of capacitance between the vibrating object and a test probe. The details of the method vary among investigators (von Békésy, 1960; Fischler, Frei, Spira, & Rubinstein, 1967; LePage & Johnstone, 1980; Møller, 1963; Wilson, 1973). To measure basilar membrane vibrations, the capacitive probe is placed close to the membrane after draining the fluid in the scala tympani. This technique of measurement has two problems associated with it: (i) Draining of perilymph was shown to produce a loss in sensitivity and the frequency selectivity of the cochlear neurons in the sharply tuned tip region (Robertson, 1974). Sharply tuned basilar membrane responses have not been observed with the capacitive probe. It is likely that draining of the perilymph alters the normal mechanical response of the cochlea. (ii) The measuring probe applies a strong radio frequency (rf) field to the organ of Corti. The magnitude of the rf current flowing into the tissue through the measuring tip is highly variable. It is dependent upon the type of probe used, on the capacitance between the probe and the tissue, and on the amplitude, frequency, and impedance of the rf source. At the very minimum, the current density in the tissue may be of the order of 60 mA/cm^2. It is likely that this would damage hair cells in the vicinity of the probe. If, during the measurements, the fluid level increased and contacted the probe, the current would increase dramatically and produce extensive damage of the tissue near the probe.

Interferometry

A variety of interferometric techniques are now available and have been applied to the vibration measurement of biological structures (Hill, Schubert, Nokes, & Michelson, 1977; Khanna, 1983; Khanna, Tonndorf, & Walcott, 1968; Nokes, Hill, & Barelli, 1978). Of these techniques, only one (Khanna) has been applied to the basilar membrane measurements in living animals (cats). This technique requires the placement of a mirror on the basilar membrane. The mirrors used were gold crystals roughly $70\mu m^2$ in area and weighing about 10^{-8} g. The weight of the mirrors and the source used in the Mössbauer experiments are comparable. The placement of a mirror seems to alter the response of the inner ear system as seen in the sound pressure changes in the ear canal before and after the placement of the mirror (Khanna & Leonard, unpublished observations). The other problem with this method is the uncertainty that the mirror will vibrate with the same amplitude as the basilar membrane. Of all the methods available at present this is the most sensitive and has been used to measure basilar membrane vibration amplitude as low as 10^{-9} cm (20 dB s/n) in living animals (Khanna & Leonard, 1982a).

Speckle Interferometry

In this technique, incident light from a He Ne laser is scattered from the basilar membrane and the resultant speckle pattern is utilized for vibration measurement. In the earliest application of this technique the eye was used as a detector and, therefore, the sensitivity of vibration detection was quite low (Kohllöffel, 1972a,b,c). A more modern technique based on light scattering was described by Dragsten, Webb, Paton, & Capranica (1974a,b, 1976). This technique was applied to the measurement of acoustic receptors in crickets (Paton, Capranica, Loftus-Hill, Dragsten, & Webb, 1974). An electronic speckle pattern interferometric method developed by Lockberg and his associates was utilized to measure the basilar membrane vibrations in human cadaver ears by Neiswander and Slettemoen (1981).

A fiberoptic technique was used by Albe, Schwab, Smigielski, and Dancer (1982) to measure basilar membrane vibrations in guinea pig ears. These speckle techniques are highly desirable as they do not require placement of a mirror on the basilar membrane. Their vibration sensitivity is, however, low at present as compared to the methods utilizing mirrors. This loss of sensitivity occurs because the basilar membrane is nearly transparent. This low reflectivity leads to a second complication; the light intensity required for measurements is much higher, and high light intensity produces damage to the cochlea.

In spite of the availability of so many measuring techniques, at present none of them is quite satisfactory; all produce trauma and introduce artifact into the measurements.

BASILAR MEMBRANE MECHANICAL RESPONSE MEASURED BY LASER INTERFEROMETER

Vibration amplitude of the basilar membrane (BM) was measured at the basal end of the cochlea in living cats using a round window approach (Khanna & Leonard, 1980b, 1981a, 1982a,b). The theoretical basis of interferometry is discussed by Khanna (1983) and the technical details of the method and hardware used are described elsewhere (Khanna, Johnson, & Jacobs, 1983).

In the course of our initial basilar membrane experiments it was discovered that procedures employed to gain access to the basilar membrane were producing trauma to the organ of Corti; some of these problems have been discussed above. The observations of cochlear damage prompted the introduction of new experimental procedures which emphasize extreme caution to minimize cochlear damage. After the introduction of these improvements, basilar membrane measurements using a round window approach showed a different frequency response curve (Khanna & Leonard, 1981a, 1982a) as compared to those obtained previously (Khanna & Leonard, 1981b).

SHARP TUNING OF THE BASILAR MEMBRANE RESPONSE AND ITS SUSCEPTIBILITY TO TRAUMA

In most experiments the basilar membrane tuning curve could be repeated at least twice with good agreement. However, from experiment to experiment the tuning curves obtained varied considerably. Representative tuning curves obtained from three different animals are shown in Figure 6-1. The sound pressure level (SPL) required to obtain a basilar membrane vibration amplitude of 10^{-8} cm is plotted as a function of frequency (Khanna & Leonard, 1982a.) These isoresponse curves show a shallow minimum in the frequency region of 0.25–3 kHz, a relatively flat (plateau) region between 5 and 14 kHz, and a sharply tuned negative peak (tip) at approximately 23 kHz. The presence of such a sharply tuned tip in the mechanical frequency response was quite surprising. Tuning curves with tip-to-tail ratios exceeding 25 dB (center frequency [CF] to 1 kHz) were observed in at least five experiments. A similar sharply tuned region in the guinea pig basilar membrane response has since been shown by Sellick and colleagues (1982).

There is excellent agreement in data below 2 kHz from the three animals. The largest differences are seen in the sharply tuned tip region. The observed variability in the tip region is due to variable damage to the cochlea. Animals in which higher SPL was required to produce the index mechanical response also showed a higher degree of histological damage (Leonard & Khanna, 1984).

The sharply tuned tip region in the guinea pig basilar membrane frequency response was also found to be highly susceptible to trauma. Increased sound pressure levels were required to obtain an index basilar membrane response, as the condition of the cochlea (measured by click evoked action potentials) deteriorated with time (Sellick et al., 1982).

After the loss of sharp tuning due to cochlear damage, the basilar membrane response exhibits the characteristics of a low-pass filter. This type of response has been measured by a large number of investigators (von Békésy, 1960; Evans & Wilson, 1975, Johnstone & Boyle, 1967; Johnstone, Taylor, & Boyle, 1970; Johnstone & Yates, 1974; Kohllöffel, 1972a,b,c; Rhode, 1971, 1973, 1974, 1978, 1980; Wilson & Johnstone, 1972, 1975).[2] Vibration amplitude of the basilar membrane is shown in Figure 6-2, as a function of frequency for constant SPL at the tympanic membrane (Rhode, 1978),

---

[2]Helfenstein (1973) obtained sharply tuned basilar membrane responses. However, he had glued his radioactive source on the basilar membrane and his tuning frequency (CF) for the place of measurement was roughly half of that obtained by other investigators at that time. It was assumed that the gluing process introduced artifacts in his measurements (Evans & Wilson, 1977).

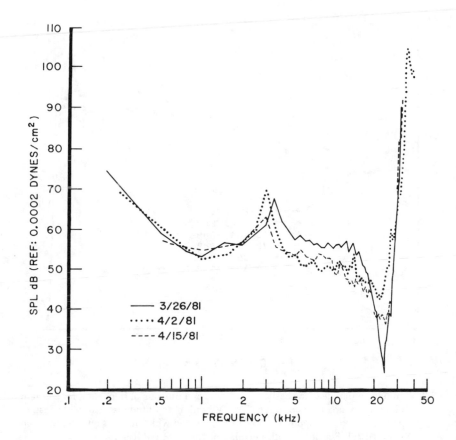

Figure 6-1. Sound pressure level at the tympanic membrane (cat) required to produce a basilar membrane displacement of 10^{-8} cm (bulla open, septum intact). Data from three animals are compared. Note that large differences occur mainly in the frequency region 15 to 25 kHz. A sharply tuned response is seen in one of the animals, 3/26/81. From Khanna and Leonard (1982). Reprinted with permission from the publisher.

and illustrates this low-pass filter characteristic. The remnants of the sharply tuned response are visible at approximately 7 kHz.

Extensive theoretical work has been carried out and at this point the low-pass characteristics of the basilar membrane response are well understood in terms of the mechanical and hydrodynamic properties of the system (Allen, 1977; De Boer, 1979; Siebert, 1974; Sondhi, 1978; Steele, 1974; Steele & Taber, 1980; Zweig, Lipes, & Pierce, 1976; Zwislocki, 1948, 1953).

From these observations we conclude that the mechanical response observed at the basilar membrane consists of two components: (i) *a low-pass filter type of response*

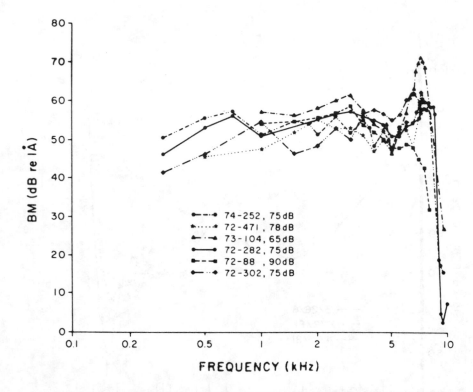

Figure 6-2. Vibration amplitude of the basilar membrane as a function of frequency, for constant SPL at the tympanic membrane (TM). Vibration amplitude is relatively constant up to a frequency of approximately 8 kHz, beyond which it drops off steeply. From Rhode (1978). Reprinted with permission from the publisher.

which is dependent mainly on the basilar membrane mechanical properties and is relatively immune to trauma and (ii) *a sharply tuned response located near the cut-off point of the low-pass system. This later response is highly susceptible to trauma.* Due to this high susceptibility to trauma the sharply tuned part of the response was missed by most of the previous investigators.

ORIGIN OF SHARP TUNING

Where does the sharply tuned response originate? We can get some insight into it by comparing the tuning curves and other data obtained at the basilar membrane, at the hair cell, and at the auditory nerve fiber levels, and by noting their similarities and differences.

Comparison of Basilar Membrane and Neural Tuning Curves

The SPL required to obtain a basilar membrane vibration amplitude of 3×10^{-8} cm in cat was compared with a neural tuning curve obtained by Liberman from a cat primary auditory fiber at similar center frequency (Figure 6-3). The low-frequency slope of 86 dB/oct., the high-frequency slope of 538 dB/oct., and the Q_{10} of 5.0 for the mechanical tuning curve were all comparable with those seen in the neural tuning curve. The principal difference was in the tip-to-tail ratio, which was 30 dB for the mechanical tuning curve and 44 dB for the neural tuning curve (Khanna & Leonard, 1982a). Similar agreement between the basilar membrane and an auditory nerve fiber tuning curve was found in the guinea pig ear (Sellick et al., 1982). These comparisons indicate that the sharply tuned portion of the basilar membrane mechanical response is as frequency selective as the neural tuning curve. The similarity in the shape of the two curves in the tip region suggests that they have a common origin.

Effect of Trauma on the Basilar Membrane and Nerve Fiber Tuning Curves

Trauma to the cochlea alters the mechanical response in the following ways: (i) The sensitivity in the tip region is reduced. (ii) The CF of the peak moves to a lower frequency. (iii) Both the high-frequency and low-frequency slopes in the peak region become less steep (Khanna & Leonard, 1980a, 1982a; Leonard & Khanna 1984; Sellick et al., 1982). Acoustic trauma also alters the tuning of the auditory neurons in the guinea pig cochlea: (i) Neural sensitivity in the peak region is reduced by as much as 90 dB. The reduction is dependent on the intensity and duration of the traumatizing tone. (ii) The CF moved down to lower frequencies. The amount is dependent on the intensity and duration of the traumatizing tone. Frequency shifts of up to an octave are seen. (iii) Both low- and high-frequency slopes of the FTC (frequency threshold curves) are reduced (Cody & Johnstone, 1980).

These comparisons show that trauma produces basically similar changes in the basilar membrane and nerve fiber tuning curves. There are, however, notable differences in the magnitudes of these changes, which are much smaller at the basilar membrane. If these changes occurred at the basilar membrane level their magnitude at the nerve fiber level should be the same but not greater.

Comparison Between Basilar Membrane and Hair Cell Nonlinearity

The nonlinearity in the basilar membrane mechanical response was discovered by Rhode in the squirrel monkey cochlea (Rhode, 1971, 1977, 1978, 1980; Rhode & Robles, 1974; Robles & Rhode, 1974; Robles et al., 1976). This nonlinearity extended

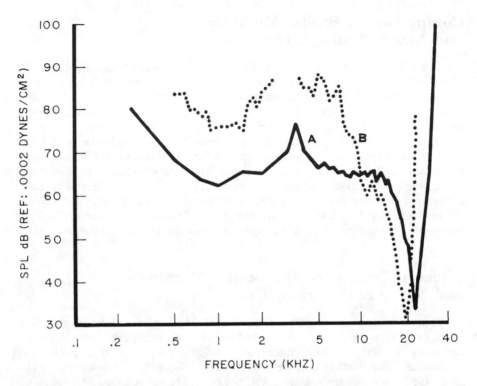

Figure 6-3. Solid line: SPL at the tympanic membrane required to produce 3×10^{-8} cm basilar membrane vibration amplitude in cat 3/26/81. Dotted line: neural tuning curve based on an isorate contour of 10 spikes per second above the spontaneous rate (Liberman, personal communication). The two curves have very similar characteristics in the peak region (20 kHz). The main difference is in the peak-to-tail (1 kHz) ratio: 44 dB for the neural tuning curve and 30 dB for the basilar membrane tuning curve. From Khanna and Leonard (1982). Reprinted with permission from the publisher.

from frequencies less than an octave below CF to frequencies in the cut-off region of the response. The responses were linear at frequencies lower than an octave below CF (Figure 6-4). These nonlinear properties of the basilar membrane response have also been seen in the guinea pig ear (Sellick et al., 1982). Basilar membrane velocity increased nonlinearly as a function of sound pressure only in the sharply tuned tip region. The nonlinearity extended from about 0.5 octave below CF to 0.5 octave above CF. The nonlinearity decreased rapidly with increasing cochlear trauma (Sellick et al., 1982) and disappeared at death (Rhode, 1973).

Nonlinearities in the dc receptor potential of the guinea pig hair cells are also located in the sharply tuned portion and the high-frequency cut-off region of the hair cell response (Figure 6-5). Damage to the cochlea results in broadly tuned hair

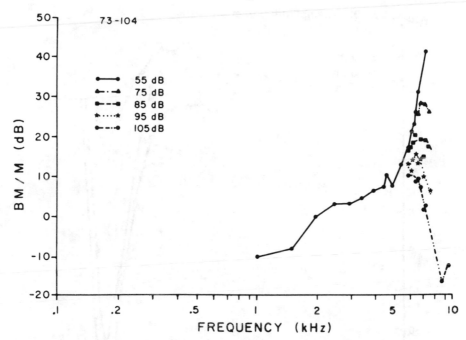

Figure 6-4. The ratio of basilar membrane and malleus vibration amplitude as a function of frequency. In the frequency region 6–8 kHz the ratio is highly dependent on the SPL used for measurement. Below 6 kHz only one curve is drawn because the results are always linear in that region. From Rhode (1980). Reprinted with permission from the publisher.

cell responses and in these traumatized cells the receptor potential rises more linearly with sound pressure level (Sellick & Russell, 1978).

Nonlinearities in the basilar membrane and hair cell responses are found only in the tip region around the center frequency. Trauma reduces nonlinearities in both basilar membrane and hair cell response. This similarity suggests that the basilar membrane and the hair cells have a common basis for nonlinear behavior. It has been shown that the mechanical response of the hair cell stereocilia bundle in guinea pig cochlea is nonlinear (Strelioff & Flock, 1982). Therefore, it is the nonlinearity of the hair cell mechanical response that is seen at the basilar membrane due to the mechanical coupling between the two.

Difference in Susceptibility to Trauma Between the Basilar Membrane and the Hair Cell Electrical Responses

The basic surgical technique of opening the cochlea is very similar in the basilar membrane measurements, in the intracellular hair cell response measurements, and

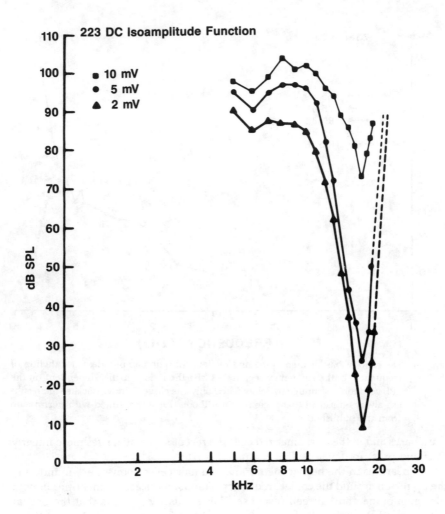

Figure 6-5. SPL required to produce 2, 5, and 10 mV dc receptor potential in an inner hair cell of a guinea pig cochlea. Note that the relationship between SPL and the receptor potential is nonlinear mainly in the sharply tuned portion of the curve. From Sellick and Russell (1978). Reprinted with permission from the publisher.

in the recording of response from the single auditory nerve fibers in the spiral ganglion. The magnitude of the trauma would be expected to be similar in these three types of experiments. Sharply tuned responses are obtained routinely for the single hair cell tuning curves (Dallos, Santos-Sacchi, & Flock, 1982; Russell & Sellick, 1977a,b,

1978; Sellick & Russell, 1978), and for the auditory nerve fibers of the spiral ganglion (Cody & Johnstone, 1980; Cody, Robertson, Bredberg, & Johnstone, 1980; Robertson, 1974; Robertson et al., 1980; Robertson & Manley, 1974), but not for the basilar membrane (Albe et al., 1982; Békésy, 1960; Evans & Wilson, 1975; Johnstone & Boyle, 1967; Johnstone et al., 1970; Johnstone & Yates, 1974; Kohllöffel, 1927a,b,c; Neiswander & Slettemoen, 1981; Rhode, 1971; Wilson & Johnstone, 1972, 1975). Therefore, the sharply tuned portion of the basilar membrane response must be much more susceptible to trauma.

If the sharp tuning originated at the basilar membrane and the trauma produced a loss of the sharp tuning, then the tuning of the hair cells and nerve fibers should be similarly affected. The difference in sensitivity to trauma, therefore, clearly indicates that the sharply tuned portion of the response does not originate at the basilar membrane.

Differences Between Hair Cell and Basilar Membrane Tuning

When the sound pressure required to produce 2 mV receptor potential in a hair cell is considered as a function of frequency (Sellick & Russell, 1978), several important features become evident (Figure 6-6). At the most sensitive frequency (CF) the SPL required to reach index is between −5 and +10 dB. An octave below CF, however, the SPL increases to about 90 dB (at frequencies below this there is no appreciable increase in SPL and the curve flattens out). The change in the SPL from an octave below CF to CF is roughly 80 dB. When similar comparisons are made for the mechanical tuning curves obtained at the basilar membrane (Khanna & Leonard, 1982a; Sellick et al., 1982), it is apparent that the increase in SPL from CF to an octave below CF is between 30 and 40 dB (Figure 6-6).

Thus, the height of the sharp part of the tuning curve seen at the hair cell is about one-hundred times larger than that seen at the basilar membrane. The height of the response is much larger at the hair cell because it originates there. This also suggests that the mechanical vibration amplitudes at the hair cell may be much higher than those observed at the basilar membrane. Due to the loose coupling between the hair cells and the basilar membrane only a small part (1%) of the hair cell mechanical response is seen at the basilar membrane. (The loose coupling may be a consequence of the cochlear damage in basilar membrane experiments.) (See chap. 7 for discussion of the importance and significance of coupling at the tectorial membrane.)

Histological Correlation Between the Condition of the Outer Hair Cells (OHC) and Basilar Membrane Tuning

The most direct evidence that hair cells affect basilar membrane mechanical response comes from the histological analysis of the cochleae used in basilar mem-

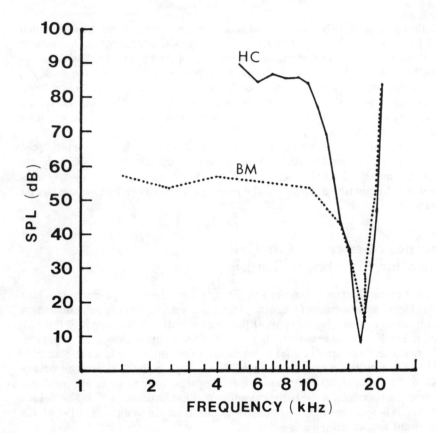

Figure 6-6. Comparison between the hair cell and basilar membrane tuning. Solid line: SPL required to produce 2 mV dc receptor potential in an inner hair cell of a guinea pig cochlea (from Sellick & Russell, 1978). Dotted line: SPL required to produce basilar membrane vibration amplitude of 3.5×10^{-8} cm in the basal turn of the guinea pig cochlea. Note differences between the two curves below 14 kHz. From Sellick et al. (1982). Reprinted with permission from the publisher.

brane experiments. (i) The SPL required to produce 10^{-8} cm basilar membrane vibration amplitude at CF, plotted as a function of percentage of damaged OHC (hair cell damage is measured in a region $\pm 5\%$ distance from the point of measurement) shows that the SPL increases with increased OHC damage (Leonard & Khanna, 1984). (ii) The CF of the basilar membrane mechanical tuning curves, plotted as a function of percentage of OHC damage, shows that the CF decreases as the damage increases (Leonard & Khanna, 1984). These observations demonstrate that both the sensitivity and the tuning of the basilar membrane are related to the condition of the outer hair cells.

In the histological study by Leonard and Khanna it was not possible to evaluate the condition of the basilar membrane and the supporting cells using optical microscopy. It is possible that these structures were also damaged along with the hair cells. The observed CF and sensitivity changes may then be explained in terms of changes in the basilar membrane mechanical properties.

The cochleae used for the interferometric studies of basilar membrane mechanics were examined with a transmission electron microscope and their ultrastructure was compared to that of the control cochlea on the contralateral side. The structures most severely damaged in the experimental cochleae are the outer hair cells and the radial afferent fibers to the inner hair cells. The basilar membrane, the pillar cells, and the tectorial membrane are not different in the experimental and control cochleae. The basilar membrane and the supporting cells are morphologically normal (Kelly & Khanna, 1984). These observations support the view that the mechanical changes seen at the basilar membrane are due to damage to the outer hair cells.

TUNING IN INNER EARS WITHOUT BASILAR MEMBRANE

The animal species without a basilar membrane include frogs, toads, salamanders, apodans, and caecilians. Amphibians, in general, have two auditory organs, an amphibian and a basilar papilla. These are shown in Figures 6-7 and 6-8, respectively (Wever, 1984).

The amphibian papilla is located at the octocranial septum and is seated on a limbic plate attached to a bony shelf. The limbic plate has holes in it and a single hair cell is supported in each hole. Ciliary tufts attached to the end of the hair cells extend out of these holes. These hair cells are supported by completely stationary structures and only their cilia are movable. The transfer of vibratory motion of the fluid to the ciliary tufts is accomplished in two ways: (i) tectorial tissue attached to the ciliary tufts pick up the vibration from the fluid; (ii) a thin sheet of tectorial tissue (sensing membrane) extends from a rigid attachment along one edge. The medial edge of this tissue is attached to the hair tufts. The fluid vibrations are thus sensed by this membrane and transmitted to the hair cells (Wever, personal communication).

The location of the basilar papilla varies with the species but is always found in a cavity that may be derived from the saccule (frog), lagena (salamander), or utricle (caecilian). The hair cells in the basilar papilla of all amphibians are supported by the limbic plate in a manner similar to that of the amphibian papilla. The bony support of the limbic plate in this case, however, is relatively thin as compared to that for the amphibian papilla (Wever, personal communication).

It is clear that in the case of the amphibian papilla the only stimulus acting on the hair cells is the mechanical stimulation of the stereocilia. There is no other means of transmitting mechanical stimuli to the hair cells. Similar considerations apply to the basilar papilla.

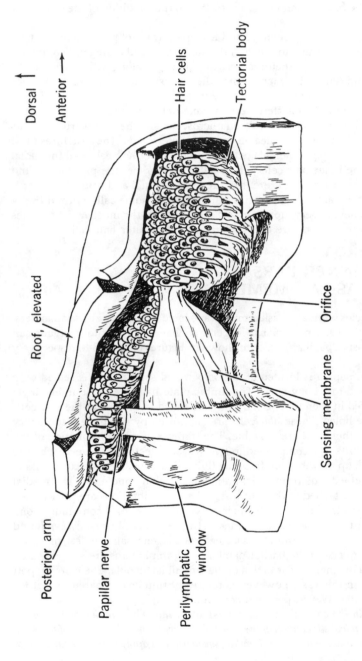

Dorsal ↑

Anterior →

Hair cells

Tectorial body

Roof, elevated

Orifice

Sensing membrane

Posterior arm

Papillar nerve

Perilymphatic window

Amphibian papilla (rana pipiens)

Figure 6-7. The hair cells in the amphibian papilla of frog hang from a stationary bony surface (roof). Stimulation of these hair cells occurs via the tectorial tissue attached to the hair cell cilia. From Wever (1973). Reprinted with permission from the publisher.

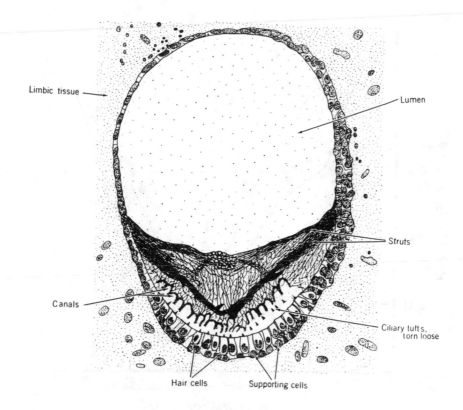

Basilar papilla   (rana pipiens)

Figure 6-8. The hair cells in the basilar papilla of frog are also seated on the stationary surface. There is no basilar membrane and the stimulation of the hair cells is via the tectorial tissue attached to the hair cell cilia. From Wever (1973). Reprinted with permission from the publisher.

NERVE FIBER TUNING IN THE PAPILLA OF AMPHIBIANS

Tuning of the auditory nerve fibers arising from the amphibian and basilar papilla have been measured in the leopard frog, tree frog, Puerto Rican tree frog, bull frog, bufonid toad, and spadefoot toad (Axelrod, 1960; Capranica & Moffat, 1974a,b, 1975; Frishkopf & Goldstein, 1963; Moffat & Capranica, 1974; Liff, 1969; Narins & Capranica, 1976). The responses show typical sharp v-shaped tuning curves (Figure 6-9),

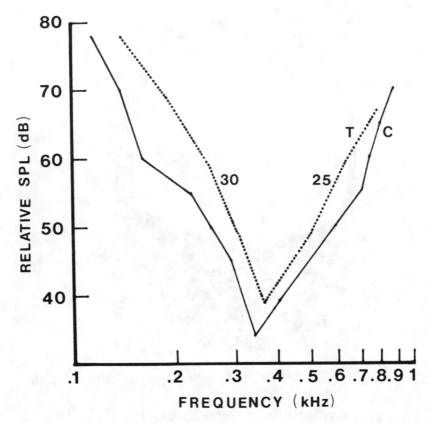

Figure 6-9. Comparison of frequency tuning curves of a single auditory nerve fiber from the amphibian papilla of *Bufo americanus* (redrawn from Capranica & Moffat, 1980), with that obtained from cat (redrawn from Kiang et al., 1965). The shape of the FTC in the two cases is quite similar although their slopes at these low frequencies are shallow (30 and 25 dB/oct.).

similar to those observed in other vertebrates with Q_{10} values between 1 and 4 (Capranica & Moffat, 1975, 1980). *Since both the amphibian and the basilar papilla lack a basilar membrane and the hair cells rest on stationary supporting structures, their frequency selectivity (tuning) must be determined solely by the mechanical properties of the tectorial membrane and the hair cell cilia* (Capranica, 1978).

DIRECT MEASUREMENT OF STEREOCILIA TUNING

In the alligator lizard cochlea there is a basilar membrane and the hair cells have free-standing stereocilia. It has been shown that the basilar membrane is not sharply tuned (Weiss, Peake, Ling, & Holton, 1978). Direct measurement of vibration of the hair bundles in excised cochleae by Holton and Hudspeth has shown that "the angular displacement of hair bundles is frequency selective and tonotopically organized. Long hair bundles move selectively at low frequencies, whereas short hair bundles move selectively at high frequencies." (Holton & Hudspeth, 1983).

THE BASIS OF HAIR CELL TUNING

The stiffness and mass of the stereocilia bundle and the associated tectorial tissue are important parameters in determination of the hair cell resonance properties. From the differences in the mechanical and physical properties of the tectorial tissue and the stereocilia it is clear that stereocilia are much stiffer than the associated tectorial tissue. This concept is based on the observations of Flock (1977) that the stereocilia are brittle. The resonance of the system is, therefore, probably determined mainly by the stereocilia stiffness, mass, and the mass of the tectorial tissue and associated fluid which is coupled to the vibrating structures.

Direct determination of stereocilia stiffness has been attempted in the crista ampularis of the semicircular canal in the frog (Flock, Flock, & Murray, 1977). In the organ of Corti of the guinea pig, the stiffness is found to increase from the apex to base (Strelioff & Flock, 1982). Stereocilia height decreases from the apex to the base. Stereocilia stiffness is, therefore, related to the physical dimensions of the stereocilia. There is growing evidence that the physical dimensions of the stereocilia are tonotopically organized along the cochlea. For example, in neonatal chicks the stereocilia height was shown to be inversely related to the frequency of tuning (Tilney & Saunders, 1982a). Quantitative analysis showed that (i) stereocilia height is 5.3 μm at the distal end and 1.5 μm at the proximal end; (ii) the number of stereocilia per hair cell increased from distal end (50) to proximal end (300); and (iii) diameter of individual cilia increased from distal to proximal end (Tilney & Saunders, 1982a). The net effect of each of these changes is to increase the stiffness of the stereocilia bundle and decrease its mass from the distal (low-frequency) to the proximal (high-frequency) end.

The inverse relationship between the stereocilia height and frequency of tuning has been observed for many other species: alligator lizard (Weiss et al., 1978), granite spiny lizard (Turner, Muraski, & Nielsen, 1981), mouse (Garfinkle & Saunders, 1983), chinchilla (Lim, 1980), squirrel monkey, cat (Lim, 1982), and man (Wright, 1981).

Stereocilia dimensions are organized systematically in all species of animals studied so far. They include reptiles, birds, and mammals. *The physical dimensions of the stereocilia (diameter, height, number) are organized along the length of the auditory sensory organ in such a way that the hair cells which respond to higher frequencies have stiffer ciliary tufts. In amphibians there are no other resonant structures and it is easy to see that the mechanical resonance of the stereocilia must provide the hair cell tuning. Similar conclusions were reached for an animal with basilar membrane, with respect to the tuning of the free-standing hair cells in the basilar papilla of an alligator lizard* (Weiss et al., 1978). *The systematic tonotopic organization of stereocilia in reptiles, birds, and mammals strongly suggests that the stereocilia provide the tuning of the hair cells in these animals.*

MECHANICAL PROPERTIES OF THE STEREOCILIA RELATED TO THEIR INTERNAL MICROSTRUCTURE

The finding of actin filaments in the stereocilia of vestibular hair cells (Flock, 1977) and the description of their precise structural organization in the stereocilia of the hair cells in the inner ear (De Rosier, Tilney, & Egelman, 1980; De Rosier & Tilney, 1982; Tilney et al., 1980) has been a major breakthrough in understanding the microstructural properties of stereocilia. These findings indicate that in each cilia there are thousands of double helical actin filaments which lie parallel to each other. The spacing between these filaments is precisely determined and the cross over points of their helices are in register. Adjacent filaments are connected by cross bridges at specific sites along the filament. These bridges are perpendicular to the axis of actin filaments. The presence of the cross bridges increases the stiffness of the structure (Tilney et al., 1980). The rigidity of a cilium is thus basically determined by the length and number of the actin filaments and the number of cross bridges (Tilney et al., 1983). The actin filaments decrease in number near the base at its junction with cuticular plate. In the alligator lizard a single stereocilium may contain as many as 3000 actin filaments at the tip; however, these reduce to only 25 filaments at the base (Tilney et al., 1982b).

EFFECT OF TRAUMA ON STEREOCILIA MICROSTRUCTURE

Organization of actin filaments of the cilia is a sensitive indicator of lesions in the cochlea. Tilney and colleagues (1982b) studied the effect of acoustic trauma (105 dB for 24 hr.) on the stereocilia of the alligator lizard. The trauma produced changes in the organization of actin filaments. The most common lesion found was depolymerization of actin filaments at the base of the stereocilium where it is the weakest. The other type of lesion seen less frequently was loss in cross bridges between adjacent actin filaments. Both these effects were found mainly in the tallest stereocilia. These stereocilia are commonly found displaced laterally relative to the rootlet, and while remaining perfectly straight, are inclined at an angle different from the rest of the stereocilia. Acoustic trauma thus dramatically reduces the rigidity of the tallest stereocilia either by uprooting them or by destroying the cross bridges between the actin fibers.

There may be some repair mechanism present because 10 days after the noise exposure the round window N_1 thresholds had returned nearly to normal control values. In these animals the lesions of the actin filaments were not seen (Tilney et al., 1982b). (However, the authors recognize the difficulty of knowing whether the stereocilia seen at 10 days were on hair cells showing damage immediately after removal from the noise. The issue of actin repair requires additional study.)

Trauma reduces the stiffness of the tallest stereocilia of the hair bundle. Reduced stiffness will lower the resonant frequency of the hair bundle. In mammalian cochleae the tallest stereocilia are attached to the tectorial membrane; loss of stereocilia stiffness will effectively decouple the hair bundle from the tectorial membrane. This should (i) produce loss in sensitivity of the hair cell response, and (ii) reduce the appearance at the basilar membrane of components of the mechanical response generated at the hair cell.

DISCUSSION

Reversible Loss in Sharp Tuning

It was proposed that stereocilia stiffness reduced by trauma should lead to loss in sensitivity, broadening of tuning curves, and downward shift in CF. A variety of other insults to cochlea are known to produce similar sets of changes. These changes, however, are reversible and raise the question of whether there is more than one mechanism by which the loss in sharp tuning takes place. (See Kim, chap. 7.)

(i) Hypoxia. Single fiber tuning curves obtained in the auditory nerve of cats before and after inducing hypoxia show reversible loss of the low-threshold sharply tuned segment of the frequency threshold curve (FTC) (Evans, 1975).

(ii) Poisoning. Short-term instillation of KCN or furosemide into scala tympani of cat produces reversible selective loss of the sharply tuned segment of FTC. The loss is accompanied in many cases by a shift in the characteristic frequency toward lower frequencies (Evans & Klinke, 1974).

(iii) Removal of perilymph from scala tympani. Removal of perilymph from scala tympani of guinea pig cochlea produces broadening of the FTC of single spiral ganglion cells. The effect is reversible. If the scala is allowed to refill, the tuning returns to nearly normal (Robertson, 1974).

Due to the nonlinearity of the stereocilia (section 5C), the shape of the hair cell tuning curves is level dependent (Figure 6-5). The tuning curves obtained for higher stereocilia amplitudes (higher SPL) are broadly tuned and less sensitive as compared to those obtained at lower amplitudes. Similar broadening may occur if the tuning curve was measured at low amplitudes but a dc component was added to shift the operating point on the nonlinear curve. Removal of perilymph from scala tympani would produce such a dc pressure on the scala media. The reversible broadening of the FTC in this case, therefore, may be explained by the mechanical nonlinearity of the stereocilia.

(iv) Effect of anoxia poisoning and acoustic trauma on the distortion products in the ear canal. A series of experiments by Kim, Molnar, and Matthews (1980) demonstrate that anoxia, KCN perfusion, and acoustic trauma all affect a nonlinear mechanical process in the inner ear. The sound pressure levels of the distortion products $(2f_1 - f_2)$

and (f_2-f_1) were measured in the ear canal of the cat and chinchilla. The SPL of the $(2f_1-f_2)$ component was found to be between 30 and 40 dB below the level of the primaries (f_1, f_2), while that of the (f_2-f_1) component was 50 dB below the primary level. These two distortion products could be reduced reversibly by anoxia, by perfusion of scala tympani with KCN, and by acoustic trauma (Kim, 1980; Kim et al., 1980). The presence of the distortion products in the ear canal sound pressure clearly points to the mechanical origin of the distortion products. Anoxia, KCN perfusion, and acoustic trauma seem to affect a nonlinear, metabolically active, and physiologically vulnerable stage which is part of the mechanical transduction process. Because of the similarity of the changes produced by anoxia, KCN perfusion, and mechanical and acoustical trauma, it is tempting to suggest that the changes in each case may be produced by the loss of stereocilia stiffness. This could account for the observed changes of loss in sensitivity, loss of sharp tuning, shift of the center frequency to lower values, and disappearance of the distortion products from the ear canal. It will be recalled, however, that each of the effects described above is reversible within a short time (minutes) and that there is no experimental evidence available at present which suggests that the actin filaments can be repolymerized or that their cross bonds can be reestablished in such a short time span.

Until now, it has been generally assumed that there is a distinct boundary between the mechanical and the electrochemical part of the transduction process at the hair cell. Under this assumption, a mechanical stimulus applied to the hair cell will produce an electrical response but an electrical signal applied to the hair cell will not produce a mechanical response of the stereocilia. A variety of recent experiments now change this view and suggest that the mechanoelectric transduction process at the hair cell works in both directions. Application of mechanical signal produces an electric response in the hair cells and application of an electric signal produces a mechanical response (Crawford & Fettiplace, 1981; Hubbard & Mountain, 1982; Mountain & Hubbard, 1982; Weiss, 1982).

The hair cell itself is physiologically vulnerable and the changes in the level of distortion products seen in the ear canal due to anoxia and poisoning (Kim et al., 1980) may be due to this electrical-to-mechanical coupling.

It is clear that our knowledge of the hair cell function is quite incomplete at present and much work needs to be done in order to clearly understand the mechanism of some of the observations described above.

The Concept of Inner Ear Damage Affecting the Mechanics of the Ear

Until now concepts of inner ear damage have been based upon the view that basilar membrane mechanics are the basis of cochlear mechanical function and that such mechanical properties are insensitive to trauma. This view is implicit in the experiments of most of the investigators in which the physiological condition of the cochlea was not determined during the basilar membrane measurements (Albe et al., 1982; Johnstone & Boyle, 1970; Johnstone & Yates, 1974; Kohllöffel, 1972c; Rhode, 1971, 1973, 1974, 1976, 1977, 1978, 1980; Rhode & Robles, 1973, 1974; Robles & Rhode, 1973, 1974). This view seemed to be supported by the uniform type of basilar membrane response seen to widely varying levels of trauma measured by N_1 response (Wilson & Johnstone, 1975). The reason for this disparity was that only the sharply tuned tip region was susceptible to trauma. The remaining response was quite robust.

The present concept of the inner ear damage is based on the mechanical and physiological condition of the hair cells in the cochlea. Under this concept, local damage to a few hair cells can alter the mechanical response seen at the basilar membrane, at a position where the mechanical resonance of the damaged hair cells will normally be seen. This concept is supported by two additional lines of evidence: (i) Local mechanical trauma to the basilar membrane was shown to alter the response only of those spiral ganglion cells that originate from the damaged region (Cody et al., 1980); (ii) Local trauma to the hair cells caused by a focused laser beam changes the mechanical response seen at the basilar membrane (unpublished observations). Under this concept it is clear how the local damage produced by the electric field of the capacitive probe and by the radiation of the Mössbauer source could alter the local mechanical response of the basilar membrane.

CONCLUDING REMARKS

In detecting an auditory signal at threshold the power reaching a single hair cell is about 10^{-20} W (Khanna & Sherrick, 1981). To detect signals of such low power it is essential that the thermal noise reaching the detector be equal to or lower than 10^{-20} W. This implies that the detector be preceded by a narrow band filter of only a few hertz bandwidth and that all mechanical signals applied to the detector enter through this filter. To cover a band of frequencies a series of such detectors and filters are needed. In the auditory system such detectors are hair cells, each tuned to a different center frequency by its own stereocilia and each covering a narrow band of frequencies.

Until recently, it was generally accepted that the sharp tuning seen in the hair cell tuning curves derived basically from the mechanical properties of the basilar membrane, however such tuning is present in primitive animals even when there is no basilar membrane or its equivalent in the inner ear. It is proposed that such tuning is a fundamental property of the auditory hair cells in all species.

REFERENCES

Albe, F., Schwab, J., Smigielski, P., & Dancer, A. (1982). Displacement measurement of the basilar membrane in guinea pigs by means of optical-fiber interferometer. In G. Von Bally & P. Greguss (Eds.) *Optics in biomedical sciences*, Berlin/Heidelberg; Springer-Verlag.

Allen, J.B. (1977). Two-dimensional cochlear fluid model: New results. *Journal of the Acoustical Society of America, 61*, 110–119.

Axelrod, F.S. As reported by Lettvin, J.Y. & Maturana, H.R., (1960). Hearing senses in the frog. *M.I.T. Research Lab Electron Quarterly Progress Report, 57*, 167–168.

Békésy, G. von (1960). *Experiments in hearing.* New York: McGraw-Hill.

Brown, M.C., Smith, D.I., Nuttall, A.L. (1983a). Anesthesia and surgical trauma: Their influence on the guinea pig compound action potential. *Hearing Research, 10,* 345-358.

Brown, M.C., Smith, D.I., Nuttall, A.L. (1983b). The temperature dependency of neural and hair cell responses evoked by high frequencies. *Journal of Acoustical Society of America, 73,* 1662-1670.

Capranica, R.R. (1978). Auditory processing in anurans. *Federation Proceedings, 37,* 2324-2328.

Capranica, R.R., & Moffat, A.J.M. (1974a). Excitation, inhibition and 'disinhibition' in the inner ear of the toad (*Bufo*). *Journal of the Acoustical Society of America, 55,* 480.

Capranica, R.R., & Moffat, A.J.M. (1974b). Frequency sensitivity of auditory fibers in the eighth nerve of the spadefood toad, *Scaphiopus couchi. Journal of the Acoustical Society of America, 55,* Supplement S85.

Capranica, R.R., & Moffat, A.J.M. (1975). Selectivity of the peripheral auditory system of spadefoot toads (*Scaphiopus couchi*) for sounds of biological significance. *Journal of Comparative Physiology, 100,* 231-249.

Capranica, R.R., & Moffat, A.J.M. (1980). Nonlinear properties of peripheral auditory system of anurans. In A.N. Popper & R.R. Fay (Eds.) *Proceedings in life science: Comparative studies of hearing in vertebrates.* New York: Springer-Verlag.

Cody, A.R., & Johnstone, B.M. (1980). Single auditory neuron response during acute acoustic trauma. *Hearing Research, 3,* 3-16.

Cody, A.R., Robertson, D., Bredberg, G., & Johnstone, B.M. (1980). Electrophysiological and morphological changes in the guinea pig cochlea following mechanical trauma to the organ of Corti. *Acta Otolaryngologica, 89,* 440-452.

Crawford, A.C., & Fettiplace, R. (1981). Nonlinearities in the responses of turtle hair cells. *Journal of Physiology, 315,* 317-338.

Dallos, P., Santos-Sacchi, J., & Flock, A. (1982). Intracellular recordings from cochlear outer hair cells. *Science, 218,* 582-584.

De Boer, E. (1979). Short-wave world revisited: Resonance in a two-dimensional cochlear model. *Hearing Research, 1,* 253-281.

De Rosier, D., Tilney, L.G., & Egelman, E. (1980). Actin in the inner ear: The remarkable structure of the stereocilia. *Nature (London), 287,* 291-296.

De Rosier, D., Tilney, L.G. (1982). How actin filaments pack into bundles. *Cold Spring Harbor Symposium, 46,* 525-540.

Dragsten, P.R., Webb. W.W., Paton, J.A., & Capranica, R.R. (1974a). Sensitive acoustic vibration measurements by optical heterodyne detection of scattered laser light. *Journal of the Acoustical Society of America, 55,* 479.

Dragsten, P.R., Webb. W.W., Paton, J.A., & Capranica, R.R. (1974b). Auditory membrane vibrations: Measurements at sub-angstrom levels by optical heterodyne spectroscopy. *Science, 185,* 55-57.

Dragsten, P.R., Webb. W.W., Paton, J.S., & Capranica, R.R. (1976). Light-scattering heterodyne interferometer for vibration measurements in auditory organs. *Journal of the Acoustical Society of America, 60,* 665-671.

Evans, E.F., & Klinke, R. (1974). Reversible effects of cyanide and furosemide on the tuning of single cochlear nerve fibers. *Journal of Physiology, 242,* 129-131.

Evans, E.F. (1975). The sharpening of cochlear frequency selectivity in the normal and abnormal cochlea. *Audiology, 14,* 419-442.

Evans, E.F., & Wilson, J.P. (1975). Cochlear tuning properties: Concurrent basilar membrane and single nerve fiber measurements. *Science, 190,* 1218-1221.

Fischler, H., Frei, E.H., Spira, D., & Rubinstein, M. (1967). Dynamic response of middle-ear structure. *Journal of the Acoustical Society of America, 41,* 1220-1231.

Flock, A. (1977). Physiological properties of sensory hairs in the ear. In E.F. Evans & J.P. Wilson (Eds.), *Psychophysics and physiology of hearing.* London/New York: Academic Press.

Flock, A., Flock, B., & Murray, E. (1977). Studies on the sensory hairs of receptor cells in the inner ear. *Acta Otolaryngology, 83,* 85-91.

Frishkopf, L.S., & Goldstein, M.H., Jr. (1963), Responses to acoustic stimuli from single units in the eighth nerve of the bullfrog. *Journal of the Acoustical Society of America, 35,* 1219-1228.

Garfinkle, T.J., & Saunders, J.C. (1983). Morphologic properties of inner hair cell stereocilia in the C57BL/6J mouse. *Journal of Otolaryngology, Head and Neck Surgery, 91,* 421-426.

Gundersen, T., Skärstein, O., & Sikkeland, T. (1978). A study of the vibration of the basilar membrane in human temporal bone preparations by the use of the Mössbauer effect. *Acta Otolaryngologica, 86,* 225-232.

Helfenstein, W.M. (1973). *Beitrag Zur Messung der Akustisch Bedingten Bewegungen und Identifikation des Mechanischen Teils des Innenohrs der Katze.* Thesis, Eidgenossischen Technischen Hochschule, Zurich, Switzerland.

Hill, B.C., Schubert, E.D., Nokes, M.A., & Michelson, R.P. (1977). Laser interferometer measurement of changes in crayfish axon diameter concurrent with action potential. *Science, 196,* 426-428.

Hillman, P., Schechter, H., & Rubinstein, M. (1964). Application of the Mössbauer technique to the measurement of small vibrations in the ear. *Review of Modern Physics, 36,* 360.

Holton, T., & Hudspeth, A.J. (1983). A micromechanical contribution to cochlear tuning and tonotopic organization. *Science,* 508-510.

Hubbard, A.E., & Mountain, D.C. (1982). Injection of ac current into scala media alters the sound pressure of the tympanic membrane: Variations with acoustical stimulus parameters. *Journal of the Acoustical Society of America, 71,* S100.

Johnstone, B.M., & Boyle, A.J.F. (1967). Basilar membrane vibrations examined with the Mössbauer technique. *Science, 158,* 390-391.

Johnstone, B.M., Taylor, K.J., & Boyle, A.J. (1970). Mechanics of the guinea pig cochlea. *Journal of the Acoustical Society of America, 47,* 504-509.

Johnstone, B.M., & Yates, G.K. (1974). Basilar membrane tuning curves in the guinea pig. *Journal of the Acoustical Society of America, 55,* 584-587.

Kelly, J.P. & Khanna, S.M. (in press). Ultrastructural damage in cochleas used for studies of basilar membrane mechanics.

Khanna, S.M. (1983a). Interpretation of the sharply tuned basilar membrane responses obtained in the cat cochlea. In R.R. Fay & G. Gourevitch (Eds.), *Hearing and other senses: Presentations in honor of E.G. Wever.* Groton, CT: Amphora Press.

Khanna, S.M. (1983b). A comparative method of interferometric measurement. Submitted for review.

Khanna, S.M., Johnson, G.A., & Jacobs, J. (1983). A comparative method of interferometric measurement: Hardware and techniques. Submitted for review.

Khanna, S.M., & Leonard, D.G.B. (1980a). Interferometric measurements of basilar membrane vibrations in cats. *Journal of the Acoustical Society of America, 67,* S46.

Khanna, S.M., & Leonard, D.G.B. (1980b). Interferometric measurements of basilar membrane vibrations in cats using a round window approach. *Journal of the Acoustical Society of America, 68,* S42.

Khanna, S.M., & Leonard, D.G.B. (1981a). Laser interferometric measurements of basilar membrane vibrations in cats using a round window approach. *Journal of the Acoustical Society of America, 69,* S51.

Khanna, S.M., & Leonard, D.G.B. (1981b). Basilar membrane response measured in damaged cochleas of cats. In M.H. Holmes & L. Rubenfeld (Eds.), *Mathematical modeling of the hearing process*. New York: Springer-Verlag.

Khanna, S.M., & Leonard, D.G.B. (1982a). Basilar membrane tuning in the cat cochlea. *Science, 215*, 305–306.

Khanna, S.M., & Leonard, D.G.B. (1982b). Laser interferometric measurement of basilar membrane vibrations in cats using a round window approach. In G. Von Bally & P. Greguss (Eds.), *Optics in biomedical science*, vol. 31. Berlin/Heidelberg: Springer-Verlag.

Khanna, S.M., & Sherrick, C. (1981). The comparative sensitivity of selected receptor systems. In T. Gualtierotti (Ed.), *The vestibular system: Function and morphology*. New York: Springer-Verlag.

Khanna, S.M., Tonndorf, J., & Walcott, W.W. (1968). Laser interferometer for the measurement of submicroscopic displacement amplitudes and their phases in small biological structures. *Journal of the Acoustical Society of America, 44*, 1555–1565.

Kiang, N.Y.S., Watanabe, T., Thomas, E.C., & Clark, L.F. (1965). *Discharge patterns of single fibers in the cat's auditory nerve*. Research Monograph No. 35. Cambridge, MA: MIT Press.

Kim, D.O. (1980). Cochlear mechanics: Implications of electrophysiological and acoustical observations. *Hearing Research, 2*, 297–317.

Kim, D.O., Molnar, C.E., & Matthews, J.W. (1980). Cochlear mechanics: Nonlinear behavior in two-tone responses as reflected in cochlear-nerve fiber responses and in ear-canal sound pressure. *Journal of the Acoustical Society of America, 67*, 1704–1721.

Kliauga, P., & Khanna, S.M. (1983). Dose rate to the inner ear during Mössbauer experiments. *Physics in Medicine and Biology, 28*, 359–366.

Kohllöffel, L.U.E. (1972a). A study of basilar membrane vibrations. I. Fuzziness detection: A new method for the analysis of microvibrations with laser light. *Acoustica, 27*, 49–65.

Kohllöffel, L.U.E. (1972b). A Study of basilar membrane vibrations. II. The vibratory amplitude and phase pattern along the basilar membrane (post-mortem). *Acoustica, 27*, 66–81.

Kohllöffel, L.U.E. (1972c). A Study of basilar membrane vibrations. III. The basilar membrane frequency response curve in the living guinea pig. *Acoustica, 27*, 82–89.

Leonard, D.G.B., & Khanna, S.M. (1984). Histological evaluation of damage in cat cochleas used for measurement of basilar membrane mechanics. *Journal of Acoustical Society of America, 75*.

LePage, E.L., & Johnstone, B.M. (1980). Nonlinear mechanical behaviour of the basilar membrane in the basal turn of the guinea pig cochlea. *Hearing Research, 2*, 183–189.

Liff, H. (1969). Responses from single auditory units in the eighth nerve of the leopard frog. *Journal of Acoustical Society of America, 45*, 512–513.

Lim, D.J. (1980). Cochlear anatomy related to cochlear micromechanics. A Review. *Journal of Acoustical Society of America, 67*, 1686–1695.

Moffat, A.J.M., & Capranica, R.R. (1974). Sensory processing in the peripheral auditory system of tree frogs (*Hyla*). *Journal of Acoustical Society of America, 55*, 480.

Moller, A.R. (1963). Transfer function of the middle ear. *Journal of Acoustical Society of America, 35*, 1526–1534.

Mountain, D.C., & Hubbard, A.E. (1982). Injection of ac current into scala media alters the sound pressure at the tympanic membrane: Variations with electrical stimulus parameters. *Journal of Acoustical Society of America, 71*, S100.

Narins, P.M., & Capranica, R.R. (1976). Sexual differences in the auditory system of the treefrog, *Eleutherodactylus coqui*. *Science, 192*, 378–380.

Neiswander, P., & Slettemoen, G.A. (1981). Electronic speckle pattern interferometric measurements of the basilar membrane in the inner ear. *Applied Optics, 20*, 4271–4276.

Nokes, M.A., Hill, B.C., & Barelli, A.E. (1978). Fiber optic heterodyne interferometer for vibration measurements in biological systems. *Reviews of Scientific Instruments, 49,* 722-728.

Paton, J.A., Capranica, R.R., Loftus-Hill, J.J., Dragsten, P.R., & Webb, W.W. (1974). Mechanical sensitivity of acoustic receptor organs in crickets. *Journal of Acoustical Society of America, 55,* 480.

Peake, W.R., & Ling, A., Jr. (1980). Basilar membrane motion in the alligator lizard: Its relation to tonotopic organization and frequency selectivity. *Journal of Acoustical Society of America, 67,* 1736-1745.

Rhode, W.S. (1971). Observations of the vibration of the basilar membrane in squirrel monkeys using the Mössbauer technique. *Journal of Acoustical Society of America, 49,* 1218-1231.

Rhode, W.S. (1973). An investigation of post-mortem cochlear mechanics using the Mössbauer effect. In A.R. Moller (Ed.), *Basic Mechanisms in Hearing* (pp. 49-68). New York/London: Academic Press.

Rhode, W.S. (1974). Measurement of vibration of the basilar membrane in the squirrel monkey. *Annals of Otology, Rhinology and Laryngology, 83,* 619-625.

Rhode, W.S. (1977). Some observations of two-tone interactions measured using the Mössbauer effect. In E.F. Evans & J.P. Wilson (Eds.), *Psychophysics and physiology of hearing* (pp. 27-38). London: Academic Press.

Rhode, W.S. (1978). Some observations on cochlear mechanics. *Journal of Acoustical Society of America, 64,* 158-176.

Rhode, W.S. (1980). Cochlear partition vibration — Recent views. *Journal of Acoustical Society of America, 67,* 1696-1703.

Rhode, W.S., & Robles, L. (1974). Evidence from Mössbauer Experiments for nonlinear vibration in the cochlea. *Journal of Acoustical Society of America, 55,* 588-594.

Robertson, D. (1974). Cochlear neurons: Frequency selectivity altered by perilymph removal. *Science, 186,* 153-155.

Robertson, D., & Manley, G.A. (1974). Manipulation of frequency analysis in the cochlear ganglion of the guinea pig. *Journal of Comparative Physiology, 91,* 363-375.

Robles, L., & Rhode, W.S. (1974). Non linear effects in the transient response of the basilar membrane. In E. Zwicker & E. Terhardt (Eds.), *Facts and models in hearing.* New York: Springer-Verlag.

Robles, L., Rhode, W.S., & Geisler, C.D. (1976). Transient response of the basilar membrane measured in squirrel monkeys using the Mössbauer effect. *Journal of Acoustical Society of America, 59,* 926-939.

Russell, I.J., & Sellick, P.M. (1977a). The tuning properties of cochlear hair cells. In E.F. Evans & J.P. Wilson (Eds.), *Psychophysics and Physiology of Hearing.* London: Academic Press.

Russell, I.J., & Sellick, P.M. (1977b). Tuning properties of cochlear hair cells. *Nature (London), 267,* 858-860.

Russell, I.J., & Sellick, P.M. (1978). Intracellular studies of hair cells in the mammalian cochlea. *Journal of Physiology, 284,* 261-290.

Sellick, P.M., & Russell, I.J. (1978). Intracellular studies of cochlear hair cells: Filling the gap between basilar membrane mechanics and neural excitation. In R.F. Naunton & C. Fernández (Eds.), *Evoked electrical activity in the auditory nervous system.* New York: Academic Press.

Sellick, P.M., Patuzzi, R., & Johnstone, B.M. (1982). Measurement of basilar membrane motion in the guinea pig using the Mössbauer technique. *Journal of Acoustical Society of America, 72,* 131-141.

Siebert, W.M. (1974). Ranke revisited — A simple short-wave cochlear model. *Journal of Acoustical Society of America, 56,* 594-600.

Sondhi, M.M. (1978). Methods for computing motion in a two-dimensional cochlear model. *Journal of Acoustical Society of America, 63,* 1468-1477.

Steele, C.R. (1974). Behavior of the basilar membrane with pure tone excitation. *Journal of Acoustical Society of America, 55,* 148-172.

Steele, C.R., & Taber, L.S. (1980). Comparison of 'WKB' calculations and experimental results for three-dimensional cochlear models. *Journal of Acoustical Society of America, 68,* 147-149.

Strelioff, D., & Flock, A. (1982). Mechanical properties of hair bundles of receptor cells in the guinea pig cochlea. *Society of Neuroscience,* (Abstract 8).

Tilney, L.G., De Rosier, D.J., & Mulroy, M.J. (1980). The organization of actin filaments in the stereocilia of cochlear hair cells. *Journal of Cell Biology, 86,* 244-259.

Tilney, L.G., & Saunders, J.C. (1982a). Actin filaments, stereocilia, and hair cells of the bird cochlea. I. The length, number, width, and distribution of stereocilia of each hair cell is related to the position of the hair cell on the cochlea. *Journal of Cell Biology, 96,* 807-821.

Tilney, L.G., Egelman, E.H., De Rosier, D.J., & Saunders, J.C. 1983). Actin filaments, stereocilia and hair cells of the bird cochlea. II. The packing of actin filaments in the stereocilia and in the cuticular plate and what happens to the organization when the stereocilia are bent. *Journal of Cell Biology, 96,* 882-834.

Tilney, L.G., Saunders, J.C., Egelman, E.H., & De Rosier, D.J. (1982b). Changes in the organization of actin filaments in the stereocilia of noise-damaged lizard cochlea. *Hearing Research, 7,* 181-197.

Turner, R.G., Muraski, A.A., & Nielsen, D.W. 1981). Cilium length: Influence on neural tonotopic organization. *Science, 213,* 1519-1521.

Wever, E.G. (1984). *The amphibian ear.* Princeton: Princeton Univ. Press.

Weiss, T.F. (1982). Bidirectional transduction in vertebrate hair cells: A mechanism for coupling mechanical and electrical processes. *Hearing Research, 7,* 353-360.

Weiss, T.F., Peake, W.T., Ling, A., Jr., & Holton, T. (1978). Which structures determine frequency selectivity and tonotopic organization of vertebrate nerve fibers? Evidence from the alligator lizard. In R.F. Naunton & C. Fernández (Eds.), *Evoked electrical activity in the auditory nervous system.* New York: Academic Press.

Wilson, J.P. (1973). A sub-miniature capacitive probe for vibration measurements of the basilar membrane. *Journal of Sound & Vibrations, 30,* 483-493.

Wilson, J.P., & Johnstone, J.R. (1972). Capacitive probe measures of basilar membrane vibration. In *Symposium on Hearing Theory,* IPO Eindhoven, the Netherlands.

Wilson, J.P., & Johnstone, J.R. (1975). Basilar membrane and middle-ear vibration in guinea pig measured by capacitive probe. *Journal of Acoustical Society of America, 75,* 705-723.

Wright, A. (1981). Scanning electron microscopy of the human cochlea – The organ of Corti. *Archives of Oto-Rhino-Laryngology, 230,* 11-19.

Yates, G.K., & Johnstone, B.M. (1979). Measurement of basilar membrane movement. In H.A. Beagley (Ed.), *Auditory investigation: The scientific and technological basis.* Oxford: Clarendon.

Zweig, G., Lipes, R., & Pierce, J.R. (1976). The cochlear compromise. *Journal of Acoustical Society of America, 59,* 975-982.

Zwislocki, J. (1948). Theorie de Schneckenmechanik Qualitative und Quantitative Analyse. *Acta Otolaryngology* (Suppl.) *72,* 1-76.

Zwislocki, J. (1953). Review of recent mathematical theories of cochlear dynamics. *Journal of Acoustical Society of America, 25,* 743-751.

Chapter 7

Functional Roles of the Inner- and Outer-Hair-Cell Subsystems in the Cochlea and Brainstem[1]

D.O. Kim

INTRODUCTION

Spoendlin's report (1966, 1969) that only about 5 to 10% of the cochlear ganglion neurons innervate the outer hair cells (OHCs) came as a great surprise (e.g., Eldredge, 1967). This marked asymmetry of afferent innervation to the OHCs still appears to be one of the most perplexing paradoxes: If Nature evolved 3.5 times as many OHCs[2] as IHCs (inner hair cells), why are the OHCs wasted by sending signals to so few cochlear neurons? One of the major classical questions in hearing science is, what are the functional roles played by the OHCs and by the IHCs of the mammalian cochlea? To date, there is no well-accepted answer to this question.

Anatomical studies have established distinct morphological features of the IHCs and OHCs and their innervations: (1) The two types of hair cells are morphologically distinct (e.g., Engstrom & Sjostrand, 1954); (2) Distinct afferent neural populations in the spiral ganglion innervate the IHCs and the OHCs, that is, Type I neurons to IHCs and Type II to OHCs (Spoendlin, 1969; Kiang, Rho, Northrup, Liberman, & Ryugo, 1982; see Figure 7-1); (3) About 93% of the cochlear spiral ganglion neurons innervate the IHCs and only about 7% of the ganglion neurons innervate the OHCs even though there are about 3.5 times as many OHCs as IHCs (Spoendlin, 1969, 1972; see Table 7-1); therefore, there is a 45:1 difference in the afferent-neuron-to-hair-cell ratios in favor of the IHCs over the OHCs; (4) Distinct efferent neural populations in the superior olivary complex send axons to the IHC and OHC regions, in other words, the small lateral olivocochlear (OC) neurons innervate nerve fibers beneath the IHCs and the large medial OC neurons innervate the OHCs (Warr, 1978; Warr & Guinan, 1979; see Figure 7-2 and Table 7-2).

[1]The substance of this chapter was presented at the 1983 Meeting of the Society for Neuroscience (Kim, 1983). Supported by Grant No. NS18426 from NINCDS, National Institutes of Health.

[2]A special type of hair cell present only in the mammalian cochlea.

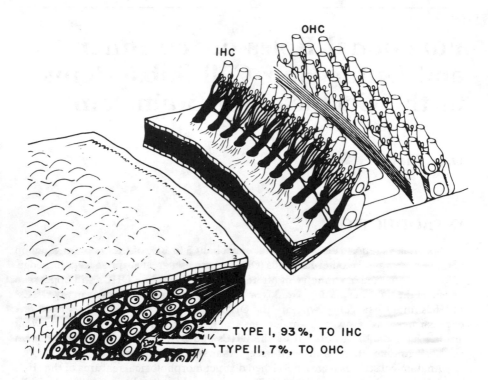

Figure 7-1. Schematic representation of the afferent innervation pattern of the organ of Corti in the cat. Most of the cochlear ganglion cells are myelinated Type I cells which innervate the IHCs and only about 7% of the ganglion cells are the unmyelinated Type II cells which innervate the OHCs. An individual Type I neuron innervates typically one IHC, and an individual Type II neuron innervates many OHCs. A particular IHC is innervated by many Type I neurons. Adapted from Spoendlin (1978); reprinted with permission from the publisher.

In contrast to the well-documented comparative anatomy of the IHC and OHC and their associated neurons, there is a paucity of related physiological data. Hence, it is difficult to form a comprehensive and thorough theory for the underlying mechanisms and functional roles played by the two types of hair cells. Nevertheless, I believe that enough indirect evidence is now available to hypothesize the existence, identification, and functional roles of two parallel subsystems that constitute the caudal part of the auditory system up to the superior olivary complex. This chapter presents such a set of working hypotheses, reviews supporting evidence, offers an integrated interpretation for some of the seemingly disjointed and perplexing facts, and highlights important missing pieces needed to complete much of the jigsaw puzzle of the auditory periphery.

TABLE 7-1.

Number of the inner and outer hair cells and their associated afferent neurons for man and cat

	Man	Cat
Hair cells		
OHC	12,000	9,900
IHC	3,500	2,600
OHC/IHC	3.4	3.8
Aff. neurons		
Type II innervating OHC	2,100 (7%)	3,500 (7%)
Type I innervating IHC	27,900 (93%)	46,500 (93%)
Aff. neuron to HC ratio		
OHC	0.18 (= 1/5.7)	0.35(= 1/2.8)
IHC	8.0	18
ratio	44	51

Notes. Assembled from Iurato (1967), Spoendlin (1972), and Kimura (1978).

A SET OF WORKING HYPOTHESES

The following set of hypotheses, some aspects of which are outlined in Figure 7-3 are proposed.

(1.) There are two distinct parallel auditory subsystems in the cochlea and the brainstem, that is, (a) the IHC subsystem, consisting of the IHCs and neural populations receiving input directly or indirectly from the IHCs, including the small lateral OC (olivocochlear) neurons projecting to the IHC region, and (b) the OHC subsystem consisting of the OHCs and neural populations receiving input directly or indirectly from the OHCs, including the large medial OC neurons whose axons make synaptic contacts with the OHCs.

(2.) The OHC has an *active bidirectional transduction* mechanism in the stereocilia and cuticular plate region. First, the mechanical energy applied to the hair bundle is transduced into electrochemical energy of receptor potential/current of the OHC; however, the electrochemical energy of endolymphatic potential and of the OHC membrane potential can also be used to drive the hair bundle mechanically. The active mechanical force at the OHC hair bundle would push against the tectorial membrane

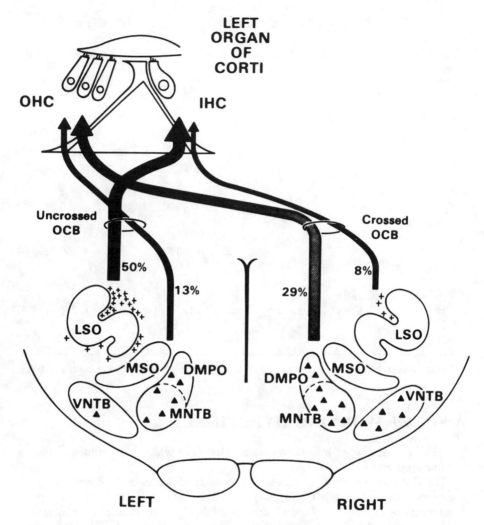

Figure 7-2. Schematic representation of the large medial (▲) and the small lateral (+) olivocochlear neurons projecting to the OHC and IHC regions, respectively. Abbreviations: LSO and MSO, lateral and medial superior olivary nuclei; MNTB and VNTB, medial and ventral nuclei of the trapezoid body; DMPO, dorsomedial periolivary nucleus. From Warr (1978); reprinted with permission from the publisher.

and drive the organ of Corti, conceivably reducing the mechanical damping associated with vibration of the organ of Corti to even negative values. This property of the OHC gives rise to *active and nonlinear* biomechanical behavior of the cochlea, and is highly vulnerable physiologically.

TABLE 7-2.

Number of the afferent and efferent cochlear neurons and myelination of their axons in cat

	Associated with OHC	Associated with IHC
Afferent	Type II (unmyelinated) 3,500 7%	Type I (myelinated) 46,500 93%
Efferent	Large medial OCN (myelinated) 520 42%	Small lateral OCN (unmyelinated) 710 58%

Notes. Assembled from Spoendlin (1972), Arnesen and Osen (1978), Warr et al. (1982), White and Warr (1983), Guinan (1983).

(3.) The function of the OHC subsystem is *not* to provide a channel for transmitting the auditory information to the brain, *but* to provide a gain control for the active and nonlinear biomechanics of the organ of Corti. (3-a.) The function of the OHCs is to enhance actively the sensitivity, tuning, and dynamic range of the mechanical response of the entire organ of Corti as stated in hypothesis 2, conferring high sensitivity, sharp tuning, and wide dynamic range to the IHC subsystem. (3-b.) The function of the Type II afferent cochlear neurons is to transmit information about the operating point associated with the motor function of the OHCs, averaged over a sizable length of the cochlear partition as well as over time. Thus the information carried by the Type II neurons is of low spatial and temporal resolution. (3-c.) The function of the large medial OC neurons is to exert a gain control upon the biomechanics of the organ of Corti by reducing the amount of mechanical energy released from the OHCs via a synaptically mediated regulation of the membrane potential and conductance of the OHCs.

(4.) The function of the IHC subsystem is to transduce the mechanical response of the cochlea ("passively" in the context of the biomechanics of the cochlear partition in that there is no active control of the biomechanics by the IHCs) into receptoneural signals, and to transmit the auditory information with high spatial and temporal resolution via the bulk of the afferent cochlear nerve channel to the higher centers of the

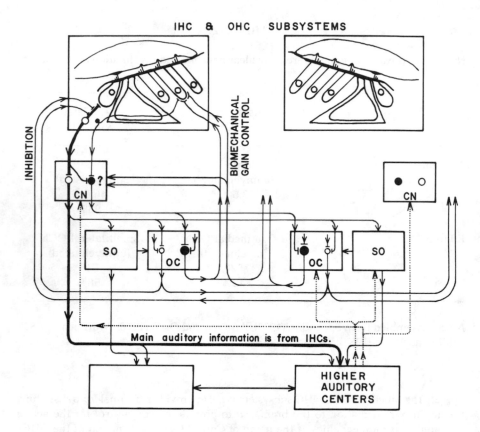

Figure 7-3. A block diagram for the hypothesized IHC and OHC subsystems in the cochlea and the brainstem up to the superior olivary complex and their connections to the remainder of the auditory system. IHC, inner hair cell; OHC, outer hair cell; CN, cochlear nucleus; SO, superior olivary complex; OC, olivocochlear neurons. Conventionally, the term superior olivary complex represents all of the nuclei at this level and includes the OC neurons besides the LSO, MSO, and so forth. In this figure, however, the OC part of the SO is taken out as a separate box for the purpose of explicitly showing the two subpopulations of the OC neurons. Thus, the SO box here represents all of the conventional superior olivary complex minus the OC neurons. The single heavy line from the IHC is intended to represent all radial afferent nerve fibers originating from the IHCs, thus including the afferent neural subpopulations with low as well as high spontaneous rates. The neurons represented by the filled circles represent those constituting the OHC subsystem loop. The question mark at the filled neuron inside the CN is intended to emphasize that such hypothesized neurons are not identified yet. For clarity, the interconnections are partly omitted on one side or the other.

brain. (4-a.) The function of the small lateral OC neurons is to inhibit the afferent cochlear neural response but not to control cochlear biomechanics.

(5.) The function of the middle-ear muscle subsystems is to provide a means of reducing the overall intensity of unwanted stimuli entering the total cochlea, operating in a simpler and cruder way and at higher stimulus levels than in the case of the OHC subsystem; the latter operates over nearly all of the stimulus levels but its involvement at the lower stimulus levels is more important.

REVIEW OF EVIDENCE

In constructing Figure 7-3, the following general references were consulted besides the specific ones cited: Adams, 1983; Farley and Warr, 1981; Fex, 1962; Hoshino, 1981; Kiang, 1975; Klinke and Galley, 1974; Kronester-Frei, 1978; Lim, 1972; Morest, 1975; Nordeen, Killackey, & Kitzes, 1983; Osen and Brodal, 1981; Warr, 1982.

Anatomical studies by Spoendlin (1966, 1969, 1972), Kiang and colleagues (1982), Warr (1978), and Warr and Guinan (1979) provide good evidence that the IHCs and OHCs have two distinct populations of afferent and efferent neurons as described above and illustrated in Figures 7-1 and 7-2. Presently unavailable is important anatomical information about the projection of the Type II cochlear neurons to the cochlear nucleus and about the projection from the cochlear nucleus directly or indirectly to the OC neurons. Thus hypothesis 1 proposed here has only incomplete support; however, the hypothesis is without contradictory evidence.

The collateral input of the Type I fibers to the "filled" neuron in the cochlear nucleus in Figure 7-3 is postulated by the author from the observation of Simmons and Liberman (1983). They showed that the central axons of the two types of the afferent cochlear neurons, originating from the two types of hair cells, travel together closely in the cochlear nerve while maintaining cochleotopic organization; the cochleotopic alignment of the Type II axons in a cross section of the cochlear nerve is the same as that of the Type I axons if the Type II fiber's cochlear position is taken at the point of its entry into the organ of Corti (i.e., the position of the IHC that the Type II fiber passes by) rather than the center of the region of the OHCs innervated by the Type II fiber. The latter position is substantially basal to the former, by as much as about 1.0 mm in the cat (Simmons & Liberman, 1983; Spoendlin, 1969). The functional significance of this peculiar anatomical arrangement of the Type II fibers is unclear, but a plausible interpretation is given later in this section. The point to note here is that the collateral input in the cochlear nucleus in Figure 7-3 is hypothesized from the closely maintained cochleotopic alignments of the two types of cochlear nerve fibers.

Using the method of retrograde labeling of neurons with the marker horseradish peroxidase (HRP) in the study of the connections of the cochlear neurons (Schmiedt and Feng, 1980), Leake-Jones and Snyder (1982) and Ruggero, Santi, & Rich (1982) have clearly shown that the Type II cochlear neurons do indeed project to the cochlear nucleus contrary to the suggestion by Spoendlin (1979) that they may not be "effectively connected" to the cochlear nucleus. From a noise-induced degeneration study, Morest and Bohne (1983) suggested that there may be a differential distribution of the thin nerve fibers of the Type II cochlear neurons in the cochlear nucleus. If, indeed, there is a well-localized region of the cochlear nucleus receiving dominant input from the Type II cochlear neurons, then the HRP method should yield results confirming such projection.

Presently, there is some strong but only indirect evidence in support of hypotheses 2 and 3. When the OHCs are selectively destroyed with ototoxic antibiotics over a sizable length in the basal region of the cochlea, leaving the IHCs seemingly intact, the behavioral threshold of hearing is elevated by about 30 to 50 dB for frequencies corresponding to the region of OHC damage (Prosen, Petersen, Moody, & Stebbins, 1978; Ryan & Dallos, 1975; Stebbins, Hawkins, Johnsson, & Moody, 1979); in addition, the responses of single cochlear nerve fibers (presumably the Type I nerve fibers from the IHC; see Liberman, 1982) associated with the region of OHC damage show threshold elevation of about 30–60 dB or more and broadening of their tuning (Dallos & Harris, 1978; Harrison & Evans, 1979; Kiang, Moxon, & Levine, 1970; Robertson & Johnstone, 1979).

Dallos and Harris (1978) suggested that there may be "frequency-dependent boost" in the IHC sensitivity contributed by the OHCs; they considered that the OHC effect on IHC may arise from electrical interaction via field currents or from an electromechanical interaction. Dallos and Harris did not elaborate on the latter possibility. Evans (1975) proposed that a physiologically vulnerable "second filter" arising from the OHCs may produce a sharp tuning and high sensitivity of the IHC response by means of certain electrical effects of the outer spiral fibers on the inner radial fibers in the vicinity of the habenula perforata. My hypothesis also suggests that the OHCs influence the IHCs, but differs in that it postulates that the OHCs influence the IHCs *mechanically* rather than *electrically* by affecting the mechanics of the *whole* organ of Corti.

Crane (1982) proposed that the OHCs may exert a mechanical influence on the IHCs by adjusting the spacing between the IHC hair bundle and the tectorial membrane (TM). There are some common elements between my hypothesis and Crane's; however, I postulate explicitly that there is an active mechanical-sensitivity enhancement for the motion of the whole partition through the OHC actions, whereas Crane's suggestion of the adjustment of the IHC–TM spacing is itself a passive mechanical effect which does not affect the sensitivity of the partition motion.

The concept of a "second filter" in the cochlea (Evans & Wilson, 1975) is contingent on the belief that the mechanics of the cochlear partition are *linear* and that the broad tuning of the mechanical response of the basilar membrane observed in earlier experiments (e.g. Evans & Wilson, 1975; Wilson & Johnstone, 1975) accurately represents the real mechanical response in the normally functioning cochlea. Opposing such a view, Kim, Molnar, and Pfeiffer (1973), Kim and Molnar (1975), Kim (1980), and Siegel, Kim, and Molnar (1982) caution that a single *nonlinear* filter could account for many of the observations used to invoke a "second filter" hypothesis. I suggest, because of the pronounced nonlinearity and physiological vulnerability in the mechanical response of the cochlear partition, that the quantitative data on basilar membrane motion such as those of Békésy (1960) and Evans and Wilson (1975) should be taken flexibly. We must allow that there may be significant differences between their measurements and the actual response of the normal cochlea. We suggest that one should give great significance to the qualitative aspects of the observations by Rhode (1971, 1973, 1978) that basilar membrane motion exhibits a frequency-dependent nonlinearity and that the mechanically manifested nonlinearity is physiologically vulnerable (LePage and Johnstone, 1980; Rhode, 1971, 1973, 1978).

Indeed, recently improved mechanical measurements of the basilar membrane motion show that the mechanical response is highly nonlinear and physiologically vulnerable (Sellick, Pattuzzi, & Johnstone, 1982b) and that it is much more sensitive and more sharply tuned than previously believed (Sellick et al., 1982b, Khanna & Leonard, 1982). There seems to be little difference between the tuning characteristics and sensitivity of an optimal basilar membrane response (at 1-nm displacement) shown in the upper panel of Figure 7-4 and those of a typical cochlear neuron located in a similar region of the guinea pig cochlea (Sellick et al., 1982b; Neely & Kim, 1983). Figure 7-4 describes the observations of Sellick et al. (1982b) which demonstrate that the sensitivity and sharp tuning of basilar membrane motion is highly vulnerable to deterioration of the physiological condition of the cochlea produced by invasive experimental procedures. The physiological condition of the cochlea was assessed with measurements of the threshold for the cochlear nerve compound action potential (N1) to tone bursts at frequencies near the characteristic frequency. The mechanical sensitivity is degraded by about 35 dB when the N1 threshold is elevated approximately 40–50 dB.

Several investigators have suggested that cochlear mechanics may indeed be *active* in the sense that the sensitivity and the frequency selectivity of the mechanical response of the cochlear partition may be substantially enhanced by means of an energy-dependent mechanism in the organ of Corti (Davis, 1983; deBoer, 1983; Gold, 1948; Kemp, 1979; Kim et al., 1980b; Neely & Kim, 1983). The lower part of Figure 7-4 shows specific results from an active model of cochlear biomechanics developed by Neely and Kim (1983) in which the model simulates a condition where mechanical energy is released from an internal source within the cochlear partition through the OHC stereocilia. Curve 1 represents the model response under a condition where a large amount of energy is released from the intracochlear source, simulating the sensitive and sharply tuned normal response; curve 2 represents the model response under a condition where the released amount of the intracochlear mechanical energy is reduced, simulating the deteriorated physiological condition; curve 3 represents the model response under a totally passive condition where the intracochlear energy source is disabled. These model results reproduce the major features of the experimental data shown in the upper panel of Figure 7-4. It appears to be difficult to account for the pronounced change of 30–40 dB in the sensitivity of the basilar membrane response with a purely passive model of cochlear mechanics.

Several studies of the cytoskeletal protein filaments in the stereocilia and the cuticular plate regions of the hair cells (Drenckhahn et al., 1982; Flock, 1983; Flock & Cheung, 1977; Hirokawa & Tilney, 1982; Macartney, Comis & Pickles, 1980; Tilney,

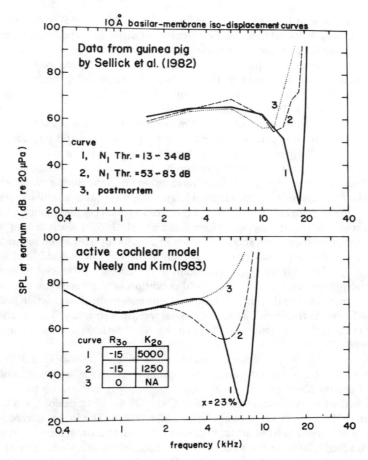

Figure 7-4. *Upper panel:* Experimental data of basilar membrane response in the guinea pig by Sellick, Patuzzi, and Johnstone (1982b) plotted as 1-nm (10-Å) isodisplacement curves for three experimental conditions in the same cochlea. Curve 1 was obtained when the cochlea showed the most sensitive neural response as indicated by the lowest threshold for the N1 compound cochlear nerve action potential measured with tone bursts at frequencies near the characteristic frequency. Curves 2 and 3, respectively, were obtained when the N1 threshold was elevated as indicated, or after death of the animal. *Lower panel:* Results from an active model for cochlear biomechanics by Neely and Kim (1983) plotted as 1-nm isodisplacement curves. Curve 1 represents the model response under a condition where a large amount of mechanical energy was released from an energy source within the cochlear partition through the OHC stereocilia. Curve 2 represents a condition of the model where the amount of energy released from the intracochlear source was reduced relative to curve 1. Curve 3 represents a totally passive condition of the model where the energy-releasing active elements were disabled.

DeRosier, & Mulroy, 1980) have provided important new details about the composition of these critical structures. Flock (1983) states that "the co-location of actin, myosin and tropomyosin at the stereocilium rootlet [in the cuticular plate] is highly suggestive in terms of active mechanical events at this point." Further experimental and theoretical works are needed to elucidate molecular mechanisms underlying the hypothesized motor function of the OHC.

Otoacoustic emission has received much attention recently since Kemp's (1978; 1979) reports of click-evoked echoes and spontaneous otoacoustic emissions (SOAE). A prominent case of SOAE in a chinchilla was reported by Zurek and Clark (1981); the SOAE signal was sufficiently strong to be audible to a listener's naked ear without any amplification and was as high as 51 dB re: 20 μPa in the occluded ear canal. This animal was subsequently studied extensively in otoacoustic and cochlear morphological examinations (Clark, Kim, Bohne, & Zurek, 1983; Kim et al., 1983). The SOAE signal exhibited a sharp suppression-tuning characteristic resembling a cochlear nerve fiber tuning; there was also a punctate lesion of the organ of Corti at a position closely associated with the frequency of the pure-tone-like SOAE. These points strongly support the notion that the SOAE in this ear was produced by a mechanical vibration of a localized region of the cochlear partition; certain elements, most likely the OHC stereocilia, in that region may have mediated a "reverse transduction" of electrochemical energy into mechanical energy. It is highly implausible that such an intense and sustained acoustic signal could emanate from a passive mechanical system.

A number of other observations suggest the possibility of bidirectional (i.e., between mechanical and electrochemical) coupling and transduction in cochlear hair cells. These observations show the consistent and pronounced vulnerability of cochlear nonlinear phenomena to virtually any alteration of the functional state of the organ of Corti, including exposure to moderate levels of acoustic stimulation, anoxia, cyanide poisoning, organ of Corti damage from intense sounds or ototoxic drugs (Anderson & Kemp, 1979; Dallos, Harris, Relkin, & Cheatham, 1980; Kim, 1980; Kim et al., 1980a; Siegel et al., 1982; Zurek, Clark, & Kim, 1982). Bidirectional transduction is also suggested from modeling considerations (Weiss, 1982). The following observations provide further support for bidirectional transduction of hair cells: Hubbard and Mountain (1983) observed that alternating electric current delivered into the scala media alters sound pressure in the ear canal; Brownell (1983) observed that the cell membrane in the supranuclear region of dissociated OHCs exhibited a motile response to electrical stimulus or iontophoretic application of acetylcholine, but he did not determine whether the OHC stereocilia would also show a motile response.

Dallos and colleagues (1982) succeeded in making the difficult intracellular recordings from the OHCs as well as from the IHCs in the third turn of chinchilla cochlea. A striking feature of the Dallos et al. OHC data is that the sensitivity of the accomponent of the receptor potential (RP) of the OHC is nearly the same as or about 10 dB *less* (not greater) than that of the IHC. Although this is consistent with the present hypothesis, this direct observation from OHCs and IHCs clearly contradicts two common notions: (a) that the OHC is approximately 30 to 40 dB more sensitive than the IHC (e.g., Dallos & Wang, 1974), and (b) that there are separate operating ranges for the two populations of hair cells such that the OHCs mediate the behaviorally measured hearing for the lower 50 dB sensation level and the IHCs take over above that level (Stebbins et al., 1979).

These erroneous conclusions are based on the assumption made by many investigators that cochlear mechanics are unaffected by a widespread degeneration of the OHCs. The present hypothesis predicts that the absence of the OHCs leads to a reduction of 30 - 50 dB in the sensitivity of the mechanical response of the whole partition, which in turn should be reflected in a shift of the response of the the surviving IHCs and Type I cochlear neurons (Dallos & Wang, 1974), in an elevation of the threshold for compound action potential (e.g., Aran, 1981), and in an elevation of the behaviorally measured hearing of the animal. This prediction is testable in the sense that the high sensitivity and sharp tuning of the basilar membrane response as shown in Figure 7-4 should be absent in a cochlea with widespread OHC loss such as the kanamycin-damaged cochleae, or in the sense that the basilar membrane response should be affected by electrical stimulation of the olivocochlear bundle. The limiting factor expected in such experiments is the great practical difficulty of making measurements of basilar membrane motions of about 1-nm amplitude with adequate speed and reliability and without damaging the vulnerable cochlear biomechanical mechanisms.

The ac component of RP of both OHC and IHC (Dallos et al., 1982) showed similar tuning characteristics which in turn resembled single cochlear nerve fiber tuning. It is intriguing to note that the dc component of the RP of an OHC is more sharply tuned than its ac component, and that the dc RP of an OHC is *hyperpolarizing* for stimulus frequencies somewhat below the characteristic frequency (CF). This *hyperpolarizing* characteristic contrasts with the finding that the dc RPs of an IHC (Dallos, et al., 1982; Russell & Sellick, 1978, 1983) or of undifferentiated hair cells in the non-mammalian hearing organs (Crawford & Fettiplace, 1981; Weiss, Mulroy, & Altman, 1974) are always *depolarizing*. The hair-bundle displacement versus membrane potential of the frog's saccular hair cell observed by Hudspeth and Corey (1977) shows an asymmetrical curve; there is a greater magnitude of depolarization than hyperpolarization. Thus, in such hair cells, a sinusoidal displacement of the hair bundle, even without any dc component, is not expected to produce any dc RP for a small-amplitude stimulus or a consistently depolarizing dc RP following a large-amplitude stimulus. In this regard, the hyperpolarizing dc RP of the OHC is highly unusual.

The stimulus-induced hyperpolarizing dc RP of the OHC at stimulus frequencies below the CF may turn out to be an important correlate for the hypothesized motor function of the OHCs. The hyperpolarization of the OHC may signify a "reverse" transduction of electrochemical energy into mechanical energy such that a mechanical correlate is produced as a baseline shift of the cochlear partition. It has been observed that application of a low-frequency biasing stimulus has powerful effects on cochlear nerve fiber responses to tones near the fiber CF (LePage, 1981; Schmiedt, 1982; Sellick et al., 1982a). In this regard, producing a mechanical baseline shift of the partition by the OHC in the region basal to the characteristic place (i.e., the place of maximum response for a particular frequency of a low-level tone stimulus) is of considerable importance. In the active cochlear biomechanical model of Neely and Kim (1983) and Kim and colleagues (1980b), a particular frequency of tonal stimulus leads to a response profile where the intracochlear energy release occurs in a region which is *not exactly centered at the characteristic place*. The apical boundary of this energy-releasing region is near or basal to the characteristic place such that the center of the region is noticeably basal to the characteristic place. Thus for a particular position on the cochlear partition, as in an OHC, I predict that the stimulus frequencies at which the OHCs release mechanical energy should be in a range below the CF. More electrophysiological data from the OHCs should be helpful, but ultimately direct mechanical data in this regard should confirm or refute this prediction.

The basal shift of the active energy-releasing region relative to the characteristic place for a single tone stimulus offers a plausible functional interpretation for the peculiar anatomy of the outer spiral fibers; these travel a substantial distance in the *basal* direction after entering the organ of Corti before making synaptic contacts with the OHCs. I suggest that the combined information about the response level at the characteristic place (via the IHC/Type-I fibers) and the operating point of the OHC's motor function located more basally (via the OHC/Type-II fibers) are used by brainstem mechanisms to regulate the cochlear response via the OC neurons. This postulate is represented by the collateral input to the "filled" neuron in the CN from the Type I fibers in Figure 7-3. The operating-point information from the OHCs in the *active region* (rather than that of the OHCs located right across the tunnel of Corti) does indeed accompany the response-level information of the IHCs in the more apically located characteristic place for a particular stimulus frequency.

The observations of Brown, Nuttal, & Masta (1983), that the IHC response is attenuated by electrical shock stimulation of the crossed olivocochlear bundle (COCB) and that this COCB effect is dependent upon the acoustic stimulus frequency (i.e., maximal attenuation of the response near the CF of the IHC), are of great significance. Since there are few efferent synaptic contacts directly on the cell membrane of the IHCs relative to the efferent synapses on the OHC membrane, the demonstration of the COCB effect on the IHC response is strong evidence for an influence by the OHCs on the IHCs. Major aspects of the IHC data as well as analogous data from single cochlear nerve fibers obtained with COCB stimulation (Gifford & Guinan, 1983, Wiederhold, 1970) are consistent with the present hypothesis; the large medial OC neurons affect the OHCs, which in turn increase the effective mechanical damping of the cochlear partition and produce the frequency-dependent reduction in the mechanical response of the partition (see lower panel of Figure 7-4).

Crucial evidence for Hypotheses 2 and 3 comes from observations by Mountain (1980) and by Siegel and Kim (1982) that electrical shock stimulation of the COCB at the floor of the fourth ventricle affects the otoacoustic distortion signal $(2f_1 - f_2)$ monitored in the ear canal. Figure 7-5 depicts the experimental procedure and the observation of Siegel and Kim. The COCB effect of influencing the otoacoustical signal is blocked by curare (lower right panel of Figure 7-5), supporting the interpretation that the COCB effect is synaptically mediated, most likely at the OHCs. This observation provides important support for the occurrence of the flow of signal in the direction opposite to the usual one in the cochlea, that is, from neuroelectric to mechanical

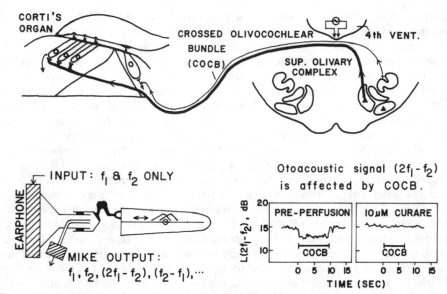

Figure 7-5. Description of experimental procedures and observations demonstrating that the crossed olivocochlear bundle (COCB) can affect the otoacoustic signal $(2f_1-f_2)$. The upper part indicates the COCB was electrically stimulated at the floor of the fourth ventricle and that the axons of the large medial olivocochlear neurons make synaptic contacts with the OHCs. The lower left panel shows that application of two tones at frequencies f_1 and f_2 into the earphone leads to a generation of nonlinear distortion signals at frequencies $(2f_1-f_2)$, (f_2-f_1), and so on in the region of the cochlea where responses to the primary frequencies f_1 and f_2 overlap. The distortion signals are mechanically propagated along the cochlea, through the middle ear, and into the ear canal; the distortion signals are observed in the sound pressure in the ear canal through a probe microphone (see Kim, 1980, for details). The lower right panel displays the observation of Siegel and Kim (1982) that COCB stimulation affected the level of the otoacoustic signal $(2f_1-f_2)$ and that this COCB effect is blocked by curare in the artificial perilymph perfused through the scala tympani. This observation supports the concept that the central nervous system can exert a control on the biomechanics of the organ of Corti through the OHCs.

rather than vice versa, and suggests that, indeed, the central nervous system may exert a significant control on the biomechanics of the organ of Corti.

There is a prominent but peculiar electrical polarization of the cochlear scala media, approximately $+100$ mV re scala tympani (Davis, 1957; Sohmer, Peake, & Weiss, 1971) called the endocochlear potential; it is peculiar because there is a near absence of electrical polarization of the endolymph in the vestibular organs despite the near uniformity of the chemical composition of endolymph in all parts of the membranous labyrinth (Eldredge, Smith, Davis, & Gannon, 1961; Smith, Davis, Deatherage, & Gessert, 1958). The function of the unusual endocochlear potential remains unclear. The motor action of the OHCs in the present hypothesis needs a power supply in order to mechanically drive the cochlear partition, and I suggest that the energy associated with the endocochlear potential/current may be the source of energy powering the motor action of the OHCs. My related explanation for the near absence of an electrical polarization in the vestibular organs is that, unlike the cochlea, the vestibular organs have no active biomechanical mechanism nor any need for increasing the sensitivity of their mechanical response. From a teleological point of view, a sufficient amount of stimulus energy seems to be readily available in our normal environment to drive the hair cells in the vestibular organs in the form of the gravitational force or the acceleration produced by the whole head motion. In contrast, acoustic stimuli, below about 30–40 dB re 20 μPa, provide an inadequate amount of energy to drive the hair cells in the hearing organs without a special mechanism for sensitivity enhancement. The hearing organs of the birds (Smith & Takasaka, 1971) and the caiman (Klinke & Pause, 1980; von Düring, Karduck & Richter, 1974) appear to have some hair cells and the associated innervation which may be the primitive counterpart of the mammalian OHC subsystem. The OHC subsystem may have evolved in the mammalian cochlea as an advanced mechanism for enhancing and controlling the biomechanics of the hearing organ.

INTERPRETATION OF CERTAIN OBSERVATIONS

The present set of hypotheses offers plausible teleological interpretations for the following major features of the auditory system.

(1.) The functional reason for the presence of so many OHCs is to deliver sufficient mechanical force and energy to drive the whole organ of Corti mechanically, thereby conferring the benefits to the IHCs.

(2.) Few of the Type II cochlear neurons receive signals from the OHCs since the information carried by Type II neurons is of low spatial and temporal resolution. This spatially and temporally averaged information about the operating point associated with the motor action of the OHCs reflects the mechanical baseline shift of the cochlear partition. Thus a large channel capacity is not needed for transmission of such a gain-control signal.

(3.) The majority of cochlear neurons innervate the IHCs to transmit auditory information to the brain with high spatial and temporal resolution. The IHCs are the primary receptor cells which transduce cochlear mechanical responses into receptor potentials conveying auditory information.

(4.) The medial OC neurons have large somata and axons in order to exert direct biomechanical influence on the motor function of the OHCs.

(5.) The lateral OC neurons have small somata and axons because they are not involved in biomechanical gain control but only in neural inhibition.

(6.) The anatomical difference between the attachments of the hair bundles of the OHCs and the IHCs, that is, the very firm attachments of the tallest row of the OHC hair bundle to the tectorial membrane, in contrast to the loose or absent contact between the IHC hair bundle and the tectorial membrane (e.g., Lim, 1972; Hoshino, 1981), reflect the active mechanical role of the OHC hair bundle. A firm anchor is needed against which to exert a mechanical force to drive the organ of Corti vis a vis the more passive mechanical role of the IHC in transduction of the partition motion into the receptoneural signal.

(7.) The basal travel of the outer spiral fibers prior to innervation of the OHCs provides an alignment of the cochleotopic organizations of the Type I and Type II cochlear nerve fibers. The more basally located active region (where the OHCs release mechanical energy) is aligned with the characteristic place (whose response level is conveyed via the IHC/Type I fibers), affording a convergence of the inputs from the two types of cochlear afferents onto neurons of the cochlear nucleus. This alignment may mediate a descending regulation of the cochlear response via the olivocochlear neurons.

(8.) The paradoxical existence of the endocochlear potential (about +100 mV in scala media re scala tympani) is to supply energy for the motor action of the OHCs, enhancing the mechanical response of the cochlear partition, whereas no such electrical polarization is needed in the endolymph of the vestibular organs for increasing the sensitivity of the vestibular mechanical response.

SUMMARY

(1.) A set of internally consistent hypotheses is proposed here for the existence, identification, and functional roles of two distinct parallel IHC and OHC subsystems in the caudal part of the auditory system up to the superior olivary complex; Table 7-3 describes an outline of the comparison of the two subsystems.

(2.) The set of hypotheses provides a theoretical framework for integrating coherently a number of seemingly disjointed and some perplexing results from anatomical, physiological, and modeling studies of the auditory system.

(3.) Some of the still-missing pieces include (a) a direct proof of the reverse transduction of the OHC by means of an experimental determination of whether or not the OHC hair bundle moves in response to an intracelluarly applied electrical stimulus; further refinements are needed in the type of experiment reported by Brownell (1983); (b) elucidation of molecular mechanisms underlying the hypothesized bidirectional transduction of the OHCs; (c) identification of the cell type and location of the target neurons in the cochlear nucleus receiving projection of the Type II cochlear afferents from the OHCs and determination of other possible ascending and descending inputs to such target neurons; (d) neuroanatomical description of the ascending and descending inputs to the two types of OC neurons, especially a determination of the way the large medial OC neurons receive input from the OHCs (via directly from the cochlear nucleus and/or via other superior olivary neurons); (e) physiological characterization of the afferent cochlear nerve fibers from the OHCs; all reported physiological data from single cochlear nerve fibers are believed to be recorded from the Type I nerve fibers originating from the IHCs (Liberman, 1982); (f) physiological characterization of the two types of the efferent OC neurons/fibers under unanesthetized conditions and of the nature and magnitude of their selective influences on the cochlear response in normal hearing; (g) further theoretical works refining and producing test-

TABLE 7-3.

Comparison of the OHC and the IHC subsystems in the caudal part of the auditory system from the cochlea up to the superior olivary complex

	OHC subsystem	IHC subsystem
Function	Biomechanical gain control	Usual sensory transduction
Role in cochlear biomechanics	Active	Passive
Enhanced sensitivity, tuning, dynamic range, & nonlinearity	Source	Beneficiary
Hair bundle re tectorial membrane	Firm attachment	Loose or no attachment
Hair cells	Many (12,000)	Few (3,500)
Afferent neurons	Few (2,100)	Many (27,900)
Efferent neurons	Large, myelinated	Small, unmyelinated
Afferent signal	Low spatial & temporal resolutions	High spatial & temporal resolutions
Efferent effect	Attenuation of cochlear mechanical response	Inhibition of radial nerve fibers
Physiological vulnerability	Highly vulnerable	Less vulnerable
Spont. rate (SR) of aff. neurons	Unknown	Bimodal distribution: 35%, SR 15 spikes/s 65%, SR 15 spikes/s

Note. The numbers for hair cells and neurons are for the human species.

able predictions from specific hypotheses about yet unknown molecular mechanisms underlying the OHC motor function using active-and-nonlinear models for cochlear biomechanics.

An ultimate integration of such models with basic neurobiology of the cochlea, the brainstem, and indeed all of the auditory nervous system appears to be necessary even if the objective is to understand only the mechanical behavior of the basilar membrane; all the subsystems are intimately and functionally interconnected in vivo.

REFERENCES

Adams, J.C. (1983). Cytology of periolivary cells and the organization of their projections in the cat. *Journal of Comparative Neurology, 215*, 275-289.

Aran, J.-M. (1981). Electrophysiology of cochlear toxicity. In C.J. Matz, S. Lerner, & J.E. Hawkins (Eds.), *Aminoglycoside ototoxicity* (pp. 31-47). Chicago: Little, Brown.

Anderson, S.D., & Kemp, D.T. (1979). The evoked cochlear mechanical response in laboratory primates: A preliminary report. *Archives of Otorhinolaryngology, 224*, 47-54.

Arnesen, A.R., & Osen, K.K. (1978). The cochlear nerve in the cat: Topography, cochleotopy and fiber spectrum. *Journal of Comparative Neurology, 178*, 661-678.

Békésy, G. von (1960). *Experiments in hearing.* New York: McGraw-Hill.

Brown, M.C., Nuttall, A.L., & Masta, R.I. (1983). Intracellular recordings from cochlear inner hair cells: Effects of stimulation of the crossed olivocochlear efferents. *Science, 222*, 69-72.

Brownell, W.E. (1983). Observations on a motile response in isolated outer hair cells. In W. Webster & L. Aitkin (Eds.), *Neural Mechanisms of Hearing* (pp. 5-10), Monash University.

Clark, W.W., Kim, D.O., Bohne, B.A., & Zurek, P.M. (1983). Spontaneous otoacoustic emissions from chinchillas: Comparison of otoacoustic observations with cochlear histopathology. *Association for Research in Otolaryngology, Meeting Abstracts*, 106.

Crane, H.D. (1982). IHC-TM connect-disconnect and efferent control. V. *Journal of Acoustical Society of America, 72*, 93-101.

Crawford, A.C., & Fettiplace, R. (1981). Nonlinearities in the responses of turtle hair cells. *Journal of Physiology, 315*, 317-338.

Dallos, P., & Harris, D. (1978). Properties of auditory nerve responses in absense of outer hair cells. *Journal of Neurophysiology, 41*, 365-383.

Dallos, P., Harris, D.M., Relkin, E., & Cheatham, M.A. (1980). Two-tone suppression and inter-modulation distortion in the cochlea: Effect of outer hair cell lesions. In G. van den Brink & F.A. Bilsen (Eds.), *Psychophysical, Physiological and Behavioural Studies in Hearing* (pp. 242-252). Noordwijkerhout, Netherlands: Delft Univ.

Dallos, P., Santos-Sacchi, J., & Flock, A. (1982). Intracellular recordings from cochlear outer hair cells. *Science, 218*, 582-584.

Dallos, P., & Wang, C-Y. (1974). Bioelectric correlates of kanamycin intoxication. *Audiology, 13*, 277-289.

Davis, H. (1957). Biophysics and physiology of the inner ear. *Physiological Reviews, 1957*, 1-49.

Davis, H. (1983). An active process in cochlear mechanics. *Hearing Research, 9*, 79-90.

de Boer, E. (1983). No sharpening? A challenge for cochlear mechanics. *Journal of the Acoustical Society of America, 73*, 567-573.

Drenckhahn, D., Keller, J., Mannherz, H.G., Groschel-Stewart, U., Kendrick-Jones, J., & Scholey, J. (1982). Absence of myosin-like immunoreactivity in stereocilia of cochlear hair cells. *Nature (London), 300*, 531-532.

Eldredge, D.H. (1967). Book review of Spoendlin, H. (1966). In Ruedi (Ed.), *The organization of the cochlear receptors, Vol. 13: Advances in Oto-Rhino-Laryngology, L.* Basel, Switzerland: Karger. (From *Journal of the Acoustical Society of America,* 1967, 1386–1388).

Eldredge, D.H., Smith, C.A., Davis, H., & Gannon, R.P. (1961). The electrical polarization of the semicircular canals (guinea pig). *Annals of Otology Rhinology and Laryngology, 70,* 1024–1036.

Engstrom, H., & Sjostrand, F.S. (1954). The structure and innervation of the cochlear hair cells. *Acta Otolaryngology, 44,* 490–501.

Evans, E.F. (1975). The sharpening of cochlear frequency selectivity in the normal and abnormal cochlea. *Audiology, 14,* 419–442.

Evans, E.F., & Wilson, J.P. (1975). Cochlear tuning properties: Concurrent basilar membrane and single nerve fiber measurements. *Science, 190,* 1218–1221.

Farley, G.R., & Warr, W.B. (1981). Some recurrent projections of the superior olive to anteroventral and dorsal cochlear nuclei in cat. *Neuroscience Abstracts, 7,* 56.

Fex, J. (1962). Auditory activity in centrifugal and centripetal cochlear fibers in cat: A study of a feedback system. *Acta Physiologica Scandinavica, 55,* Suppl. 189.

Flock, A. (1983). Hair cells, receptors with a motor capacity? In R. Klinke, & R. Hartman (Eds.), *Symposium on Hearing–Physiological Bases and Psychophysics* (pp. 1–6). Bad Nauheim, Germany: Springer-Verlag.

Flock, A., & Cheung, H.C. (1977). Actin filaments in sensory hairs of inner ear receptor cells. *Journal of Cell Biology, 75,* 339–343.

Gifford, M.L., & Guinan, J.J. (1983). Effects of crossed-olivocochlear-bundle stimulation on cat auditory nerve fiber responses to tones. *Journal of the Acoustical Society of America, 74,* 115–123.

Gold, T. 1948). Hearing II. The physical basis of the action of the cochlea. *Proceedings of the Royal Society of London [B], 135,* 492–498.

Guinan, J.J. (1983). The physiology and morphology of the efferent auditory system of the cat. *Society for Neuroscience Abstracts, 9,* 890.

Harrison, R.V., & Evans, E.F. (1979). Cochlear fibre responses in guinea pigs with well defined cochlear lesions. *Scandinavian Audiology [Suppl. 9],* 83–92.

Hirokawa, N., & Tilney, L. (1982). Interactions between actin filaments and membrane in quick-frozen and deeply etched hair cells of the chick ear. *Journal of Cell Biology, 95,* 249–261.

Hoshino, T. (1981). Imprints of the inner sensory cell hairs on the human tectorial membrane. *Archives of Otolaryngology, 232,* 65–71.

Hubbard, A.E., & Mountain, D.C. (1983). Alternating current delivered into the scala media alters sound pressure at the eardrum. *Science, 222,* 510–512.

Hudspeth, A.J., & Corey, D.P. (1977). Sensitivity, polarity, and conductance change in the response of vertebrate hair cells to controlled mechanical stimuli. *Proceedings of the National Academy of Science USA, 74,* 2407–2411.

Iurato, S. (1967). *Submicroscopic structure of the inner ear.* New York: Pergamon.

Kemp, D.T. (1978). Stimulated acoustic emissions from within the human auditory system. *Journal of the Acoustical Society of America, 64,* 1386–1391.

Kemp, D.T. (1979). Evidence of mechanical nonlinearity and frequency selective wave amplification in the cochlea. *Archives of Otorhinolaryngology, 224,* 37–45.

Khanna, S.M., & Leonard, D.G.B. (1982). Basilar membrane tuning in the cat cochlea. *Science, 215,* 305–306.

Kiang, N.Y.S. (1975). Stimulus representation in the discharge patterns of auditory neurons. In D.B. Tower (Ed.), *The Nervous System, Vol. 3: Human Communication and its Disorders* (pp. 81–97). New York: Raven Press.

Kiang, N.Y.S., Moxon, E.C., & Levine, R.A. (1970). Auditory-nerve activity in cats with normal and abnormal cochleas. In G.E.W. Wolstenholme & J. Knight (Eds.), *Sensorineural Hearing Loss* (pp. 241–267). London: Churchill.

Kiang, N.Y.S., Rho, J.M., Northrup, C.C., Liberman, M.C., & Ryugo, D.K. (1982). Hair-cell innervation by spiral ganglion cells in adult cats. *Science, 217,* 175–177.

Kim, D.O., (1980). Cochlear mechanics: Implications of electrophysiological and acoustical observations. *Hearing Research, 2,* 297–317.

Kim, D.O. (1983). The inner-hair-cell (IHC) and outer-hair-cell (OHC) subsystems in the cochlea and the brainstem. *Society of Neuroscience Abstracts, 9,* 43.

Kim, D.O., Clark, W.W., & Zurek, P.M. (1983). Spontaneous otoacoustic emissions in chinchillas: Changes in level and frequency of the emission by application of an external tone. *Association for Research in Otolaryngology Meeting Abstracts,* 107.

Kim, D.O., & Molnar, C.E. (1975). Cochlear mechanics: Measurements and models. In D.B. Tower (Ed.), *The nervous system, Vol. 3, Human communication and its disorders,* pp. 57–68. New York: Raven Press.

Kim, D.O., Molnar, C.E., & Matthews, J.W. (1980a). Cochlear mechanics: Nonlinear behavior in two-tone responses and in ear-canal sound pressure. *Journal of the Acoustical Society of America, 67,* 1704–1721.

Kim, D.O., Molnar, C.E., & Pfeiffer, R.R. (1973). A system of nonlinear differential equations modeling basilar-membrane motion. *Journal of the Acoustical Society of America, 54,* 1516–1529.

Kim, D.O., Neely, S.T., Molnar, C.E., & Matthews, J.W. (1980b). An active cochlear model with negative damping in the partition: Comparison with rhode's anti- and post-mortem observations. In G. van den Brink & F.A. Bilsen (Eds.), *Psychophysical, physiological and behavioural studies in hearing* (pp. 7–15). Noordwijkerhout, The Netherlands: Delft Univ. Press.

Kimura, R. (1978). Differences in innervation of cochlear inner and outer hair cells. *Association for Research in Otolaryngology Meeting Abstracts.*

Klinke, R., & Galley, N. (1974). Efferent innervation of vestibular and auditory receptors. *Physiological Reviews, 54,* 316–357.

Klinke, R., & Pause, M. (1980). Discharge properties of primary auditory fibers in Caiman crocodilus: Comparisons and contrasts to the mammalian auditory nerve. *Experiments in Brain Research, 38,* 137–150.

Kronester-Frei, A. (1978). Ultrastructure of the different zones of the tectorial membrane. *Cell and Tissue Research, 193,* 11–23.

Leake-Jones, P.A., & Snyder, R.L. (1982). Uptake and transport of horseradish peroxidase by cochlear spiral ganglion neurons. *Hearing Research, 8,* 199–223.

LePage, E.L. (1981). *The role of nonlinear mechanical processes in mammalian hearing.* PhD thesis, University of Western Australia, Nedlands.

LePage, E.L., & Johnstone, B.M. (1980). Nonlinear mechanical behavior of the basilar membrane in the basal turn of the guinea pig cochlea. *Hearing Research, 2,* 183–189.

Liberman, M.C. (1982). Single-neuron labeling in the cat auditory nerve. *Science, 216,* 1239–1241.

Lim, D.J. (1972). Fine morphology of the tectorial membrane. *Archives of Otolaryngology, 96,* 199–215.

Macartney, J.C., Comis, S.D., & Pickles, J.O. (1980). Is myosin in the cochlea a basis for active motility? *Nature (London), 28,* 491–492.

Morest, D.K. (1975). Structural organization of the auditory pathways. In D.B. Tower (Ed.), *The nervous system, Vol. 3: Human Communication and its Disorders* (pp. 19–30). New York: Raven Press.

Morest, D.K., & Bohne, B.A. (1983). Noise-induced degeneration in the brain and representation of inner and outer hair cells. *Hearing Research, 9,* 145–151.

Mountain, D.C. (1980). Changes in endolymphatic potential and crossed olivocochlear bundle stimulation alter cochlear mechanics. *Science, 210,* 71–72.

Neely, S.T., & Kim, D.O. (1983). An active cochlear model showing sharp tuning and high sensitivity. *Hearing Research, 9,* 123–130.

Nordeen, K.W., Killackey, H.P., & Kitzes, L.M. (1983). Ascending auditory projections to the inferior colliculus in the adult gerbil, Meriones unguiculatus. *Journal of Comparative Neurology, 214,* 131–143.

Osen, K.K., & Brodal, A. (1981). The auditory system. In A. Brodal (Ed.), *Neurological anatomy* (3rd ed., pp. 602–639). New York: Oxford Univ. Press.

Prosen, C.A., Petersen, M.R., Moody, D.B., & Stebbins, W.C. (1978). Auditory thresholds and kanamycin-induced hearing loss in the guinea pig assessed by a positive reinforcement procedure. *Journal of the Acoustical Society of America, 63,* 559–566.

Rhode, W.S. (1971). Observations of the vibration of the basilar membrane in squirrel monkeys using the Mössbauer technique. *Journal of the Acoustical Society of America, 49,* 1218–1231.

Rhode, W.S. (1973). An investigation of post-mortem cochlear mechanics using the Mössbauer effect. In A.R. Moller (Ed.), *Basic mechanisms of hearing* (pp. 49–67). New York: Academic Press.

Rhode, W.S. (1978). Some observations on cochlear mechanics. *Journal of the Acoustical Society of America, 64,* 158–176.

Robertson, D., & Johnstone, B.M. (1979). Aberrant tonotopic organization in the inner ear damaged by kanamycin. *Journal of the Acoustical Society of America, 66,* 466–469.

Ruggero, M.A., Santi, P.A., & Rich, N.C. (1982). Type II cochlear ganglion cells in the chinchilla, *Hearing Research, 8,* 339–356.

Russell, I.J., & Sellick, P.M. (1978). Intracellular studies of hair cells in the mammalian cochlea. *Journal of Physiology, 284,* 261–290.

Russell, I.J., & Sellick, P.M. (1983). Low-frequency characteristics of intracellular recorded receptor potentials in guinea-pig cochlear hair cells. *Journal of Physiology, 338,* 179–206.

Ryan, A., & Dallos, P. (1975). Effect of absence of cochlear outer hair cells on behavioral auditory threshold. *Nature (London), 253,* 44–46.

Schmiedt, R.A., & Feng, A.S. (1980). Method for tracing single fibers in the organ of Corti with horseradish peroxidase. *Hearing Research, 2,* 79–85.

Schmiedt, R.A. (1982). Effects of low-frequency biasing on auditory-nerve fiber activity. *Journal of the Acoustical Society of America, 72,* 142–150.

Sellick, P.M., Patuzzi, R., & Johnstone, B.M. (1982a). Modulation of responses of spiral ganglion cells in the guinea pig cochlea by low frequency sound. *Hearing Research, 7,* 199–221.

Sellick, P.M., Patuzzi, R., & Johnstone, B.M. (1982b). Measurement of basilar membrane motion in the guinea pig using the Mössbauer technique. *Journal of the Acoustical Society of America, 72,* 131–141.

Siegel, J.H., & Kim, D.O. (1982). Efferent neural control of cochlear mechanics? Olivocochlear bundle stimulation affects cochlear biomechanical nonlinearity. *Hearing Research, 6,* 171–182.

Siegel, J.H., Kim, D.O., Molnar, C.E. (1982). Effects of altering organ of Corti on cochlear distortion products f_2-f_1 and $2f_1-f_2$. *Journal of Neurophysiology, 47,* 303–328.

Simmons, D.D., & Liberman, M.C. (1983). Afferent innervation of outer hair cells in the adult cat. *Society of Neuroscience Abstracts, 9,* 44.

Smith, C.A., & Takasaka, T. (1971). Auditory receptor organs of reptiles, birds and mammals. In W.D. Neff (Ed.), *Contributions to Sensory Physiology, Vol. 5* (pp. 129–178). New York: Academic Press.

Smith, C.A., Davis, H., Deatherage, B.H., & Gessert, C.F. (1958). DC potentials of the membraneous labyrinth. *American Journal of Physiology, 193,* 203–206.

Sohmer, H.S., Peake, W.T., & Weiss, T.F. (1971). Intracochlear potential recorded with micropipets. I. Correlations with micropipet location. *Journal of the Acoustical Society of America, 50,* 572–586.

Spoendlin, H. (1966). The organization of the cochlear receptor. In Dr. L. Ruedi (Ed.), *Advances in Oto-Rhino-Laryngology* (Vol. 13). New York: Karger.

Spoendlin, H. (1969). Innervation patterns in the organ of Corti of the cat. *Acta Otolaryngology, 67,* 239–254.

Spoendlin, H. (1972). Innervation densities of the cochlea. *Acta Otolaryngology, 73,* 235–248.

Spoendlin, H. (1978). The afferent innervation of the cochlea. In R.F. Naunton & C. Fernandez (Eds.), *Evoked electrical activity in the auditory nervous system* (pp. 21–41). New York: Academic Press.

Spoendlin, H. (1979). Neural connections of the outer haircell system. *Acta Otolaryngology, 87,* 381–387.

Stebbins, W.C., Hawkins, J.E., Johnsson, L-G, & Moody, D.B. (1979). Hearing thresholds with outer and inner hair cell loss. *American Journal of Otolaryngology, 1,* 15–27.

Tilney, L.G., De Rosier, D.J., & Mulroy, M.J. 1980). The organization of actin filaments in the stereocilia of cochlear hair cells. *Journal of Cell Biology, 86,* 244–259.

von Düring, M., Karduck, A., & Richter, H.G. (1974). The fine structure of the inner ear in Caiman crocodilus. *Zeitschrift für Anatomie und Entwicklungsgeschichte, 145,* 41–65.

Warr, W.B. (1978). The olivocochlear bundle: its origins and terminations in the cat. In R.F. Naunton & C. Fernandez (Eds.), *Evoked electrical activity in the auditory nervous system.* New York: Academic Press.

Warr, W.B. (1982). Parallel ascending pathways from the cochlear nucleus. *Contributions to Sensory Physiology, 7,* 1–38.

Warr, W.B., & Guinan, J.J., Jr. (1979). Efferent innervation of the organ of Corti: Two separate systems. *Brain Research, 173,* 152–155.

Warr, W.B., White, J.S., & Nyffeler, M.J. (1982). Quantitative comparison of the lateral and medial efferent systems in adult and newborn cats. *Neuroscience Abstracts, 8,* 346.

Weiss, T.F. (1982). Bidirectional transduction in vertebrate hair cells: A mechanism for coupling mechanical and electrical processes. *Hearing Research, 7,* 353–360.

Weiss, T.F., Mulroy, M.J., & Altman, D.W. (1974). Intracellular responses to acoustic clicks in the inner ear of the alligator lizard. *Journal of the Acoustical Society of America, 55,* 606–619.

White, J.S., & Warr, W.B. (1983). The dual origins of the olivocochlear bundle in the albino rat. *The Journal of Comparative Neurology, 219,* 203–214.

Wiederhold, M.L. (1970). Variations in the effects of electric stimulation of the crossed olivocochlear bundle on cat single auditory nerve fiber responses to tone bursts. *Journal of the Acoustical Society of America, 48,* 966–977.

Wilson, J.P., & Johnstone, J.R. (1975). Basilar membrane and middle-ear vibration in guinea pig measured by capacitive prove. *Journal of the Acoustical Society of America, 57,* 705–723.

Zurek, P.M., Clark, W.W., & Kim, D.O. (1982). The behavior of acoustic distortion products in the ear canals of chinchillas with normal or damaged ears. *Journal of the Acoustical Society of America, 72,* 774–780.

Zurek, P.M., & Clark, W.W. (1981). Narrow-band acoustic signals emitted by chinchilla ears after noise exposure. *Journal of the Acoustical Society of America, 70,* 446–450.

Chapter 8

Speech Encoding in the Auditory Nerve

Murray B. Sachs

INTRODUCTION

Between the early 1940's and middle 1970's, many studies explored the responses of auditory-nerve fibers to "simple" stimuli such as tones, sums of two tones, and clicks and noise; these studies enabled us to describe in detail the auditory-nerve encoding of such "simple" stimuli. Among the characteristics of fiber responses most frequently studied were frequency selectivity as measured by tuning curves (Kiang & Moxon, 1974), phase locking in response to one- and two-tone stimuli (Abbas, 1978; Brugge, Anderson, Hind, & Rose, 1969; Javel, 1981; Rose, Brugge, Anderson, & Hind, 1967), rate-saturation and limited dynamic range in responses to tones (Palmer & Evans, 1980; Sachs & Abbas, 1974; Schalk & Sachs, 1980; Smith & Brachman, 1980a), and, nonlinear interactions in responses to two-tone stimuli such as two-tone suppression (Abbas & Sachs, 1976; Arthur, Pfeiffer, & Suga, 1971) and combination-tone generation (Goldstein & Kiang, 1968; Kim, Siegel, & Molnar, 1979). This data base then led to the development of a number of models which could predict at least qualitatively many of the aspects of the auditory-nerve discharge patterns (Hall, 1977; Kim, Molnar, & Pfeiffer, 1973; Sachs & Abbas, 1976; Weiss, 1966).

Although many aspects of the responses to one- and two-tone stimuli remained to be worked out (see, for example, Liberman, 1978; Sachs & Hubbard, 1981; Sokolich, Hamernik, Zwislocki, & Schmeidt, 1976), it seemed appropriate to consider how well responses to more complex stimuli, specifically speech, could be predicted on the basis of our knowledge of the responses to the simpler stimuli. Thus, simultaneously, a number of groups began detailed analysis of the encoding of speech in the auditory nerve (Delgutte, 1980; Hashimoto, Katayama, Murato, & Taniguchi, 1975; Reale & Geisler, 1980; Sachs & Young, 1979).

This chapter reviews the recent studies of speech encoding with an emphasis on how a number of speech features might be represented in auditory-nerve discharge patterns. We begin with steady-state vowels to illustrate the experimental paradigms and data processing techniques commonly used in the speech studies. We then illustrate how results for steady vowels have been extended to stimuli with time-varying spectra such as stop consonants and fricatives. We conclude with a discussion of the peripheral encoding of pitch.

REPRESENTATION OF VOWELS

In processing any stimulus, the central nervous system has available to it the spike discharge patterns of the entire population of auditory-nerve fibers. By the nature of its pattern of innervation of cochlear hair cells, the auditory nerve is strictly tonotopically organized (Sando, 1965); that is, fibers in the auditory nerve are arranged according to their most sensitive frequency or characteristic frequency (CF). Such organization according to frequency is also maintained at higher levels of the central auditory system (Merzenich, Knight, & Roth, 1975). It is therefore appropriate to consider how responses to a stimulus like speech are distributed across characteristic frequency in the auditory-nerve fiber population. According to what have classicially been called "place" theories of hearing (Helmholtz, 1863), peaks in the acoustic spectrum of a sound (e.g., formant peaks of a speech sound) would result in peaks in response in the population of auditory-nerve fibers at places along the basilar membrane where characteristic frequencies correspond with the peak (formant) frequencies. An example of this scheme is shown in Figure 8-1. At the top is shown the spectrum of a synthesized steady-state vowel /ɛ/ whose first three formant frequencies are 512, 1792, and 2432 Hz, respectively. This vowel has a fundamental frequency (pitch) of 128 Hz. Because the stimulus is perfectly periodic, it has energy only at the fundamental frequency and its harmonics. The center plot shows tuning curves from three auditory-nerve fibers. The characteristic frequencies (CFs) of the fibers are close to the formant frequencies of the vowel. Because the vowel has more energy in the vicinity of their CFs, these fibers should begin to respond to the vowel at lower sound levels than fibers with CFs between the formants and should respond more vigorously at moderate vowel levels.

Thus far we have been purposefully vague about how we define a fiber "response." Two types of response measures have been used as the basis for two very different representations of complex spectra in the auditory nerve. The basis of the *rate place* representation is simply average discharge rate. The basis of the *temporal-place* representation is a measure of the phase-locking (Rose et al., 1967) of auditory-nerve fibers to the complex stimulus. The computation of phase-locking measures for a temporal-place representation is illustrated below; the bottom plot of Figure 8-1 shows an example of the rate-place representation. The data shown here come from one experiment in which 269 fibers were studied in the auditory nerve of a single cat. The goal of such an experiment is to get a good sample of the responses of the entire auditory-nerve fiber population (Pfeiffer & Kim, 1975). Data are shown in Figure 8-1 for the /ɛ/ presented at a stimulus level of 38 dB SPL. Each data point comes from a different fiber. As discussed below, there is some evidence that auditory-nerve fibers with very low rates of spontaneous activity form a separate population. For this reason data from fibers with spontaneous rates less than 1/s are plotted with open square symbols, whereas fibers with higher spontaneous rates are plotted with Xs. Each fiber is plotted at an abscissa value equal to its CF. The ordinate is average discharge rate normalized in such a way that each fiber's rate increase (above spontaneous rate) to the vowel is plotted as a fraction of its maximal (saturation) rate increase to CF tones. The solid line is a windowed average of the data points; this average includes

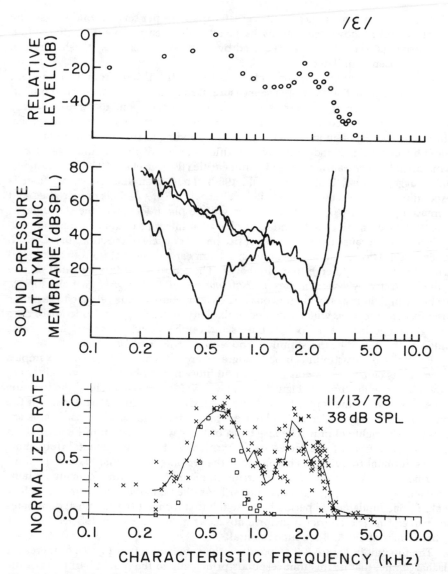

Figure 8-1. Top: Amplitude spectrum of /ɛ/. Middle: Tuning curves from three auditory-nerve fibers whose characteristic frequencies are close to the formant frequencies of /ɛ/ (from Eaton–Peabody Laboratory). Bottom: Plot of normalized rate versus characteristic frequency for population of fibers studied with /ɛ/ as the stimulus. X's represent data from fibers with spontaneous rates greater than one/second; open square symbols are from fibers with lower spontaneous rates. Solid line is a moving window average of the data points for high spontaneous fibers. (From Sachs & Young, 1980.)

only the fibers with spontaneous rates greater than one per second. In this case, the rate-place profile shows peaks of discharge rate at CFs corresponding with the first three formants of the vowel, as required by a rate-place scheme. We shall return to this representation later.

The development of a temporal-place representation differs from the rate-place scheme primarily in that the response measure used is based on phase-locked properties of the fiber discharge pattern. Auditory nerve fibers respond to stimuli in a way that is temporally locked to the stimulus waveform. The instantaneous rate (or probability of discharge) of auditory nerve fibers responding to stimuli with frequencies below about 6 kHz is modulated by a rectified version of the stimulus waveform, as modified by cochlear filtering and nonlinearities (Brugge et al., 1969; Hind, Anderson, Brugge, & Rose, 1967; Rose et al., 1967). Thus, if an auditory-nerve fiber is responding to a 1-kHz tone, there will be alternate 0.5-ms periods of increased and decreased probability of discharge which will be phase-locked to the stimulus; as a consequence, the fiber will tend to discharge at intervals of about 1 ms and multiples of 1 ms (because the fiber will not fire on every cycle of the stimulus). Considerable information about the stimulus spectrum can be derived from the temporal structure of auditory nerve fiber discharge. The existence of this information can be demonstrated by several means: *poststimulus time (PST) histograms* which estimate discharge probability or instantaneous rate as a function of time relative to stimulus onset; *period histograms* which estimate probability of discharge as a function of time through one period of a periodic stimulus and can be thought of as PST histograms folded at the period of the stimulus; and *interspike interval histograms.*

Examples of poststimulus time histograms are shown in Figure 8-16; examples of period histograms of responses of four auditory nerve fibers to the vowel /ɛ/ are shown in the left column of Figure 8-2. The waveform of one cycle of the periodic vowel is shown at the top of the column. The CFs of the fibers are shown in the center and the magnitudes of the Fourier transforms of the period histograms are shown in the right column. The spectrum of the vowel is shown in Figure 8-1; in this case the formant frequencies are at harmonics of the fundamental frequency: the first formant frequency is harmonic 4, the second is harmonic 14, and the third is harmonic 19. As shown by the spectrum in Figure 8-1, the first formant contains considerably more energy than the others. Thus, the temporal waveform shows four peaks in one fundamental period because the first formant (harmonic 4) dominates this waveform. The Fourier transform abscissae in Figure 8-2 are labeled in terms of harmonics of the 128-Hz fundamental.

The top unit in Figure 8-2 responds to the vowel with four phases of increased discharge rate; that is, this unit responds principally to the fourth harmonic of the vowel. The frequency of the fourth harmonic, 0.512 kHz, is near the fiber's CF (0.46 kHz). The second unit in Figure 8-2 has a CF near the 14th harmonic of the vowel and its response contains 14 peaks, indicating that it is responding to the 14th harmonic. Such responses, in which one frequency component dominates, are seen most often in fibers whose CFs are near a formant frequency. They are quite similar to period histograms of responses to pure tones at the same frequencies. The Fourier

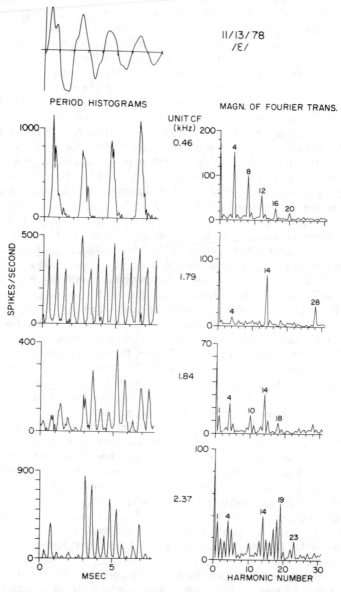

Figure 8-2. Period histograms (left column) and amplitude spectra of Fourier transforms of the period histograms (right column). One pitch period of the stimulus (vowel /ɛ/) is shown at the top of the left column; time scale is same as those of period histograms. (From Young & Sachs, 1981.)

transforms of these two period histograms (right column) have a large component at the frequency of the dominant harmonic (4 in the top histogram and 14 in the second histogram). They also have significant energy at integer multiples (harmonics) of the dominant harmonic (8, 12, 16, 20 in the top histograms and 28 in the second histogram). The components at integer multiples of the dominant harmonic arise, at least in part, from the rectification inherent in the fact that auditory nerve fibers cannot discharge at negative rates; the inhibitory half cycles of period histograms such as these are therefore clipped at zero rate, resulting in the production of frequency components in the response histogram at harmonics of the actual stimulus frequency (Goldstein, 1972; Johnson, 1974; Littlefield, 1973; Molnar, 1974; Young & Sachs, 1979). This distortion must be kept in mind when considering the results to be presented later; it will be referred to as *rectifier distortion*. Responses to frequency components not present in the stimulus can also be produced by *combination tones*, which are generated by cochlear nonlinearities and produce stimulus-like propagating excitation patterns in the population of auditory nerve fibers (Kim et al., 1979).

The third and fourth histograms in Figure 8-2 show examples of fibers which respond significantly to more than one stimulus component. The third histogram has 14 peaks which are strongly modulated in amplitude. Its Fourier transform has a large component at the 14th harmonic and a component almost as large at the 4th harmonic (first formant). Two of the remaining peaks (10th and 18th harmonics) are probably difference and sum distortion products of the two large response components. The CF of the bottom unit is near the third formant (2.432 kHz); its response shows a large third formant (19th harmonic) component, as well as first and second formant components (harmonics 4 and 14) and various distortion products.

We can use the magnitudes of the Fourier transform components of the period histograms as a measure of the phase-locked response of auditory-nerve fibers to the corresponding frequency components. Figure 8-3 shows how the responses to three stimulus harmonics were distributed across the population of auditory-nerve fibers, again with /ɛ/ as the stimulus. Each column shows the distribution of temporal response to one of three harmonics, the 4th (first formant) in the left column, the 10th in the center column, and the 14th (second formant) in the right column. Each row shows the responses to the three harmonics at one of three different sound levels (38, 58, or 78 dB SPL, indicated at the right). The plots were constructed in the same way as that at the bottom of Figure 8-1; there is one point for each unit, which shows the amplitude of the appropriate harmonic (ordinate; normalized by average discharge rate) plotted against the unit's CF (abscissa). Symbols and lines are as in Figure 8-1. The arrow in each graph points to the CF, which is equal to the frequency of the harmonic plotted in that graph; this CF will be referred to below as the place of that harmonic.

The temporal response distributions in Figure 8-3 illustrate the behavior of responses to all harmonics. At the lowest stimulus level (38 dB, top row) the response to each harmonic is maximum in the vicinity of its place; that is, the largest amount of response to each harmonic is found among those fibers whose CFs are approximately equal to the frequency of that harmonic. As stimulus level is increased, the

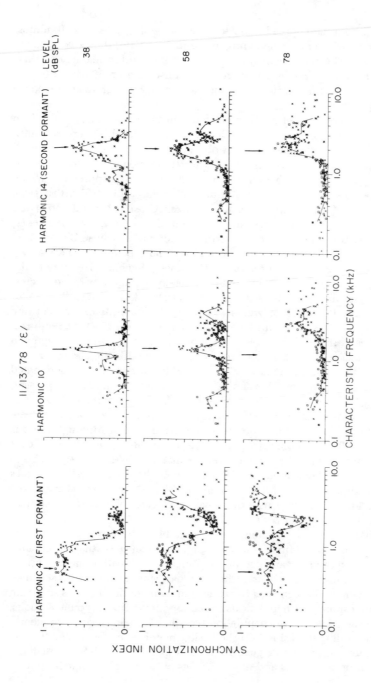

Figure 8-3. Distribution of synchronization as a function of CF for a population of fibers with /ε/ as the stimulus. Synchronization is defined in the text. Each plot shows synchronization to one harmonic of /ε/. Arrow points to the CF, which is equal to the frequency of the harmonic (i.e., place of the harmonic). Symbols and lines as in Figure 8-1 bottom.

response to the first formant spreads over a wide range of CFs. At 78 dB, almost the entire population of fibers is responding to the first formant; the exceptions are those fibers whose CFs lie in the vicinity of the second and third formants. Response to the second formant near its place stays roughly constant from 38 to 58 dB SPL. At 78 dB the response to this formant is reduced slightly, but significant response to this harmonic remains.

In contrast to the behavior of the formant harmonics, the response to the 10th harmonic near its place decreases monotonically as sound level is increased until at 78 dB there is no sign of the peak that was observed at 38 dB. Instead, units with CFs near the 10th harmonic's place respond to the 4th harmonic, the first formant. This behavior is similar to the behavior of two-tone synchrony suppression which has been described previously in detail (Arthur, 1976; Bernardin, 1979; Brugge et al., 1969; Johnson, 1974; Kim et al., 1979; Rose, Kitzes, Gibson, & Hind, 1974) and is illustrated in Figure 8-4. Fourier transform magnitude (unnormalized, spikes/s) is plotted versus overall level of a two-tone stimulus for a fiber whose CF was 1.90 kHz. One tone is at fiber CF; the other (suppressing) tone is below CF and its level is fixed relative to the CF tone (suppressor 15 dB greater). Synchronized rate to the CF alone is shown by Xs, to the CF in the two-tone combination by filled circles, and to the suppressor in the combination by open circles. At low overall levels of the two-tone stimulus, the synchronized rate to the CF tone approximates the value to the CF presented alone. At about the level where synchronized rate to the suppressor begins to increase, the rate locked to the CF in the two-tone stimulus begins to decline. As level is increased further, synchronized rate to the CF ultimately decreases to the noise level of the measurements. At high levels this unit's response is dominated by the low-frequency suppressor. This dominance by the low-frequency suppressor, which is similar to the dominance of harmonic 10 by the first formant in Figure 8-3, has also been observed in responses to two-tone approximations to vowels by Reale and Geisler (1980) and in multitone complexes by Evans (1980). Although there is no response to the 10th harmonic near its place (Figure 8-3) there is significant response to this harmonic at CFs between approximately 2.5 and 5.0 kHz. This is the CF region where units are responding strongly to both the 4th and 14th harmonics and where the distribution of the 10th harmonic has roughly the same shape as the distribution of the 14th harmonic. This is the behavior expected of a rectifier distortion product (difference tone; Young & Sachs, 1979).

The fact that the formant harmonics (4th and 14th) dominate the temporal responses of the population of fibers shown in Figure 8-3 suggests that a good idea of the spectrum of a speech stimulus could be gained by comparing the amount of temporal response at various harmonics of the stimulus. Figure 8-5 illustrates schematically one method which has been used to extract a measure of the stimulus spectrum from the temporal responses of populations of auditory nerve fibers (Young & Sachs, 1979). Fibers are ordered within the population according to characteristic frequency, in other words, according to position on the basilar membrane. (Characteristic frequency is represented vertically in Figure 8-5). The responses of each fiber are determined by the filtering properties and nonlinearities of the cochlea (first column of

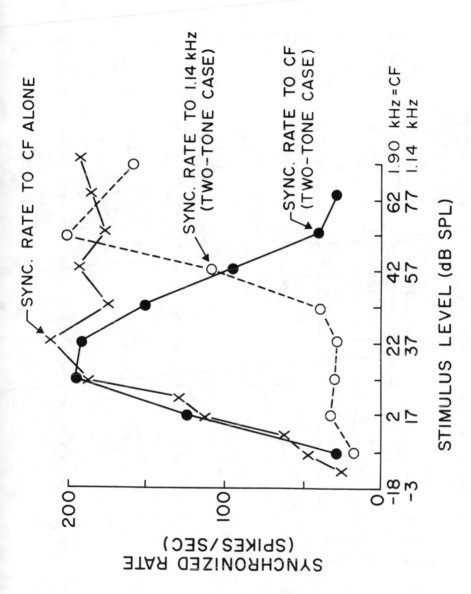

Figure 8-4. Synchronized rate versus level functions for a single fiber with two-tone stimulus. (From Bernardin, 1979.)

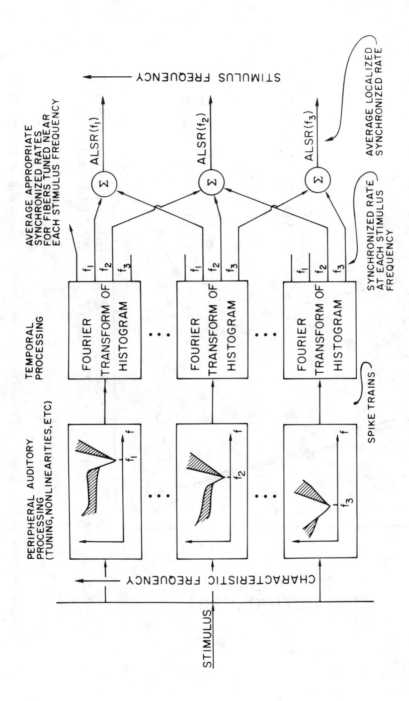

Figure 8-5. Schematic representation of the construction of the average localized synchronized rate (ALSR) temporal profile. (From Sachs et al., 1982b.)

boxes). From the responses of each fiber a histogram (period, interval or PST) and its discrete Fourier transform are computed (second column of boxes). The result for each unit is the amplitude of its temporal response as a function of stimulus frequency (equal to the Fourier transform magnitudes). The response of the population of fibers to each stimulus frequency is then obtained by averaging the responses to that frequency of all fibers whose CFs are within a range of either one-half or one-quarter octave of that stimulus frequency. The resulting measure has been called average localized synchronized rate (ALSR; Young & Sachs, 1979). ALSR (f) is the *average* of the responses of fibers whose CFs are *localized* to the vicinity of frequency f; *synchronized rate* is the amplitude of a fiber's Fourier transform at frequency f in units of spikes per second. The ALSR measure gives a temporal-place representation because it reflects both place (CF) in the population and temporal response (synchronized rate).

Figure 8-6 shows ALSR plots for the vowel /ɛ/ presented at seven stimulus levels. The spectrum of this vowel has been compensated for the effects of the external ear of human beings (Young & Sachs, 1981). This compensation increases the amplitudes of the second and third formants by about 8 and 17 dB, respectively. The points at the first three formants frequencies have been plotted with filled circles. Notice that the ALSR is always largest at the first formant frequency. At lower sound levels the profile of the ALSR is a good reflection of the spectrum of the /ɛ/ (Figure 8-1) with local maxima at the first three formant frequencies. The only serious deviation is the slightly elevated response at the second harmonic of the first formant (harmonic 8, 1024 Hz). At higher levels the first three formants continue to stand out, although the second and third formant peaks are slightly reduced at the highest level used. This reduction is greater if the vowel spectrum is not compensated for external ear effects, a finding which could indicate an important role for the external ear resonance in speech encoding. Responses to the second and third harmonics of the first formant (8th and 12th harmonics of the fundamental) grow considerably at higher levels until they are larger than the second formant response at the highest level. Except for these two distortion products related to the first formant, however, all response components between the first and second formants are suppressed at higher levels (as in the case of harmonic 10 in Figure 8-3).

The lines drawn through some of the points in Figure 8-6 are meant to show the extent to which the ALSR resembles the stimulus spectrum if presumed distortion components are ignored. The lines are drawn through all the points except those at the second and third harmonics of the first formant and the first sum and difference tone of the first two formants. The similarity of these plots to the spectrum of the stimulus (Figure 8-1) is clear.

Having illustrated the computation of both rate-place and temporal-place representations, let us turn now to the question of how vowel features can be encoded in these representations. Figure 8-7 shows the spectra of three synthesized vowels which have been considered in the early studies of Sachs and Young (1979). The vowels /I/ (bit) and /ɛ/ (bet) are both front vowels (Gleason, 1961; Jacobson, Fant, & Halle, 1963) and thus have a concentration of energy in the vicinity of the second and third

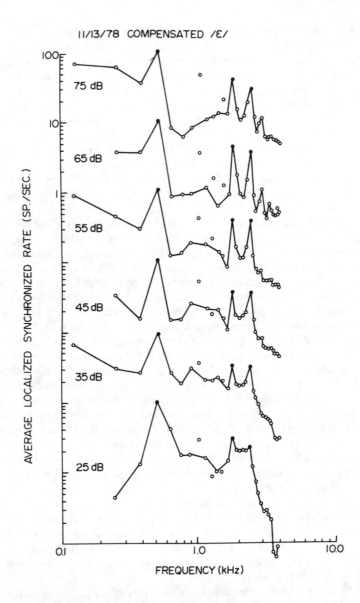

Figure 8-6. Average localized synchronized rate (ALSR) for /ɛ/ presented at seven levels. The vowel spectrum has been compensated for human external ear characteristics. See text for definition of ALSR and explanation of lines. Each plot shifted vertically from previous one by one order of magnitude; ordinate labels refer to top plot only. (From Young & Sachs, 1981.)

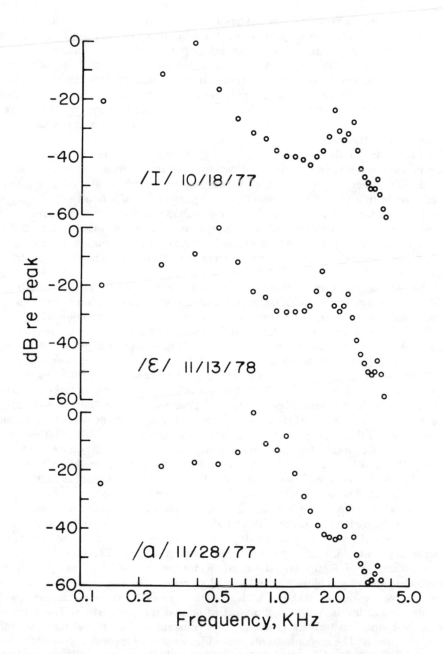

Figure 8-7. Spectra of three vowels considered in this section. (From Young & Sachs, 1979.)

formants. The back vowel /a/ (father) has a second formant at a low frequency and thus lacks the high-frequency peak seen in the other two. The very low first formant of /I/ and the high first formant of /a/ reflect the fact that these are "high" and "low" vowels, respectively. The resulting spectrum is "compact" for /a/ and diffuse for /I/.

These vowel features could be represented in the auditory nerve by any faithful reproduction of the formant structure of the vowel. Figure 8-8 shows that at stimulus levels below about 50 dB SPL normalized rate-versus-place profiles provide a representation for the first two formant frequencies. The figure shows normalized rate plotted versus CF for three levels of /I/ and /a/. Average curves only are shown. (Data for /ɛ/ are similar to those for /I/.) For both /I/ and /a/ there are peaks in the rate profiles in the vicinity of the first two formant frequencies and thus the rate-place profiles seem to preserve at least these first two formants at moderate sound levels. (Indeed, a clear third formant peak is present for /ɛ/ when the stimulus is compensated for the external ear.) However, as shown in Figure 8-9, as sound level is increased these formant-related peaks disappear from the rate profiles. This disappearance of formant peaks can be explained in terms of rate saturation (Evans, 1980; Sachs & Abbas, 1974) and two-tone suppression (Abbas & Sachs, 1976; Sachs & Kiang, 1968).

The average rate profiles shown in Figures 8-8 and 8-9 do not include data from fibers with spontaneous rates less than one per second (see discussion of Figure 8-1). Fibers with low spontaneous rates appear to form a separate population within the auditory nerve on both morphological (Liberman, 1982) and physiological grounds (Liberman, 1978; Schalk & Sachs, 1980). These fibers, which form about 15% of the population, have higher thresholds (Figure 8-10) and wider dynamic ranges (Figure 8-11) than do the higher spontaneous-rate units. Sachs and Young (1979) have suggested that this small population might play a role in preserving formant peaks in rate profiles at high stimulus levels. Figure 8-12 shows that formant-related peaks are observed in rate profiles for the low-spontaneous population at levels higher than those at which the high-spontaneous group has saturated. At 78 dB SPL there are no peaks in rate profiles for high spontaneous units in this population (see Sachs & Young, 1979). Although the data are sparse in Figure 8-12, there are clearly formant-related peaks in these profiles at 78 dB SPL. Thus, the low-spontaneous units could extend the range of levels over which formant-related peaks occur.

The data in Figures 8-8, 8-9, and 8-12 show that the rate-place representation of vowels changes dramatically with stimulus level; maintenance of formant peaks at high levels, if possible, seems to depend on the low-spontaneous-rate fibers as a separate population. The temporal-place profiles, on the other hand, are quite stable with stimulus level. Figure 8-13 shows ALSRs for the vowels /I/, /ɛ/, and /a/ whose spectra are shown in Figure 8-7. In these plots presumed distortion products have been removed as discussed above. Each set of three plots shows data from one vowel at three sound levels, with the plots superimposed for comparison. The average response to the first formant grows or stays constant as sound level increases for all three vowels. The response to the second formant may grow monotonically (for /I/) with level or may be suppressed somewhat at the highest level (for /a/ and /ɛ/;

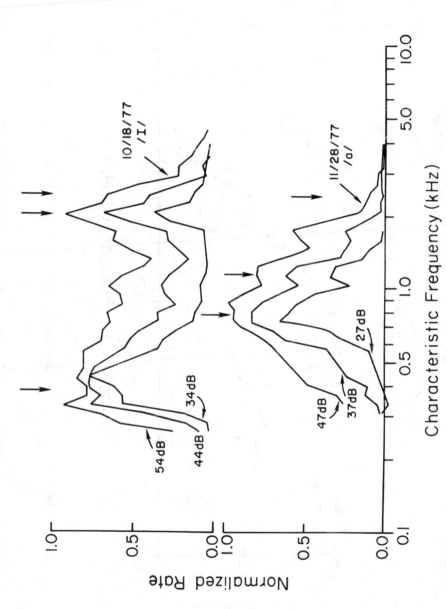

Figure 8-8. Normalized average rate profiles for /I/ and /a/ presented at three stimulus levels. (From Sachs et al., 1982b.)

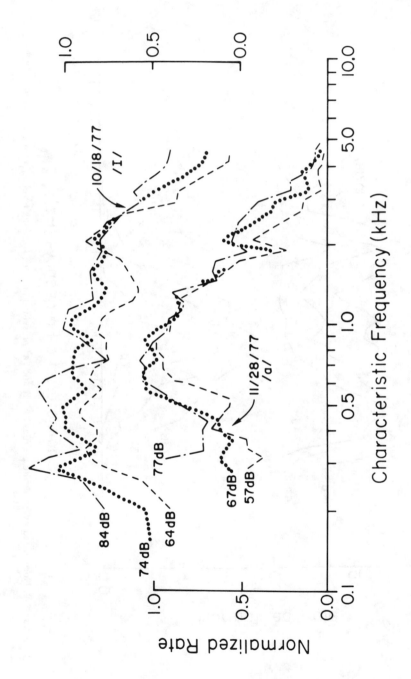

Figure 8-9. Normalized average rate profiles for /I/ and /a/ are presented at three levels. (From Sachs et al., 1982b.)

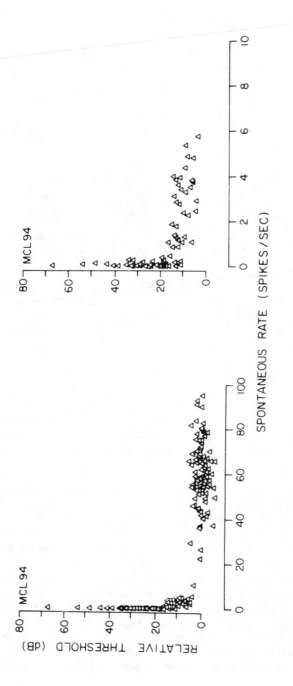

Figure 8-10. Relation between spontaneous rate and relative threshold in one cat reared in a low-noise chamber. The relative threshold of each unit is the difference between the threshold at CF and the average threshold at CF of all units from the same ear with similar CFs and rates of spontaneous activity greater than 18 spikes/s. In the right panel the data from the low-rate units are displayed on an expanded horizontal scale. (From Liberman, 1978.)

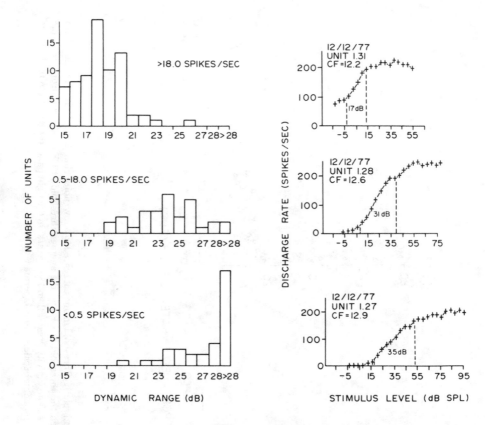

Figure 8-11. Histograms of dynamic ranges for CF tones grouped by spontaneous rates and a typical rate-level function for each group. (From Schalk, 1979.)

but recall that compensation for the external ear transfer function removes the suppression for /ɛ/, as in Figure 8-6). Responses to stimulus components between the first and second formants are always suppressed at the highest level. This suppression is sufficient to maintain a local maximum at the second formant frequency even at the highest levels used. In all three cases, the response to components between the first and second formants is lowest at the highest stimulus level. Because of this synchrony suppression, the representation of the first two formant frequencies is well maintained in these temporal-place representations. Although the third formant is suppressed at the highest levels, the human external ear can be expected to overcome this suppression (as, for example, in Figure 8-6).

There are those who argue that the perception of vowels need not depend on extraction of formant frequencies (see, for example, Bladon & Lindblom, 1981). Vowel discrimination certainly need not depend on preservation of well-defined formant

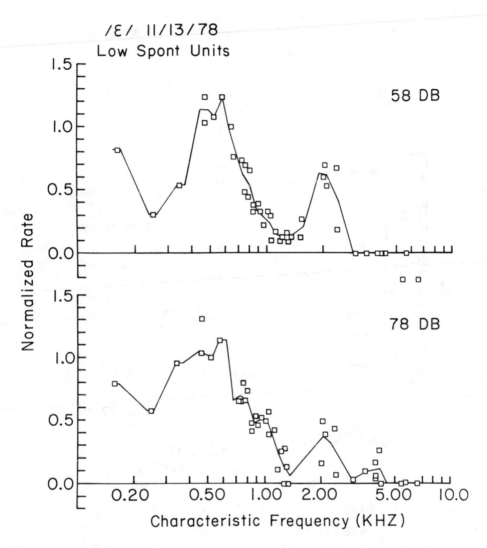

Figure 8-12. Normalized rate versus CF for low-spontaneous-rate units (less than 1/s) for one cat studied with /ɛ/ as the stimulus. (From Sachs & Young, 1979.)

peaks in rate- or temporal-place profiles (Sachs & Young, 1979). In Figure 8-7, for instance, even though there are no formant peaks in the rate profiles for /a/ and /I/, these two vowels could easily be discriminated on the basis of the gross shapes of the profiles. These gross shapes reflect important spectral differences between the two vowels. The high front vowel /I/ has a low first- and high second-formant frequency; its spectrum is diffuse with energy at high as well as low frequencies. The

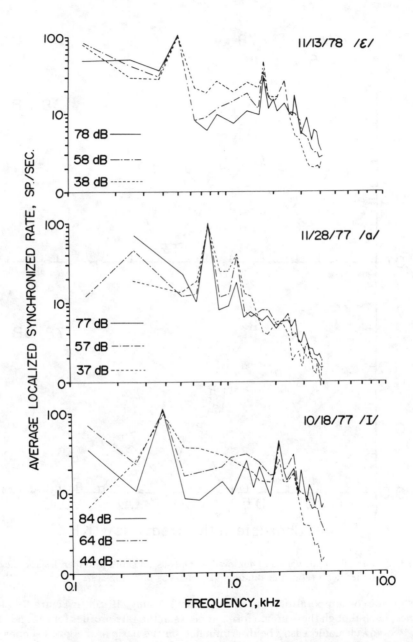

Figure 8-13. Average localized synchronized rate profiles for the vowels /ɛ/, /I/, and /a/. Each
plot shows ALSR at three sound levels for one vowel. Plots are superimposed on
same ordinate for comparison. (From Young & Sachs, 1979.)

low back vowel /a/ has a high first- and low second-formant frequency which results in a compact spectrum with a peak of energy in the region of the first two formants. The gross shapes of the rate-place profiles clearly reflect this difference in vowel spectra. Whereas the rate profile for /I/ is spread diffusely across the characteristic frequency dimension, the profile for /a/ has a peak in the region of the places of the first two formants and remains more compact than the profile for /I/ even at the highest sound levels used. Sachs and Young (1979) have argued that the compactness of the /a/ profile is maintained at high stimulus levels by two-tone rate suppression (see also Sachs, Young, & Miller, 1982b). Thus even at levels where saturation and suppression effects have eliminated formant peaks in the rate profiles, the gross spectral features of the stimulus are preserved. These features are, of course, also preserved in the temporal-place ALSR plots in Figure 8-13, which provide a more detailed representation of the stimulus spectrum.

In summary, formant frequencies in vowels are well preserved in a temporal-place representation. Formant structure is preserved at high stimulus levels in a rate-place representation if low-spontaneous, high-threshold fibers are considered as a separate population. Gross spectral features of vowels are well preserved in both representations.

REPRESENTATION OF STOP CONSONANTS

The steady-state vowels considered in the previous section have spectra which do not vary with time. On the other hand, much of the information conveyed by speech is carried by consonants, many of which involve rapid spectral changes. For example, stop consonants are characterized by a very brief burst of noise at release from the stop, followed by a rapid formant frequency transition as the articulators move from the stop configuration to that for the following vowel (see, for example, Stevens & Blumstein, 1978). A number of questions arise when one thinks about extending results for steady-state vowels to consonants with time-varying stimuli. For example, á priori it is not clear how well a temporal representation, which did a good job with perfectly periodic vowels, will work for aperiodic stop consonants whose spectra are changing rapidly. Second, Smith and Brachman (1980a) have shown that the dynamic range of auditory-nerve fiber rate responses is considerably larger when rate is measured over short intervals near stimulus onset than when it is measured in the steady state. This dynamic range expansion could be important for the encoding of consonants, especially stop consonants in the initial position. For example, it could extend the range of levels over which formant peaks are maintained in rate profiles.

The discharge patterns of single auditory nerve fibers can follow the instantaneous frequency of a frequency modulated tone, if that frequency is within the phase-locking range (less than about 5.0 kHz). An example from a recent study by Sinex and Geisler (1981) is shown in Figure 8-14. The stimulus in this case was an FM tone in which the instantaneous frequency ascended linearly from 20 to 690 Hz between 50 and

710 ms and descended from 690 to 20 Hz between 800 and 1460 ms. The figure plots all of the interspike intervals that occurred during several repetitions of the frequency sweep. The abscissa gives the mean time of occurrence of the interval relative to the period of modulation. The stimulus period changes as the reciprocal of the instantaneous frequency, so that when the frequency changes linearly the instantaneous period follows a hyperbolic trajectory. The data show that as time increases the intervals first decrease (as frequency increases) and then increase (as frequency decreases). The intervals follow the hyperbolic trajectory of the stimulus period. At a given peristimulus time, corresponding to a constant stimulus period, the intervals cluster around multiples of that period just as they would for a pure tone. Kiang (1980) shows the same effect in a PST histogram for responses to a swept tone. Peaks in the PST histogram are separated by a time which changes in proportion to the instantaneous stimulus period.

These results suggest that a temporal measure can be used to represent the spectra of the formant transitions in a consonant-vowel syllable as well as in the steady vowel. Figure 8-15 shows an example of stimuli used in a recent study of the encoding of such syllables (Miller & Sachs, 1983). The trajectories of the first three formants used to produce the syllable /da/ are shown at the left in Figure 8-15A; fundamental frequency (pitch) as a function of peristimulus time is also shown here. The plot at right in Figure 8-15A shows that sound level increases from a value of about 65 dB SPL near the consonant onset to a value of 69 dB SPL in the steady-state vowel. The entire time waveform is shown in Figure 8-15B. The largest peaks occur at the frequency of glottis excitation (pitch); the damped oscillations between these peaks reflect the response of the vocal tract to the glottis excitation. Figure 8-15C shows expanded waveforms for the first and last 20 ms of the stimulus. During the first 20 ms the pitch frequency is 120 Hz and there are four peaks in the waveform per pitch period. These peaks result from the fact that the first formant dominates the temporal pattern (it has the greatest energy). During this 20-ms interval the first formant is at about 500 Hz or about four times the pitch; thus, there are four peaks per pitch period. During the last 20 ms the first formant has moved to 700 Hz or roughly six times the pitch frequency. Correspondingly there are six peaks in the waveform per pitch period. The features of time-varying stimuli such as this stop consonant are commonly displayed in short-time spectra computed over time intervals shorter than the transition time. The short-time spectra of these two short stimulus segments are shown in Figure 8-15D. These spectra show formant peaks at frequencies corresponding with the formant trajectories shown in Figure 8-15A.

Responses of auditory nerve fibers to these time-varying stimuli can also be analyzed over corresponding short-time segments. These responses are best analyzed with poststimulus time (PST) histograms. Figure 8-16 shows PST histograms computed from the responses of one fiber to the stimulus illustrated in Figure 8-15. The top row shows data from the first 20 ms of the stimulus; the bottom row shows data from the last 20 ms. The left column shows the stimulus waveform for the corresponding time segment; the middle column shows PST histograms computed over the same segments; and the right column shows the Fourier transforms of these histograms.

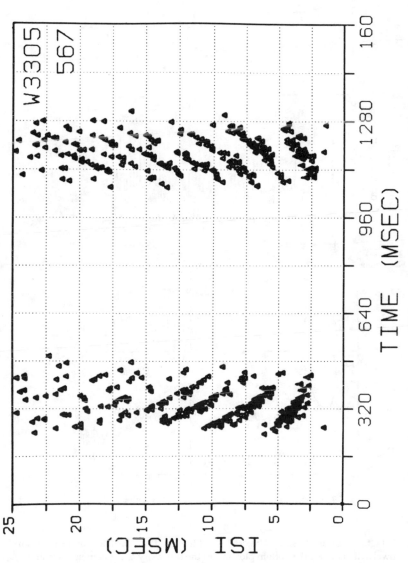

Figure 8-14. Time course of interspike intervals (ISIs) in response to a frequency-modulated tone. ISIs occurring over 26 repetitions of modulation are plotted against their mean times of occurrence during the modulation cycle. The instantaneous frequency of the tone changed linearly from 20 to 690 Hz between 50 and 710 ms, and from 690 to 20 Hz between 800 and 1460 ms. The sweep tone was presented at a 1.0 kHz/s modulation rate at 95 dB SPL. (From Sinex & Geisler, 1981.)

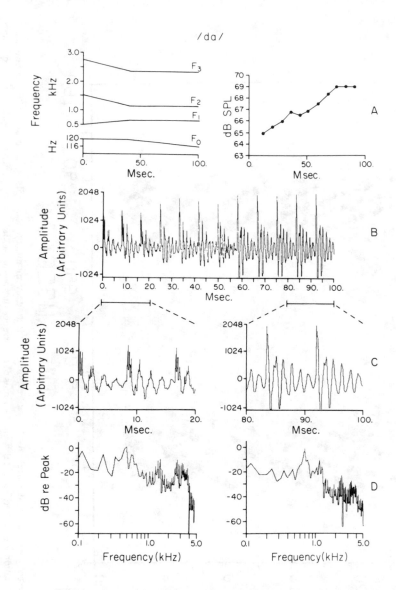

Figure 8-15. (A) Left: Top three plots show trajectories of the first three formants of the constant-vowel syllable /da/; the bottom plot shows the trajectory of fundamental frequency. Right: Stimulus level as a function of time after stimulus onset. (B) Stimulus waveform. (C) Expanded versions of first and last 20-ms segments of the stimulus waveform. (D) Power spectra derived from the two segments shown in (C) (From Miller & Sachs, 1983.)

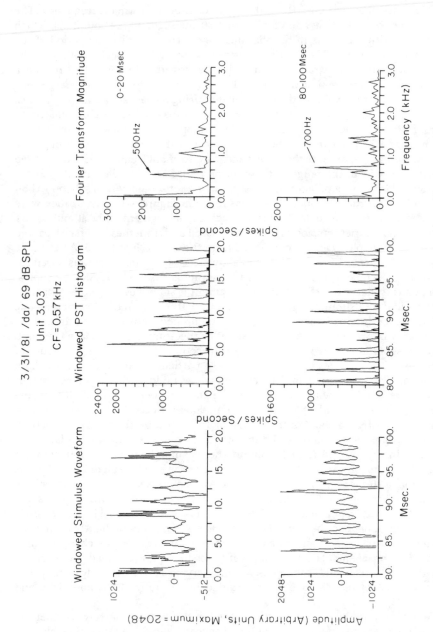

Figure 8-16. PST histograms and their Fourier transforms computed over first 20-ms segment of the /da/ stimulus (top) and last 20-ms segment (bottom). Corresponding stimulus waveforms in left column. (From Miller & Sachs, 1983.)

The CF of this fiber was 0.5 kHz in the range of the first formant frequency. The spacing of peaks in the histogram for the first 20-ms segment is about 2 ms, which corresponds with the peaks in the stimulus waveform and with the period of the first formant frequency. The Fourier transform shows a large peak at 500 Hz. The peaks in the bottom histogram have moved closer together in a way that reflects a similar change in the stimulus waveform. The Fourier transform shows a large peak at 700 Hz, which is the value of the first formant during the last 20 ms of the stimulus. Thus the responses of this fiber during the first 20-ms segment are dominated by the first formant, which is near fiber CF. These responses, as measured by Fourier transforms of PST histograms, follow the motion of the first formant through the stimulus. Similar responses to the second and third formant frequencies are observed in fibers with CFs in the range of these formants (Miller & Sachs, 1983).

To summarize the population response to such a consonant-vowel syllable, ALSR plots can be constructed from data such as those in Figure 8-16, just as they were for the steady-state vowel data. That is, for each 20-ms segment of the stimulus, PST histograms and Fourier transforms can be computed and from these average localized synchronized rate plots can be constructed from these as in Figure 8-5. An example is shown in Figure 8-17. The plot at top shows the short-time stimulus spectrum computed for the time segment 20–40 ms after stimulus onset. The ALSR for a population of auditory-nerve fibers for this same segment is shown below. Note, here, that both the ALSR and stimulus spectrum are plotted at 50-Hz frequency increments, which is the resolution of a Fourier transform computed from a 20-ms data sample. The similarity between the ALSR and the stimulus spectrum indicates that a temporal-place representation (ALSR) does a good job in coding the short-time spectrum of a consonant. Two features of the similarity are particularly important. First, both spectrum and ALSR have a component which varies rapidly with frequency, super-imposed on a slowly varying envelope. As we shall see below, the rapidly varying part is related to stimulus pitch while the envelope reflects the formant structure (vocal tract transfer function) of the stimulus. To emphasize the formant structure, both stimulus and ALSR plots can be smoothed to eliminate the rapid variations in frequency. In Figure 8-18 the left column shows smoothed spectra and the right column shows smooth ALSR plots corresponding to the spectra at left. Each plot was derived from a 20-ms segment of the data. The ALSR plots clearly resemble the stimulus spectrum throughout. The dashed lines superimposed on the ALSR plots show the locations of the first three formant frequencies taken from the plot in Figure 8-15A. The close correspondence between these trajectories and peaks in the ALSRs indicate that a temporal-place representation can follow the kinds of spectral changes which occur in stop consonants. That is, the answer to the first question posed in this section is that a temporal-place code can represent time-varying as well as steady-state speech signals. Consistent results have been obtained by Delgutte (1981) and Sinex and Geisler (1983).

We turn next to the second question posed in this section, namely whether the dynamic range extension seen at stimulus onset can extend the range of levels over which formant-related peaks occur in rate profiles for stop consonants. Figure 8-19

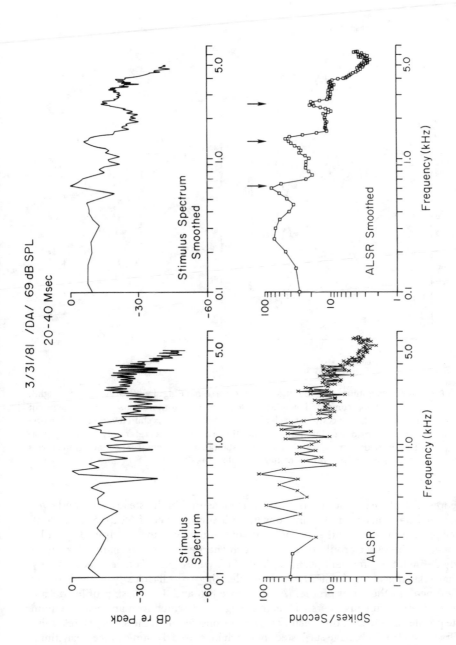

Figure 8-17. Spectrum and average localized synchronized rate profile for one 20-ms segment of /da/, computed from PST histograms.

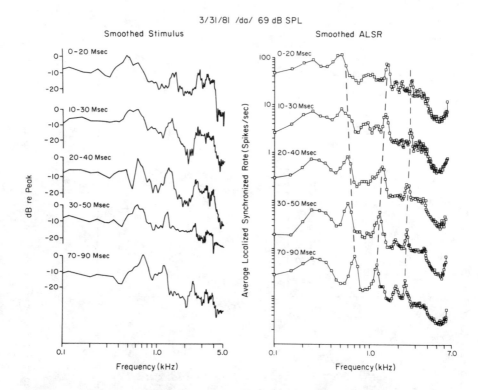

3/31/81 /dɑ/ 69 dB SPL

Figure 8-18. Smooth stimulus power spectra (left) and corresponding smoothed ALSR plots (right).
Each plot was computed over 20-ms segment after stimulus onset; time of segment
is given in the left corner of each plot. Each plot on right is shifted vertically from previous one by one order of magnitude; the ordinate labels refer only to the top plot.
The dashed lines indicate the three instantaneous formant frequency trajectories
of the synthesizer. (From Miller & Sachs, 1983.)

compares rate-place profiles for the vowel /ɛ/ measured in the steady state and over
the interval 5–10 ms after stimulus onset. At a sound level of 58 dB SPL there is
a small peak at the place of the second formant frequency in the steady-state profile.
However, in the onset profile there is a much sharper second formant peak and a
clearly defined third formant peak. At 78 dB SPL where there is no evidence of any
formant-related peaks in the steady-state profiles, there is still a clearly defined second
formant peak in the onset profile. (As in Figure 8-8 and 8-9, these profiles do not
include low-spontaneous fibers.) Thus the range over which formant peaks remain
in rate profiles is considerably greater at stimulus onset than in the steady state. Smith
and Brachman (1980a,b) have suggested that such increased dynamic range near stimulus onset may be related to adaptation of the auditory-nerve fibers. Near stimulus

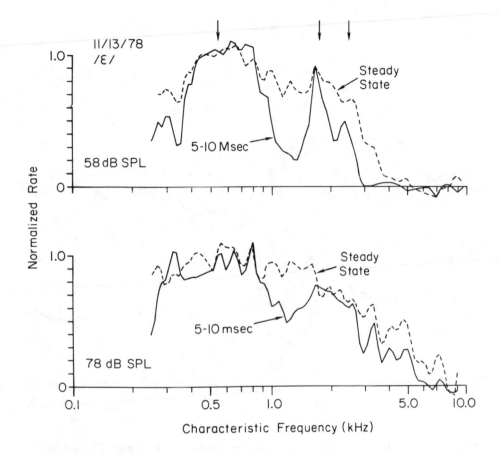

Figure 8-19. Normalized rate plotted versus CF for fibers in one cat with /ɛ/ as stimulus at 58 and 78 dB SPL. Only the average of the high-spontaneous fibers is shown. Dashed curves show rate computed over the interval 20–40 ms after stimulus onset ("steady-state"). Solid curves show rate computed over the 5–10-ms interval after onset. (From Sachs et al., 1982a.)

onset fibers are in an unadapted state, whereas in the steady state they are subject to adapation effects. However, for vowels presented in continuous background noise, these onset effects are not present (Delgutte, 1981; Sachs, Voigt, & Young, 1983).

Figure 8-20 shows that this extended dynamic range may be quite important in the encoding of stop consonants (Miller & Sachs, 1983). The figure shows rate profiles computed over 20-ms segments of the /da/ syllable. During the formant transition (first 50 ms; i.e., near the onset of the stimulus) there are clear peaks at places corresponding to formants 2, 3, and 4 and a broad, less well-defined peak in the range of the first formant. In the steady state, however, these peaks are replaced by a broad

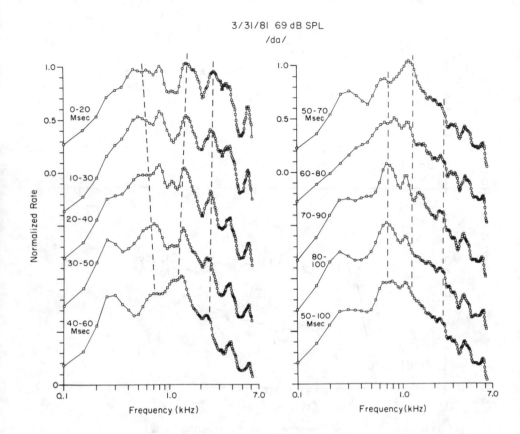

Figure 8-20. Smoothed average rate plots for one cat with /da/ as the stimulus. The time during which average rate was computed is given in the upper left corner of each plot. The dashed lines show the instantaneous formant frequency trajectories of the first three formant frequencies. (From Miller & Sachs, 1983.)

single peak in the vicinity of the first and second formants (50- to 100-ms segment at lower right). The steady-state profiles are similar to those shown for the steady-state vowel /a/ in Figure 8-9. Thus, even at stimulus levels where there are no formant peaks in rate profiles for the steady-state vowel, at least the second, third, and fourth formant peaks are preserved during the consonant transition. Again, this difference in preservation of spectral features is likely the result of short-term adaptation effects.

Delgutte (1981) has further emphasized the importance of such short-term adaptation on auditory-nerve responses to speech. For example, he considers speech stimuli in which there is a rapid spectral change that can be preceded by a number of different contexts and shows that the auditory-nerve fiber responses to the spectral change can be very sensitive to the context. Figure 8-21 shows one example. The stimuli, shown in the bottom traces, have in common steady-vowel segment /a/ and a transition during which the first formant increases from 0.3 to 0.65 kHz while the second formant increases from 0.9 to 1.1 kHz. The transition occurs at about the 100-ms point on the abscissa. In isolation (right column) this stimulus sounds like /ba/. When the transition is preceded by a steady nasal segment containing only low frequencies the result is /ma/. Figure 8-21 shows PST histograms for these stimulu from five fibers whose CFs are given in the left column. All five fibers shows a large increase in discharge rate during the transition interval for the /ba/. However, the fibers with the lower CFs respond strongly to the preceding nasal. These fibers show much less, if any, rate change during the transition, again a clear effect of short-term adaptation. For fibers with higher CFs that do not respond much to the nasal, the response to the transition is roughly the same for /ba/ and /ma/. Delgutte suggests that the distribution of the discharge rates to the transition across CF could cue the /ba/-/ma/ distinction. Similar examples for a /da/ transition in various contexts are shown by Delgutte (1981).

Delgutte suggests that short-term adaptation might operate to enhance spectral contrasts between adjacent speech signals in rate versus CF profiles. According to this idea, at the beginning of a speech segment fibers with CFs near major peaks in the preceding segment will discharge at relatively low rates because they will be in an adapted state. Fibers with CFs near the new peaks in the current segment would not have responded to the preceding stimulus and thus would not be adapted. Their responses at the onset of the new segment would be correspondingly larger than those of fibers responding to the preceding segment.

REPRESENTATION OF FRICATIVE CONSONANTS

The speech stimuli we have considered thus far have all been generated by exciting a model of the vocal tract with a periodic (glottal) pulse train or with a pulse train whose frequency varied only slowly with time. Furthermore, the formant frequencies of these stimuli have all been at relatively low frequencies (less than 3 kHz). In contrast to these vowels and voiced stop consonants are the unvoiced fricatives which generally have their major energy at higher frequencies and are generated by a noise excitation of the vocal tract (Heinz & Stevens, 1961; Strevens, 1960). The nature of these sounds raises a number of questions about how they might be represented in the auditory nerve. It was shown above that a temporal place code can represent quite precisely the spectral structure of both vowels and consonants. One might question whether or not such a temporally based representation can encode spectral features of a speech sound generated from a random noise excitation. Secondly, the kinds of synchrony measures we have discussed above decrease in proportion to stimulus frequency (Johnson, 1980). Whether or not a temporally based measure can represent the high-frequency spectral features of fricatives is a serious question.

The most extensive study of auditory nerve fiber responses to fricatives is that of Delgutte (1980, 1981). Figure 8-22 shows the spectra of four "steady-state" fricatives

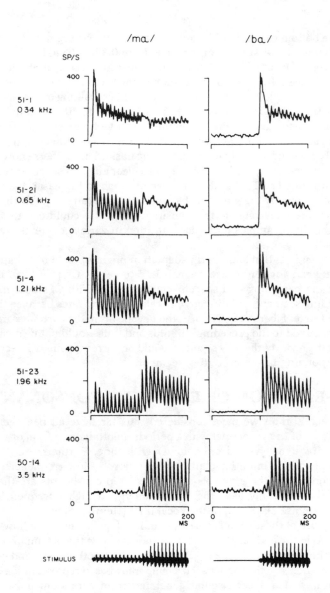

Figure 8-21. PST histograms showing response patterns of five auditory-nerve fibers to /ma/
and /ba/ synthetic stimuli. Stimuli have in common the steady-vowel segment /a/
and a transition during which the first and second formants increase in frequency.
In isolation this stimulus sounds like /ba/; when preceded by a steady nasal segment
it sounds like /ma/. (From Delgutte, 1980.)

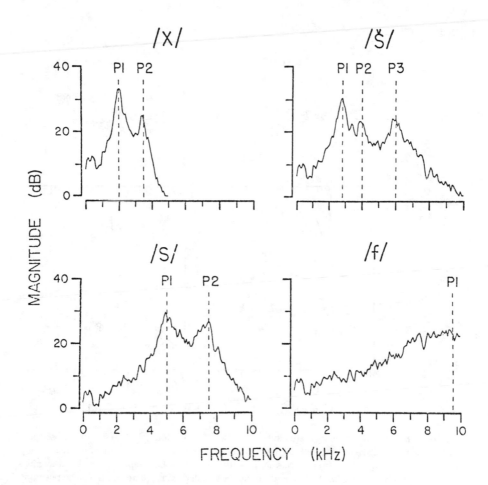

Figure 8-22. Power spectra of four fricative stimuli. Vertical dashed lines mark the positions of the formant frequencies P1, P2, P3. (From Delgutte, 1981.)

used in that study. The stimuli were generated by adding the outputs of noise-excited bandpass filters. The formants (filter center frequencies) are indicated by P_1, P_2, P_3 in the figure. Figure 8-23 shows average rate versus CF profiles for responses to these four stimuli. The profiles for /s/ and /f/ show clear peaks in the CF regions near the formant frequencies. For /X/ (as in German "Ba*ch*" and /š/ (sh), on the other hand, there are no clear peaks at the places of the formant frequencies. Note, however, that these two profiles can be distinguished on the basis of their cut-offs at high CFs and this limited set of four fricatives could certainly be discriminated on the basis of these rate profiles. Thus, the only existing data suggest that fricatives can at least be discriminated on the basis of a rate-place code.

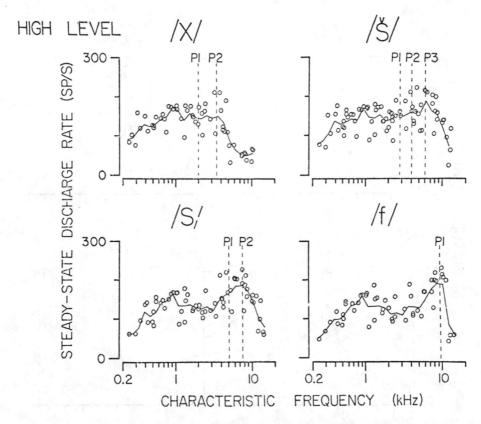

Figure 8-23. Steady-state discharge rate plotted against CF for the four fricative stimuli whose spectra are shown in Figure 8-22. Each circle represents the discharge rate for one auditory
nerve fiber. Data from 17 cats are pooled. Continuous lines represent the band-average
discharge rates for 0.55-octave CF bands sampled every quarter octave. The positions
of the formant frequencies are marked by dashed lines. (Delgutte, 1981.)

Voigt, Sachs, and Young (1984) have clearly demonstrated that speech stimuli
generated with a random noise excitation of the vocal tract can be encoded by a
temporal-place representation. They recorded responses to stimuli which were approximations to whispered vowels. Figure 8-24 shows the spectrum of the vowel they
used; it has formant frequencies appropriate to the vowel /ɛ/. Interval histograms
were computed for the responses of a population of fibers to this vowel; from the
Fourier transforms of these histograms temporal profiles (ALSRs) were computed.
Figure 8-25 shows temporal profiles based on interval histograms for the whispered
/ɛ/ at two sound levels. The profiles show clear peaks at the formant frequencies and
indicate that a temporal measure is certainly capable of encoding such noise-excited
speech sounds.

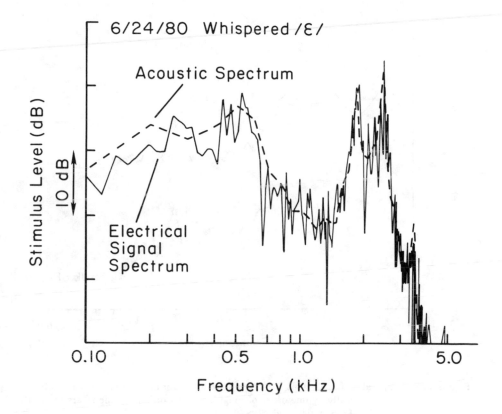

Figure 8-24. The spectrum of electrical signal applied to the earphone (solid line) and acoustic signal (dashed line) for synthesized whispered /ε/.

The formant frequencies of the whispered vowel of Figure 8-25 are lower than most of those in the fricatives shown in Figure 8-22. In fact, with the exception of the formants for /X/ and the first formant for /š/, the remaining fricative formant frequencies in Figure 8-22 are close to or above the upper bound of significant phase locking (5–6 kHz; Johnson, 1980). To determine whether a temporal measure could represent such high frequencies, Delgutte (1981) has computed Fourier transforms of PST histograms for the stimuli whose spectra are shown in Figure 8-22. From these transforms he plotted a measure similar to the ALSR discussed above. As might be expected, only the two /X/ formants and the first formant of /š/ led to peaks in his temporal profiles; the higher formant frequencies were not represented by significant peaks.

Finally, Delgutte (1981) has shown that short-term adaptation effects can be important in the representation of certain fricative features. For example, the fricative /š/ (as in sha) and the affricate /č/ (cha) have similar spectra but differ in the duration

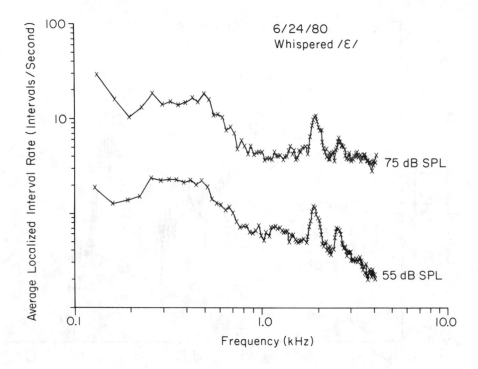

Figure 8-25. Temporal profile for whispered /ɛ/ at two levels for fibers from one cat. Plots are shifted vertically by one order of magnitude; the ordinate scale refers to 75-dB data only. (From Voigt et al., 1982.)

of the rise in amplitude at stimulus onset. Stimuli with rise times less than about 40 ms are heard as /č/; stimuli with longer rise times are heard as /š/ (Cutting & Rosner, 1974). Delgutte synthesized these stimuli by filtering broadband noise to obtain a spectrum similar to those of /š/ and /č/. He presented the stimuli as 200-ms bursts which differed only in the rise–fall times, which for /č/ was 10 ms and for /š/ was 75 ms. For fibers with CFs near the peak of the spectra for both stimuli (3–6 kHz) PST histograms for /č/ presented at 45 dB SPL show a sharp peak immediately after the onset of the stimulus. This sharp peak corresponds with the rapid rise of the /č/ stimulus. The histogram for /š/ has a broad peak occurring at least 20 ms after stimulus onset, reflecting the gradual onset of the /č/. At 60 dB SPL, however, PSTs for both stimuli show a peak at simulus onset. At this higher level, then, the /š/–/č/ difference cannot be carried by fibers with CFs in the region of the stimulus energy peak. On the other hand, Delgutte shows that fibers with CFs removed from this region do show the /š/–/č/ differences. He suggests that the difference between onset and steady-state rates across the population could be signaling this phonetic distinction. As Delgutte points out, these onset effects are related to short-term adaptation.

REPRESENTATION OF PITCH

Estimation of the pitch of complex sounds has occupied auditory theorists for many years (see de Boer, 1976, for review) and a number of recent theories have sought to explain psychophysically measured pitch discrimination. Some of these theories have been based on hypothesized neural representations of pitch (Goldstein, 1973; Terhardt, 1980; Wightman, 1973). In this section we explore what information exists in auditory-nerve discharge patterns that can be used to represent the pitch of speech sounds.

Steady-state vowels are periodic at the fundamental frequency; as indicated by the waveform at the top of Figure 8-2, each period consists of a damped oscillation which is dominated by the large first formant frequency. The voiced stop consonants shown in Figures 8-15 and 8-16 have envelopes which repeat at the fundamental frequency. The phase-locked responses of auditory-nerve fibers reflect this stimulus pattern. Figure 8-26 shows a number of examples (Delgutte, 1980). The stimulus, shown below each column, was an 0.8-kHz single formant stimulus presented at a level of about 60 dB SPL. The fundamental frequency of the stimulus was 100 Hz. Shown above the stimuli are histograms showing two cycles of fibers' responses to the stimulus. The horizontal markers above the histograms indicate a time interval equal to the reciprocal of fiber CF. For all but the top two units in the left column, the histograms show peaks spaced at $1/F_1$, the stimulus formant frequency. The response of the upper left unit is dominated by the fundamental frequency as does the stimulus envelope. Note, however, that the units tuned most closely to the formant frequency show the smallest envelope fluctuations. In fact, Delgutte (1980) shows several examples of responses of fibers to single formant vowels in which the formant is at the CF of the fibers. At 60 dB SPL, a moderate speech level, fibers with CFs below about 1.0 kHz show little, if any, envelope fluctuation. Delgutte (1980) associates this behavior with saturation of discharge rate. As indicated in Figure 8-26, units with CFs considerably above the formant frequency have large envelope fluctuations at 60 dB SPL. Thus, pitch information could be conveyed by the response envelope fluctuations of these high-CF fibers. However, Kiang and Moxon (1974) and Delgutte (1980) have shown that such envelope-related pitch information carried by the high-CF fibers deteriorates badly in background noise. Coding schemes based on envelope fluctuations of individual neurons may thus be inadequate to represent the pitch of speech signals.

Schemes which would extract pitch from the envelope fluctuations such as those in Figure 8-26 work directly on the time domain waveform of individual auditory nerve fiber responses (see, for example, de Boer, 1976). Goldstein (1973), on the other hand, has argued that the nervous system extracts pitch on the basis of spectral patterns displayed across the population of auditory nerve fibers. Let us explore this possibility in terms of the auditory nerve data available. Consider a speech sound which has a pitch of frequency f_0. The spectrum of such a sound will have a broad envelope with peaks at the formant frequencies. Superimposed on the envelope there will be large rapid fluctuations in which peaks occur at harmonics of the pitch frequency; these peaks reflect the pitch excitation function. An example of such a

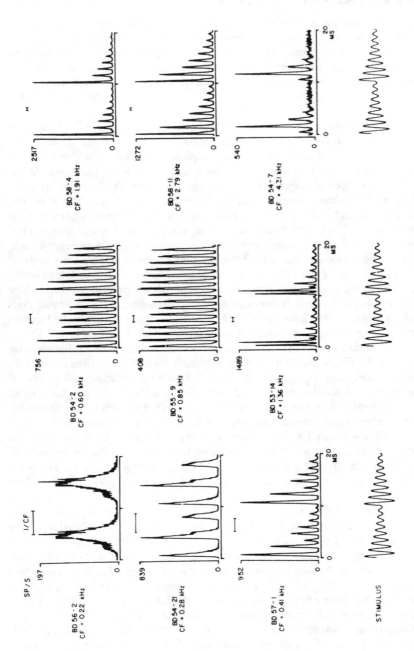

Figure 8-26. PST histograms of responses of nine auditory nerve fibers to a single formant stimulus. The stimulus has a 0.8-kHz formant frequency, a fundamental frequency of 100 Hz, and a formant bandwidth of 70 Hz. The horizontal markers over the histograms indicate an interval of 1/CF. (From Delgutte, 1980.)

spectrum is shown at the top left in Figure 8-27 (from Miller & Sachs, 1983). This spectrum was computed over the interval 20–40 ms after the onset of the /da/ stimulus illustrated in Figure 8-15. The envelope of the spectrum peaks at the formant frequencies. There are, in addition, rapid spectral variations in which peaks and troughs are spaced roughly at 120 Hz (within the 50-Hz resolution of the 20-ms transform used to compute the spectrum). The peaks occur at harmonics of the pitch (120 Hz). Pitch can be extracted from such spectra by a signal processing technique called cepstral analysis (Bogert, Healy, & Tukey, 1963; Oppenheim & Schafer, 1968; Schafer & Rabiner, 1970). The result of this analysis, when applied to the spectrum of a signal whose fundamental frequency is f_0, is a time-domain function with a peak at a time equal to $1/f_0$. The upper right plot in Figure 8-27 shows the cepstrum computed from the spectrum shown at upper left. There is a sharp peak at 8.3 ms which is the reciprocal of 120 Hz, the stimulus fundamental during this 20-ms segment of the /da/.

The plot at lower left in Figure 8-27 is the ALSR computed from the responses of a population of fibers over this 20-ms stimulus segment. The ALSR shows a structure quite similar to the stimulus spectrum. Specifically, there is an envelope with peaks at the formant frequencies. Superimposed on this envelope is a rapidly varying component with peaks and troughs roughly corresponding to the peaks and troughs in the stimulus spectrum. This correspondence is demonstrated quantitatively at lower right in Figure 8-27. Here we show the cepstrum computed from the ALSR at left. This cepstrum has a sharp peak at 8.36 ms, which is the reciprocal of 119.6 Hz. Thus, the rapid variations in the ALSR with frequency reflect the pitch of the speech stimulus in the same way as does the stimulus spectrum.

This cepstral analysis is used only to quantify the relation of the rapid spectral and ALSR fluctuations to the stimulus pitch. One certainly would not suggest that the central nervous system performs such an analysis to extract pitch. What the analysis does show is that there is enough information in the temporal-place representation from which a precise measure of pitch can be extracted. The temporal patterns of the auditory-nerve fibers are dominated by responses to harmonics of the pitch. The ALSR simply illustrates the fact that responses to most pitch harmonics are large near the place (CF) in the population appropriate to the harmonic. How the central nervous system might extract this information is a matter of speculation at this time.

Miller and Sachs (1983) have shown that average rate profiles for a population of fibers do not appear to contain features related to fundamental pitch frequency. That is, even when rate profiles contain a good representation of the formant structure of the stimulus (e.g., Figure 8-20), there are no clear peaks and troughs corresponding to the harmonics of pitch.

SUMMARY OF CURRENT ISSUES

The question of whether the central nervous system uses the fine temporal details of auditory nerve discharge patterns or relies entirely on measures of average firing rates in extracting spectral information about a stimulus has been the focus of considerable interest in recent years (e.g., Goldstein, 1973; Goldstein & Srulovicz, 1977; Siebert,

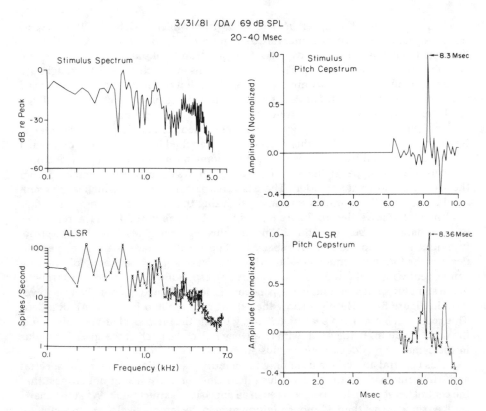

Figure 8-27. Top: Spectrum of the 20- 40-ms segment of /da/ and the cepstrum computed from it. The first 6.0 ms of the cepstrum has been set to zero. Below: Corresponding ALSR profile and the cepstrum computed from it. (From Miller & Sachs, 1983.)

1970). While the studies of speech encoding reviewed in this chapter have not entirely resolved this question, they have brought the issues involved into somewhat clearer perspective. As a summary we highlight the issues that are now being faced.

Although it is possible that, for speech perception, formant peaks need not be maintained in a neural representation of vowels (Bladon & Lindblom, 1981), there is evidence that even small spectral peaks can strongly affect vowel quality (Chisto-vich, Seikin, & Lubinska, 1979), and that small changes in formant frequency can be detected (Mermelstein, 1978). The temporal-place representation maintains a pre-cise definition of formant peaks across a wide range of stimulus levels. There are clear formant peaks in a rate-place profile at low stimulus levels but these are main-tained at high levels only by the small population of low-spontaneous fibers. Thus, a crucial issue in the quest for the peripheral speech code is: *What is the role of the low-spontaneous-rate, high-threshold fibers in representation of speech at high stimulus levels?*

Some data that we have not reviewed are pertinent here. Sachs and associates (1983) have shown that rate-place profiles for vowels presented in background noise show no second formant peak at signal/noise ratios where small changes in second formant frequency can be detected by human subjects. In this case there is no second formant peak even for the low spontaneous-rate fibers considered as a separate population. Temporal-place representations, on the other hand, are robust with respect to background noise (Delgutte, 1981; Voigt et al., 1980). Interpretation of these noise results leads to a second important issue with regard to the peripheral encoding of complex stimuli. There is a significant and apparently highly organized efferent innervation of the cochlea (Rasmussen, 1960; Warr, 1980). Although the function of this efferent innervation is not known, Dewson (1968) has shown that monkeys whose crossed olivocochlear bundle (one component of the efferent system) has been cut do not discriminate noise-masked vowels as well as do intact monkeys. A second major question is this: *What role do the cochlear efferents play in the peripheral encoding of speech?* These efferents are likely to be inactive in the anesthetized preparations used to study auditory nerve encoding. It is possible that in an awake performing animal the efferents could operate to preserve rate profiles in background noise or at high stimulus levels. A closely related question is: *What is the role of the middle ear muscles in speech encoding?* Simmons (1959, 1964) has shown that the middle ear muscles can produce large decreases in sound transmission through the ear. These muscles could act in a similar way to preserve rate profiles.

Considerable attention has been given to temporal representations of frequency information in the auditory nerve (Delgutte, 1981; Goldstein & Srulovicz, 1977; Reale & Geisler, 1980; Siebert, 1970; Young & Sachs, 1979). There is, however, no direct evidence that the central nervous system is able to extract such temporally coded spectral information. Probably the strongest evidence that the central nervous system can use temporally coded information at all comes from studies of binaural lateralization. An interaural phase of two equal-intensity, simultaneously presented tones determines the perceived location of the binaurally fused tone within the head. Interaural phase difference is effective in moving the position of a tone for frequencies up to at least 2.0 kHz (Yost, 1974). Average rate measures by nature average out such phase effects and one is forced to consider a temporal-based central processing for such binaural effects (Colburn, 1973).

There are a number of models that explore the ways in which an optimum processor could extract spectral cues from auditory-nerve temporal patterns (Colburn, 1973; Goldstein & Srulovicz, 1977; Siebert, 1970). However, there have been few attempts to develop quantitative models of how a real neural system would operate on the auditory-nerve input (Merzenich, Loeb, & White, 1980). *Another current challenge is thus the task of developing some quantitative hypotheses about how spectral information might be extracted from temporal patterns with real neural "hardware."*

With these issues in mind, we can summarize our current knowledge of speech encoding in the auditory nerve briefly as follows. Vowels and stop consonants are well represented by a temporally based encoding scheme. Detailed formant structure of vowels is present in a rate-place code at moderate stimulus levels, but is maintained at high levels only in the small population of low-spontaneous fibers. Some formant structure of stop consonants may be preserved at higher stimulus levels in a rate-place code. Formant structure of fricatives may be represented in a rate-place scheme but probably not adequately represented in a temporal code. Voice pitch is well preserved in a temporal code but not in a rate-place code. This summary leads us to suggest that the central nervous system may well need to utilize both rate-place and temporal-place information in extracting all perceptually relevant features from speech.

REFERENCES

Abbas, P.J. (1978). Effects of frequency on two-tone suppression: A comparison of physiological and psychophysical results. *Journal of the Acoustical Society of America, 63,* 1878–1886.

Abbas, P.J. & Sachs, M.B. (1976). Two-tone suppression in auditory-nerve fibers: Extension of a stimulus–response relationship. *Journal of the Acoustical Society of America, 59,* 112–122.

Arthur, R.M. (1976). Harmonic analysis of two-tone discharge patterns in cochlear nerve fibers. *Biological Cybernetics, 22,* 21-31.

Arthur, R.M., Pfeiffer, R.R., & Suga, N. (1971). Properties of "two-tone inhibition" in primary auditory neurons. *Journal of Physiology, 212,* 593–609.

Bernardin, C.P. (1979). *Two-tone interactions in auditory-nerve fibers: Synchrony suppression and rate suppression.* Doctoral dissertation, Johns Hopkins University.

Bladon, R.A.W., & Lindblom, B. (1981). Modeling the judgment of vowel quality differences. *Journal of the Acoustical Society of America, 69,* 1414–1422.

Bogert, B.P., Healy, M.J.R., & Tukey, J.W. (1963). The frequency analysis of time series of echoes: Cepstrum, pseudo-autocovariance, cross-cepstrum, and saphe cracking. In M. Rosenblatt (Ed.), *Proceedings of the Symposium on Time Series Analysis.* New York: Wiley.

Brugge, J.F., Anderson, D.J., Hind, J.E., & Rose, J.E. (1969). Time structure of discharges in single auditory-nerve fibers of the squirrel monkey in response to complex periodic sounds. *Journal of Neurophysiology, 32,* 386–401.

Chistovich, L.A., Seikin, R.L., & Lubinska, V.V. (1979). Centres of gravity and spectral peaks as the determinants of vowel quality. In B. Lindblom & S. Ohman (Eds.), *Frontiers of Speech Communication Research.* London: Academic Press.

Colburn, H.S. (1973). Theory of binaural interaction based on auditory-nerve data. I. General strategy and results on interaural discrimination. *Journal of the Acoustical Society of America, 54,* 1458–1470.

Cutting, J.E., & Rosner, B.S. (1974). Categories and boundaries in speech and music. *Perception and Psychophysics, 16,* 564–570.

de Boer, E. (1976). On the "residue" and auditory pitch perception. In W.D. Keidel & W.D. Neff (Eds.), *Handbook of Sensory Physiology (Vol. V). Auditory System, Part 3: Clinical and Special Topics.* New York: Springer-Verlag.

Delgutte, B. (1980). Representation of speech-like sounds in the discharge patterns of auditory-nerve fibers. *Journal of the Acoustical Society of America, 68,* 843–857.

Delgutte, B. (1981). *Representation of speech-like sounds in the discharge patterns of auditory-nerve fibers.* Doctoral dissertation, Massachusetts Institute of Technology.

Dewson, J.H., III (1968). Efferent olivocochlear bundle: Some relationships to stimulus discrimination in noise. *Journal of Neurophysiology, 31,* 122–130.

Evans, E.F. (1980). Phase-locking of cochlear fibers and the problem of dynamic range. In G. van den Brink & F.A. Bilsen (Eds.), *Psychophysical, physiological and behavioral studies in hearing*. Delft: Delft Univ. Press.

Gleason, H.A. (1961). *Introduction to descriptive linguistics*. New York: Holt, Rinehart, Winston.

Goldstein, J.L. (1972). Neural phase locking to combination tones predicted by simple transducer models. *Journal of the Acoustical Society of America, 52*, 142, (Abstract).

Goldstein, J.L. (1973). An optimum processor theory for the central formation of the pitch of complex tones. *Journal of the Acoustical Society of America, 54*, 1496–1516.

Goldstein, J.L., & Kiang, N.Y.S. (1968). Neural correlates of the aural combination tone $2f_1 - f_2$. *Proceedings of the IEEE, 56*, 981–992.

Goldstein, J.L., & Srulovicz, P. (1977). Auditory-nerve spike intervals as an adequate basis for aural analysis. In E.F. Evans & J.P. Wilson (Eds.), *Psychophysics and physiology of hearing*, New York: Academic Press.

Hall, J.L. (1977). Two-tone suppression in a nonlinear model of the basilar membrane. *Journal of the Acoustical Society of America, 61*, 520–524.

Hashimoto, T., Katayama, Y., Murato, K., & Taniguchi, L. (1975). Pitch synchronout response of cat cochlear nerve fibers to speech sounds. *Japanese Journal of Physiology, 25*, 633–644.

Heinz, J.M., & Stevens, K.N. (1961). On the properties of voiceless fricative consonants. *Journal of the Acoustical Society of America, 34*, 179–188.

Helmholtz, H.L.F. von. (1863). On the sensations of tone as a physiological basis for the theory of music. (A.J. Ellis, trans.) New York: Dover, 1954. (Originally published, 1863).

Hind, J.E., Anderson, D.J., Brugge, J.F., & Rose, J.E. (1967). Encoding of information pertaining to paired low-frequency tones in single auditory-nerve fibers of the squirrel monkey. *Journal of Neurophysiology, 30*, 794–816.

Jacobson, R., Fant, C.G.M., & Halle, M. (1963). *Preliminaries to Speech Analysis*. Cambridge, MA: MIT Press.

Javel, E. (1981). Suppression of auditory-nerve responses. I. Temporal analysis, intensity effects and suppression contours. *Journal of the Acoustical Society of America, 69*, 1753–1745.

Johnson, D.H. (1974). *The responses of single auditory-nerve fibers in the cat to single tones: Synchrony and average discharge rate*. Doctoral dissertation, Massachusetts Institute of Technology.

Johnson, D.H. (1980). The relationship between spike rate and synchrony in responses of auditory-nerve fibers to single tones. *Journal of the Acoustical Society of America, 68*, 1115–1122.

Kiang, N.Y.S. (1980). Processing of speech by the auditory nervous system. *Journal of the Acoustical Society of America, 68*, 830–842.

Kiang, N.Y.S., & Moxon, E.C. (1974). Tails of tuning curves of auditory-nerve fibers. *Journal of the Acoustical Society of America, 55*, 620–630.

Kim, D.O., Molnar, C.E., & Pfeiffer, R.R. (1973). A system of nonlinear differential equations modelling basilar membrane motion. *Journal of the Acoustical Society of America, 54*, 1517–1529.

Kim, D.O., Siegel, J.H., & Molnar, C.E. (1979). Cochlear nonlinear phenomena in two tone responses. *Scandinavian Audiology (Suppl. 9)*, 63–82.

Liberman, M.C. (1978). Auditory-nerve responses from cats raised in a low-noise chamber. *Journal of the Acoustical Society of America, 63*, 442–455.

Liberman, M.C. (1982). Single neuron labelling in the cat auditory nerve. *Science, 216*, 1239–1241.

Littlefield, W.M. (1973). *Investigation of the linear range of the peripheral auditory system*. Doctoral dissertation, Washington University.

Mermelstein, P. (1978). Difference limens for formant frequencies of steady-state and consonant-sound vowels. *Journal of the Acoustical Society of America, 63*, 572–580.

Merzenich, M.M., Knight, P.L., & Roth, G.L. (1975). Representation of the cochlea within primary auditory cortex in the cat. *Journal of Neurophysiology, 38,* 231–249.

Merzenich, M.M., Loeb, G.E., & White, M.W. (1980). Extraction of spectral information in auditory brainstem nuclei; hypothesis and experimental observations. *Journal of the Acoustical Society of America, 68,* S19 (Abstract).

Miller, M.I., & Sachs, M.B. (1983). Representation of stop consonants in the discharge patterns of auditory-nerve fibers. *Journal of the Acoustical Society of America, 74,* 502–517.

Molnar, C.E. (1974). Analysis of memoryless polynomial nonlinearities. *Journal of the Acoustical Society of America, 56,* 531. (abstract)

Oppenheim, A.V., & Schafer, R.W. (1968). Homomorphic analysis of speech. *IEEE Transactions on Audio and Electroacoustics, AU-16,* 221–226.

Palmer, A.R., & Evans, E.F. (1980). Cochlear fiber rate-intensity functions: No evidence for basilar membrane nonlinearities. *Hearing Research, 2,* 319–326.

Pfeiffer, R.R., & Kim, D.O. (1975). Cochlear nerve fiber responses: Distribution along the cochlear partition. *Journal of the Acoustical Society of America, 58,* 867–869.

Rasmussen, G.L. (1960). Efferent fibers of the cochlear nerve and cochlear nucleus. In G.L. Rasmussen & W.F. Windle (Eds.), *Neural mechanisms of auditory and vestibular systems.* Springfield, Ill.: Thomas.

Reale, R.A., & Geisler, C.D. (1980). Auditory-nerve fiber encoding of two-tone approximations to steady-state vowels. *Journal of the Acoustical Society of America, 67,* 891–902.

Rose, J.E., Brugge, J.F., Anderson, D.J., & Hind, J.E. (1967). Phase-locked response to low frequency tones in single auditory nerve fibers of the squirrel monkey. *Journal of Neurophysiology, 30,* 769–793.

Rose, J.E., Kitzes, L.M., Gibson, M.M., & Hind, J.E. (1974). Observations on phase-sensitive neurons of anteroventral cochlear nucleus of the cat: Nonlinearity of cochlear output. *Journal of Neurophysiology, 37,* 218–253.

Sachs, M.B., & Abbas, P.J. (1974). Rate versus level functions for auditory-nerve fibers in cats: Tone burst stimuli. *Journal of the Acoustical Society of America, 56,* 1835–1847.

Sachs, M.B., & Abbas, P.J. (1976). Phenomenological model for two-tone suppression. *Journal of the Acoustical Society of America, 60,* 1157–1163.

Sachs, M.B., & Hubbard, A.E. (1981). Responses of auditory-nerve fibers to characteristic-frequency tones and low-frequency suppressors. *Hearing Research, 4,* 309–324.

Sachs, M.B., & Kiang, N.Y.S. (1968). Two-tone inhibition in auditory-nerve fibers. *Journal of the Acoustical Society of America, 43,* 1120–1128.

Sachs, M.B., Voigt, H.F., & Young, E.D. (1983). Auditory nerve representation of vowels in background noice. *Journal of Neurophysiology, 50,* 27–45.

Sachs, M.B., & Young, E.D. (1979). Encoding of steady-state vowels in the auditory nerve: Representation in terms of discharge rate. *Journal of the Acoustical Society of America, 66,* 470–479.

Sachs, M.B., & Young, E.D. (1980). Effects of nonlinearities on speech encoding in the auditory nerve. *Journal of the Acoustical Society of America, 68,* 858–875.

Sachs, M.B., Young, E.D., & Miller, M.I. (1982a). Speech encoding in the auditory nerve: Implications for cochlear implants. *Annals of the New York Academy of Science, 405,* 94–113.

Sachs, M.B., Young, E.D., & Miller, M.I. (1982b). Encoding of speech features in the auditory nerve. In R. Carlson & B. Granstrom (Eds.), *The representation of speech in the peripheral auditory system* (pp. 115–130). Amsterdam: Elsevier.

Sando, I. (1965). The anatomical interrelationships of the cochlear nerve fibers. *Acta Oto-laryngology, 59,* 417–436.

Schafer, R.W., & Rabiner, L.R. (1970). System for automatic formant analysis of voiced speech. *Journal of the Acoustical Society of America, 47,* 634–648.

Schalk, T.B. (1979). *Nonlinearities in auditory-nerve fiber responses to bandlimited noise. An experimental study and a model.* Doctoral dissertation, Johns Hopkins University.

Schalk, T.B., & Sachs, M.B. (1980). Nonlinearities in auditory-nerve fiber responses to band-limited noise. *Journal of the Acoustical Society of America, 67,* 903–913.

Siebert, W.M. (1970). Frequency discrimination in the auditory system: Place or periodicity mechanisms? *Proceedings of the IEEE, 58,* 723–730.

Simmons, F.B. (1959). Middle ear muscle activity at moderate sound levels. *Annals of Otology, Rhinology and Laryngology, 68,* 1126–1143.

Simmons, F.B. (1964). Perceptual theories of middle ear muscle function. *Annals of Otology, Rhinology and Laryngology, 73,* 724–739.

Sinex, D.G., & Geisler, C.D. (1981). Auditory-nerve fiber responses to frequency-modulated tones. *Hearing Research, 4,* 127–148.

Sinex, D.G., & Geisler, C.D. (1984). Responses of auditory-nerve fibers to consonant–vowel syllables. *Journal of the Acoustical Society of America, 73,* 602–615.

Smith, R.L., & Brachman, M.L. (1980a). Dynamic responses of single auditory-nerve fibres: Some effects of intensity and time. In G. van den Brink & F.A. Bilson (Eds.), *Psychophysical, physiological and behavioral studies in hearing.* Delft: Delft Univ. Press.

Smith, R.L., & Brachman, M.L. (1980b). Operating range and maximum response of single auditory-nerve fibers. *Brain Research, 183,* 499–505.

Sokolich, W.G., Hamernik, R.P., Zwislocki, J.J., & Schmeidt, R.T. (1976). Inferred response properties of cochlear hair cells. *Journal of the Acoustical Society of America, 59,* 963–974.

Stevens, K.N., & Blumstein, S.E. (1978). Invariant cues for place of articulation in stop consonants. *Journal of the Acoustical Society of America, 64,* 1358–1368.

Strevens, P. (1960). Spectra of fricative noise in human speech. *Language and Speech, 3,* 32–49.

Terhardt, E. (1980). Toward understanding pitch perception: Problems, concepts and solutions. In G. van den Brink and F.A. Bilsen (Eds.), *Psychophysical, physiological and behavioral studies in hearing.* Delft: Delft Univ. Press.

Voigt, H.F., Sachs, M.B., & Young, E.D. (1980). Effects of masking noise on the representation of vowel spectra in the auditory nerve. In J. Syka & L. Aitkins (Eds.), *Neuronal mechanisms of hearing.* New York: Plenum.

Voigt, H.F., Sachs, M.B., & Young, E.D. (1982). Representation of whispered vowels in discharge patterns of auditory-nerve fibers. *Hearing Reseaarch, 8,* 49–58.

Warr, W.B. (1980). Efferent components of the auditory system. *Annals of Otology, Rhinology, and Laryngology (Suppl. 74), 89,* 114–120.

Weiss, T.F. (1966). A model of the peripheral auditory system. *Kybernetic, 3,* 153–175.

Wightman, F.L. (1973). The pattern transformation model of pitch. *Journal of the Acoustical Society of America, 54,* 407–416.

Yost, W.A. (1974). Discriminations of interaural phase differences. *Journal of the Acoustical Society of America, 55,* 1299–1303.

Young, E.D., & Sachs, M.B. (1979). Representation of steady-state vowels in the temporal aspects of the discharge patterns of populations of auditory-nerve fibers. *Journal of the Acoustical Society of America, 66,* 1381–1403.

Young, E.D., & Sachs, M.B. (1981). Processing of speech in the peripheral auditory system. In T. Myers, J. Laver, & J. Anderson (Eds.), *The cognitive representation of speech.* New York: North-Holland.

Chapter 9

Cochlear Implants[1]

Josef M. Miller
Bryan E. Pfingst

Sensorineural hearing loss is an area of communication disorders that has received a great deal of attention and effort in recent years. One's first response to this is "It's about time!" The problems of sensorineural hearing loss have been well recognized and well defined for many years and the effect of the disability is certainly of major proportion. Yet historically, major clinical efforts and research have been directed towards problems of conductive loss. At one level, this emphasis may simply be attributed to the view that conductive loss is a disorder we can do something about. Habilitation and therapeutic strategies for dealing with receptor dysfunction have been weak, at best. The development of the cochlear prosthesis has changed this view and has encouraged efforts to understand and deal with profound sensorineural loss.

Attempts to identify appropriate candidates for cochlear implants have added emphasis to clinical audiological research on identification of hearing loss specific to receptor pathology. This is particularly true in the case of patients with profound hearing loss (e.g., Owens & Telleen, 1981). It has motivated work on alternative prostheses for the profoundly deaf, for example, tactile devices as well as hearing aids (Collins, 1979; Levitt, Pickett, & Houde, 1980; Shiff & Foulke, 1982; Sparks, Ardell, Bourgois, Wiedmer, & Kuhl, 1979). It has raised a variety of questions regarding rehabilitation of the sensorineural profoundly deaf. At a basic level, development of a device such as the cochlear prosthesis has motivated fundamental research on histopathology of the temporal bone (e.g., Bergstrom, 1975; Hinojosa & Marion, 1983; Nadol, 1984; Otte, Schuknecht, & Kerr, 1978), and on mechanisms of hair-cell pathology related to development of animal models of sensorineural deafness (Leake-Jones, Vivion, & O'Reilly, & Merzenich, 1982; Leake-Jones, Walsh, & Merzenich, 1981), and it has helped to specify more precisely questions regarding the physiology of the normal and pathological auditory system. Thus, research directly reflecting a concern for development of the cochlear prosthesis has been performed on electroanatomy of the cochlea (Black & Clark, 1980; Black, Clark, & Patrick, 1981; Spelman et al.,

[1]We gratefully acknowledge the financial support of the National Institutes of Health (Grants NS13056 and RR00166) and the Deafness Research Foundation. We also thank Marcy Brooks, Trudy Schleicher, and Kathleen Schmitt for preparation of the manuscript and invaluable editorial assistance.

1979; Spelman, Clopton, Pfingst, & Miller, 1980a; Spelman et al., 1980b, 1982) on transduction and encoding of complex acoustic and electrical signals by the auditory periphery (Clopton, et al., 1983; Glass, 1983; Kiang & Moxon, 1972; Kiang et al., 1979, 1983; Merzenich, Michelson, Pettit, Schindler, & Reid, 1973; Moxon, 1971, Schindler, Merzenich, White, & Bjorkroth, 1977), and on the psychophysics of such signals (Eddington, Dobelle, Brachmann, Mladejovsky, & Parkin, 1978a,b; Helmerich & Edgerton, 1982; Herndon, 1981; Muller, 1971; Pfingst et al., 1979, 1983; Schubert, 1983; Shannon, 1983, 1984; Simmons, 1966; Simmons et al., 1965; Tong & Clark, 1983; Tong et al., 1983a,b; Walker, 1978). Finally, the cochlear prosthesis has led directly to basic work on the electronics of implanted devices with questions ranging from circuitry, connector development, and packaging, to tissue tolerance (Brummer & Turner, 1977a,b; Gheewala, Melen, & White, 1975; Loeb, McHardy, Kelliher, & Brummer, 1982; Loeb et al., 1983a,b; Shamma, May, & White, 1980; Spelman, Pfingst, & Miller, 1978; Soma, May, Duvall, & White, 1980; Sonn, 1974; Vurek, White, Fong, & Walsh, 1981; White, 1977, 1980, 1982; White et al., 1983).

Simmons (1966, 1976) has provided excellent reviews of the early history of research on electrical stimulation of the inner ear and the early findings on the hearing capabilities provided by simple electrical signals. Since then major developments have occurred that are well beyond the scope of this chapter. One view of the developments is provided by the statistics that by the end of the 1960s, about 10 patients had been chronically implanted with various inner ear devices by one of three clinical-investigative groups. During the following 6 to 7 years, the number of patients increased by one to two dozen, and the number of facilities doubled. During the last 6 to 7 years, over 200 additional patients have been implanted and the facilities are worldwide.

To optimize the utility and comfort of the prosthesis we must address engineering questions of design and packaging, psychological questions of tolerance, acceptance, fatigue, and annoyance, and questions of habilitation. One set of questions within this area concerns the kind and amount of acoustic information to be provided by the prosthesis. While all agree that the most desirable goal of the cochlear prosthesis would be to permit speech reception and understanding, the available data have led many investigators to conclude that an appropriate immediate goal is to assist lipreading and provide environmental contact. The strategy of research concerned with the development of the optimal prosthesis will vary depending on the immediate and long-term goals that we specify.

CLINICAL APPROACHES

A review of the approaches and principal devices currently offered by clinical researchers in this area may provide a perspective on these questions. (For a detailed review see Spelman, 1982.)

(1) The cooperative program directed by House (House & Berliner, 1982; House, Berliner, Eisenberg, Edgerton, & Thielemeir, 1981) utilizes a single platinum–iridium electrode placed in the basal turn of the scala tympani. Stimulation occurs between

this active scala tympani electrode and an indifferent electrode in the middle ear. The intended electrical stimulus is a direct analog of the relatively unfiltered acoustic signal provided as an amplitude modulation of a 16-kHz carrier.

(2) The so-called Vienna device (Burian, Hochmair, Hochmair-Desoyer, & Lessel, 1980; Hochmair & Hochmair-Desoyer, 1981) is based on a multi-electrode system implanted in the scala tympani which has been used as either a single- or a four-channel system. Basically, this system uses an amplitude-compressed and equalized analog signal. In the single-channel mode, this system is applied to the "best" electrode (defined on the basis of psychophysical tests and subjective patient evaluation). When used as a multichannel system, the acoustic signal is divided by a bank of four band-pass filters; the output of each of these is treated as in the unfiltered system and applied to individual electrodes. The matching of filtered output to electrode is based on pitch-matching,[2] that is, that electrode eliciting the highest perceived pitch with a fixed stimulus is assigned the output of the filter with the highest center frequency.

(3) The Utah device (Eddington et al., 1978b) is a multichannel system, analogous to the four-channel Viennese system. An analog output of each filter is applied directly to each electrode, with highest frequency assigned to the most basal electrode. The current waveform varies directly with the filter output.

(4) The San Francisco device (Michelson, Merzenich, Schindler, & Schindler, 1975; Michelson & Schindler, 1981), while varying in detail, is analogous to the Vienna and Utah systems. It is based on an analog processor in which the spectral outputs of bandpass filters are distributed as modulated constant currents to pairs of electrodes located under the osseous spiral lamina and basilar membrane.

(5) The implant system developed in Duren, Germany (Banfai, Hortmann, Wustrow, Kubik, & Zeisberg, 1981) also uses a modified vocoder strategy, employing eight bandpass filters ranging from 300 to 3600 Hz center frequency. However, the eight electrodes are introduced into the membranous labyrinth, presumably without opening the cochlear scali, by drilling holes in the bony wall of the cochlea at various points over the three cochlear turns (Banfai, Hortmann, Kubik, & Wustrow, 1980).

By contrast to the five systems described above, the following systems incorporate an aspect of speech processing in their design. That is, they selectively extract one or more features of the acoustic signal thought to be relevant to speech perception, and apply each feature to the cochlea in a unique fashion.

(6) The implant system developed in England (Douek, Fourcin, Moore, & Clarke, 1977; Douek et al., 1983; Fourcin et al., 1979) extracts the fundamental frequency of speech and uses this to modulate a current driving an electrode located in the middle ear. Vocal tract frequencies of female and child speakers are transposed downward to the male F_0 range, where the psychophysical characteristics for electrical stimulation are most desirable.

(7) The Stanford system (Simmons et al., 1965; Simmons, 1966, 1976; White, 1980) as used in humans has consisted of four electrodes implanted in the modiolus and driven as a single-channel or three-channel system. In the multichannel formant tracking mode, two channels deliver downward-transposed pulses, with frequencies in

---

[2]The term "pitch" corresponds only in the most general sense to psychoacoustic pitch (see Schubert, 1983). The term "timbre" might be more appropriate to describe the sensation associated with electrode place. The Australian group of investigators has found it most useful to describe the sensations along a continuum of sharpness and dullness (Tong et al., 1983a).

a fixed ratio to F_1 and F_2 of the speech signal. The third electrode receives a noise signal which indicates the presence or absence of sibilance.

(8) The Australia implant is a 22-electrode system, typically driven as a 20-channel device (Clark et al., 1977; Clark & Tong, 1982; Patrick et al., 1984). Each channel is driven with current pulses at a rate equal to F_0; the electrode pair stimulated varies with the principal frequency of the second formant of the speech signal. High-frequency F_2 signals activate basal electrodes and, with a decrease in F_2 frequency, more apical electrodes are individually activated. Only one electrode is activated at any time. Pulse amplitude varies with sound intensity.

ANALYSIS OF CURRENT APPROACHES

Given these strategies, there are at least three practical questions we may raise: (1) Which is better — one channel or more than one? (2) Should electrodes be implanted *on* or *in* the cochlea? (3) Does it help to shape the driving signal on each electrode according to some speech processor algorithm or according to a physiological model? Unfortunately, the answers to these questions are not yet available. Obviously it is difficult to compare the performance of subjects implanted with different electrode systems by different groups and tested in different manners to answer such basic questions. In part, however, it is also clear that such questions could be largely answered with appropriate efforts (e.g., see Bilger, 1977). There have not been adequate efforts to perform cooperative and collaborative testing and evaluation of patients among clinical investigative groups.

It is also clear that there are a variety of basic questions regarding the implant that cannot be addressed in humans regardless of investigator concern and effort. For example, evaluation of histopathological changes of inner ear tissue that may be associated with the implant is difficult at best in human material, in which implant-induced pathology is compounded by the preexisting and, in some cases, ongoing disease processes that underlie the deafness responsible for the patient's implantation. Obviously, basic studies requiring invasive procedures aimed at analysis of neurophysiological response features elicited by electrical stimulation are not possible. Such information is fundamental to our understanding of the mechanisms of electrically induced hearing and to evaluation of proposed processor models for providing physiologically useful information via the prosthesis. The alternative is trial-and-error research in humans in which the occasional surprising and gratifying response of the patient occurs but cannot be evaluated in any systematic way. By and large, the latter strategy has been followed in this field; it has led to the diversity of current approaches, and to developments which leap-frog into new areas based on guesses by well-intentioned individuals, but not on empirical or theoretical foundations.

SINGLE- VERSUS MULTICHANNEL IMPLANTS

A fundamental question that is receiving the concern, time, and effort of many laboratories relates to the utility of single- versus multichannel implants. This question may be addressed at a variety of levels. At the most obvious level, comparison may be made between one patient implanted with a single-electrode system and another implanted with a multichannel system; however, many factors may influence the results. Obviously, the system selected may influence the results of such a comparison at a variety of levels. A comparison between the Australian multichannel system and a House single-channel system may yield very different results than a comparison between the Australian system and a Douek round window implant. Moreover, we expect such comparisons to be influenced by the characteristics of the individual implant patient. Thus, for example, a patient who has a large complement of remaining eighth nerve fibers, was recently deafened, is highly motivated, and has marked discrimination skills and the ability to use subtle discrimination cues (of an auditory or nonauditory nature) may, with a multichannel implant, demonstrate greater electrical hearing capacity than the patient who has been deaf since birth, has few neural elements, is poorly motivated, has few developed skills for recognition of cues related to discrimination of auditory information, and has a single-channel drive. Obviously, observed differences in performance may have little to do with differences between prostheses in such cases. Individual patient-related characteristics are somewhat difficult to assess and very difficult to control.

One alternative is to assess multichannel performance versus single-channel performance in the same patient. Schindler (1983) observed improved performance in a set of discrimination tests when the information was bandpass filtered and introduced via a four-channel system, compared with the case in which all information was led to all active electrodes of the implant in parallel. Similar results were obtained by Hochmair and Hochmair-Desoyer (1984). The differences were statistically significant, but relatively small. These authors noted that interpretation of their results is difficult since duration of each patient's experience with each processor (single- versus multichannel) was not equal, and equal levels of device optimization are difficult to ensure.

In a pilot study concerned with this question, the ability of animals to discriminate between two different two-sinusoidal complexes (representing two vowels) was compared under single- and two-channel stimulation strategies (Pfingst, Glass, Spelman, & Sutton, 1984). This study showed a slight improvement in discrimination with the multichannel system (different stimulus components to different channels) compared with the single-channel system (whole stimulus to one electrode pair). Even with this rather simplified approach, a number of interpretations of the results are possible, and further experiments are needed to parcel out which aspects of the multichannel stimulation schemes contribute to the subject's performance with a particular encoding scheme. One factor that may contribute to a difference in single- versus multichannel performance was addressed in the study by Pfingst and associates (1984). A comparison of performance was made with the complex signal imposed across a single electrode pair versus both electrode pairs (a localized versus distributed, single-channel system). Performance was slightly better with the distributed system, although not as good as in the multichannel case. Other factors, whose contributions have not been evaluated, include use of a strict-place pitch code, loudness compensation for various frequency components, and distributed temporal characteristics. Thus, some of the more beneficial features of the multichannel encoding schemes may be applicable to the single-electrode implant, once their utility is understood.

It must be noted that while there are many areas of disagreement in this field, most investigators assume that, with development, the multichannel system will prove superior to a single-channel device in providing discriminative hearing capabilities for at least some patients. The most receptive patient population will probably be characterized by the number and distribution of surviving eighth nerve fibers and perhaps by their past experience with sound.

In spite of the complications of comparing performance in humans, there are and will be enough humans implanted with multichannel devices that, with some care for experimental design, the questions posed here can be answered. Perhaps the primary contribution that animal investigations can make to this question concerns the mechanisms that underlie multichannel activation and optimization of electrode implants. As previously noted, basic to multichannel strategies is the necessity to activate subgroups of eighth nerve elements; in other words, differential stimulation should be used, electrode pairs should be placed near excitable elements and, if possible, shunting fluids of the cochlea should be minimized. Loeb and associates (1983a) suggested a molded silicone rubber carrier that displaces most perilymph with electrodes located in more or less radially oriented pairs, one electrode just under the basilar membrane and the other under the osseous spiral lamina, close to the spiral ganglion cells. In acute studies of cats with "drained" cochleae, White and Merzenich (1983) demonstrated that such electrode placement yielded isolated neural responses with as little as 1.5 mm separating the electrode pairs.

The relevance of the perilymph as a shunting medium is well demonstrated by the findings of Spelman and associates (1982). With pairs of electrodes in a tubular silicone carrier, which displaced approximately 50% of the scala tympani fluid, they found that when the intrascalar electrodes were driven, 75% of the current remained in the scala tympani. The fluid provided a sufficiently low resistance pathway that only 25% of the current reached excitable elements within the modiolus. Moreover, observations by Clopton and Spelman (1982) indicate a relatively low-resistance path to the structures of the modiolus at the base of the cochlea compared with that in other regions. Thus, perilymph tends to shunt current within the scala tympani, and the current that does enter the modiolus tends to do so in a selective region at the cochlear base. Such conditions well account for the single-unit electrophysiological findings at the level of the inferior colliculus which indicate that selective stimulation of single cells is possible when excitation is restricted to near-threshold currents but that when currents are 2-3 dB above threshold, a broad region of the cochlea is activated (Clopton & Silverman, 1978; Merzenich et al., 1973). Obviously, these conditions are less than desirable if selective multichannel excitation is the goal.

It must also be noted that very little perilymph is necessary to provide a shunt. Thus, a molded silicone rubber carrier must be able to displace essentially all fluid and place electrodes in electrically firm contact with tissues of the cochlea. Obviously, a trade-off of selective activation versus cochlear trauma must be considered (see

Morbidity section below). Finally, while physiological measures suggest that differential electrode activation of cochlear segments may be difficult to obtain, human data indicate that some degree of differential stimulation is certainly possible. Thus Eddington (1980), using a four-channel system consisting of "free"-ball electrodes (no carrier), obtained evidence of place-pitch responses for at least one patient. A similar result was obtained with multiple electrodes in a tubular silicone rubber carrier by Hochmair, Hochmair-Desoyer, & Burian (1979) and with ring electrodes mounted in a carrier which only partially displaces scala tympani perilymph (Tong et al., 1982).

Clearly, there is a need for a more rigorous evaluation of the degree of channel separation provided by the various types of implants. Using a two-channel, phase-reversal paradigm in cats, White and Merzenich (1983) showed that the suppression of an electrically evoked auditory brainstem response (EABR) obtained by interacting stimulation at adjacent sites along the osseous spiral lamina varies with stimulation level. With rich innervation and low stimulation levels, different subgroups of eighth nerve fibers are activated and little interaction of evoked EABRs occurs; but with low innervation density (and thus the need to use higher intensity levels to achieve a response) interaction is great. Shannon (1984) has proposed a psychophysical analog to the EABR interaction studies based on peripheral (electrical interaction) versus central (neural interaction) summation of loudness. These electrophysiological and psychophysical techniques may be used as quantifiable measures to supplement objective perceptual responses used to select individual electrodes of a multichannel system and to set stimulation parameters in multichannel devices.

INTRA- VERSUS EXTRACOCHLEAR DEVICES

Given the resistive characteristics of the perilymph and presumed moderately low impedance of the round window membrane, a single electrode on or adjacent to the round window should be nearly as effective as a single electrode introduced into the scala tympani for distributed activation of the peripheral auditory system. However, initial observations indicated such was not the case. While details of the electrode placement, number of subjects, and evaluation performed were not presented, it was suggested that thresholds of hearing were higher and dynamic ranges smaller in patients stimulated via middle ear and round window electrodes than in other patients stimulated with scala tympani electrodes (Brackmann & Selters, 1978). Presumably, the limiting conditions reflected current spread to nonauditory structures. For example, the facial nerve might be activated at current levels just above those required to elicit hearing, or in some cases, below the hearing threshold.

In England, promontory stimulation has been applied to a group of patients with open middle ears. A removable "spring-loaded" electrode system is placed on the promontory through an open ear canal (see Fourcin et al., 1983, Figure 1). Because of processor differences, it is not possible to compare performance of these patients with that of patients implanted with scala tympani electrodes by other groups. However, it appears that with careful placement, stimulation of nonauditory structures can be minimized and a sufficient dynamic range made available, at least at low frequencies of sinusoidal stimulation, to allow the implant to function as a significant lipreading aid that is generally comparable to intracochlear prostheses.

Hochmair and Hochmair-Desoyer (1984) report more direct comparisons between patients implanted with multielectrode systems and those with one electrode placed on the round window using similar processors in the same laboratory. A comparison of reception and discrimination performance elicited by stimulation of an intracochlear electrode versus a round window electrode yielded few differences.

Pfingst (1983) is investigating this question in psychophysical studies in a neomycin-deafened nonhuman-primate model. The first observations with electrodes placed on the promontory yielded threshold values that were above the upper limit of the range of thresholds observed in other subjects implanted with scala tympani electrodes. Moreover, the dynamic range of hearing in these promontory-implanted subjects was correspondingly low, particularly at high frequencies, and damage considerations limited the operating range at low frequencies.

In the second set of subjects, electrodes were placed in recesses drilled at sites overlying the lateral wall of various cochlear turns. In this procedure an attempt was made to avoid invasion of the membraneous labyrinth. Thresholds and dynamic ranges for these subjects were compared with those of subjects who had scala tympani implants. Lowest threshold and largest dynamic ranges were seen with the best scala tympani implants. However, values for middle ear electrodes placed in recesses were in the range of many scala tympani cases.

Histology has not yet been performed on these subjects, but presumably the potential morbidity associated with a middle ear or round window electrode is significantly less than that associated with a scala tympani chronic implant. Extracochlear prostheses would seem to be a most feasible alternative approach to intracochlear electrodes, particularly in young patients, and particularly during this period of rapid development and change in prosthesis design.

Perhaps the greatest potential reservation regarding future development of middle ear implants lies in their utility as a multichannel device. Assuming that the minimal requirement of a multichannel system is that stimulation of different implant sites should evoke different perceptions, one can approach this question in the animal model. Following the elimination of other stimulus cues, ability to discriminate between different sites of stimulation may be tested. Loudness differences can be eliminated by using stimuli matched for similar positions within the dynamic range of hearing and by presenting different intensities of stimulation which vary systematically on a trial-by-trial basis so that this cue cannot be used in any consistent fashion as a basis for discrimination. Under these conditions, Pfingst (1983) has demonstrated in preliminary experiments that subjects can discriminate among round window promontory and apical stimulation sites with electrodes placed in the drilled bony recesses. Banfai and associates (1981), using this technique in human patients, have reported some place-pitch effects. If small amounts of perilymph are a limiting condition on the channel independence that can be obtained in multichannel devices, then the middle ear multichannel system may provide a comparable approach with reduced morbidity. The threshold for place discrimination versus separation of middle ear stimulation sites must yet be determined. Such factors may limit the number of useful channels of information that can be provided with this approach. In addition, it must be noted that the surgery involved and the technology of fixing more than a few electrodes via this approach are significantly more demanding than the techniques involved in placing a multichannel system within the scala tympani.

PROCESSOR STRATEGIES

Specific processor schemes should be viewed in terms of the assumptions that underlie their particular development. When so viewed, categories of processor schemes become clear; more important, fundamental questions amenable to experimental evaluation also become clear. Most processor designs are based on one or more of three general approaches. The first approach stresses our knowledge of speech reception and discrimination and emphasizes the extraction of specific features of acoustic signals thought to be important for speech recognition or to aid lipreading. The second and perhaps most fundamental approach is the attempt to mimic the "normal" physiological response characteristics of the auditory system, and in this approach emphasis is placed on the form and distribution of currents delivered to the inner ear. The third approach focuses on the selected features of the response of the auditory nervous system to electrical stimulation and seeks to determine empirically what types of electrical stimuli are most effective and safe for transfer of information. Data obtained from studies using this approach provide a basis for the reduction of environment and speech signals to a form that is effectively transmitted by electrical stimulation and applied to most effective regions of the inner ear.

Obviously, these three approaches are not mutually exclusive. Indeed, all prostheses employed today or under discussion combine some measure of each. Furthermore, each is influenced not only by physiological and performance capabilities, but by safety factors, engineering considerations, and patient preference.

Speech Models

Speech perception scientists have described in some detail the features of speech that determine its detection, discrimination, and recognition. Distinctive characteristics of speech sound have been characterized in a variety of ways (e.g., segmental features versus suprasegmental ones), each of which has been defined in terms of physical characteristics of the acoustic energy (e.g., spectral content, amplitude features, short-term transitions between energies, long-term temporal and envelope features), and related physiological and anatomical features of the vocal tract (e.g., rate of vocal cord vibration, position and change in position of lips, tongue).

Certain sets of these observations are of particular interest for the cochlear prosthesis. Suprasegmental cues provide information regarding the temporal and waveform pattern of running speech (Stevens, 1983), which in turn yield information on word stress and boundaries, and syntactic structure (Cooper, 1983). Such information provided in a weighted-center frequency representation of a speech sound presented as a single cue has been found to provide a significant cue for closed set word discriminations (Risberg & Agelfors, 1982).

Many of the cues related to suprasegmental information are contained in the fundamental frequency (F_0) of speech sounds (Stevens, 1983) and provide prosodic, low-frequency temporal information. F_0 is generated by the frequency of vibration of the vocal cords. As such, it is information that is not readily available to the lipreader. Aids to the profoundly deaf that provide cues about prosodic information have been demonstrated to be effective. Fourcin and colleagues (1979) have extracted a measure of larynx frequency, related to F_0, and have shown that this is a significant aid when presented tactically or when presented electrically to the promontory or round window of the deaf lipreader. This would seem a simple and effective approach for aiding the profoundly deaf via an implant. The high-frequency cutoff of information to be transmitted is typically restricted to less than 300 Hz. This is the frequency range of the prosthesis where hearing sensitivity and dynamic range are greatest and frequency discrimination is best. It avoids problems associated with restricted stimulation of cochlear segments and draws on the most clearly documented physiological strength of the prosthesis, that is, its ability to elicit synchronous periodic excitation of eighth nerve fibers. Reservations regarding this approach are based on the same features that form some of its strength. Only one channel of information is provided, and it provides little high-frequency information. Hochmair-Desoyer, Hochmair, & Stiglbrunner (1984) have reported that in patients with single-channel stimulation where the bandwidth of the excitatory stimulus was varied, speech discrimination was significantly better with a bandwidth extending to several kilohertz than when the speech signal was low-pass filtered at 300 Hz.

This consideration forms, in part, the basis for the speech processing scheme used by the Australian group (see above). For the discrimination of some speech sounds (e.g., vowels) higher-frequency information is distinctively useful; thus the second formant is particularly important. The Australian processor uses a bandpass filter to extract spectral energy related to this feature (specifically, it is related to the volume of air anterior to the tongue: the front cavity resonance) and presents this information across 20 channels of their multielectrode system. The electrode (channel) activated varies with frequency of the second formant, thus, it is hoped, providing place-pitch information. The pulse rate varies with fundamental frequency of the signal. Thus, their processor attempts to provide prosodic information superimposed on a "place" cue reflecting F_2 information.

Physiological Considerations

In the various speech processor schemes described above, we see reflected a concern for mimicking what is thought to be normal function of the cochlea with some fairly clear deviations. We know that basal-turn fibers of the cochlea can be activated by low-frequency stimuli (Evans, 1975; Kiang, Keithley, & Liberman, 1983). We know that such low-frequency activation of these fibers can provide temporal, suprasegmental-like information regarding speech-like sounds and melodies (Burns & Viemeister,

1981). It has been proposed that such information accounts for the much-better-than-expected speech of profoundly deaf patients with an isolated island of ultra-high-frequency hearing (Berlin, Wexler, Jerger, Halperin, & Smith, 1978). Acoustic activation of these fibers presumably provides cues in the form of periodicity-pitch precepts (Plomp & Smoorenburg, 1970). Inadequate study has been done to date on the characteristics of prosthesis hearing versus periodicity-pitch hearing to establish the relationship between the two. It would seem clear that the existence of facilities for synthesis and control of speech sounds with nearly any characteristics desired would enable investigators to study hearing based on a "restricted-periodicity" model, a multichannel "phase-normalized" model, or any other number of reduced-hearing models, and to compare such hearing with that obtained by the cochlear prosthesis (Blamey, Dowell, Tong, & Clark, 1983).

At a physiological level, electrically elicited periodic-pitch information presumably is encoded in terms of phase-locking characteristics of the discharge of eighth nerve fibers. Basic neurophysiological information is necessary to evaluate this suggestion. Recently Glass (in press) found evidence that cells of the cochlear nucleus demonstrate a higher degree of phase locking in response to sinusoidal electrical stimulation than in response to acoustic stimulation — with examples indicating phase locking above 10 kHz. Thus phase locking provides a powerful neurophysiological mechanism that most certainly accounts for the pitch-like perceptual changes observed with variation in stimulation rate in implant patients (Eddington et al., 1978a; Mathews, 1978).

The neurophysiological studies of Glass and Clopton (Clopton et al., 1983; Clopton & Glass, submitted for publication; Glass, 1983) also indicate that (1) in the recently deafened ear, little or no spontaneous activity is seen in cells of the cochlear nucleus; (2) cochlear nucleus cells show a highly uniform frequency-response field to electrical stimuli with all of the cells tuned to approximately 100 Hz and showing symmetric slope values of 3–4 dB per octave on the low- and high-frequency limb; and (3) dynamic ranges for electrical stimuli are limited to 2–15 dB throughout the receptive field, and the slopes of these functions are relatively variable. In general, these findings are consistent with the observations in studies of eighth nerve fiber responses to round window stimulation (Kiang & Moxon, 1972; Moxon, 1971) and in studies of cochlear nucleus activity with intracochlear stimulation (Loeb et al., 1983b).

These studies shed some light on the characteristics of the system's response to simple sinusoidal stimulation. For a multichannel system to be developed, we must determine the manner in which currents interact in the periphery and the way resultant complex stimuli determine evoked activity. To date, our information is limited to two studies. Clopton and associates (1983) and Clopton and Glass (submitted for publication) have reported first observations with two-sinusoid complexes near the best frequency of neurons for electrical stimuli. They found that responses to such signals are phase-locked to the maximum-amplitude spectral component and thus largely reflect the envelope of the stimulus. Glass (submitted for publication) has studied the influence of sinusoidal stimulation at constant frequency when provided simultaneously to two separated bipolar pairs of electrodes within the scala tympani. He examined the effect of phase reversal of stimulus current provided at one electrode pair relative to the other. The resultant activity is consistent with a model of simple summation of sinusoidal current in a relatively isotropic medium. Characteristics of evoked activity were predicted by a current waveform reflecting a simple summation.[3]

In the normal cochlea, place and periodicity mechanisms are coordinated in that for a given frequency, nerve fibers innervating the cochlear place at which the basilar membrane is displaced maximally also exhibit the strongest phase locking to that frequency (Young & Sachs, 1979). In the ideal cochlear prosthesis, therefore, rate information should be presented at the appropriate cochlear place. With current prosthesis designs in which implants are inserted through the round window into the basal turn of the cochlea, there are certain physical limitations on this ideal since no electrodes are located in the low-frequency (apical) region of the cochlear spiral. In fact, there have been few, if any, attempts by current cochlear implant programs to match rate pitch with place pitch. This may account for some of the difficulties in achieving higher-frequency rate pitch and in transmitting speech signals to the patient.

On the basis of the above considerations, we propose the following scheme for implant-processor design. The frequency range covered by a prosthesis selected on the basis of speech discrimination considerations might range from 50 Hz to at least 3.2 kHz, thus permitting first- and second-formant information to be encoded. The frequency of each band of information delivered to each electrode should be equally spaced within this range on a logarithmic scale (see Greenwood, 1961). The most basal pair of electrodes should receive the highest-frequency information, and so on. Stimuli should be delivered in charge-balanced, biphasic pulses, in which information on each channel would be reflected as a change in activity superimposed upon a Poisson-like distribution of pulses providing a spontaneous rate of activity, as in the intact system. Loudness may be encoded by an increase in current amplitude, leading to greater current spread and the recruitment of a larger pool of activated fibers. This approach is more appropriate than increasing stimulation rate with increased stimulus intensity, since the latter has been shown in psychophysical studies to provide a minimal cue for loudness. Across channels, mean pulse rate should vary in a systematic fashion, with average rates higher at basal electrodes reflecting resonant characteristics of the normal cochlea. However, a range of variation about this mean rate must be available to reflect periodic pitch features of the acoustic signal.

Many reservations need to be considered in regard to such a model. The model assumes not only a significant independence of the individual channels, but also linear interaction between them as simultaneous currents are applied to the individual channels. It is assumed that the system will be capable of extracting frequency information of signals on the basis of different rates of stimulation at different places in spite of ongoing rate changes introduced by loudness changes – all of which is superimposed on a randomly varying spontaneous activity. Given the compelling nature of electrical stimuli, as demonstrated by evoked activity and a limited dynamic range, it would not be surprising to find that any scheme for introducing a background spontaneous rate may result in "jamming" of the system. Thus, by contrast with the normal system

---

[3]Interestingly, this appeared to hold sufficiently that one may be able to predict the location of the active elements relative to two pairs of electrodes (but there has been no anatomical study to verify this).

in which background spontaneous activity provides a bias upon which signals may be superimposed in some probabilistic manner, in the sensorineurally defeaned system that is activated electrically we are dealing with a system that is normally turned off. We might expect that lack of such biasing of baseline activity may decrease the overall sensitivity of the system to change. Moreover, given the very limited dynamic range of electrical stimuli to which units are differentially sensitive, it may be necessary to model the system as a set of elements, any one of which is either completely off or completely on.

For the encoding of simple information based on a strategy of mimicking normal auditory system function, a compromise must be made between the subtle complexities of the normal physiological processes of the auditory system and the limitations of the electrically activated system. We must define a few important categories of information we wish to transfer and then attempt to assign quantitative values to these characteristics based on electrophysiological features of the auditory system with acoustic stimulation (see Evans, 1978, 1984). To do this we need additional basic information on the neurophysiological response characteristics of the system with electrical stimulation and on the relation of these response features to electrically elicited hearing.

Psychophysical Considerations

The psychophysics of simple sinusoidal and pulsatile stimuli have been studied sufficiently that a basic picture emerges with some implications for processor strategies. The most extensive study has concerned the measurement of detection thresholds. A consistent result is seen in virtually all of these studies, in that the shapes of the threshold contours measured under a wide variety of conditions are quite similar, although absolute levels can vary considerably from case to case. For sinusoidal stimuli, thresholds are almost always lowest at low frequencies (below 100 Hz). Thresholds rise as a function of frequency above 100 Hz, initially at rates of 5–15 dB per octave (see review by Pfingst, 1984). Thus, for near-threshold stimuli, the system looks to incoming stimuli like a low-pass filter and frequency equalization is necessary if higher frequencies of electrical stimulation are to be represented equally. Hochmair-Desoyer and associates (1983) showed that this equalization is important for speech comprehension with cochlear implants. At higher stimulus amplitudes, the slopes of the equal-loudness countours are less steep than those of the threshold contours, and at the upper limit of the dynamic range the slope lessens to about 3 dB per octave, so the frequency equalization must be specific to sensation level.

The slope of the threshold contour above 100 Hz is much steeper than the slope of the higher intensity equal-loudness contours in this frequency region, and the dynamic ranges for lower-frequency stimuli are larger than for higher-frequency sinusoids. Typical values are 20–40 dB at low frequencies and 10–25 dB at higher frequencies (Pfingst, 1984). To understand the real significance of these dynamic range differences, however, one must know the number of discriminable steps within the dynamic range in each frequency region. Amplitude-difference limens measured in monkeys and human patients indicate a decrease in difference limens as a function of frequency at a constant sensation level (Pfingst et al., 1983; Shannon, 1983). Thus, the number of discriminable steps in the dynamic range may be similar at low and high frequencies, despite the differences in dynamic range.

Frequency-difference limens are also frequency specific, a factor of major importance for processor design. Although the data on frequency-difference limens are sparce, there is a consistent indication that frequency discrimination or pulse-rate discrimination, while reasonably good at frequencies below 300 Hz, is poor or non-existent at frequencies above 300 Hz (Merzenich et al., 1973; Mathews, 1978). This result is rather puzzling since electrophysiological data seem to indicate that phase locking in single neurons occurs at frequencies well above 300 Hz (Glass, 1983). There are indications that the situation may improve as the patient gains experience with electrical stimulation (Hochmair-Desoyer, personal communication). The Hochmairs report that after a year or two of experience with a cochlear prosthesis, their patients are able to discriminate frequencies and make pitch matches for stimuli in the 1-kHz range. Even so, there seems at present little hope for using a rate code for higher frequencies of stimulation and so emphasis for encoding these frequencies has been on a place code.

There have been a number of reports of place-specific pitch in patients with multi-electrode implants (Eddington, 1980; Tong et al., 1982). Pitch differences between electrodes spaced a few millimeters apart are not large and the pitch percept is highly dependent on the rate of stimulation delivered to the electrode (Eddington, 1980), but if stimulation rate is held constant, an orderly progression of pitches (or perhaps, more correctly, "timbres") corresponding to the tonotopic organization of the cochlea can be observed. Using a 22-electrode array, for example, Tong and associates (1983a) found that patients could consistently rank the electrodes on a continuum from sharp to dull over a range that has proved useful for encoding F_2 information.

Tong and colleagues (1982) have, moreover, evaluated the comparative effectiveness of changing site of stimulation versus rate of stimulation at a fixed site, on implant patients' ability to perceive a frequency change. Their findings indicate that (1) percepts elicited by pulse-rate changes are different from those elicited by changing stimulation site (Tong et al., 1983a) and (2) changing site of stimulation more effectively encodes a rapid change in frequency than does changing the pulse rate (Tong et al., 1982). Given that rapid frequency transitions provide a major segmental cue for CV discriminations, they suggest that this finding provides support for encoding F_2 on the basis of place of stimulation.

Mechanisms of Prosthesis Function

Throughout these studies on the psychophysics of hearing with the implant there is an obvious concern for the identification of physiological mechanisms that underlie a given hearing feature. Optimization of the implant will surely depend on such an understanding. At the beginning of this section we suggested that one approach to development of the prosthesis might be based on a definition of the speech elements to be encoded. In the second section, consideration was given to models, primarily those mimicking normal auditory system function, that may provide a basis for encoding this information. In the third section the characteristics of hearing with the prosthesis were described. These characteristics should be viewed as setting the limits on which features of speech or any acoustic signal may be reasonably encoded.

The psychophysical data also establish a number of questions and experimental problems that must be answered at a mechanistic level. Indeed they provide the basis for an alternative and somewhat more classic strategy for studies of the mechanisms of prosthesis hearing. Historically in studies of the mechanisms of perception we define a perceptual feature of interest as rigorously as possible and then attempt to identify neurophysiological correlates that may underlie the characteristics of this perception. To date, our approach to development of a prosthesis has appropriately drawn upon our knowledge of auditory system function with acoustic stimuli and applied these concepts of system function to electrical stimuli. However, now we are beginning to acquire data on the extent to which these "normal" response features are available with electrical stimulation. Such evaluation and the formulation of appropriate neurophysiological questions and models for prosthesis development must be based on psychophysical characteristics of prosthesis hearing. Studies based upon such strategy are just beginning, but it offers great potential for contributing to the development of a scientific base from which an improved prosthetic device will evolve.

Such an approach can be illustrated by consideration of the absolute sensitivity of prosthesis hearing. As noted above, on the basis of human and animal psychophysical studies, we know that absolute sensitivity is greatest and relatively constant at low frequencies, up to approximately 100 Hz. Above 100 Hz, sensitivity decreases at a rate of approximately 9 dB per octave to 700–1000 Hz in monkeys or to 300 Hz in humans and then increases at approximately 3–4 dB per octave beyond. Though interactive mechanisms presumably underlie this function, certainly it is not surprising to see greatest sensitivity at low frequencies. On the basis of our knowledge of the resistive–capacitative characteristics of neural membranes, we would expect thresholds to be lowest for lower frequencies of stimulation. Physiologically this is supported by the observations of Glass (1984) demonstrating a uniform low best frequency for cells excited by sinusoidal electrical stimulation. These single-unit studies do suggest that the hearing threshold should rise at frequencies below approximately 100 Hz, an anticipated result which is not observed behaviorally to the degree expected. Similarly for very low frequencies, adaption mechanisms (Guttman & Hachmeister, 1971) should lead to some elevation in threshold of excitation. At lowest frequencies there is, on occasion, some increase in behavioral threshold; however, it is typically for frequencies below 30 Hz.

Presumed membrane characteristics would lead to a slope of threshold versus frequency of approximately 6 dB per octave (Butikofer & Lawrence, 1978; Frankenhaeuser & Huxley, 1964). Guttman and Hachmeister's data on squid axons indicate that the relation of threshold to frequency is not linear; one can obtain almost any value of slope desired for whatever model is preferred. Frankenhaeuser and Huxley's model of activity at the nodal membrane would suggest a slope of 6 dB per octave. Clopton and associates (1983) and Glass (1984) provided data from cochlear nucleus cells in mammals with electrical stimulation indicating a slope of approximately 3 to 4 dB per octave. If this is an appropriate slope value, then it would appear to account well for the high-frequency (>1 kHz) rise in behavioral detection function observed in humans and monkeys, leaving a second mechanism to provide an additional 6-dB/octave change for frequencies between 100 and 1000 Hz. If the higher 6-dB/octave change in membrane characteristics determines threshold change, we must then hypothesize one mechanism to add 3 dB/octave between 100 and 1000 Hz and another mechanism to subtract 3 dB/octave between 100 and 1000 Hz and another mechanism to subtract 3 dB/octave between 100 and 1000 Hz and another mechanism to subtract 3 dB/octave above 1 kHz.

While the data to support such a notion are scarce, one proposal is that a membrane sensitivity change of 3 dB per octave accounts for the high-frequency limb of the behavioral sensitivity function, and that a central mechanism based on an autocorrelator function accounts for the change in sensitivity between 100 and 1 kHz. This central mechanism introduced for frequencies below 1 kHz would improve detection sensitivity at a rate of an additional 6 dB per octave. These two mechanisms based on independent physiological characteristics of the system are then additive. Such a mechanism, based on phase-locking characteristics of auditory system neurons, has been proposed to account for acoustic perceptions – particularly those related to periodicity-pitch and acoustic distortion products (e.g., Goldstein, 1978). Obviously a number of analytic psychoacoustic as well as neurophysiological studies may be proposed to evaluate such a suggestion directly.

At this time, data are inadequate to propose, quantitatively and confidently, specific neurophysiological models to account for prosthesis hearing features. However, it is important to recognize that, at least to date, this strategy of approach to prosthesis hearing has been largely ignored. Certainly it has proven fruitful and powerful in the analysis of acoustic hearing. While it has been most reasonable, in the absence of rigorous psychophysical data, to borrow models based on acoustic response characteristics, it is undoubtedly time to generate our neurophysiological questions and models on the basis of electrically induced hearing.

CANDIDATE SELECTION

A most basic statement of the purpose of the cochlear prosthesis is that it provides some hearing capacity to the profoundly sensorineural deaf patient, and it is reasonably assumed that these patients must exhibit a sufficient population of excitable eighth nerve fibers to mediate system activation. The first requirements concerning the selection of candidates for a cochlear prosthesis, then, involve tests to identify profound sensorineural deafness and to determine the presence of viable eighth nerve fibers.

While the general identification of a profound sensorineural hearing loss is readily accomplished, the means for systematic classification of differences in hearing performance among the profoundly deaf have not been developed. Until recently, subtle differences have been unimportant from a practical point of view since there was little one could do with this knowledge. Owens, Kessler & Schubert (1981, 1982) have developed a comprehensive set of audiological tests referred to as the Minimum Auditory Capabilities (MAC) Test, which provides a means for developing selection standards for prosthesis candidates. These tests range from relatively simple tasks, such as recognition of whether an utterance is a question or a statement or whether a sound is noise or voice, to tests involving open-set recognition of everyday sentences. Intermediate tests include vowel recognition, initial and final consonant recognition, and spondee recognition in closed and open sets.

Recently the Iowa Cochlear Implant Battery was developed as an extension and supplement to the MAC Test. It includes speechreading tests (with and without context), tests of initial and final vowel recognition, a test of speaker-gender recognition, and it has extended the test of environmental sounds, including a test of warning sounds. These tests may be used as well to provide a base line against which postimplant performance may be evaluated. Continued development of these tests is important, including collection of normative data in deaf populations that will permit further definition of the reliability of each measure and quantification of its validity.

In general there are two primary audiometric criteria for implant candidates: (1) profound deafness, which usually means no detection of pure-tone stimuli at the limits of the audiometer, typically 90–110 dB; and (2) some indication that the patient can respond to electrical stimulation of the cochlea. The latter criterion has proved difficult to apply consistently. The rationale underlying this criterion is that a minimum number of nerve fibers is necessary for cochlear implant function. Moreover, as noted previously, there is evidence indicating that implant function will vary with the number of surviving nerve fibers (see Pfingst et al., 1984). Thus, the goals set for a particular implant candidate and the rehabilitative strategy to be used might be determined more appropriately if it were possible, before implantation, to estimate the percentage and distribution of nerve fibers in the patients' cochleae.

One approach to determining eighth nerve survival is based on temporal bone studies. From such studies information has been provided regarding the pathological state of the eighth nerve with various diseases that underlie profound hearing loss. Bergstrom (1975) and Otte and colleagues (1978) have provided comprehensive studies of the relative sensory and neural pathology associated with deafness of various etiologies. They found that recent trauma yielded the highest values of surviving eighth nerve elements while, as may be expected, acoustic neuromas yielded one of the lowest. Nadol (1984) has outlined considerations of temporal bone pathology that are important in such studies. Clearly, variability is a major consideration and problem with this strategy. In a study of 15 temporal bones from profoundly deaf patients, Hinojosa and Marion (1983) found it impossible to predict nerve survival on the basis of etiology. Interestingly, in a number of cases in which, from other studies, we might have predicted few surviving neural elements, he observed a rather extensive surviving population. The observed variability in this area may in part reflect the inadequacy of our current data base. Further study of additional material may enable us to better account for this variability, and thus lead to development of a catalog of the probability of eighth nerve survival associated with the various durations and various etiologies. Regardless, functional measures that can be applied to the individual candidate would be preferred.

Assumptions regarding the necessity of a minimum population of eighth nerve fibers for function of the prosthesis are supported by the study of Dobie and Kimm (1980). Auditory brainstem responses (ABRs) elicited by electrical stimulation via an electrode in the scala tympani were unaffected by section of the vestibular and seventh nerves, but were abolished by section of the auditory division of the eighth nerve at its medial exit from the internal auditory meatus. In all human (Johnsson, House, & Linthicum, 1982) and animal (Pfingst, Sutton, Miller, & Bohne, 1981b; Pfingst & Sutton, 1983) studies in which histological data as well as behavioral measures are available, results indicate that at least some spiral ganglion cells and eighth nerve axons were present in all cases in which electrically elicited hearing capacity was demonstrated, although in some cases the number of surviving neural elements was certainly few.

Two measures have been proposed that may aid in confirmation of the presence of excitable eighth nerve fibers in the implant candidate. Both are based on promontory or round window electrical stimulation. The first is based on hearing perceptions and the second on electrically evoked auditory brainstem responses (EABR). These tests, quite simply, consist of stimulating the promontory under local anesthesia in prospective candidates to see if a hearing percept or an EABR can be elicited. Presumably a positive response indicates excitable auditory nerves are present. While the hearing measure was originally suggested with some enthusiasm (House & Brackmann, 1974), it is not used routinely now. Apparently this is due to the number of false negatives generated with this test, a problem that has been attributed to inadequate test sensitivity.

There is a clear need to obtain systematic data on the relation between these test results and the eventual implant performance. It would seem appropriate to do this within the context of a rigorously designed experimental protocol in which relatively objective measures of responses to promontory stimulation are correlated with specified measures of postimplant performance. Psychophysical measures that seem promising on the basis of current work include detection thresholds, the detection of periodic versus aperiodic signals, gap detection, and temporal discrimination.

The use of threshold measures for evaluating nerve survival seems promising on the basis of studies in monkey subjects and human patients using multichannel scala tympani implants. Work in monkeys has shown that sensitivity to low-frequency sinusoids (approximately 100 Hz) is directly correlated with nerve survival (Pfingst & Sutton, 1983). Over the range of pathologies that might be expected in cochlear implant patients, these thresholds can vary over a range of 37 dB or more (Pfingst et al., 1984). Low-frequency sinusoidal thresholds for cochlear implant patients vary over a similar range, and Shannon (1983; personal communication) has found in a small sample that threshold level is reasonably predictive of patient performance in more complex perceptual tasks. On the other hand, it must be pointed out that

Fourcin and associates (1979) have found thresholds for round window stimulation to be a poor predictor of patient performance. One reason for this poor correlation may be variability in electrode placement. Before a threshold task can be accepted as a predictor of nerve survival in implant candidates, further study is needed in at least two areas. First, it must be demonstrated in animals that thresholds for *extra-cochlear* electrodes are correlated with nerve survival, and second, data should be obtained from carefully documented stimulation sites in patients to see if thresholds are a useful predictor of implant performance when obtained from a constant stimulation site across patients or when obtained from some "optimal" site that may vary across patients.

One measure that Fourcin and co-workers (1979) have found useful for predicting the patients' ability to use an extracochlear device as an aid to lipreading is a test of discrimination of periodic (sinusoidal) versus aperiodic (band-limited noise) signals. Fourcin and associates (1979) and Hochmair-Desoyer and associates (1984) found psychophysical measures of gap detection and temporal discrimination to be useful as well. These tests may be less sensitive to electrode position on the cochlea and therefore may be more robust measures if consistent electrode placement proves to be problematic.

Another potential measure of nerve survival that offers some promise is the EABR. Starr and Brackmann (1979) have demonstrated that EABRs may be elicited in humans using promontory stimulation. Smith and Simmons (1983) studied EARBs evoked by round window stimulation in cats following experimental destruction of spiral ganglion cells. While threshold of the EABR did not change in a consistent fashion with the percentage of surviving spiral ganglion cells, the slopes of the amplitude input–output functions did vary in a systematic way with damage: the fewer the surviving spiral ganglion cells, the lower the slope. This observation in cats has been corroborated by work in guinea pigs (Allegra & Dobie, 1982).

Although the determination of the presence or absence of viable eighth nerve fibers may provide a sufficient minimum indication for implantation, we hope that decisions regarding the best implant for an individual patient and an optimal rehabilitation program will be based on measures of the percentage of surviving neural elements and their distribution. To obtain such measures, we must examine the response characteristics of groups of eighth nerve fibers with restricted differential stimulation of points along the cochlea. Thus, if an area of the osseous spiral lamina is devoid of viable fibers we may expect restricted stimulation to elicit no response, or a response of higher threshold or reduced magnitude, compared with responses obtained by stimulation at a richly innervated point. Such tests may evolve from continued studies in damaged animal models in which neural response characteristics evoked by restricted intracochlear stimulation are compared with those elicited by stimulation of the middle ear at various sites.

MORBIDITY

Clinical morbidity associated with cochlear implants has included transient vertigo and infection. Neither of these effects is typical, but certainly the transient vestibular disorder is not unusual either (Black, 1977, 1978). At times infection has been sufficient to require explantation, although this condition is unusual. In all cases, clinical morbidity has been readily reversible. At the histological level, implant morbidity is irreversible; sufficient data now exist to indicate that some histological change must be associated with implantation of a cochlear prosthesis in the inner ear. We must yet determine how great the changes are, what the mechanisms are that underlie these changes, to what extent they can be controlled, and to what extent the benefits obtained with the prosthesis outweigh the histological changes.

A fundamental issue that allows us to define risk versus benefit ratios in objective terms is: Will the implant cause so much damage that it will no longer be functional? While there are data indicating this is certainly possible, the evidence to date would indicate that it is not probable. If only to give credit to the brief history of this field, a discussion of morbidity must begin with the findings of Johnsson and associates (1982) — the first and, so far, only detailed and comprehensive published report on histopathological changes in the sensorineural epithelium and neural tissue of the temporal bone that may occur in the human with implantation and chronic stimulation. Johnsson found mechanical trauma associated with electrode insertion in both ears of this bilaterally implanted subject, and a marked reduction in the spiral ganglion cell population of both ears; in one the total appeared from representative illustrations to be about 1% of the normal population.[4] Extensive bone growth was found in one cochlea that had been implanted with a multielectrode system and showed marked mechanical trauma, while no bone growth was found in the contralateral ear with a single-electrode implant, although new bone growth was observed in the vestibular labyrinth. Interpretation of these findings is difficult. Obviously the pathological state of the temporal bone at the time of implantation was unknown. Interpretations of the data range from those suggesting that the implant and chronic stimulation had little or no effect (i.e., that the observed pathology all reflected preexisting pathological processes) to the view that the spiral ganglion cell population would have been much more extensive in the absence of an implant. While sufficient retrospective human material may become available to permit us to make more educated guesses as to the nature of prosthesis-induced changes in the presence of cochlear pathology, prospective controlled investigations using animal models clearly would be of substantial help in resolving this issue.

Initial investigations with animals included the chronic implantation of single-ball electrodes in the base of the scala tympani of normal cats (Simmons, 1967), and the implantation of multielectrode prostheses in a Silastic carrier molded to fit the scala tympani in normal and kanamycin-treated cats (Leake-Jones et al., 1981; Schindler, 1976; Schindler & Bjorkroth, 1979; Schindler & Merzenich, 1974). In normal material, in the absence of infection and mechanical trauma, degeneration was relatively small: with single-wire implants it was almost nonexistent; with the molded prostheses in both treated and untreated cochleae, relatively long-term survival of spiral ganglion cells on the order of 40–50% was reported. Such observations in cats have been corroborated in nonhuman primates (Sutton & Miller, 1983a). In monkey or cat cochleae in which infection was associated with the implant, massive degenera-

---

[4]However, recent reevaluation of this material (Burgio, 1983) indicated that as many as 1,650 spiral ganglion cells (about 5.5% of the average normal population) remained in this temporal bone.

tion was observed. In those cases in which direct mechanical trauma to the membranous labyrinth occurred, sensory and neural elements were absent in the vicinity of the damage. In other nonhuman-primate studies, greater degeneration of neural elements was observed with multichannel scala tympani implants (Miller & Sutton, 1980; Pfingst & Sutton, 1983; Sutton & Miller, 1983b; Sutton, Miller, & Pfingst, 1983). However, in these investigations in monkeys the implants were introduced into ears that had been topically treated with neomycin. It is clear that the neomycin alone may cause massive loss of sensory and neural elements (Duckert, 1983; Sutton & Miller, 1983a). Indeed it would appear that this toxic effect may be a direct one on the neural elements of the modiolus rather than mediated by damage to sensory and supporting structures (Clopton et al., submitted for publication; Duckert, 1983).

In a comparison of damage with molded versus tubular scala tympani implants in the monkey, it was found that the molded prosthesis invariably produced greater damage. This sometimes occurred in the absence of direct mechanical damage to tissues of the membranous labyrinth and was interpreted as presumably reflecting the occlusion of vessels in the endosteum of the lateral wall of the scala tympani and perhaps under the basilar membrane (Sutton et al., 1980). However, in addition, greater incidence of mechanical damage to soft tissue was found with the molded prosthesis. O'Reilly (1981), in a study of human cadaver temporal bones, observed that mechanical trauma following insertion of molded implants was rare. Although one must thus question the extent to which postmortem changes in the mechanical characteristics of scala tympani tissues may influence this finding and the extent to which it can be generalized to the implant candidate, support for this notion is provided by observations in living cats in which molded prostheses usually do not produce mechanical damage (Leake-Jones et al., 1981). It is to be hoped that, in spite of the larger relative diameter of the basal scala tympani of the cat, this preparation will serve as an adequate model for man.

In the case of these latter investigations, no electrical stimulation was provided. And while other factors related to infection and mechanical damage can be avoided (for example, with a single-ball electrode introduced but a few millimeters into the scala tympani or placed on the round window), by definition electrical stimulation cannot be avoided in cochlear prostheses. One of the first clear demonstrations of the influence of electrical stimulation in controlled animal experiments was provided by Walsh and Leake-Jones (1982). With 100-μs current pulses at levels of 2, 4, and then 8 mA, for 300–500 hr, damage was done. On the basis of real surface area estimations from geometric surface area measurements a threshold for damage of 40 μC/cm^2/phase was suggested. Clearly a definition of the threshold for damage with variation in parameters and duration of stimulation is necessary. More important, analyses must be performed to define the mechanisms involved.

Duckert and Miller (1982) demonstrated damage in an acute investigation of guinea pigs following 3 hr of continuous 1-kHz sinusoidal stimulation at 70 μC/cm^2/phase and above (based on real surface area measurements). In an extension of this investigation to four weekly 3-hr stimulation sessions, the threshold for damage was found to be reduced to 15–20 μC/cm^2/phase.

In the acute investigation, damage was observed at 400 μA rms. In a similar investigation but with 100-Hz stimulation, damage was observed at 200 μA rms. This comparative study was done to elucidate the mechanism that might be involved with electrically induced damage. If simple electrochemical mechanisms underlie damage, the threshold current for damage should vary at 6 dB per octave, with the charge density remaining constant. The comparative observations at 100 Hz and 1 kHz indicate a change in the damage threshold of 6 dB per *decade.* At 100 Hz the charge density was approximately at the level of theoretical nongassing limit for platinum–iridium electrodes (Brummer & Turner, 1977a), that is, approximately 300 μC/cm^2/phase, but at 1 kHz it was substantially less. Duckert suggests that for low-frequency stimuli an electrochemical process related to gassing may account completely for the threshold for damage, while at higher frequencies other mechanisms contribute to lowering the damage threshold. Obviously, these studies must be expanded to include other frequencies of stimulation. Furthermore, on the basis of these studies it is suggested that the investigation of pH changes, toxic by-products, and other biochemical changes in the fluid and tissues surrounding a stimulated electrode should be evaluated, particularly at higher frequencies of stimulation.

Some of the implications of nerve loss for cochlear prosthesis function are obvious from psychophysical studies in monkeys, as noted repeatedly. In ears with very low nerve survival, thresholds for low-frequency sinusoids can be as much as 36 dB higher than thresholds from implanted ears with high nerve survival (Pfingst & Sutton, 1983; Pfingst et al., 1984). These higher thresholds lead to higher current requirements for perceivable stimulation and a reduced operating range for the implant. A further consequence of nerve damage is its impact on channel separation. Electrophysiological studies of channel interaction in cats (Vivion, Merzenich, Leake-Jones, White, & Silverman, 1981; White & Merzenich, 1983) indicate increased channel interaction with reduced neural innervation of the cochlea. These findings are supported by studies in monkeys which indicate that a minimal number of nerve fibers must be present to permit electrode-place discrimination along the scala tympani (Pfingst et al., 1981a; Pfingst, 1984).

Recently, animal studies have revealed a temporary-threshold-shiftlike effect with continuous electrical stimulation. In studies designed to evaluate the functional significance of continuous moderate level stimulation, Miller and colleagues (1984a,b) observed changes in the threshold for the EABR. These studies were performed in guinea pigs with chronic electrodes implanted in the scala tympani, on the round window, or on the promontory. Threshold elevations of 300–500% were observed. The magnitude of the threshold change was found to be correlated with intensity of stimulation and site of implant: greater threshold shifts were seen with scala tympani electrodes than with extracochlear placements. In general, the effects on suprathreshold characteristics of the response (such as the slope of the amplitude-intensity growth function) were greater than the effects seen on threshold. This observation is in agreement with the findings of Smith and Simmons (1983) and Allegra and Dobie (1982), noted above, in their studies on EABR responses following destruction of spiral-ganglion cells. Miller and associates (1984a,b), using stimulus intensities that produced clear and reliable threshold changes, found that repeated stimulation was associated with histological changes in the inner ear. Similar changes were not found where stimulation levels produced small and inconsistent elevation in EABR threshold. The fact that the EABR response demonstrated complete recovery following weekly stimulation in spite of histological change would indicate that this measure, when elicited with monopolar stimulation, is not sensitive to restricted histological damage.[5]

Preliminary studies of this temporary threshold shift effect have been initiated in trained monkeys. Such shifts have been observed to result from 15-min exposures to moderate intensities of electrical stimulation (Miller et al., 1984a). In addition to these temporary threshold changes, some small permanent threshold changes have been observed to result from repeated exposures.

These data suggest that moderate levels of stimulation well within the dynamic range of use of the prosthesis may cause functional changes, albeit often reversible, in system function. The possible mechanisms underlying these changes range from electrode tissue interface changes, through variation in phase-locking characteristics of essential auditory fibers, to effects on descending systems. Implant patients do report that with prosthesis use, fatigue and changes in the characteristics of sensation are observed. For these reasons, as well as the fact that these changes may provide early signs for more permanent changes in function, it would seem appropriate to evaluate these effects further.

CONCLUSION

The cochlear prosthesis is gaining wide acceptance as the therapy of choice for the sensorineural profoundly deaf patient. This acceptance seems to be based on the patients' enthusiasm for receiving a device that will restore to them some sort of sound perception, the lack of obvious signs of serious morbidity in patients implanted for many years, demonstrable benefits to the patients in terms of contact with the environment, and some improvement of lipreading ability. The hope of most investigators is that the prosthesis will be developed to the point that it can reliably restore perception of running speech without the aid of lipreading. While this goal has been achieved to a limited degree in a few "star" patients from some laboratories, the vast majority of cochlear implant wearers fall far short of this goal. Furthermore, the reasons for success in the "star" patients are unknown.

Although a number of "obvious" implant designs and encoding schemes have been tested in patients, typically all fall short of reliably providing recognizable speech information to the patient. Star patients are well distributed across implant designs, including single- and multichannel implants. Perhaps this reflects the rather sparse scientific data base underpinning these prosthesis designs. A significant scientific base of knowledge regarding implantation of the cochlea and the effects of electrical stimulation on the auditory nervous system has just begun to develop. At the same time, significant strides are being made in our understanding of the neural processing of speech information in the auditory pathway. We hope that experimental studies described in this chapter will be extended, providing in the near future the foundation

---

[5]In these cases, damage was less than 10% of the cochlea; thus, this finding in no way stands in contrast to the findings and clinical implications of the studies of Smith and Simmons (1983) and Dobie and Allegra (1982).

upon which significantly improved cochlear prostheses will be based – prostheses that will safely overcome speech communication deficits in the sensorineural profoundly deaf patient.

REFERENCES

Allegra, L.A., & Dobie, R.A. (1982). Electrically evoked ABR in the guinea pig following drug-induced deafness. *Abstracts of the Fifth Midwinter Research Meeting, Association for Research in Otolaryngology,* 4–5.

Banfai, P., Hortmann, G., Kubik, S., & Wustrow, F. (1980). Projection of the spiral cochlear canal on the medial wall of the tympanic cavity with regard to the cochlear implant. *Scandinavian Audiology Supplement 11,* 157–162.

Banfai, P., Hortmann, G., Wustrow, F., Kubik, S., & Zeisberg, B. (1981). Mebdaten und Psycho-Akustische Auswertung mit 8-Kanal-Horprothese, HNO, 29, 22–26.

Bergstrom, L. (1975). Some pathologies of sensory and neural hearing loss. *Canadian Journal of Otolaryngology Supplement 2, 4,* 1–28.

Berlin, C.I., Wexler, K.F., Jerger, J.F., Halperin, H.R., & Smith, S. (1978). Superior ultra-audiometric hearing: A new type of hearing loss which correlates highly with unusually good speech in the "profoundly deaf." *Otolaryngology, 86,* 111–116.

Bilger, R.C. (1977). Evaluation of subjects presently fitted with implanted auditory prostheses. *Annals of Otology, Rhinology and Laryngology (St. Louis) Supplement 38, 86,* 176 pages.

Black, F.O. (1977). Present vestibular status of subjects implanted with auditory prostheses. *Annals of Otology, Rhinology and Laryngology (St. Louis) Supplement 38, 86,* 49–56.

Black, F.O., (1978). Value determination of inner ear prosthetic implants. In R.F. Naunton & C. Fernandez (Eds.), *Evoked electrical activity in the auditory nervous system* (pp. 323–333). New York: Academic Press.

Black, R.C., & Clark, G.M. (1980). Differential electrical excitation of the auditory nerve. *Journal of the Acoustical Society of America, 67,* 868–874.

Black, R.C., Clark, G.M., & Patrick, J.F. (1981). Current distribution measurements within the human cochlea. *IEEE transactions on Biomedical Engineering, 28,* 721–725.

Blamey, P.J., Dowell, R.C., Tong, Y.C., & Clark, G.M. (1983). Psychophysical matching of sensations produced by acoustic and electrical stimulation of the auditory nerve. In W.R. Webster & L.M. Aitkin (Eds.), *Mechanisms of Hearing.* Clayton: Monash Univ. Press.

Brackmann, D.E., & Selters, W.A. (1978). Sensorineural hearing impairment: Clinical differentiation. *Otolaryngologic Clinics of North America, 11,* 195–199.

Brummer, S.B., & Turner, M.J. (1977a). Electrical stimulation with pt electrodes: II – Estimation of maximum surface redox (theoretical non-gassing) limits. *IEEE Transactions of Biomedical Engineering, BME-24,* 440–443.

Brummer, S.B., & Turner, M.J. (1977b). Electrochemical considerations for safe electrical stimulation of the nervous system with platinum electrodes. *IEEE Transactions of Biomedical Engineering, BME-24,* 59–63.

Burgio, P. (1983). Presented at the tenth anniversary conference on cochlear implants, San Francisco, June.

Burian, K., Hochmair, E., Hochmair-Desoyer, I., & Lessel, M.R. (1980). Electrical stimulation with multichannel electrodes in deaf patients. *Audiology, 19,* 128.

Burns, E.M., & Viemeister, N.F. (1981). Played-again sam: Further observations on the pitch of amplitude-modulated noise. *Journal of the Acoustical Society of America, 70,* 1655–1660.

Butikofer, R., & Lawrence, P.D. (1978). Electrocutaneous nerve stimulation: I. Model and experiment. *IEEE Transactions of Biomedical Engineering, BME-25,* 526–531.

Clark, G.M., Black, R., Dewhurst, D.J., Forster, I.C., Patrick, J.F., & Tong, Y.C. (1977). A multiple-electrode hearing prosthesis for cochlear implantation in deaf patients. *Medical Progress through Technology, 5,* 127–140.

Clark, G.M., & Tong, Y.C. (1982). A multiple-channel cochlear implant: A summary of results for two patients. *Archives of Otolaryngology, 108,* 214–217.

Clopton, B.M., & Glass, I. Unit responses at cochlear nucleus to electrical stimulation through a cochlear prosthesis. Submitted for publication.

Clopton, B.M., & Silverman, M.S. (1978). Central correlates of intracochlear electrical stimulation determined by single-unit recording. *Abstracts of the First Midwinter Research Meeting, Association for Research in Otolaryngology,* 23.

Clopton, B.M., & Spelman, F.A. (1982). Neural mechanisms relevant to the design of an auditory prosthesis. Location and electrical characteristics. *Annals of Otology, Rhinology and Laryngology (St. Louis) Supplement 98, 91,* 9–14.

Clopton, B.M., Spelman, F.A., Glass, I., Pfingst, B.E., Miller, J.M., Lawrence, P.D., & Dean, D.P. (1983). Neural encoding of electrical signals. *Annals of the New York Academy of Sciences, 405,* 146–158.

Collins, M.J. (1979). Clinical and laboratory use of a wearable master hearing aid. In D.L. McPherson (Ed.), *Advances in prosthetic devices for the deaf: A technical workshop (pp. 168–176).* Rochester: National Tech. Inst. Deaf.

Cooper, W.E. (1983). The perception of fluent speech. *Annals of the New York Academy of Sciences, 405,* 48–63.

Dobie, R.A., & Kimm, J. (1980). Brainstem responses to electrical stimulation of the cochlea. *Archives of Otolaryngology, 106,* 573–577.

Douek, E., Fourcin, A.J., Moore, B.C.J., & Clarke, G.P. (1977). A new approach to the cochlear implant. *Proceedings of the Royal Society of Medicine, 70,* 379–383.

Douek, E., Fourcin, A.J., Moore, B.C.J., Rosen, S., Walliker, J.R., Frampton, S.L., Howard, D.M., & Abberton, E. (1983). Clinical aspects of extracochlear electrical stimulation. *Annals of the New York Academy of Sciences, 405,* 332–336.

Duckert, L.G. (1983). Morphological changes in the normal and neomycin-perfused guinea pig cochlea following chronic prosthetic implantation. *Laryngoscope, 93,* 841–855.

Duckert, L.G., & Miller, J.M. (1982). Acute morphological changes in guinea pig cochlea following electrical stimulation. A preliminary scanning electron microscope study. *Annals of Otology, Rhinology and Laryngology (St. Louis), 91,* 33–40.

Eddington, D.K. (1980). Speech discrimination in deaf subjects with cochlear implants. *Journal of the Acoustical Society of America, 68,* 885–891.

Eddington, D.K., Dobelle, W.H., Brackmann, D.E., Mladejovsky, M.G., & Parkin, J.L. (1978a). Place and periodicity pitch by stimulation of multiple scala tympani electrodes in deaf volunteers. *Transactions—American Society for Artificial Internal Organs, 24,* 1–5.

Eddington, D.K., Dobelle, W.H., Brackmann, D.E., Mladejovsky, M.G., & Parkin, J.L. (1978b). Auditory prosthesis research with multiple channel intracochlear stimulation in man. *Annals of Otology, Rhinology and Laryngology (St. Louis) Supplement 53, 87,* 5–39.

Evans, E.F. (1975). The cochlear nerve and cochlear nucleus. In W.D. Keidel & W.D. Neff (Eds.), *Handbook of sensory physiology (pp. 1–108).* Heidelberg: Springer-Verlag.

Evans, E.F. (1978). Peripheral auditory processing in normal and abnormal ears: Physiological considerations for attempts to compensate for auditory deficits by acoustic and electrical prostheses. *Sensorineural Hearing Impairment and Hearing Aids (Scandinavian Audiology Suppl. 6)*, 9–44.

Evans, E.F. (1984). Dimension of the problem: An overview – How to provide speech through an implant device. In R.A. Schindler & M.M. Merzenich (Eds.), *Tenth anniversary conference on cochlear implants: An international symposium.* New York: Raven Press.

Fourcin, A.J., Douek, E.E., Moore, B.C.J., Rosen, S., Walliker, J.R., Howard, D.M., Abberton, E., & Frampton, S. (1983). Speech perception with promontory stimulation, *Annals of the New York Academy of Sciences, 405*, 280–294.

Fourcin, A.J., Rosen, S.M., Moore, B.C.J., Douek, E.E., Clarke, G.P., Dodson, H., & Bannister, L.H. (1979). External electrical stimulation of the cochlea: Clinical, psychophysical, speech-perceptual and histological findings. *British Journal of Audiology, 13*, 85–107.

Frankenhaeuser, B., & Huxley, A.F. (1964). The action potential in the myelinated nerve fibre of Xenopus laevis as computed on the basis of voltage clamp data, *Journal of Physiology (London), 171*, 302–315.

Gheewala, T.R., Melen, R.D., & White, R.L. (1975). A CMOS implantable multi-electrode auditory stimulator for the deaf. *IEEE Journal of Solid State Circuits, SC-10*, 472–479.

Glass, I. Responses of cochlear nucleus units to electrical stimulation through a cochlear prosthesis: Channel interaction. Submitted for publication.

Glass, I. (1983). Tuning characteristics of cochlear nucleus units in response to electrical stimulation of the cochlea. *Hearing Research, 12*, 223–237.

Glass, I. (in press). Phase-locked responses of cochlear nucleus units to electrical stimulation through a cochlear implant. *Experimental Brain Research* in press.

Goldstein, J.L. (1978). Mechanisms of signal analysis and pattern perception in periodicity pitch. *Audiology, 17*, 421–445.

Greenwood, D.D. (1961). Critical bandwidths and the frequency coordinates of the basilar membrane. *Journal of the Acoustical Society of America, 33*, 1344–1356.

Guttman, R., & Hachmeister, L. (1971). Effect of calcium, temperature, and polarizing currents upon alternating current excitation of space-clamped squid axons. *Journal of General Physiology, 58*, 304–321.

Helmerich, L.F., & Edgerton, B.J. (1982). Psychoelectric measurements and results from cochlear implant patients. *Annals of Otology, Rhinology and Laryngology (St. Louis) Supplement 91, 91*, 35–40.

Herndon, M.K. (1981). *Psychoacoustics and speech processing for a modiolar auditory prosthesis.* Stanford: Integrated Circuits Laboratory.

Hinojosa, R., & Marion, M. (1983). Histopathology of profound sensorineural deafness. *Annals of the New York Academy of Sciences, 405*, 459–484.

Hochmair, E.S., & Hochmair-Desoyer, I.J. (1981). An implanted auditory 8-channel stimulator for the deaf. *Medical and Biological Engineering and Computing, 19*, 141–148.

Hochmair, E.S., & Hochmair-Desoyer, I.J. (1984). Aspects of sound signal processing using the vienna intra- and extracochlear implants. In R.A. Schindler & M.M. Merzenich (Eds.), *Tenth anniversary conference on cochlear implants: An international symposium.* New York: Raven Press.

Hochmair, E.S., Hochmair-Desoyer, I.J., & Burian, K. (1979). Investigations towards an artificial cochlea. *The International Journal of Artificial Organs, 2*, 255–261.

Hochmair-Desoyer, I.J., Hochmair, E.K., & Burian, K. (1983). Design and fabrication of multi-wire scala tympani electrodes. *Annals of the New York Academy of Sciences, 405*, 173–182.

Hochmair-Desoyer, I.J., Hochmair, E.S., & Stiglbrunner, H.K. (1984). Psychoacoustic temporal processing and speech understanding in cochlear implant patients. In R.A. Schindler & M.M. Merzenich (Eds.), *Tenth anniversary conference on cochlear implants: An international symposium.* New York: Raven Press.

House, W.F., & Berliner, K.I. (1982). Cochlear implants: Progress and perspectives. *Annals of Otology, Rhinology and Laryngology (St. Louis) Supplement 91,* 1–124.

House, W.F., Berliner, K.I., Eisenberg, L.S., Edgerton, B.J., & Thielemeir, M.A. (1981). The cochlear implant: 1980 update. *ACTA Otolaryngologica (Stockholm), 91,* 457–462.

House, W.F., & Brackmann, D.E. (1974). Electrical promontory testing in differential diagnosis of sensori-neural hearing impairment. *Laryngoscope, 84,* 2163–2171.

Johnsson, L.-G., House, W.F., & Linthicum, F.H., Jr. (1982). Otopathological findings in a patient with bilateral cochlear implants. *Annals of Otology, Rhinology and Laryngology (St. Louis) Supplement 91, 91,* 74–89.

Kiang, N.Y.S., Eddington, D.K., & Delgutte, B. (1979). Fundamental considerations in designing auditory implants. *ACTA Otolaryngologica (Stockholm), 87,* 204–218.

Kiang, N.Y.S., Keithley, E.M., & Liberman, M.C. (1983). The impact of auditory nerve experiments on cochlear implant design. *Annals of the New York Academy of Sciences, 405,* 114–121.

Kiang, N.Y.S., & Moxon, E.C. (1972). Physiological considerations in artificial stimulation of the inner ear. *Annals of Otology, Rhinology and Laryngology (St. Louis), 81,* 714–730.

Leake-Jones, P.A., Vivion, M.C., O'Reilly, B.F., & Merzenich, M.M. (1982). Deaf animal models for studies of a multichannel cochlear prosthesis. *Hearing Research, 8,* 225–246.

Leake-Jones, P.A., Walsh, S.M., & Merzenich, M.M. (1981). Cochlear pathology following chronic intracochlear electrical stimulation, *Annals of Otology, Rhinology and Laryngology (St. Louis) Supplement 82, 90,* 6–8.

Levitt, H., Pickett, J.M., & Houde, R.A. (1980). *Sensory aids for the hearing impaired.* New York: IEEE Press.

Loeb, G.E., Byers, C.L., Rebscher, S.J., Casey, D.E., Fong, M.M., Schindler, R.A., Gray, R.F., & Merzenich, M.M. (1983a). Design and fabrication of an experimental cochlear prothesis. *Medical and Biological Engineering and Computing, 21,* 241–254.

Loeb, G.E., McHardy, J., Kelliher, E.M., & Brummer, S.B. (1982). Neural prostheses. In D.F. Williams (Ed.), *Biocompatibility in clinical practice* (pp. 123–149). Boca Raton, Florida: CRC Press.

Loeb, G.E., White, M.W., & Jenkins, W.M. (1983b). Biophysical considerations in electrical stimulation of the auditory nervous system. *Annals of the New York Academy of Sciences, 405,* 123–136.

Mathews, R.G. (1978). *Sound processing for an auditory prosthesis (Technical Report No. 5306-3).* Palo Alto: Stanford University.

Merzenich, M.M., Michelson, R.P., Pettit, C.R., Schindler, R.A., & Reid, M. (1973). Neural encoding of sound sensation evoked by electrical stimulation of the acoustic nerve. *Annals of Otology, Rhinology and Laryngology (St. Louis), 82,* 486–503.

Michelson, R.P., Merzenich, M.M., Schindler, R.A., & Schindler, D.N. (1975). Present status and future development of the cochlear prosthesis. *Annals of Otology, Rhinology and Laryngology (St. Louis), 84,* 494–498.

Michelson, R.P., & Schindler, R.A. (1981). Multichannel cochlear implants. Current status and future developments. *Laryngoscope, 91,* 886–888.

Miller, J.M., Duckert, L., Malone, M., & Pfingst, B.E. (1984a). Cochlear prosthesis: Stimulation induced damage. *Annals of Otology, Rhinology and Laryngology (St. Louis), 92,* 599–609.

Miller, J.M., Duckert, L., Sutton, D., Pfingst, B.E., & Malone, M. (1984b). Animal models: Relevance to implant use in humans. In R.A. Schindler & M.M. Merzenich (Eds.), *Tenth anniversary conference on cochlear implants: An international symposium.* New York: Raven Press.

Miller, J.M., & Sutton, D. (1980). Cochlear prosthesis: Morphological considerations. *Journal of Laryngology and Otology, 94,* 359–366.

Moxon, E.D. (1971). *Neural and mechanical responses to electric stimulation of the cat's inner ear.* Cambridge: Massachusetts Institute of Technology.

Muller, C. (1981). Survey of cochlear implant work. *Journal of the Acoustical Society of America, 70,* S52.

Nadol, J.B., Jr. (1984). Histological considerations in implant patients. *Archives of Otolaryngology, 110,* 160–163.

O'Reilly, B.F. (1981). Probability of trauma and reliability of placement of a 20mm long model human scala tympani multielectrode array, *Annals of Otology, Rhinology and Laryngology (St. Louis) Supplement 82, 90,* 11–12.

Otte, J., Schuknecht, H.F., Kerr, A.G. (1978). Ganglion cell populations in normal and pathological human cochleae. Implications for cochlear implantation. *Laryngoscope, 88,* 1231–1246.

Owens, E., Kessler, D.K., & Schubert, E.D. (1981). The minimum auditory capabilities (MAC) battery. *Hearing Aid Journal, 34,* 9–34.

Owens, E., Kessler, D.K., & Schubert, E.D. (1982). Interim assignment of candidates for cochlear implants. *Archives of Otolaryngology, 108,* 478–483.

Owens, E., & Telleen, C.C. (1981). Speech perception with hearing aids and cochlear implants. *Archives of Otolaryngology, 107,* 160–163.

Patrick, J.F., Crosby, P.A., Hirshorn, M.S., Kuzma, J.A., Money, D.K., Ridler, J., & Seligman, P.M. (1984). The Australian multichannel implantable hearing prosthesis. In R.A. Schindler & M.M. Merzenich (Eds.), *Tenth anniversary conference on cochlear implants: An international symposium.* New York: Raven Press.

Pfingst, B.E. (1983). Initial psychophysical results from multi-electrode middle-ear cochlear prostheses in monkeys. *Abstracts of the Sixth Midwinter Research Meeting, Association for Research in Otolaryngology,* 28–29.

Pfingst, B.E. (1984). Operating ranges and intensity psychophysics for cochlear implants. Implications for speech processing strategies. *Archives of Otolaryngology, 110,* 140–144.

Pfingst, B.E., Burnett, P.A., & Sutton, D. (1983). Intensity discrimination with cochlear implants. *Journal of the Acoustical Society of America, 73,* 1283–1292.

Pfingst, B.E., Donaldson, J.A., Miller, J.M., & Spelman, F.A. (1979). Psychophysical evaluation of cochlear prostheses in a monkey model. *Annals of Otology, Rhinology and Laryngology (St. Louis), 88,* 613–625.

Pfingst, B.E., Glass, I., Spelman, F.A., & Sutton, D. (1984). Psychophysical studies of cochlear implants in monkeys: Clinical implications. In R.A. Schindler & M.M. Merzenich (Eds.), *Tenth anniversary conference on cochlear implants: An international symposium.* New York: Raven Press.

Pfingst, B.E., & Sutton, D. (1983). Relation of cochlear implant function to histopathology in monkeys. *Annals of the New York Academy of Sciences, 405,* 224–239.

Pfingst, B.E., Sutton, D., & Miller, J.M. (1981a). Electrode-place discrimination by monkeys with cochlear and modiolar implants. *Abstracts of the Fourth Midwinter Research Meeting, Association for Research in Otolaryngology,* 64.

Pfingst, B.E., Sutton, D., Miller, J.M., & Bohne, B.A. (1981b). Relation of psychophysical data to histopathology in monkeys with cochlear implants. *Acta Otolaryngologica, 92,* 1–13.

Plomp, P., & Smoorenburg, G.F. (1970). *Frequency analysis and periodicity detection in hearing.* Leiden: Sijthoff.

Risberg, A., & Agelfors, E. (1982). Speech perception based on non-speech signals. In R. Carlson & B. Granstrom (Eds.), *The representation of speech in the peripheral auditory system* (pp. 209–215). New York: Elsevier.

Schindler, R.A. (1976). The cochlear histopathology of chronic intracochlear implantation. *Journal of Laryngology and Otology, 90,* 445–457.

Schindler, R.A. (1983). Presented at the tenth anniversary conference on cochlear implants, San Francisco, June.

Schindler, R.A., & Bjorkroth, B. (1979). Traumatic intracochlear electrode implantation. *Laryngoscope, 89,* 752–758.

Schindler, R.A., & Merzenich, M.M. (1974). Chronic intracochlear electrode implantation: Cochlear pathology and acoustic nerve survival. *Annals of Otology, Rhinology and Laryngology (St. Louis), 83,* 202–216.

Schindler, R.A., Merzenich, M.M., White, M.W., & Bjorkroth, B. (1977). Multielectrode intracochlear implants: Nerve survival and stimulation patterns. *Archives of Otolaryngology, 103,* 691–699.

Schubert, E.D. (1983). Use of the pitch response in assessing cochlear implants. *Abstracts of the Sixth Midwinter Research Meeting, Association for Research in Otolaryngology,* 127.

Shamma, S.A., May, G.A., & White, R.L. (1980). Photolithographic fabrication of microelectrode arrays for an auditory prosthesis. In: *IEEE 1980 frontiers of engineering in health care* (pp. 108–111). New York: IEEE Press.

Shannon, R.V. (1983). Electrical stimulation of the auditory nerve in Man. I. Basic Psychophysics. *Hearing Research, 11,* 157–189.

Shannon, R.V. (1984). Loudness summation as a measure of channel interaction in a cochlear prosthesis. In R.A. Schindler & M.M. Merzenich (Eds.), *Tenth anniversary conference on cochlear implants: An international symposium.* New York: Raven Press.

Shiff, W., & Foulke, E. (1982). *Tactual perception: A sourcebook.* Cambridge: Cambridge Univ. Press.

Simmons, F.B. (1966). Electrical stimulation of the auditory nerve in man. *Archives of Otolaryngology, 84,* 24–76.

Simmons, F.B. (1967). Permanent intracochlear electrodes in cats, tissue tolerance and cochlear microphonics. *Laryngoscope, 77,* 171–186.

Simmons, F.B. (1976). Electrical stimulation of the ear in man. In W.D. Keidel & W.D. Neff (Eds.), *Handbook of sensory physiology: Volume V. Auditory system, Part 3, Clinical and special topics* (pp. 417–429). New York: Springer-Verlag.

Simmons, F.B., Epley, J.M., Lummis, R.C., Guttman, N., Frishkopf, L.S., Harmon, L.D., & Zwicker, E. (1965). Auditory nerve: Electrical stimulation in man. *Science, 148,* 104–106.

Smith, L., & Simmons, F.B. (1983). Estimating eighth nerve survival by electrical stimulation. *Annals of Otology, Rhinology, and Laryngology (St. Louis), 92,* 19–23.

Soma, M., May, G.A., Duval, F., & White, R.L. (1980). Fabrication and packaging of an implantable multichannel auditory prosthesis. In: *IEEE 1980 Frontiers of engineering in health care* (pp. 105–107). New York: IEEE Press.

Sonn, M. (1974). An artificial cochlea for the sensory deaf: Presurgical development. *Journal of Auditory Research, 14,* 89–108.

Sparks, D.W., Arell, L.A., Bourgois, M., Wiedmer, B., & Kuhl, P.K. (1979). Investigating the MESA (multipoint electrotactile speech aid): The transmission of connected discourse. *Journal of the Acoustical Society of America, 65,* 810–815.

Spelman, F., Pfingst, B., Powers, W., Miller, J., Hassul, M., & Clopton, B. (1979). Biophysics of the implanted ear: Electrical parameters. In D.L. McPherson (Ed.), *Advances in prosthetic devices for the deaf: A technical workshop* (pp. 312–323). Rochester: National Technical Institute for the Deaf.

Spelman, F.A. (1982). The cochlear prosthesis: A review of the design and evaluation of electrode implants for the profoundly deaf. *CRC Critical Reviews in Bioengineering, 8*, 223–252.

Spelman, F.A., Clopton, B.M., & Pfingst, B.E. (1982). Tissue impedance and current flow in the implanted ear: Implications for the cochlear prosthesis. *Annals of Otology, Rhinology and Laryngology (St. Louis) Supplement 98, 91*, 3–8.

Spelman, F.A., Clopton, B.M., Pfingst, B.E., & Miller, J.M. (1980a). Design of the cochlear prosthesis: Effects of the flow of current in the implanted ear. *Annals of Otology, Rhinology and Laryngology (St. Louis) Supplement 66, 89*, 8–10.

Spelman, F.A., Pfingst, B.E., & Miller, J.M. (1978). A constant-current stimulator for use with chronic cochlear implants. *Proceedings of the San Diego Biomedical Symposium, 17*, 1–3.

Spelman, F.A., Pfingst, B.E., Miller, J.M., Hassul, M., Powers, W.E., & Clopton, B.M. (1980b). Biophysical measurements in the implanted cochlea. *Otolaryngology, Head and Neck Surgery, 88*, 183–187.

Starr, A., & Brackmann, D.E. (1979). Brain stem potentials evoked by electrical stimulation of the cochlea in human subjects. *Annals of Otology, Rhinology and Laryngology (St. Louis), 88*, 550–556.

Stevens, K.N. (1983). Acoustic properties used for the identification of speech sounds. *Annals of the New York Academy of Sciences, 405*, 2–17.

Sutton, D., & Miller, J. (1983a). Intracochlear implants: Potential histopathology. *Otolaryngologic Clinics of North America, 16*, 227–232.

Sutton, D., & Miller, J.M. (1983b). Cochlear implant effects on the spinal ganglion. *Annals of Otology, Rhinology and Laryngology (St. Louis), 92*, 53–58.

Sutton, D., Miller, J.M., & Pfingst, B.E. (1980). Comparison of cochlear histopathology following two implant designs for use in scala tympani. *Annals of Otology, Rhinology and Laryngology (St. Louis) Supplement 66, 89*, 11–14.

Tong, Y.C., Blamey, P.J., Dowell, R.C., & Clark, G.M. (1983a). Psychophysical studies evaluating the feasibility of a speech processing strategy for a multiple-channel cochlear implant. *Journal of the Acoustical Society of America, 74*, 73–80.

Tong, Y.C., & Clark, G.M. (1983). Percepts from scala tympani stimulation. *Annals of the New York Academy of Science, 405*, 264–267.

Tong, Y.C., Clark, G.M., Blamey, P.J., Busby, P.A., & Dowell, R.C. (1982). Psychophysical studies for two multiple-channel cochlear implant patients. *Journal of the Acoustical Society of America, 71*, 153–160.

Tong, Y.C., Dowell, R.C., Blamey, P.J., & Clark, G.M. (1983b). Two-component hearing sensations produced by two-electrode stimulation in the cochlea of a deaf patient. *Science, 219*, 993–994.

Vivion, M.C., Merzenich, M.M., Leake-Jones, P.A., White, M., & Silverman, M. (1981). Electrode position and excitation patterns for a model cochlear prosthesis. *Annals of Otology, Rhinology and Laryngology (St. Louis) Supplement 82, 90*, 19–20.

Vurek, L.S., White, M., Fong, M., & Walsh, S.M. (1981). Optoisolated stimulators used for electrically evoked BSER. Some observations on electrical artifact. *Annals of Otology, Rhinology and Laryngology (St. Louis) Supplement 82, 90*, 21–24.

Walker, M.G. (1978). *Sound professors for an auditory prosthesis (Technical Report no. 5306-4)*. Stanford University: Integrated Circuits Laboratory.

Walsh, S.M., & Leake-Jones, P.A. (1982). Chronic electrical stimulation of auditory nerve in cat: Physiological and histological results. *Hearing Research, 7,* 281–304.

White, M.W., & Merzenich, M.M. (1983). Multichannel electrical stimulation of the auditory nerve: Channel interaction and processor design. *Abstracts of the Sixth Midwinter Research Meeting, Association for Research in Otolaryngology,* 128.

White, R.L. (1977). Electronics and electrodes for sensory prostheses. In F.T. Hambrecht & J.B. Reswick (Eds.), *Functional electrical stimulation* (pp. 485–498). New York: Dekker.

White, R.L. (1980). Microelectronics and neural prostheses. *Annals of Biomedical Engineering, 8,* 317–332.

White, R.L. (1982). Review of current status of cochlear prostheses. *IEEE Transactions on Biomedical Engineering, BME-29,* 233–239.

White, R.L., Roberts, L.A., Cotter, N.E., & Kwon, O.H. (1983). Thin-film electrode fabrication techniques. *Annals of the New York Academy of Sciences, 405,* 183–190.

Young, E.D., & Sachs, M.B. (1979). Representation of steady-state vowels in the temporal aspects of the discharge patterns of populations of auditory nerve fibers. *Journal of the Acoustical Society of America, 66,* 1381–1403.

Chapter 10

Neurotransmitters of the Auditory Nerve and Central Auditory System

Robert J. Wenthold

Michael R. Martin

INTRODUCTION

The study of central auditory neurotransmitters is a relatively new and largely unexplored field. The information we have about the nature and function of central auditory neurotransmitters is scattered throughout the neurobiological literature of the past two decades. This review brings together what is known of the auditory nerve and central auditory system neurotransmitters, considers possible functions of these neurotransmitters, and suggests areas of research which need further exploration and show greatest promise. For the many auditory researchers unfamiliar with the pharmacology and biochemistry of neurotransmitters, we briefly review the criteria for neurotransmitter identification and the methods employed in this effort. This is followed by sections on the neurotransmitter of the auditory nerve, other cochlear nucleus neurotransmitters, and neurotransmitters in higher auditory nuclei.

Identification of a neurotransmitter utilized at a particular synapse is a complex undertaking involving the techniques of anatomy, biochemistry, pharmacology, and physiology. To identify a substance as a neurotransmitter, two primary criteria must be fulfilled: The putative transmitter must be released from the presynaptic terminal under normal conditions of action potential-activated synaptic release, and its interaction with the postsynaptic receptor must produce a response identical to that of the synaptically released transmitter. Realistically, these events can only be studied indirectly. Consequently, scientists have generally agreed on several criteria that should be met to identify a substance as a neurotransmitter. These criteria include the mechanism to produce and the presence of the substance in the presynaptic element, the presence of an inactivating system, presynaptic release with appropriate stimulation, and the pharmacological and physiological interchangeability of the candidate substance and the neurotransmitter. The presence of a substance, the mechanism of production, and an inactivating system are experimentally the most accessible and provide a means of screening candidates for further characterization. In fact, most of what we know about neurotransmitters in the mammalian central nervous system is based on these three less rigorous criteria. This should always be kept in mind in our thinking of neurotransmitters in the central nervous system. For example, several recent reports demonstrate the presence of two or more putative neurotransmitters in the same neuron yet only one may be released or only one may interact with the postsynaptic receptor.

Demonstration of the presynaptic presence of a substance is traditionally done by measuring the neurotransmitter candidate itself or an enzyme known to be specifically linked to the neurotransmitter. Coupled with selective lesions, the pathways containing various neurotransmitters can be identified. The recent development of immunocytochemistry has revolutionized the field of biochemical anatomy. Substances to which antibodies can be produced, including, for example, neuroactive peptides, neurotransmitter-related enzymes, receptors, and some smaller neurotransmitters such as serotonin, can be directly localized. Neurotransmitters for minor pathways as well as major pathways can be studied. Unfortunately, not all neurotransmitters can be localized in this way, including the class of α-amino acid putative neurotransmitters, glutamate, aspartate, and glycine. We are optimistic that recent work aimed at characterizing the biosynthesis of glutamate and aspartate will provide an immunocytochemical marker for neurons using these neurotransmitters (Altschuler, Neises, Harmison, Wenthold, & Fex, 1981).

The ability of some presynaptic terminals to take up and concentrate some putative neurotransmitters has been used as a way to identify possible neurotransmitters. It is believed that high-affinity uptake is part of the neurotransmitter inactivation and reutilization system. Although uptake has been successfully applied, its reliability as a criterion appears to depend on the neurotransmitter used, the tissue studied, and the conditions under which the study is carried out. For substances like amino acids, some of the problems may be due to metabolism of the original molecule. For localizing aspartergic neurons, nonmetabolizable D-aspartate has recently been used to show selective uptake and subsequent transport (Beaudet, Burkhalter, Reubi, & Cuenod, 1981; Rustioni & Cuenod, 1982; Streit, 1980).

Demonstration of release in vivo in the central nervous system has been limited for most neurotransmitters. Since the site of collection is usually relatively far from the point of actual release, these studies require prior blocking of the neurotransmitter inactivation system. Consequently, only a very few neurotransmitters can be studied in this way. Alternatively, release has been studied in vitro by measuring the release of endogenous, or more frequently, preloaded radioactive substances from slices or synaptosomes after chemical or electrical stimulation. It is generally considered that release from presynaptic terminals is calcium dependent (Rubin, 1970) and this fact is often used to differentiate between specific release of neurotransmitters and nonspecific release from other metabolic pools. While it remains to be determined if the in vitro studies accurately reflect in vivo mechanisms, most putative neurotransmitters in the central nervous system are released under these conditions.

Ideally, to demonstrate that a putative transmitter and the natural transmitter have identical pharmacological and physiological actions, an intracellular recording electrode and a means of applying the putative transmitter (or some other drug such as an antagonist) equally to all of the receptors and only those receptors, activated by a given input, are needed. Intracellular recording is a difficult task on its own in many regions of the central nervous system. Additionally, within this vast matrix of neurons and glia, the requisite precision application of drugs and putative transmitters is not yet technically possible. A workable compromise is microiontophoresis. This technique involves the application of discrete quantities of putative transmitters and other drugs in a localized region around a neuron with simultaneous monitoring of changes in the neuron's activity. With microiontophoresis it is possible to define the pharmacological sensitivity of the neuron, and the sensitivity of physiologically defined synaptic inputs as well.

THE AUDITORY NERVE

Introduction

Morphologically, the cell bodies of the auditory nerve, the spiral ganglion cells, can be divided into two groups: Type I cells, which make up 90–95% of the total, and Type II cells, which make up the remaining 5–10% (Spoendlin, 1971; 1975, 1979a, 1981). The most common characteristics of Type II cells in all species are their smaller size and lighter, more filamentous cytoplasm with fewer ribosomes or Nissl substance. Type II cells frequently, but not always, lack a myelin sheath (Spoendlin, 1981). Present evidence suggests that the two types of ganglion cells differ in their innervation patterns of the organ of Corti (Kiang, Rho, Northrup, Liberman, & Ryugo, 1982; Morrison, Schindler, & Wersall, 1975; Spoendlin, 1971, 1975, 1979a,b; 1981). The evidence indicates that Type I cells innervate inner hair cells and Type II cells innervate outer hair cells. The fact that Type II cells apparently do not degenerate after section of the auditory nerve has prompted suggestions that these cells do not extend past the cochlea (Spoendlin, 1981). However, recent studies using tracing techniques suggest that these cells project at least to the cochlear nucleus (Jones, Oliver, Potashner, & Morest, 1982; Ruggero & Santi, 1981). And, studies have shown that destruction of outer hair cells does lead to degeneration in the cochlear nucleus (Webster & Webster, 1978).

The cochlear nucleus receives the terminals of the auditory nerve. The nucleus has been broken down morphologically into parcels in many ways by investigators, but there is agreement that in mammals there are three general divisions: the anteroventral (AVCN), posteroventral (PVCN), and dorsal (DCN) cochlear nuclei (Merzenich, 1970; Merzenich, Kitzes, & Aitkin, 1973). The auditory nerve bifurcates in the interstitial region separating the AVCN and PVCN (Ramon y Cajal, 1909). Most of the auditory nerve fibers terminate on the neurons of these two regions, but some continue posterior and dorsal to end in the DCN.

Each of the three divisions of the nucleus has been further divided on the basis of internal variations observed with Nissl, Protargol, and Golgi preparations (Brawer, Morest, & Kane, 1974; Harrison & Irving, 1965, 1966; Harrison & Warr, 1962; Lorente de Nó, 1933; Martin, 1981a; Moore & Osen, 1979; Osen, 1969). In particular the DCN is covered by a superficial molecular layer, and has an underlying pyramidal or fusiform layer and a deep region. The auditory nerve fibers of the DCN terminate within the deep region. There is a number of cell types within the ventral nucleus. Globular cells are concentrated in the caudal pole of the PVCN and in the rostral pole of the AVCN are the spherical cells, or bushy cells as they appear in Golgi preparations. The calyceal end-bulbs of bulbs of Held form the terminals of the auditory nerve on this latter cell type. Between the rostral and caudal pole, there is a variety of cell types including small, multipolar, giant, and granule cells. The organization of these neurons within the nucleus and their innervation by auditory nerve and central afferents are discussed elsewhere in this book (Cant & Morest, chapter 11).

The auditory nerve has been extensively studied with respect to the biochemistry and pharmacology of its neurotransmitter. Glutamate and aspartate are at present the best candidates for the auditory nerve neurotransmitter. Evidence supporting this falls into four areas: presence of glutamate and aspartate in terminals of the auditory nerve, presence of enzymes capable of catalyzing the synthesis of these amino acids in these terminals, release of glutamate and aspartate from auditory nerve terminals, and pharmacological similarity of the auditory nerve neurotransmitter to glutamate and aspartate. There are considerable data tentatively ruling out most other putative neurotransmitters, including acetylcholine (Fex & Wenthold, 1976; Godfrey, Williams, & Matschinsky, 1977b; Godfrey & Matschinsky, 1981a; Osen & Roth, 1969; Rasmussen, 1967; Wenthold & Gulley, 1978), GABA (Fex & Wenthold, 1976; Fisher & Davies, 1976; Godfrey et al., 1977a, 1978; Wenthold & Morest, 1976), catecholamines (Fex, Fuxe, & Lennerstrand, 1965; Fex & Wenthold, 1976; Fuxe, 1965; Kromer & Moore, 1980; Levitt & Moore, 1980; Swanson & Hartman, 1975), serotonin (Fuxe, 1965), glycine (Godfrey et al., 1978; Wenthold & Gulley, 1977), taurine (Wenthold & Gulley, 1977), enkephalin (Altschuler, 1979; Hökfelt, Elde, Johansson, Terenius, & Stein, 1977; Uhl et al., 1979a), substance P (Ljungdahl, Hökfelt, & Nilsson, 1978), somatostatin (Shiosaka et al., 1981; Tachibana, Rothman, & Guth, 1979), and neurotensin (Uhl et al., 1979b).

Biochemistry

The first suggestion that an amino acid may be the neurotransmitter of the auditory nerve came from Godfrey and associates (1977a), who measured the levels of glutamate, aspartate, GABA, and glycine in subdivisions of the cochlear nucleus and auditory nerve of the cat. They found that the distribution of aspartate somewhat followed that of auditory nerve terminals and fibers while the distribution of glutamate was more uniform. Similar distributions of these amino acids have been reported in rat and guinea pig cochlear nucleus (Godfrey et al., 1978; Wenthold, 1978). More direct evidence showing that glutamate and aspartate are concentrated in terminals and fibers of the auditory nerve was obtained by correlating the degeneration of auditory nerve fibers with the specific loss of these amino acids in the cochlear nucleus (Wenthold & Gulley, 1977; Wenthold, 1978). After destruction of the auditory nerve by cochlear ablation or after spiral ganglion cell degeneration in the genetically deaf waltzing guinea pig, glutamate and aspartate decreased in a way paralleling the loss of auditory nerve input. Although the percent decrease was greater for aspartate, reflecting the lower levels of aspartate compared to glutamate in the cochlear nucleus, absolute changes, expressed in nanomoles, were the same for both amino acids.

Although suggestive, these results did not conclusively demonstrate that the pool of glutamate and aspartate lost from the cochlear nucleus originated from terminals of the auditory nerve. It is conceivable that the decrease in the amino acid could be secondary to the loss of auditory nerve terminals and caused by major metabolic changes in areas of the cochlear nucleus. This can be addressed by directly visualizing the substance in the presynaptic terminal as has been done for the monoamines. Terminals containing a specific neurotransmitter have also been identified by localizing an enzyme involved in the metabolism of that substance as for acetylcholine and GABA. Although no enzyme was known to be specifically associated with the neurotransmitters glutamate and aspartate, results showed that aspartate aminotransferase and glutaminase were enriched in the auditory nerve (Wenthold, 1980). Production of antibodies to these enzymes and subsequent immunocytochemical localization shows they are concentrated in auditory nerve fibers and terminals as well as in spiral ganglion cell bodies (Altschuler et al., 1981; Fex, Altschuler, Wenthold, & Parakkal, 1982). Nonprimary terminals did not contain these enzymes, suggesting that the presence of aspartate aminotransferase and glutaminase may serve as a marker for synapses releasing glutamate and aspartate. Subsequent studies in other areas of the central nervous system have supported this hypothesis (Altschuler, Mosinger, Harmison, Parakkal, & Wenthold, 1982). The localization of aspartate aminotransferase and glutaminase in the terminals of the auditory nerve provides the first direct evidence of these terminals' capability to synthesize and metabolize glutamate and aspartate.

One of the most critical, and also most difficult, aspects of identifying a neurotransmitter for a population of neurons is to demonstrate the release of the substance from the presynaptic terminal after appropriate stimulation. Three laboratories have studied release of glutamate and aspartate from auditory nerve terminals. Wenthold (1979) studied the release of endogenous glutamate and aspartate from slices of the cochlear nucleus and found that the calcium-dependent release of these amino acids is selectively reduced by prior lesion of the auditory nerve. The release of glutamate was reduced by nerve lesion more than the release of aspartate. Similar results were obtained by measuring the release of radioactive glutamate after incubation of cochlear nucleus slices with labeled glutamate or aspartate (Canzek & Reubi, 1980). After labeling with radioactive glutamate and aspartate in vivo, Hansson, Karlstedt, & Sellstrom, (1980) reported that both amino acids were released from the cochlear nucleus with sound stimulation. However, it was not determined if the radioactivity was associated with the original compound at the time of release.

It has been shown that several putative neurotransmitters can each be taken up and concentrated in terminals from which they are released by a high-affinity process. Using labeled substances and autoradiography, synaptic terminals capable of taking up specific neurotransmitters have been identified. Although the technique has been useful for studying catecholamines and some amino acids, results with glutamate and aspartate have not been straightforward. In some cases, these amino acids may be taken up into nerve terminals, but in others they are found mostly in glial cells. These differences may be explained by regional variations in uptake or rapid metabolism of glutamate and aspartate. It has been suggested that the use of the D-isomer of glutamate or aspartate may circumvent the latter problem because they are not appreciably metabolized. Results show an uptake of D-aspartate into neurons purportedly using glutamate or aspartate as a neurotransmitter and also both retrograde and anterograde transport of label after uptake (Beaudet et al., 1981; Rustioni & Cuenod, 1982; Streit, 1980). This technique has been recently applied to the auditory nerve (Jones et al., 1982; Oliver, Jones, Potashner, & Morest, 1981). After injection of D-aspartate into the cochlear nucleus, spiral ganglion cell bodies and dendrites in the cochlea were labeled. In this study both types of spiral ganglion cells were labeled, suggesting that terminals of both cell types may release glutamate or aspartate.

Pharmacology

The N-methyl-D-aspartate, kainate, and quisqualate receptor types. Advances in our understanding of glutamate and aspartate in the mammalian central nervous system have come from research on the pharmacology of their receptors. In the early 1970s, research on the pharmacology of excitatory amino acids progressed along two parallel, yet interdependent avenues. Investigation along the first avenue examined structure–activity relationships with a view towards defining the structural requirements of the postsynaptic receptor. A series of analogs of glutamate and aspartate with agonist properties has been described, including N-methyl-D-aspartate (NMDA; Curtis & Watkins, 1963), kainic acid (KA; Johnston, Curtis, Davies, & McCullock, 1974), and quisqualate (QA; Biscoe, Evans, Headley, Martin, & Watkins, 1975). At the same time a number of possible excitatory amino acid antagonists were being reported, including glutamate diethylester (GDEE; Haldeman, Huffman, Marshall, & McLennan, 1972; Haldeman & McLennan, 1972), HA-966 (Davies & Watkins, 1973), and Mg^{+2} in low concentrations (Davies & Watkins, 1977). Each of these antagonists depressed glutamate- and aspartate-evoked responses. However, acetycholine (ACH)-evoked responses were also affected, suggesting that the specificity of these antagonists for excitatory amino acid receptors is low.

Following the suggestion of Hall, McLennan, and Wheal (1977) that D-α-aminoadipate (DAA), an amino acid containing one more carbon group than glutamate, might be an antagonist, Biscoe and associates (1977) demonstrated that DAA abolished responses evoked by NMDA, reduced aspartate-evoked more than glutamate-evoked responses, and had no effect on KA-evoked responses. Moreover, DAA did not affect ACH-evoked responses. In addition, DAA greatly reduced the dorsal root evoked excitation of Renshaw cells without affecting the ventral root excitation. For the first time, there was clear pharmacological evidence that a physiologically identified synapse used an excitatory amino acid as a transmitter.

Since the actions of DAA were initially described, a number of other compounds related to glutamate and aspartate have been shown to possess antagonist properties (for review of the literature, see McLennan, 1981; Watkins, 1981a,b). To summarize, three receptor types are currently recognized and named according to the agonist which preferentially interacts with each. The first is the NMDA receptor type. The NMDA receptor is particularly sensitive to the antagonists DAA, HA-966, Mg^{+2}, 2-amino-5-phosphonovalerate and γ-D-glutamylglycine. The QA receptor, on the other hand, is blocked by GDEE. KA preferentially activates the third receptor type. Unlike the other NMDA receptor antagonists mentioned, γ-D-glutamylglycine also depresses KA-evoked responses. And finally, cis-2,3-piperidine dicarboxylate reduces responses evoked by all three agonists; NMDA, QA, and KA.

While certain antagonists show preferential depression of responses evoked by either glutamate or aspartate (e.g., DAA reduces aspartate more than glutamate and GDEE reduces glutamate more than aspartate-evoked responses), all of the antagonists mentioned depress responses to both of these amino acids to some degree. Two conclusions can be drawn from this. First, glutamate and aspartate act as "universal" agonists capable of interacting with all three receptor types. The fact that aspartate-evoked responses are more sensitive to DAA might suggest that aspartate preferentially interacts with the NMDA receptor type. The same is true for glutamate and the QA receptor. Secondly, there is no evidence for receptors that are specific for either aspartate or glutamate. For instance, the notion that KA interacts with glutamate receptors is incorrect. Aspartate and glutamate may interact with KA receptors, for example, but not all receptors that respond to aspartate and glutamate interact with KA.

The pharmacology of auditory nerve transmission. Although a large body of information exists concerning excitatory amino acids in the CNS, there are relatively few reports describing their action in the cochlear nucleus and their possible auditory nerve transmitter function. Whitfield and Comis (1966) were the first to report the excitatory effects of locally applied glutamate on cochlear nucleus neurons responsive to tone stimuli. The precise locations of the units were not indicated. The units initially showed a lowering of threshold to tone stimuli, accompanied by an increase in the spontaneous firing of the unit.

Martin and Adams (1979) gave the first detailed description of the response of cochlear nucleus neurons to excitatory amino acids and the antagonist DL-α-aminoadipate (DLAA), the racemic mixture of α-aminoadipate. Recordings were confined to the AVCN. Two categories of units could be recognized physiologically: prepotential and nonprepotential. In the AVCN prepotential units show a characteristic waveform associated with unit action potentials (Bourk, 1976; Pfeiffer, 1966). Preceding each action potential by approximately 0.5 ms is a "prepotential" that has been shown to be presynaptic. These prepotential waveforms are associated with cells that receive large calyceal endings on their somata, the large spherical or bushy cells of the anterior AVCN with their tightly compacted dendritic tree (Brawer & Morest, 1975; Tolbert & Morest, 1978). This indicates that units which have prepotentials correspond to cells with auditory nerve terminals concentrated on their somata. The remaining cells of the AVCN have long branching dendrites (Brawer and Morest, 1975; Tolbert & Morest, 1978). Units with auditory nerve terminals scattered along these long dendrites then correspond to nonprepotential units.

Prepotential and nonprepotential units respond differently to excitatory amino acids (Martin & Adams, 1979). Nonprepotential units behave like most other neurons in the CNS; they are readily excited by glutamate, aspartate, NMDA, and KA. Prepotential units, on the other hand, are rarely excited. Usually, they do not respond at all or they appear to become overdepolarized and their firing rate decreases. Spinal motoneurons show a similar response (Zieglgansberger & Puil, 1973). The mechanism of depolarization block is not fully understood, but is believed to result from an abnormally large increase in the conductance of the soma membrane in a localized area which leads to shunting and sodium inactivation.

In studying DLAA, the specificity of the antagonist was determined against a series of excitatory compounds, including glutamate, aspartate, NMDA, KA, and (ACh) on nonprepotential units. DLAA was shown to block NMDA, reduce aspartate more than glutamate, and to have no effect on KA- or ACh-evoked responses. The effects of DLAA on tone-evoked excitation was then tested. On prepotential units, DLAA was a potent antagonist. On nonprepotential units, however, DLAA had very little effect. This apparent discrepancy was probably due to the low stimulus intensities used for nonprepotential units, as will be discussed below.

In a follow-up study, Martin (1980) reported the effects of a series of antagonists, including DAA, HA-966, Mg^{+2}, and GDEE, on excitatory amino acid- and tone-evoked excitations of AVCN units. Once again DAA, HA-966, and MG^{+2} proved to be effective antagonists of NMDA, and reduced aspartate- more than glutamate-evoked responses on nonprepotential units. In contrast, GDEE had no effect on NMDA-evoked responses and reduced response to glutamate more than to aspartate. DAA, HA-966, and Mg^{+2} consistently reduced tone-evoked responses of both nonprepotential and prepotential units. GDEE had no effect. Stimulus intensities used for nonprepotential units were 20 and 30 dB above threshold compared to 0 to 20 dB for the earlier study (Martin & Adams, 1979).

The earlier study (Martin & Adams, 1979) suggested that DLAA was not effective against tone-evoked excitation of nonprepotential units because many of the auditory nerve terminals along the long branching dendrites would be located some distance from the site of application of the antagonist near the somata. This view is strengthened by Martin (1980); by increasing the stimulus intensity there is an increased probability of auditory nerve terminals being active near the recording electrode.

The facts that AVCN units respond to KA (Martin & Adams, 1979), that GDEE reduced glutamate more than aspartate (and has no effect on NMDA-evoked responses), and that DAA (and DLAA, HA-966, and Mg^{+2}) blocks NMDA-evoked responses (Martin, 1980), suggest that all three of the currently known excitatory amino acid receptor types – KA, QA, and NMDA – are present on AVCN units. The fact that NMDA receptor antagonists block tone-evoked excitations indicates that the NMDA receptor is probably the postsynaptic receptor at the auditory nerve–cochlear nucleus synapse.

Caspary, Havey, and Faingold (1981) have reported data from the PVCN corroborating the findings of Martin and Adams (1979) and Martin (1980). PVCN units responded to microiontophoretic applications of glutamate, aspartate, and NMDA. DLAA effectively reduced responses to the excitatory amino acids as well as tone-evoked excitation. Also, in the in vitro mouse cochlear nucleus slice preparation, DAA blocked the excitatory actions of NMDA on AVCN units (Martin, 1983).

In addition to the studies on single units, pharmacological manipulations of audiogenic seizures and the brainstem auditory evoked potential (BAEP) also indicate that an excitatory amino acid is the transmitter of the auditory nerve. 2-Amino-7-phosphonoheptanoic acid, a potent amino acid antagonist whose specificity of action is similar to that of DAA, is an effective anticonvulsant for audiogenic seizures in mice (Croucher, Collins, & Meldrum, 1982). Baclofen, an antispastic drug which occasionally produces auditory side effects (Ashby & White, 1973; Pedersen, Arlien-Soberg, Grynderup, & Hendriksen, 1970), is believed to block the release of excitatory amino acid neurotransmitters from presynaptic terminals (Curtis, Lodge, Bornstein, & Peet, 1981; Davies, 1981; Potashner, 1978). Peak 1 of the BAEP is associated with the auditory nerve compound action potential and Peak 2, the field potential arising from the cochlear nucleus (Achor & Starr, 1980; Buchwald & Huang, 1975). Intravenous baclofen (2–3 mg/kg, cat) has no effect on Peak 1 but strongly suppresssed Peak 2 and subsequent peaks, indicating that release of an excitatory amino acid neurotransmitter from the auditory nerve terminal has been blocked (Martin, 1982). This provides evidence for the site and mechanism of anticonvulsant action of baclofen on audiogenic seizures in mice (Meldrum, Pedley, Horten, Anlezark, & Franks, 1980).

Summary

At present, we must entertain the possibility that both glutamate and aspartate are neurotransmitters of the auditory nerve, bearing in mind that it could also be either amino acid or some unidentified substance metabolically and pharmacologically related to glutamate and aspartate. With the present data, we can construct a model of the auditory nerve synapse (Figure 10-1), in which glutamate, aspartate, or both could be the neurotransmitter. In this model, glutamine from excellular fluid is the major precursor of glutamate, although both glutamate and aspartate can be taken up directly into the presynaptic terminal to a limited extent. Inside the terminal, glutamine is rapidly converted to glutamate, consistent with a small presynaptic pool of glutamine. To produce aspartate, it is necessary to go through the citric acid cycle and finally oxaloacetate is converted to aspartate by aspartate aminotransferase (ATT). Therefore, if aspartate is the neurotransmitter, the high levels of AAT and glutaminase in the presynaptic terminal can be explained since both enzymes would be necessary to produce aspartate from glutamine. On the other hand, if glutamate is the neurotransmitter, it could be synthesized from both glutamine and α-ketoglutarate, with AAT catalyzing the production of glutamate from α-ketoglutarate, since glutamate dehydrogenase is not enriched in auditory nerve terminals. Alternatively, most glutamate could be synthesized from glutamine and AAT would provide a sensitive mechanism for regulating the amount of glutamate within the terminal. This model may also serve if both glutamate and aspartate are neurotransmitters released from the same terminal.

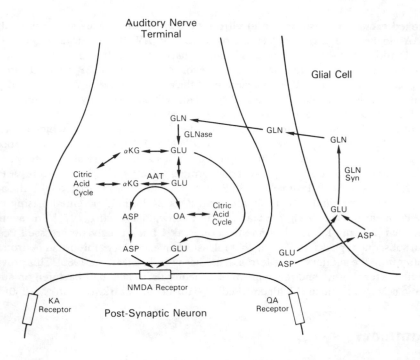

Figure 10-1. Model of the auditory nerve synapse. Glutamine from the extracellular fluid is the major precursor of glutamate. Inside the terminal, either glutamate or aspartate can be produced for release as a neurotransmitter. The postsynaptic neuron contains three different excitatory amino acid receptors of which only the NMDA receptor forms the postsynaptic element of the auditory nerve–cochlear nucleus neuron synapse. Abbreviations: AAT, aspartate aminotransferase; GLNase, glutaminase; GLN syn, glutamine synthetase; ASP, aspartic acid; GLU, glutamic acid; GLN, glutamine; αKG, α-ketoglutarate; OA, oxaloacetate; KA, kainic acid; NMDA, N-methyl-D-aspartate; QA, quisqualic acid.

The released aspartate or glutamate produces an excitatory response in the post-synaptic neuron. Three amino acid receptors exist on the postsynaptic neuron; the NMDA, KA, and QA receptors. Of these, the NMDA receptor, which is sensitive to both glutamate and aspartate, forms the postsynaptic element of the auditory nerve–cochlear nucleus neuron synapse. The remaining two receptor types are not associated with this receptor. Their functional significance is not known; they may be extrasynaptic receptors or receptors associated with other synaptic inputs. As in other systems, the major route of inactivation of glutamate and aspartate appears to be uptake into glial cells. Glia are enriched in glutamine synthetase (Norenberg & Martinez-Hernandez, 1979) and contain aspartate aminotransferase (Altschuler et al., 1981) to allow the synthesis of glutamine from glutamate and aspartate.

Several major questions remain concerning the auditory nerve neurotransmitter and excitatory amino acid neurotransmitters in general. Is glutamate or aspartate the auditory nerve transmitter? Do the two populations of spiral ganglion cells utilize different neurotransmitters at their terminals? What is the molecular basis for the different populations of receptors? Do these different receptors normally interact with different neurotransmitters? What are the ionic components and reversal potentials for the auditory nerve transmitter-evoked response? And how is the transmitter inactivated in vivo and recycled to the presynaptic element? Although the auditory nerve–cochlear nucleus synapse may be one of the best-documented examples of an excitatory amino acid synapse known today, we still have much to learn.

OTHER COCHLEAR NUCLEUS NEUROTRANSMITTERS

Acetylcholine

Biochemical assays for choline acetyltransferase and acetylcholinesterase (AChE), enzymes associated with the metabolism of acetylcholine, have found both enzymes to be distributed throughout the cochlear nucleus of the cat (Godfrey et al., 1977b), guinea pig (Wenthold & Morest, 1976), and rat (Godfrey et al., 1981a). In all cases the auditory nerve root contained the least of either enzyme. Godfrey and Associates (1977b, 1981a) have found several differences in the distributions of the two enzymes between cat and rat. Both enzymes had a more uniform distribution in the rat cochlear nucleus and the high level of both enzymes found in the cat granule cell regions were not found in corresponding regions of the rat nucleus. In the rat, generally high values of both enzymes were found throughout the ventral cochlear nucleus. In a recent study in which virtually all central inputs to the cochlear nucleus were cut, almost all the choline acetyltransferase activity in the cochlear nucleus was eliminated (Godfrey et al., 1981b). Most remaining activity was in the granule cell region of the AVCN and this was attributed to interneurons.

The distribution of AChE-positive fibers in the cochlear nucleus has been described for the cat (McDonald & Rasmussen, 1971; Osen & Roth, 1969; Rasmussen, 1964, 1967), rat (Brown & Howlett, 1972), mouse (Martin, 1981b) and chinchilla (McDonald & Rasmussen, 1971; Rasmussen, 1967). The fibers are associated with the olivocochlear bundle and project to a number of regions within the nucleus. The two principal projections are to the granule cell layer covering the ventral cochlear nucleus and the interstitial region of the AVCN. A few fibers enter the deep DCN and terminate in the granule cell layer. There is a large projection to all areas of the PVCN but a differential distribution within the AVCN. Although there is a major AChE-positive projection to the caudal two-thirds of the AVCN, the projection to the rostral third is strictly limited to the granule cell layer and the most medial edge of the nucleus. AChE-positive fibers only very rarely enter the spherical cell region proper. In contrast, in the most rostral pole of the cat AVCN, there are numerous AChE-positive fibers (Adams, 1982; Adams, personal communication). This highlights the known anatomical differences between the cat and mouse and is consistent with the absence of large spherical cells in the rostral pole of the mouse AVCN (Martin, 1981a).

Two classes of ACh receptors are recognized in the CNS based on their sensitivity to cholinomimetics and antagonists, nicotinic and muscarinic (for review see Krnjević, 1974). Both receptor types appear to be present on cholinoceptive neurons with Renshaw cells being predominantly nicotinic and cerebral cortical neurons muscarinic. Nicotinic responses are typically rapid in onset and offset and are sensitive to the antagonist dihydro-β-erythroidine. Muscarinic receptor responses, which are antagonized by atropine, are more gradual in both onset and offset.

Many cochlear nucleus units respond to locally applied ACh in a manner typical of excitatory muscarinic receptors (Martin & Adams, 1979; Whitfield & Comis, 1966). As mentioned above, the prepotential units of the AVCN are typically noncholinoceptive (Martin & Adams, 1979). The response of cholinoceptive units to ACh is gradual both in onset and offset. However, the sensitivity of ACh-evoked response to atropine and dihydro-β-erythroidine have not been tested. Cholinoceptive cochlear nucleus neurons are more sensitive to the muscarinic agonist acetyl-β-methylcholine than to nicotine, and physostigmine, an AChE inhibitor, increases spontaneous activity in low concentrations (Whitfield & Comis, 1966). High binding of α-bungarotoxin, a ligand for the peripheral nervous system nicotinic cholinergic receptor, has been demonstrated in the cochlear nucleus, suggesting the presence of nicotinic receptors (Hunt & Schmidt, 1978). However, although α-bungarotoxin may be specific for the nicotinic receptor in electric organ and neuromuscular junction, this specificity has not been as rigorously established for the mammalian central nervous system. On the other hand, binding of labeled quinuclidynl benzilate, a muscarinic agonist, demonstrates high binding levels over the nucleus (Wamsley, Lewis, Young, & Kuhar, 1981).

It is of interest to note that while cholinomimetics increase the sensitivity of cholinoceptive cochlear nucleus neurons to sound stimulation, the antagonists atropine and, to a lesser degree, dihydro-β-erythroidine have the opposite effect, suggesting a tonic or acoustically evoked ACh-excitatory input (Whitfield & Comis, 1966). The input is unlikely to be tonic since transection of the auditory nerve abolishes virtually all spontaneous activity in the ventral cochlear nucleus (Koerber, Pfeiffer, Warr, & Kiang, 1966). Also, because there is no evidence to support an auditory nerve transmitter role for ACh, the origin of the cholinergic antagonist-sensitive acoustically evoked activity may be from a positive feedback system. The origin of such a system could be the superior olivary complex. Electrical stimulation of the medial aspect of the ipsilateral lateral superior olive produces an excitatory response from AVCN units that can be antagonized by locally applied atropine (Whitfield & Comis, 1966), and to a lesser extent, dihydro-β-erythroidine and gallamine (Comis & Whitfield, 1968). Hemicholinium, which inhibits the synthesis of acetylcholine, also blocks the excitatory effects of olivary stimulation (Comis, 1970). Also, ACh is released from the dorsal bundle (Comis & Guth, 1974).

Inhibitory Amino Acids

Studies of GABA in the subdivision of cat and rat cochlear nucleus showed a 40-fold range in concentrations with highest levels in the dorsal cochlear nucleus and lowest in the auditory nerve root (Godfrey et al., 1977a; 1978). Intermediate levels were found in the AVCN and PVCN. Distributions of glutamate decarboxylase (GAD; Wenthold & Morest, 1976) and GABA-transaminase (GABA-T; Davies, 1975) generally follow the distribution of GABA in the cochlear nucleus. Shortly after cochlear abla-tion, GAD is slightly decreased in the cochlear nucleus, but later returns to normal or slightly above normal levels (Fisher & Davies, 1976). These results and the distribu-tion studies rule out an association of auditory nerve fibers with most cochlear nucleus GABA. The fact that GAD levels are affected by cochlear ablation suggests that changes take place in GABA neurons after loss of primary innervation. The identity of neurons containing GABA in the cochlear nucleus is not known. Lesions of the trapezoid body did not cause a decrease in GAD in the cochlear nucleus (Fisher & Davies, 1976). Lesioning the dorsal acoustic stria leads to a decrease of about 30% of the cochlear nucleus GAD (Davies, 1977). Results of uptake and autoradiographic studies have led Schwartz (1981) to suggest that GABA may be associated with granule cell axons, the parallel fibers. GABA-T has been shown to be associated with fusiform cells using histochemical methods (Davies, 1975).

Like GABA, glycine also shows a marked regional distribution in the cochlear nucleus (Godfrey et al., 1977a, 1978). Highest levels in the cat are in the deep and fusiform cell layers of the DCN and the lowest levels are in the auditory nerve root. Glycine levels in the cochlear nucleus are similar to those found in the spinal cord gray matter where there is considerable evidence that glycine is a neurotransmitter. Godfrey and colleagues (1977a) have suggested that glycine may be associated with small cells scattered throughout the cochlear nucleus, many of which appear to be interneurons. Schwartz (1981) found uptake of glycine into synaptic boutons in all layers of the DCN, with some terminals being on fusiform cells. Tritiated strychnine binding has localized glycine-like receptors by autoradiography to the dorsal cochlear nucleus in the rat (Zarbin, Wamsley, & Kuhar, 1981). Binding in the ventral cochlear nucleus is very low.

Bicuculline is an antagonist of GABA-like compounds and strychnine an antago-nist of glycine-like compounds (Curtis & Johnson, 1974). Pharmacologically, there appear to be two differentially distributed bicuculline-sensitive receptors in the mam-malian CNS, suggesting two types of GABA receptors. In cortical regions GABA-, muscimol-, taurine-, and β-alanine-evoked responses are bicuculline-sensitive (Curtis, Duggan, Felix, Johnston, & McLennan, 1971; Curtis & Tebecis, 1972; Krnjević & Puil, 1976). In the spinal cord only GABA and muscimol are bicuculline sensitive (Curtis, Hösli, & Johnston, 1968; Curtis et al., 1971). Strychnine-sensitive receptors are typi-cally confined to spinal cord and brainstem (Bruggencate & Sonnhof, 1971; Curtis et al., 1968; Curtis et al., 1971; Denavit-Saubie & Champagnat, 1975; Haas & Hösli, 1973; Hösli & Tebecis, 1970). Within these regions glycine-, taurine- and β-alanine-evoked responses are strychnine sensitive.

Whitfield and Comis (1966) first reported that cochlear nucleus neurons were readily depressed by local application of GABA; an observation confirmed by Caspary and colleagues (1979) and Martin and colleagues (1982). Caspary and associates (1979) also reported that this depression was strychnine insensitive. Martin and co-workers (1982) have conducted a more detailed study of agonist–receptor interactions on AVCN units. GABA- and muscimol-evoked responses are bicuculline sensitive, strychnine insensitive. Conversely, glycine-, taurine-, and β-alanine-evoked responses are strychnine sensitive and bicuculline insensitive. Thus, there are at least two inhibitory amino acid receptor types in the cochlear nucleus, glycine-like and GABA-like, corresponding to those found on other brain stem and spinal cord neurons, but differing from those found in the cerebrum and cerebellum. The sensitivity of cochlear nucleus units to GABA-like agonists may account for their anticonvulsant action in audiogenic seizures (Meldrum et al., 1980).

It is well documented that strychnine, whether applied intravenously, topically, or by micropressure or microiontophoresis, has no effect on electrically or ipsilateral tone-evoked activity in the cochlear nucleus (Caspary et al., 1979; Martin et al, 1982; Pirsig, Pfalz, & Sandanaga, 1968; Watanabe, 1979; Whitfield & Allanson, 1958; Whitfield & Comis, 1966). Bicuculline and picrotoxin (a GABA antagonist less specific than bicuculline) also have no effect on tone-evoked activity in the cochlear nucleus (Martin et al., 1982, Watabane, 1971). Thus GABA and glycine are unlikely to be involved in the generation of cochlear nucleus unit responses to tones at characteristic frequencies.

The suppression of a cochlear nucleus unit's response to a tone at its characteristic frequency by a second superimposed tone at a higher or lower frequency is generally referred to as two-tone interaction. The unit's response pattern most likely results from a nonsynaptic biophysical property of the basilar membrane in the cochlea (c.f. Hall, 1980; Sachs & Abbas, 1976). Nonetheless, Watanabe (1971) has reported that iontophoretically applied picrotoxin reduces the two-tone interaction response of cochlear nucleus units. This is contrary to the earlier report by Whitfield & Comis (1966). In agreement with Whitfield & Comis (1966), bicuculline, given intravenously, or by micropressure or microiontophoresis, has no effect on the two-tone interaction response (Comis, personal communication; Martin et al., 1982). The singular report by Watanabe (1971) may be due to picrotoxin's poor specificity as a GABA antagonist (Curtis & Johnston, 1974; Hill, Simmonds, & Straughan, 1976; Krnjević, 1974). It must be noted that the iontophoretic dose of picrotoxin used by Watanabe (1971) was excessively large and prolonged, and that its specificity of action against a series of agonists was never tested. Strychnine also appears to have no effect on the two-tone interaction response (Martin et al., 1982; Watanabe, 1979; Whitfield & Allanson, 1958; Whitfield & Comis, 1966).

Stimulation of the lateral part of the lateral superior olive inhibits neurons in the ipsilateral dorsal and ventral cochlear nuclei (Comis, 1970). Locally applied strychnine has no effect on this inhibition (Comis, 1970). Unfortunately, the effects of GABA antagonists on this inhibition have not been reported.

Amongst the numerous negative reports on the effect of inhibitory amino acid antagonists is one possible positive note. Pirsig and associates (1968) electrically stimulated the cochlea; the resulting field potential in the ventral cochlear nucleus was depressed by a 1,000-Hz tone applied to the contralateral ear. Intravenous strychnine readily blocked the tone-evoked depression. Unfortunately, neither the mechanism of the depression nor the site of action of the strychnine can be deduced from this study. The antagonism of the depression may have occurred on the ventral cochlear nucleus neurons. There is an alternative explanation. As suggested by Comis (1973), Pickles and Comis (1973), and Pickles (1976a), axons from neurons in the lateral superior olive terminate on cochlear nucleus neurons, possibly forming a positive feedback loop to enhance signals. Neurons of the lateral superior olive are inhibited by tones presented to the contralateral ear through a strychnine-sensitive glycinergic input (Moore, Caspary, & Havey, 1981). Thus, the intravenous strychnine given by Pirsig and associates (1968) may have blocked the inhibition of lateral superior olive neurons, resulting in the increased amplitude of ventral nucleus field potential as a result of the positive feedback loop. This ambiguity should serve as an example of the necessity to study the pharmacological properties of synaptic inputs as close to the cellular level as possible. Nevertheless, these results are of interest and further research is warranted.

Catecholamines and Serotonin

Catecholamine-containing fibers innervating the cochlear nucleus have been studied in some detail. Based on the relative levels of norepinephrine and dopamine present in the cochlear nucleus, it is suggested that norepinephrine is likely to be the neurotransmitter of these fibers (Kromer & Moore, 1976). Lesion studies show that most of these fibers originate in the locus coeruleus and innervate the cochlear nucleus bilaterally via two pathways, the rostral coeruleocochlear bundle and the caudal coeruleocochlear bundle (Kromer & Moore, 1980; Levitt & Moore, 1980). All subdivisions of the cochlear nucleus receive catecholamine-containing fibers based on dopamine-β-hydroxylase localization and the Falck–Hillarp histochemical method of catecholamine localization, with densest projections to the anteroventral cochlear nucleus and posteroventral cochlear nucleus (Kromer & Moore, 1980; Swanson & Hartman, 1975). Heaviest innervation in dorsal cochlear nucleus is in the deep layers. The catecholamine-containing fibers appear to terminate on most neuronal cell types in the cochlear nucleus.

Classically, there are two types of noradrenergic receptors, the α and β types, which can be differentiated by the sensitivity to various agonists and antagonists (Krnjević, 1974). Propranolol is a β-blocker and phentolamine an α-blocker. Intravenous injections of these compounds affect local glucose utilization. The depressant effects of propranolol may be due to its membrane-stabilizing properties since the more specific β-blocker, sotalol, does not affect glucose utilization in the cochlear nucleus. The increase in local glucose utilization might therefore indicate blockade of an inhibitory α-noradrenergic pathway with increased neuronal activity as the end result.

Locally applied norepinephrine and, to a lesser extent, adrenaline depress spontaneous and acoustically evoked activity in the cochlear nucleus (Whitfield & Comis,
1966). Norepinephrine, topically applied through an indwelling cannula, impairs the
ability of freely behaving cats to distinguish signals in noise and produces large shifts
in the auditory threshold (Pickles, 1976b). Stimulation of the locus coeruleus depresses
auditory nerve-evoked activity in the dorsal cochlear nucleus (Chikamori, Sasa, Fujimoto, Takaori, & Matsuoka, 1980; Matsuoka, Chikamori, Sasa, & Takaori, 1978). In
reserpine-treated animals, locus coeruleus stimulation does not affect dorsal cochlear
nucleus activity (Chikamori et al., 1980). Reserpine also affects brainstem auditory
evoked potentials (Bhargava & McKean, 1977). Peak 2, and to a lesser extent, Peak
3, are generated by potentials in the cochlear nucleus (Achor & Starr, 1980). Peak
2 is unaffected by reserpine treatment, but Peak 3 is greatly enhanced.

Fluorescence studies suggest the presence of serotonin in the dorsal cochlear
nucleus (Fuxe, 1965). Whitfield and Comis (1966) reported that some neurons in the
nucleus could be excited by local application of serotonin. However, neither the origin
of the serotonin-positive fibers nor the position of the serotonin-sensitive cochlear
nucleus units is known. Injections of p-chlorophenylalanine, which depletes serotonin
in neurons in the brain, and 5-hydroxytryptophan, a serotonin precursor, affect brainstem auditory evoked potentials (Bhargava & McKean, 1977). As mentioned above,
Peak 2, and to a lesser extent, Peak 3 are generated by the cochlear nucleus.
p-Chlorophenylalanine increases and 5-hydroxytryptophan decreases Peak 4, but
neither has an effect on Peak 2. The studies by Whitfield and Comis (1966) suggest
that serotonin may play a role as an excitatory transmitter in the dorsal cochlear
nucleus, but the studies by Bhargava and McKean (1977) indicate that serotonin may
actually decrease auditory evoked activity. Clearly, further studies on single-unit activity are required to resolve this issue.

Neuroactive Peptides

A number of peptides with possible neurotransmitter or neuromodulator roles have
been reported in the cochlear nucleus. Enkephalin-containing cells and fibers are present
in the cochlear nucleus with cells concentrated in the deeper layers of the dorsal cochlear
nucleus (Altschuler, 1979; Hökfelt et al., 1977; Uhl et al., 1979a). Receptors for opiates
have also been reported in the dorsal cochlear nucleus (Herkenham & Pert, 1980). Substance P-containing (Ljungdahl et al., 1978) and neurotensin-containing (Uhl, Goodman,
& Snyder, 1979b) cells and fibers have also been localized in the cochlear nucleus by
immunocytochemistry. Somatostatin has been shown to be present in the cochlear
nucleus by radioimmunoassay (Tachibana et al., 1979) and immunocytochemistry
(Shiosaka et al., 1981). In the rat cochlear nucleus, as in other places in the brainstem,
somatostatin is rather abundant in cells and fibers of the DCN and VCN of immature
animals, but these diminish as the animal matures, suggesting somatostatin may play
a role in development of the auditory system (Shiosaka et al., 1981).

In a microiontophoresis study, Caspary and associates (1981) were unable to
demonstrate any effect of substance P on a small sample of units. However, the

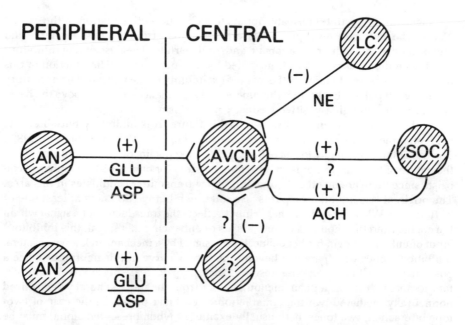

Figure 10-2. Hypothetical circuit diagram of four inputs to units in the caudal part of the antero-ventral cochlear nucleus (AVCN). These include two inputs of peripheral origin and two inputs of central origin. The inputs of peripheral origin consist of the excitatory (+) primary afferent input where either glutamate or aspartate may be the transmitter ($\frac{GLUT}{ASP}$), and an indirect lateral inhibitory (−) input of unknown origin (?) using an unidentified transmitter. The inputs of central origin are from the locus coeruleus (LC) and superior olivary complex (SOC). The inhibitory (−) LC input is mediated by norepinephrine (NE). The excitatory (+) cholinergic (ACH) input from the SOC is part of the a positive feedback loop.

location of these units within the cochlear nucleus was not reported. If the number of substance P-containing neurons is small, it may prove to be difficult to study their pharmacology.

Summary

Several possible neurotransmitters in the cochlear nucleus have been described. Of these, acetylcholine, and possibly serotonin, are excitatory and norepinephrine, GABA, and glycine inhibitory. It is difficult to discuss the functional significance of each input in a unifying way since a variety of methods have been used to identify these pathways and different types of neurons studied. However, one population of neurons in the caudal AVCN, many of which are cholinoceptive, seem to have been studied sufficiently to generate some speculation about the roles of the certain inputs.

Figure 10-2 illustrates probable inputs to a cholinoceptive neuron in the caudal AVCN. The neuron receives primary afferent terminals from the auditory nerve and the excitatory transmitter is glutamate and/or aspartate. The descending inhibitory input from the locus coeruleus is mediated by norepinephrine. The function of this pathway may be modulation of the level of excitability of the neuron. The excitatory cholinergic input, probably from the superior olive, enhances a signal above the background noise through a positive feedback mechanism.

A third centrifugal input is shown in this figure. It is inhibitory but all efforts to identify the nature of the transmitter have failed to date (Martin & Dickson, 1983). The transmitter is unlikely to be GABA, glycine, enkephalin, or norepinephrine. Thus the nature of this transmitter is an intriguing mystery for biochemists and pharmacologists since there are no other known inhibitory transmitter candidates in this area. The origin of this inhibitory input is also unknown but we do know at least one of its functions. While the auditory nerve input reflects the transduction of a signal within the cochlea and the cholinergic input assists in enhancing this signal, this inhibitory input of unknown origin further delineates the signal by a mechanism known as lateral inhibition. Tones which are just beyond the tuning curve of this neuron produce a postsynaptic inhibitory response, resulting in a sharp decrease in activity. It is important to note that this is a phenomenon distinct from the more generally recognized nonneurally mediated two-tone interaction of cochlear origin. In the case of two-tone interaction, two tones, both usually excitatory when presented alone, must be presented together to observe the phenomenon. In the case of lateral inhibition in the cochlear nucleus, only the single side band tone is presented, and this results in a neuronally mediated postsynaptic inhibitory response in neurons of this region.

Thus, it appears that there is a constant interplay of inputs to neurons in the caudal AVCN, shaping and modifying their activity. The same is certainly true of the other neurons within this nucleus. Efforts to identify neurotransmitter-specific inputs and understand their functional significance have only just begun. Clearly not only are such studies of importance in defining how signals are processed within central auditory structures, but predicting the functional consequences of clinical drug therapies.

OTHER AUDITORY NUCLEI

The Superior Olive

Cell bodies containing enkephalin and acetylcholinesterase have been described in the lateral superior olive and these may be the source of the cochlear efferents (Altschuler, Fex, & Parakkal, 1980). Choline acetyltransferase has also been reported to be enriched in the superior olive relative to elsewhere in the auditory system (Contreras & Bachelard, 1979). It is interesting to note that there is virtually no quinuclidynl benzilate binding in the superior olive (Wamsley et al., 1981). Only one brief note has been published on the pharmacology of units in the superior olive (Moore et al., 1981). Units excited by ipsilateral tones and inhibited by contralateral tones can be depressed by glycine and GABA. The glycine-evoked depressions are strychnine sensitive and bicuculline resistant. The opposite is true for GABA-evoked depressions. The inhibition produced by contralateral tones are strychnine sensitive and bicuculline resistant, strongly suggesting that the inhibition is mediated by a glycinergic pathway. Binding of [H^3]strychnine is high in this nucleus (Zarbin et al., 1981).

Inferior Colliculus

Amino acids. The inferior colliculus has been subdivided and levels of several neurotransmitters and neurotransmitter-related enzymes have been measured (Adams & Wenthold, 1979). All substances measured showed a nonuniform distribution with the distribution of glycine being the most striking. Lesions of inputs from the auditory cortex or cochlear nucleus failed to show consistent changes in any of the substances measured. Glutamate and aspartate excite and glycine and GABA depress virtually all collicular neurons (Curtis & Koizumi, 1961; Watanabe & Simada, 1973). Microiontophoretic application of the glycine antagonist strychnine has no effect on tone-evoked activity (Watanabe & Simada, 1973). Binding of [H^3]strychnine is low in the inferior colliculus (Zarbin et al., 1981). Picrotoxin, a compound which is a relatively nonspecific antagonist of GABA-evoked responses, reportedly causes a disinhibition of "on-type" collicular neuron responses, prompting Watanabe and Simada (1971, 1973) to suggest a GABAergic tone-evoked suppression of these units. Further studies with the GABA antagonist bicuculline will be needed to confirm these observations.

Acetylcholine. The inferior colliculus has been shown to have exceptionally high levels of nicotinic cholinergic receptor based on α-bungarotoxin binding and intermediate levels of muscarinic cholinergic receptor based on quinuclidynl benzilate binding (Kobayashi et al., 1978; Morley et al., 1977; Schechter, Handy, Peggemonte, & Schmidt, 1978; Wamsley et al., 1981). This appears inconsistent with the relatively low levels of choline acetyltransferase and acetylcholinesterase in the inferior colliculus measured biochemically (Adams & Wenthold, 1979; Ramon-Moliner, 1972). ACh produces excitatory effects with a gradual onset and offset typical of muscarinic responses on a number of collicular neurons (Curtis & Koizumi, 1961; Watanabe & Simada, 1973). Curtis and Koizumi (1961) tested a series of nicotinic antagonists including dihydro-β-erythroidine, D-tubocurarine, and gallamine and found all to be ineffective against ACh- and glutamate-evoked responses and synaptically evoked activity. Watanabe and Simada (1973) confirmed this observation on synaptically evoked activity with D-tubocurarine. Farley, Morley, Javel, and Gorda (1982) also found α-bungarotoxin to be ineffective but suggest that D-tubocurarine has an excitatory action. According to Watanabe and Simada (1970, 1973), dihydro-β-erythroidine reduced synaptic activity. Unfortunately, they did not test the specificity of the drug or control for current artifacts. Curtis and Koizumi (1961) observed that whenever dihydro-β-erythroidine reduced auditory evoked activity, it reduced both ACh- and glutamate-evoked responses equally, indicating a current artifact.

Watanabe and Simada (1973) also claimed that atropine readily blocked tone-evoked activity, but again did not test the specificity of the antagonists. Farley and colleagues (1982) suggest that atropine is excitatory. While it appears that ACh receptors in the inferior colliculus may be of the muscarinic type, a more detailed analysis of its role in synaptic transmission in this structure is needed. It is of interest to note that neostigmine, a cholinesterase inhibitor, prolongs ACh-evoked responses in the colliculus without influencing auditory evoked activity (Curtis & Koizumi, 1961).

Catecholamines and serotonin. Neither norepinephrine or serotonin have any effect when applied microiontophoretically to inferior colliculus units (Curtis & Koizumi, 1961; Watanabe & Simada, 1973). Monoamine fibers are present, however (Dahlstrom & Fuxe, 1964).

Medial Geniculate

Amino acids. There are scattered reports in the literature that cat medial geniculate units are excited by glutamate and DL-homocysteate (Tebecis, 1967; 1970a; b; c; Torda, 1978). Medial geniculate units are also depressed by GABA, β-alanine, and glycine (Tebecis, 1967; 1970a; 1973) with glycine-evoked responses being particularly sensitive to microiontophoretically applied strychnine (Tebecis, 1970a). There have not been any pharmacological studies aimed at defining the types of amino acid receptors present or their possible role in synaptic transmission.

Acetylcholine. Medial geniculate units have a mixture of cholinergic receptor types with the muscarinic type predominating (Tebecis, 1970b). The muscarinic agonists carbamylcholine and acetyl-β-methylcholine were more potent than nicotine. Atropine was more effective against ACh-evoked responses than the nicotinic antagonists dihydro-β-erythroidine and D-tubocurarine. The cholinesterase inhibitors physostigmine and neostigmine potentiated ACh-evoked responses. Approximately twice as many units were excited by ACh as were depressed (Tebecis, 1970b; Torda, 1979).

Many cat medial geniculate neurons can be activated by electrical stimulation of the auditory cortex, inferior colluculus, or reticular formation (Tebecis, 1970c). Atropine, but not dihydro-β-erythroidine or D-tubocurarine, blocked portions of the excitatory responses evoked from each of these regions, suggesting a mixture of muscarinic cholinergic and noncholinergic inputs.

Catecholamines and serotonin. The response of medial geniculate units to norepinephrine and serotonin are mixed, but predominantly they act as depressants (Tebecis, 1967; 1970a; 1973; Torda, 1978). Dopamine, however, is almost always a depressant on responsive units (Tebecis, 1970a; Torda, 1978). Studies with α- and β-antagonists, or other agents which modify monoamine transmission, on chemically or synaptically evoked medial geniculate unit responses have not been conducted.

Auditory Cortex

Very little is known about the specific pharmacology of auditory cortex units. Spontaneous and evoked activity are depressed by locally applied GABA and norepinephrine and potentiated by ACh (Foote, Freedman, & Oliver, 1975). There are no other pharmacological data relating to their possible role in synaptic transmission in the auditory cortex.

FINAL COMMENTS

A major objective of studying auditory system neurotransmitters is to provide information about the molecular organization of the auditory system that will eventually aid in the understanding of normal speech processing and the treatment of human hearing disorders. It is apparent that the general field of neuroscience also benefits from the biochemical and pharmacological dissection of auditory pathways. Visualization of specific molecules through immunocytochemistry and enzyme histochemistry has already provided new dimensions for neuroanatomy in the description of several neurotransmitter-specific pathways. Pharmacological manipulations of neuronal activity have enabled us to develop theories on how central auditory structures detect and enhance signals in noise. Although the use of the microiontophoretic techniques in neurophysiological studies is new, one of its most potentially powerful uses lies in this area. When neurotransmitters of more auditory pathways are known, it is expected that we will be better equipped to explain the neurophysiological response of central auditory neurons to acoustic stimuli.

Although in many hearing disorders affecting humans, the primary pathology is in the organ of Corti, the importance of understanding the molecular organization of the central auditory system is emphasized by recent developments in designing a cochlear prosthesis. (See chap. 9 by Miller & Pfingst.) Although such a device may circumvent faulty or missing hair cells, it does require that the auditory nerve and central auditory structures be functional. In genetic disorders this may not always be the case. For example, in the Reeler mutant mouse, the cholinergic input to the cochlear nucleus and the granule cells within this nucleus is severely affected (Martin, 1981a,b). This emphasizes the importance of understanding developmental and degenerative changes and the interaction of various pathways in signal processing.

The consideration of causes and treatments of tinnitus must also encompass the auditory nerve and central auditory system. The fact that tinnitus is frequently associated with hearing loss suggests that the disorder may be connected with the degeneration or abnormal regeneration of auditory neurons. Since hair cell loss leads to spiral ganglion cell degeneration, which can then cause transneuronal changes in other auditory neurons, damage to a hair cell can be manifested in the cochlear nucleus or higher auditory structures. It was recently shown that activity of cochlear nucleus neurons, as measured by the uptake of $[^{14}C]$deoxyglucose, decreases after cochlear ablation but later increases to near normal levels (Sasaki, Kauer, & Babitz, 1980). Although tinnitus is a symptom with many causes, these findings suggest that changes may occur in central auditory structures under conditions that can cause tinnitus in humans. A knowledge of the neuronal pathways involved and their pharmacology should provide a basis for the design of drugs for treatment.

Much more research directed at understanding synaptic transmission in the auditory system must be done. Certainly we have made progress but as we learn more about the auditory system, we also discover its complexities. Many of the newer biochemical techniques, developed over the past 12 years, including immunocytochemistry, monoclonal antibody production, and electrophoretic ways of analyzing complex protein mixtures, should allow us to extend our characterization of neurons of the auditory system to very sophisticated levels. We fully expect that our knowledge of the auditory system at the molecular level will increase dramatically over the next several years.

REFERENCES

Achor, L.J., & Starr, A. (1980). Auditory brainstem responses in the cat. I. Intracranial and extracranial recordings. *E.E.G. Clinical Neurophysiology 48*, 154–173.

Adams, J.C. (1982). Collaterals of labyrinthine efferent axons. *Neuroscience Abstracts, 8*, 149.

Adams, J.C., & Wenthold, R.J. (1979). Distribution of putative amino acid transmitters, choline acetyltransferase and glutamate decarboxylase in the inferior colliculus. *Neuroscience 4*, 1947–1951.

Altschuler, R.A. (1979). Met-enkephalin positivity in the small cells of the deep dorsal cochlear nucleus and posteroventral cochlear nucleus of the rat. *Neuroscience Abstracts, 5*, 15.

Altschuler, R.A., Fex, J., & Parakkal, M. (1980). Combined met-enkephalin-like immunoreactivity and acetylcholinesterase staining in neurons in the lateral superior olive of the guinea pig. *Neuroscience Abstracts, 6*, 617.

Altschuler, R.A., Mosinger, J.L., Harmison, G.G., Parakkal, M.H., & Wenthold, R.J. (1982). Aspartate aminotransferase-like immunoreactivity as a marker for aspartate/glutamate in guinea pig photoreceptors. *Nature (London), 298*, 657–659.

Altschuler, R.A., Neises, G.R., Harmison, G.G., Wenthold, R.J., & Fex, J. (1981). Immunocytochemical localization of aspartate aminotransferase immunoreactivity in cochlear nucleus of the guinea pig. *Proceedings of the National Academy of Sciences USA, 78*, 6553–6557.

Ashby, P., & White, D.G. (1973). "Presynaptic" inhibition in spasticity and the effect of beta (4-chlorophenyl) GABA. *Journal of Neurological Science, 20*, 329–338.

Beaudet, A., Burkhalter, A., Reubi, J.C., & Cuenod, M. (1981). Selective bidirectional transport of [^{3}H] D-aspartate in the pigeon retino-tectal pathway. *Neuroscience, 6*, 2021–2034.

Bhargava, V.K., & McKean, C.M. (1977). Role of 5-hydroxytryptamine in the modulation of acoustic brainstem (far-field) potentials. *Neuropharmacology, 16*, 447–449.

Biscoe, T.J., Evans, R.H., Francis, A.A., Martin, M.R., Watkins, J.C., Davies, J., & Dray, A. (1977). D-alpha-Aminoadipate as a selective antagonist of amino acid-induced and synaptic excitation of mammalian spinal neurones. *Nature (London), 270*, 743–745.

Biscoe, T.J., Evans, R.H., Headley, P.M., Martin, M., & Watkins, J.C. (1975). Domoic and quisqualic acids as potent amino acid excitants of frog and rat spinal neurons. *Nature (London), 255*, 166–167.

Bourk, T.R. (1976). *Electrical responses of neural units in the anteroventral cochlear nucleus of the cat*. PhD thesis. Boston: Massachusetts Institute of Technology.

Brawer, J.R., & Morest, D.K. (1975). Relations between auditory nerve endings and cell types in the cat's anteroventral cochlear nucleus seen with the Golgi method and Nomarski optics. *Journal of Comparative Neurology, 160*, 491–506.

Brawer, J.R., Morest, D.K., & Kane, E.C. (1974) The neuronal architecture of the cochlear nucleus of the cat. *Journal of Comparative Neurology, 155,* 251–300.

Brown, J.C., & Howlett, B. (1972). The olivo-cochlear tract in the rat and its bearing on the homologies of some consistent cell groups of the mammalian superior olivary complex: A thiocholine study. *Acta Anatomy, 83,* 505–526.

Bruggencate, G. Ten, & Sonnhof, U. (1971). Glycine and GABA actions in hypoglossus nucleus and blocking effects of strychnine and picrotoxin. *Experientia (Basel), 27,* 1109.

Buchwald, J.S., & Huang, C.M. (1975). Far-field acoustic response origins in the cat. *Science, 189,* 382–384.

Canzek, V., & Reubi, J.C. (1980). The effect of cochlear nerve lesion on the release of glutamate, aspartate and GABA from cat cochlear nucleus, *in vitro. Experimental Brain Research, 38,* 437–441.

Caspary, D.M., Havey, D.C., & Faingold, C.L. (1979). Effects of microiontophonetically applied glycine and GABA on neuronal response patterns in the cochlear nuclei. *Brain Research, 172,* 179–185.

Caspary, D.M., Havey, D.C., & Faingold, C.L. (1981). Glutamate and aspartate: Alteration of thresholds and response patterns of auditory neurons. *Hearing Research, 4,* 325–333.

Chikamori, Y., Sasa, M., Fujimoto, S., Takaori, S., & Matsuoka, I. (1980). Locus coeruleus-induced inhibition of dorsal cochlear nucleus neurons in comparison with lateral vestibular nucleus neurons. *Brain Research, 194,* 53–63.

Comis, S.D. (1970). Centrifugal inhibitory processes affecting neurons in the cat cochlear nucleus. *Journal of Physiology, 210,* 751–760.

Comis, S.D. (1973). Detection of signals in noisy backgrounds: A role for centrifugal fibres. *Journal of Laryngology and Otology, 87,* 529–534.

Comis, S.D., & Guth, P.S. (1974). The release of acetylcholine from the cochlear nucleus upon stimulation of the crossed olivo-cochlear bundle. *Neuropharmacology, 13,* 633–641.

Comis, S.D., & Whitfield, I.C. (1968). Influence of centrifugal pathways on unit activity in the cochlear nucleus. *Journal of Neurophysiology, 31,* 62–68.

Contreras, N.E., & Bachelard, H.S. (1979). Some neurochemical studies on auditory regions of mouse brain. *Experimental Brain Research, 36,* 573–584.

Croucher, M.J., Collins, J.F., & Meldrum, B.S. (1982). Anticonvulsant action of excitatory amino acid antagonists. *Science, 216,* 899–901.

Curtis, D.R., Duggan, A.W., Felix, D., Johnston, G.A.R., & McLennan, H. (1971). Antagonism between bicuculline and GABA in the cat brain. *Brain Research, 33,* 57–73.

Curtis, D.R., Hösli, L., & Johnston, G.A.R. (1968). A pharmacological study of the depression of spinal neurones by glycine and related amino acids. *Experimental Brain Research, 6,* 1–18.

Curtis, D.R., & Johnston, G.A.R. (1974). Amino acid transmitters in the mammalian central nervous system. *Ergebnisse Der Physiologie Biologischen Chemie Und Experimentellen Pharmakologie, 69,* 97–188.

Curtis, D.R., & Koizumi, K. (1961). Chemical transmitter substances in brain stem of cat. *Journal of Neurophysiology, 24,* 80–90.

Curtis, D.R., Lodge, D., Bornstein, J.C., & Peet, M.J. (1981). Selective effects of (−)-baclofen on spinal synaptic transmission in the cat. *Experimental Brain Research, 42,* 158–170.

Curtis, D.R., & Tebecis, A.K. (1972). Bicuculline and thalamic inhibition. *Experimental Brain Research, 16,* 210–218.

Curtis, D.R., & Watkins, J.C. (1963). Acidic amino acids with strong excitatory actions on mammalian neurones. *Journal of Physiology, 166,* 1–14.

Dahlstrom, A., & Fuxe, K. (1964). Localization of monamines in the lower brain stem. *Experientia (Basel), 20,* 1–3.

Davies, J. (1981). Selective depression of synaptic excitation in cat spinal neurones by baclofen: An iontophoretic study. *British Journal of Pharmacology, 72,* 373–384.

Davies J., & Watkins, J.C. (1973). Microelectrophoretic studies on the depressant action of HA-966 on chemically and synaptically excited neurons in the cat cerebral cortex and cuneate nucleus. *Brain Research, 59,* 311–322.

Davies, J., & Watkins, J.C. (1977) Effect of magnesium ions on the responses of spinal neurones to excitatory amino acids and acetylcholine. *Brain Research, 130,* 364–368.

Davies, W.E. (1975). The distribution of GABA transaminase-containing neurons in the cat cochlear nucleus. *Brain Research, 83,* 27–33.

Davies, W.E. (1977). GABAergic innervation of the mammalian cochlear nucleus. In M. Portmann & J.M. Aran (Eds.), *Inner Ear Biology* (Vol. 68, pp. 155–164). Paris: INSERM.

Denavit-Saubie, M., & Champagnat, J. (1975). The effect of some depressing amino acids on bulbar respiratory and non-respiratory neurons. *Brain Research, 97,* 356–361.

Farley, G.R., Morley, B.J., Janel, E., & Gorda, M.P. (1982). Single-unit responses in rat inferior colliculus during iontophoresis of cholinergic agents. *Society of Neuroscience Abstracts, 8,* 348.

Fex, J., Altschuler, R.A., Wenthold, R.J., & Parakkal, M.H. (1982). Aspartate aminotransferase immunoreactivity in cochlea of guinea pig. *Hearing Research, 7,* 149–160.

Fex, J., Fuxe, K., & Lennerstrand, G. (1965). Absence of monoamines in olivocochlear fibers in the cat. *Acta Physiology Scandinavia, 64,* 259–262.

Fex, J., & Wenthold, R.J. (1976). Choline acetyltransferase, glutamate decarboxylase and tyrosine hydroxylase in the cochlea and cochlear nucleus of the guinea pig. *Brain Research, 109,* 575–585.

Fisher, S.K., & Davies, W.E. (1976). GABA and its related enzymes in the lower auditory system of the guinea pig. *Journal of Neurochemistry, 27,* 1145–1155.

Foote, S.L., Freedman, R., & Oliver, A.P. (1975). Effects of putative neurotransmitters on neuronal activity in monkey auditory cortex. *Brain Research, 86,* 229–242.

Fuxe, K. (1965). Evidence for the existence of monoamine neurons in the central nervous system. IV. Distribution of monoamine terminals in the central nervous system. *Acta Physiology Scandinavia, 64 (Suppl. 247),* 39–85.

Godfrey, D.A., Carter, J.A., Berger, S.J., Lowry, O.H., & Matschinsky, F.M. (1977a). Quantitative histochemical mapping of candidate transmitter amino acids in cat cochlear nucleus. *Journal of Histochemistry and Cytochemistry, 25,* 417–431.

Godfrey, D.A., Carter, J.A., Lowry, O.H., & Matschinsky, F.M. (1978). Distribution of gamma-aminobutyric acid, glycine, glutamate and aspartate in the cochlear nucleus of the rat. *Journal of Histochemistry and Cytochemistry, 26,* 118–126.

Godfrey, D.A., & Matschinsky, F.M. (1981a). Quantitative distribution of CAT and AChE activities in the rat cochlear nucleus. *Journal of Histochemistry and Cytochemistry, 29,* 720–730.

Godfrey, D.A., Park, J.L., Rabe, J.R., Dunn, J.D., Smith, J.T., & Ross, C.D. (1981b). Quantitative evaluation of centrifugal cholinergic pathways to the rat cochlear nucleus. *Neuroscience Abstracts, 7,* 56.

Godfrey, D.A., Williams, A.D., & Matschinsky, F.M. (1977b). Quantitative histochemical mapping of enzymes of the cholinergic system in cat cochlear nucleus. *Journal of Histochemistry and Cytochemistry, 25,* 397–416.

Haas, H.L., & Hösli, L. (1973). Strychnine and inhibition of bulbar reticular neurons. *Experientia (Basel), 29,* 542–544.

Haldeman, S., Huffman, R.D., Marshall, K.C., & McLennan, H. (1972). The antagonism of the glutamate induced and synaptic excitation of thalamic neurones. *Brain Research, 39,* 419–425.

Haldeman, S., & McLennan, H. (1972). The antagonistic action glutamic acid diethylester towards amino acid-induced and synaptic excitations of central neurones. *Brain Research, 45,* 393–400.

Hall, J.L. (1980). Cochlear models: Two-tone suppression and the second filter. *Journal of the Acoustical Society of America, 67,* 1722–1728.

Hall, J.G., McLennan, H., & Wheal, H.V. (1977). The actions of certain amino acids as neuronal excitants. *Journal of Physiology, 272,* 52–53.

Hansson, E., Karlstedt, J., & Sellstrom, A. (1980). Sound-stimulated ^{14}C-glutamate release from the nucleus cochlearis. *Experientia, 36,* 576–577.

Harrison, J.M., & Irving, R. (1965). The anterior ventral cochlear nucleus. *Journal of Comparative Neurology, 124,* 15–42.

Harrison, J.M., & Irving, R. (1966). The organization of the posterior ventral cochlear nucleus in the rat. *Journal of Comparative Neurology, 126,* 391–402.

Harrison, J.M., & Warr, W.B. (1962). A study of the cochlear nucleus and ascending auditory pathways of the medulla. *Journal of Comparative Neurology, 119,* 341–379.

Herkenham, M., & Pert, C.B. (1980). *In vitro* autoradiography of opiate receptors in brain suggests loci of opiatergic pathways. *Proceedings of the National Academy of Science USA, 77,* 5532–5536.

Hill, R.G., Simmonds, M.A., & Straughan, D.W. (1976). Antagonism of gamma-aminobutyric acid and glycine by convulsants in the cuneate nucleus of cat. *British Journal of Pharmacology, 56,* 9–19.

Hökfelt, T., Elde, R., Johansson, O., Terenius, L., & Stein, L. (1977). The distribution of enkephalin-immunoreactive cell bodies in the rat central nervous system. *Neuroscience Letters, 5,* 25–31.

Hösli, L., & Tebecis, A.K. (1970). Actions of amino acids and convulsants on bulbar reticular neurones. *Experimental Brain Research, 11,* 111–127.

Hunt, S., & Schmidt, J. (1978). Some observation of the binding patterns of alpha-bungarotoxin in the central nervous system of the rat. *Brain Research, 157,* 213–232.

Johnston, G.A.R., Curtis, D.R., Davies, J., & McCullock, R.M. (1974). Spinal interneurone excitation by conformationally restricted analogues of L-glutamic acid. *Nature (London), 248,* 804.

Jones, D.R., Oliver, D.L., Potashner, S.J., & Morest, D.K. (1982). Retrograde axonal transport of D-aspartate from cochlear nucleus to Type II spiral ganglion cells in the cat. *Association for Research in Otolaryngology Abstracts, 5,* 119.

Kiang, N.Y.S., Rho, J.M., Northrop, C.C., Liberman, M. C., & Ryugo, D.K. (1982). Hair-cell innervation by spiral ganglion cells in adult cats. *Science, 217,* 175–177.

Kobayashi, R.M., Palkovits, M., Hruska, R.E., Rothschild, R., & Yamamura, H.I. (1978). Regional distribution of muscarinic cholinergic receptors in rat brain. *Brain Research, 154,* 13–23.

Koerber, K.C., Pfeiffer, R.R., Warr, W.B., & Kiang, N.Y.S. (1966). Spontaneous spike discharges from single units in the cochlear nucleus after destruction of the cochlea. *Experimental Neurology, 16,* 119–130.

Krnjević, K. (1974). Chemical nature of synaptic transmission in vertebrates. *Physiology Review, 54,* 418–540.

Krnjević, K., & Puil, E. (1976). Electro-physiological studies on actions of taurine. In R. Huxtable & A. Barbeau (Eds.), *Taurine* (pp. 179–189). New York: Raven Press.

Kromer, L.F., & Moore, R.Y. (1976). Cochlear nucleus innervation by central norepinephrine neurons in the rat. *Brain Research, 118,* 531–537.

Kromer, L.F., & Moore, R.Y. (1980). Norepinephrine innervation of the cochlear nuclei by locus coeruleus neurons in the rat. *Anatomy and Embryology (Berlin), 158,* 227–244.

Levitt, P., & Moore, R.Y. (1980). Organization of brainstem noradrenaline hyperinnervation following neonatal 6-hydroxydopamine treatment in rat. *Anatomy and Embryology, 158,* 133-150.

Ljungdahl, A., Hökfelt, T., & Nilsson, G. (1978). Distribution of substance P-like immunoreactivity in the central nervous system of the rat. 1. Cell bodies and nerve terminals. *Neuroscience, 3,* 861-943.

Lorente de Nó, R. (1933). Anatomy of the eighth nerve. III. General plans of structure of the primary cochlear nuclei. *Laryngoscope, 53,* 327-350.

Martin, M.R. (1980). The effects of iontophoretically applied antagonists on auditory nerve and amino acid evoked excitation of anteroventral cochlear nucleus neurons. *Neuropharmacology, 19,* 519-528.

Martin, M.R. (1981a). Morphology of the cochlear nucleus of the normal and Reeler mutant moust. *Journal of Comparative Neurology, 197,* 141-152.

Martin, M.R. (1981b). Acetylcholinesterase-positive fibers and cell bodies in the cochlear nuclei of normal and reeler mutant mice. *Journal of Comparative Neurology, 197,* 153-167.

Martin, M.R. (1982). Baclofen and the brain stem auditory evoked potential. *Experimental Neurology, 76,* 675-680.

Martin, M.R. (1983). Preliminary observations on a tissue slice preparation of the mouse cochlear nucleus. *Journal of Physiology (London), 334,* 25-26.

Martin, M.R., & Adams, J.C. (1979). Effects of DL-alpha-amino adipate on synaptically and chemically evoked excitation of anteroventral cochlear nucleus neurons of the cat. *Neuroscience, 4,* 1097-1105.

Martin, M.R., & Dickson, J.W. (1983). Lateral inhibition in the anteroventral cochlear nucleus of the cat: A microiontophoretic study. *Hearing Research, 9,* 35-41.

Martin, M.R., Dickson, J.W., & Fex, J. (1982). Bicuculline, strychnine and depressant amino acid responses in the anteroventral cochlear nucleus of the cat. *Neuropharmacology, 21,* 201-207.

Matsuoka, I., Chikamori, Y., Sasa, M., & Takaori, S. (1978). Influence of monoaminergic neurons on the vestibular and cochlear nuclei in cats. In J.D. Hood (Ed.), *Vestibular mechanisms in health and disease* (pp. 52-58). London: Academic Press.

McDonald, D.M., & Rasmussen, G.L. (1971). Ultrastructural characteristics of synaptic endings in the cochlear nucleus having acetylcholinesterase activity. *Brain Resaaerch, 28,* 1-18.

McLennan, H. (1981). On the nature of the receptors for various excitatory amino acids in the mammalian central nervous system. In G. DiChiara & G.L. Gessa, (Eds.), *Glutamate as a neurotransmitter* (pp. 253-262).

Meldrum, B., Pedley, T., Horten, R., Anlezark, G., & Franks, A. (1980). Epiliptogenic and anticonvulsant effects of GABA agonists and GABA uptake inhibitors. *Brain Research Bulletin, 5, (Suppl. 2),* 685-690.

Merzenich, M.M. (1970). Morphological specialization of the cochlear nuclear complex in certain mammals. *Anatomy Record, 166,* 347.

Merzenich, M.M., Kitzes, L., & Aitkin, L. (1973). Anatomical and physiological evidence for auditory specialization in the mountain beaver (Aplodenita rufa). *Brain Research, 58,* 331-344.

Moore, J.K., & Osen, K.K. (1979). The cochlear nuclei in man. *American Journal of Anatomy, 154,* 393-418.

Moore, M., Caspary, D.M., & Havey, D.C. (1981). Iontophoretic application of putative inhibitory neurotransmitters onto binaural units in the superior olive. *Society for Neuroscience Abstracts, 7,* 389.

Morley, B.J., Lorden, J.F., Brown, G.B., Kemp, G.E., & Bradley, R.J. (1977). Regional distribution of nicotinic acetylcholine receptors in rat brain. *Brain Research, 134,* 161–166.

Morrison, D., Schindler, R.A., & Wersall, J. (1975). A quantitative analysis of the afferent innervation of the organ of Corti in guinea pig. *Acta Otolaryngologica, 79,* 11–23.

Norenberg, M.D., & Martinez-Hernandez, A. (1979). Fine structural location of glutamine synthetase in astrocytes of rat brain. *Brain Research, 161,* 303–310.

Oliver, D.L., Jones, D.R., Potashner, S.J., & Morest, D.K., (1981). Evidence for selective uptake, release and axonal transport of D-aspartate in the auditory system and cerebellum of cat and guinea pig. *Anatomy Record, 199,* 186A.

Osen, K.K. (1969). Cytoarchitecture of the cochlear nuclei in the cat. *Journal of Comparative Neurology, 136,* 453–484.

Osen, K.K., & Roth, K. (1969). Histochemical localization of cholinesterase in the cochlear nuclei of the cat, with notes on the origin of acetylcholinesterase-positive afferents and the superior olive. *Brain Research, 16,* 165–185.

Pedersen, E., Arlien-Soborg, P., Grynderup, V., & Hendriksen, O. (1970). GABA derivative in spasticity. *Acta Neurology, Scandinavia, 46,* 257–266.

Pfeiffer, R.R. (1966). Anteroventral cochlear nucleus: Waveforms of extracellularly recorded spike potentials. *Science, 154,* 667–668.

Pickles, J.O. (1976a). Role of centrifugal pathways to cochlear nucleus in determination of critical band width. *Journal of Neurophysiology, 39,* 394–400.

Pickles, J.O. (1976b). The noradrenaline-containing innervation of the cochlear nucleus and the detection of signals in noise. *Brain Research, 105,* 591–596.

Pickles, J.O., & Comis, S.D. (1973). Role of centrifugal pathways to cochlear nucleus in detection of signals in noise. *Journal of Neurophysiology, 36,* 1131–1137.

Pirsig, W., Pfalz, R., & Sandanaga, M. (1968). Postsynaptic auditory crossed efferent inhibition in the ventral cochlear nucleus and its blocking by strychnine nitrate (guinea pig). *Kumamoto Medical Journal, 21,* 75–82.

Potashner, S.J. (1978). Baclofen: Effects on amino acid release. *Canadian Journal of Physiology and Pharmacology, 56,* 150–154.

Ramon-Moliner, E. (1972). Acetylthiocholinesterase distribution in the brain stem of the cat. *Advances in Anatomy, Embryology, and Cell Biology, 46,* 4.

Ramon y Cajal, S. (1909). *Histologie du système nerveux de l'homme et des vertèbrès* (pp. 774–838). Paris: A. Moloine.

Rasmussen, G.L. (1964). Anatomic relationships of the ascending and descending auditory systems. In W.S. Fields & B.R. Alford (Eds.), *Neurological aspects of auditory and vestibular disorders,* (pp. 5–23). Springfield: Thomas.

Rasmussen, G.L. (1967). Efferent connections of the cochlear nucleus. In A.B. Graham (Ed.), *Sensorineural hearing processes and disorders* (pp. 61–75). Boston: Little, Brown.

Rubin, R.P. (1970). The role of calcium in the release of neurotransmitter substances and hormones. *Pharmacological Review, 22,* 389–428.

Ruggero, M.A., & Santi, P.A. (1981). Evidence for the projection of Type II spiral ganglion neurons in the cochlear nucleus of the chinchilla. *Neuroscience Abstracts, 7,* 146.

Rustioni, A., & Cuenod, M. (1982). Selective retrograde transport of D-aspartate in spinal interneurons and cortical neurons of rats. *Brain Research, 236,* 143–155.

Sachs, M.B., & Abbas, P.J. (1976). Phenomenological model for two-tone suppression. *Journal of the Acoustical Society of America, 60,* 1157–1163.

Sasaki, C.T., Kauer, J.S., & Babitz, L. (1980). Differential ^{14}C-2-deoxyglucose uptake after deafferentation of mammalian auditory pathway – a model for examining tinnitus. *Brain Research, 194,* 511–516.

Schechter, N., Handy, I.C., Peggementi, L., & Schmidt, J. (1978). Distribution of alpha-bungaro-toxin binding sites in the central nervous system and peripheral organs of the rat. *Toxicon. 16,* 245–251.

Schwartz, I.R. (1981). The differential distribution of label following uptake of ^{3}H-labeled amino acids in the dorsal cochlear nucleus of the cat. *Experimental Neurology, 73,* 601–617.

Shiosaka, S., Takatsuki, M., Sakana, M., Inagaki, S., Takagi, H., Senba, E., Kawai, Y., & Tohyama, J. (1981). Ontogeny of somatostatin-containing neuron system of the rat: Immunohisto-chemical observations. I. Lower brain stem. *Journal of Comparative Neurology, 203,* 173–188.

Spoendlin, H. (1971). Degeneration behavior of the cochlear nerve. *Arch. Klin. Exp. Ohren Nasen Kehlkopfheilkd, 200,* 275–291.

Spoendlin H. (1975). Retrograde degeneration of the cochlear nerve. *Acta Otolaryngologica, 79,* 266–275.

Spoendlin, H. (1979a). Neural connections of the outer haircell system. *Acta Otolaryngologica, 87,* 381–387.

Spoendlin, H. (1979b). Sensory neural organization of the cochlea. *Journal of Laryngology and Otology, 93,* 853–877.

Spoendlin, H. (1981). Differentiation of cochlear afferent neurons. *Acta Otolaryngologica, 91,* 451–456.

Streit, P. (1980). Selective retrograde labeling indicating the transmitter of neuronal pathways. *Journal of Comparative Neurology, 191,* 429–463.

Swanson, L.W., & Hartman, B.K. (1975). The central adrenergic system. An immunofluorescence study of the locations of cell bodies and their afferent connections in the rat utilizing dopa-mine-beta-hydroxylase as a marker. *Journal of Comparative Neurology, 163,* 467–506.

Tachibana, M., Rothman, J.M., & Guth, P.S. (1979). Somatostatin along the auditory pathway. *Hearing Research, 1,* 365–368.

Tebecis, A.K. (1967). 5-Hydroxytryptamine and noradrenaline inhibitory transmitters in the medial geniculate nucleus? *Brain Research, 6,* 780–782.

Tebecis, A.K. (1970a). Effects of monoamines and amino acids on medial geniculate neurones of the cat. *Neuropharmacology, 9,* 381–390.

Tebecis, A.K. (1970b). Properties of cholinoceptive neurones in the medial geniculate nucleus. *British Journal of Pharmacology, 38,* 117–137.

Tebecis, A.K. (1970c). Studies on cholinergic transmission in the medial geniculate nucleus. *British Journal of Pharmacology, 38,* 138–147.

Tebecis, A.K. (1973). Studies on the identity of the optic nerve transmitter. *Brain Research, 63,* 31–42.

Tolbert, L.P., & Morest, D.K. (1978). Patterns of synaptic organization in the cochlear nucleus of the cat. *Society for Neuroscience Abstracts, 4,* 11.

Torda, C. (1978). Effects of noradrenaline and serotonin on activity of single lateral and medial geniculate neurons. *General Pharmacology, 9,* 455–462.

Torda, C. (1979). Acetylcholine dependent modulation of the activities of lateral and medial geniculate neurons. *International Journal of Neuroscience, 8,* 195–203.

Uhl, G.R., Goodman, R.R., Kuhar, M.J., Childers, S.R., & Snyder, S.H. (1979a). Immunohisto-chemical mapping of enkephalin containing cell bodies, fibers and nerve terminals in the brain stem of the rat. *Brain Research, 166,* 75–94.

Uhl, G.R., Goodman, R.R., & Snyder, S.H. (1979b). Neurotensin-containing cell bodies, fibers and nerve terminals in the brain stem of the rat: Immunohistochemical mapping. *Brain Research, 167,* 77–91.

Wamsley, J.K., Lewis, M.S., Young, W.S., & Kuhar, M.J. (1981). Autoradiographic localization of muscarinic cholinergic receptors in rat brainstem. *Journal of Neuroscience, 1,* 176–191.

Watanabe, T. (1971). Effect of picrotoxin on two-tone inhibition of auditory neurons in the cochlear nucleus. *Brain Research, 28,* 586–590.

Watanabe, T. (1979). Funneling mechanism in hearing. *Hearing Research, 1,* 111–119.

Watanabe, T., & Simada, Z. (1970). Collicular auditory interneuron and its blocking by dihydro-beta-erythroidine hydrobromide. *Proceedings of the Japanese Academy, 46,* 983–988.

Watanabe, T., & Simada, Z. (1971). Picrotoxin: Effect on collicular auditory neurons. *Brain Research 28,* 582–585.

Watanabe, T., & Simada, Z. (1973). Pharmacological properties of cat's collicular auditory neurons. *Japanese Journal of Physiology, 23,* 291–308.

Watkins, J.C. (1981a). Pharmacology of excitatory amino acid receptors. In P.J. Roberts, J. Storm-Mathiesen, & G.A.R. Johnston (Eds.), *Glutamate: Transmitter in the central nervous system* (pp. 1–24). Chichester: Wiley.

Watkins, J.C. (1981b). Pharmacology of excitatory amino acid transmitters. *Advances in Biochemistry and Psychopharmacology, 29,* 205–212.

Webster, M., & Webster, D.B. (1978). Cochlear nuclear projections from outer hair cells. *Neuroscience Abstracts, 4,* 11.

Wenthold, R.J. (1978). Glutamic acid and aspartic acid in subdivision of the cochlear nucleus after auditory nerve lesion. *Brain Research, 143,* 544–548.

Wenthold, R.J. (1979). Release of endogenous glutamic acid, aspartic acid and GABA from cochlear nucleus slices. *Brain Research, 162,* 338–343.

Wenthold, R.J. (1980). Glutaminase and aspartate aminotransferase decrease in the cochlear nucleus after lesion of the auditory nerve. *Brain Research, 190,* 293–297.

Wenthold, R.J., & Gulley, R.L. (1977). Aspartic acid and glutamic acid levels in the cochlear nucleus after auditory nerve lesion. *Brain Research, 138,* 111–123.

Wenthold, R.J., & Gulley, R.L. (1978). Glutamic acid and aspartic acid in the cochlear nucleus of the waltzing guinea pig. *Brain Research, 158,* 279–284.

Wenthold, R.J. & Morest, D.K. (1976). Transmitter related enzymes in the guinea pig cochlear nucleus. *Neuroscience Abstracts, 2,* 28.

Whitfield, I.C., & Allanson, J.T. (1958). A study of the effect of some neurally active drugs on inhibition in the auditory pathway. *Archives of Italian Biology, 96,* 29–37.

Whitfield, I.C., & Comis, S.D. (1966). *The role of inhibition in information transfer: The interaction of centrifugal and centripetal stimulation on neurones of the cochlear nucleus.* Final Report (Part 2), European Office of Aerospace Research, United States Air Force, Grant 63–115.

Zarbin, M.A., Wamsley, J.K. & Kuhar, M.J. (1981). Glycine receptor: Light microscopic autoradiographic localization with [^{3}H]strychnine. *Journal of Neuroscience, 1,* 532–547.

Zieglgansberger, W., & Puil, E.A. (1973). Actions of glutamic acid on spinal neurons. *Experimental Brain Research, 17,* 35–49.

Chapter 11

The Structural Basis for Stimulus Coding in the Cochlear Nucleus of the Cat[1]

Nell B. Cant

D.K. Morest

INTRODUCTION

The purpose of this review is to assess the state of neuroanatomical knowledge of the cochlear nucleus as it relates to information processing in the auditory system. After first reviewing the status of cytoarchitectonic studies of the cochlear nuclear complex, we discuss in detail some of the main neuronal types in the nucleus and their afferent and efferent connections. Finally, the implications of the anatomy for stimulus coding in the cochlear nucleus are analyzed.

SUBDIVISIONS OF THE COCHLEAR NUCLEAR COMPLEX

Early students of the central auditory pathways recognized that the cochlear nerve terminates in several morphologically distinct regions within the brain stem (Fuse, 1913; Held, 1891; Koelliker, 1896; Ramón y Cajal, 1909; Sala, 1893; van Gehuchten, 1902, 1906; Winkler, 1921). All authors agreed in describing two major areas – known today as the ventral and dorsal cochlear nuclei – that were further subdivided in various ways.

The dorsal cochlear nucleus (DCN) of most mammals has three easily distinguished layers, although the arrangement is not so orderly in primates. Brawer,

[1]N.B. Cant was supported by USPHS Grant NS 14655 and by a grant from the Deafness Research Foundation; D.K. Morest, by USPHS Grant NS 14347. We are very grateful to Ms. Karen Thompson, who measured the areas of approximately 4,300 neurons and entered the data into the computer. We also thank Ms. Thompson and Ms. Laura Andrus for help with the illustrations and Ms. Anne Boyd for typing the manuscript.

Morest, and Kane (1974) have termed these the molecular (or superficial) layer (layer 1 of Lorente de Nó, 1933a, 1981), the fusiform cell (or granular) layer (layer 2 of Lorente de Nó), and the polymorphic (or deep) layer. The polymorphic layer can be further divided into a superficial sublayer (layer 3 of Lorente de Nó) containing the basal dendrites of the fusiform cells and a deep sublayer (layer 4 of Lorente de Nó). Lorente de Nó added a fifth layer, or central nucleus, making five layers in all, although it may be that the central nucleus is better understood as a region of the deep layer. Lorente de Nó (1933a) also divided the dorsal cochlear nucleus into five regions, but this scheme has not usually been used by subsequent investigators.

Some of the early views of the ventral cochlear nucleus have been summarized by Harrison and Irving (1966a), who point out that, since the studies of Ramón y Cajal (1909), the ventral cochlear nucleus has generally been divided into two parts, the anteroventral (AVCN) and posteroventral (PVCN) cochlear nuclei, by the entering auditory nerve fibers, although a few authors have emphasized mediolateral differences (Fuse, 1913; Winkler, 1921). Lorente de Nó (1933a, 1981) maintained that within these two major divisions eight regions could be distinguished. A detailed scheme for partitioning the ventral cochlear nucleus was presented by Harrison and his colleagues (Harrison & Warr, 1962; Harrison & Irving, 1965, 1966a,b). In the rat, they distinguished five subdivisions. They strengthened their argument that the nucleus was usefully divided into at least five parts by demonstrating that a number of neuronal types, as defined in Protargol impregnations, were found in only one or a few subdivisions. A similar parcellation of the ventral cochlear nucleus of the guinea pig was published by Pirsig (1968).

Because it is our purpose to discuss the structural basis for stimulus coding in the cochlear nucleus, further discussion of its subdivisions will be restricted to the cat, since most of the studies of the physiological properties of the constituent neurons have been done in this species (e.g., Bourk, 1976; Bourk, Mielcarz, & Norris, 1981; Britt, 1976; Britt & Starr, 1976a,b; Brugge, Javel, & Kitzes, 1978; Brugge, Kitzes, & Javel, 1981; Evans & Nelson, 1973a,b; Gibson, Hind, Kitzes, & Rose, 1977; Gisbergen, Grashuis, Johannesma, & Vendrik, 1975; Godfrey, Kiang, & Norris, 1975a,b; Goldberg & Brownell, 1973; Goldberg & Greenwood, 1966; Greenwood & Goldberg, 1970; Greenwood & Maruyama, 1965; Greenwood, Merzenich, & Roth, 1976; Kiang, Pfeiffer, Warr, & Backus, 1965; Koerber, Pfeiffer, Warr, & Kiang, 1966; Pfeiffer, 1966a,b; Pfeiffer & Kiang, 1965; Rhode, Oertel, & Smith, 1983a; Rhode, Smith, & Oertel, 1983b; Romand, 1979; Rose, 1960; Rose, Galambos, & Hughes, 1959; Rose, Kitzes, Gibson, & Hind, 1974; Voigt & Young, 1980; Young, 1980; Young & Voigt, 1982). Although a number of authors have recognized anatomical subdivisions in the cat's cochlear nucleus (Fuse, 1913; Lorente de Nó, 1933a, 1976, 1981; Powell & Erulkar, 1962; Ramón y Cajal, 1909; Rasmussen, 1967; van Noort, 1969; see Brawer et al., 1974, Table 1, for a comparison of the major cytoarchitectonic schemes in the cat), the first detailed descriptions were published by Osen (1969a) and by Brawer, Morest, and Kane (1974). Osen (1969a) described nine cell types in the cochlear nucleus based on their morphology in Nissl and reduced silver preparations and suggested a scheme for subdividing the nucleus based on the differential distribution of the cell types. Osen recognized three layers in the dorsal cochlear nucleus, which she did not parcel further. The ventral cochlear nucleus was subdivided into six cell areas, two of which – the globular cell area and the multipolar cell area – overlapped extensively and which Osen later referred to collectively as the "central region of the ventral cochlear nucleus" (Osen, 1970). The remaining cell areas – the large and small spherical cell areas, the octopus cell area, and the small cell cap – were each characterized by one predominant cell type. A detailed discussion of the cell types themselves will be included in a later section.

Brawer and associates (1974) subdivided the ventral cochlear nucleus on cytoarchitectonic grounds, using Nissl- and Protargol-stained material to examine the relative sizes, shapes, and packing density of the larger neurons in each part of the nucleus. They divided DCN into three layers, but they distinguished 13 cytoarchitectonic regions in the ventral cochlear nucleus, 5 in AVCN, 7 in PVCN, and a nucleus of the intermediate acoustic stria. In a separate part of the study, they defined cell types in the nucleus on the basis of their morphology in Golgi impregnations. When the locations of these cell types were mapped on the cytoarchitectonic atlas, it was demonstrated that some of the cell types were confined to only one or a few of the cytoarchitectonic subdivisions, whereas others had a much wider distribution.

Although Brawer and co-workers did not emphasize the distinct appearance of the axonal plexus in different parts of the nucleus, it is possible to correlate some of the regions they defined cytoarchitectonically with those distinguished on the basis of axonal branching patterns in rapid Golgi material. In studies of axonal patterns in AVCN of kittens, it was noted that the major divisions described by Brawer and colleagues could also be recognized by the distinct appearance of the plexuses formed by the axons in each (Brawer & Morest, 1975; Cant & Morest, 1978). Because different patterns of terminal arborizations among cells presumably result in distinct patterns of neuronal activity, the recognition of this different way of specifying the cytoarchitectonic areas increases our confidence that the subdivisions are functionally meaningful. It was further pointed out that, although each division of AVCN has a characteristic axonal plexus, the axonal arborization patterns of noncochlear inputs to the nucleus do not always coincide exactly with the boundaries of the subdivisions defined cytoarchitectonically (Cant & Morest, 1978). For example, within the anterior division of the AVCN (AVCN-A), the differences in the axonal plexus divide it into dorsal and ventral parts (which would coincide with high- and low-frequency parts, respectively – see below). Thus, the spatial organization of the inputs to the cells of the nucleus may add an additional basis for distinguishing functionally important areas.

In broad outline, the results of the studies of Osen and of Brawer and associates are similar. In AVCN, there is a clear correspondence between the large and small spherical cell areas of Osen and the anterior division (AVCN-A) of Brawer and colleagues (Brawer et al., 1974; Cant & Morest, 1979a). It further appears that the large spherical cell area corresponds to the anterior subdivision (AA of Brawer et al.) and the small spherical cell area, to the posterior (AP) and possibly also the posterodorsal (APD) subdivisions. It is not possible to be certain on this last point, however, since no extensive quantitative data are available on the sizes of the spherical cells in various parts of the nucleus. As an addition to previous definitions of the subdivisions of the anterior division we suggest that the anterior subdivision (AA) consists almost exclusively of one cell type, the spherical bushy cell (this being especially true if the smaller marginal cells are ignored), whereas the posterior subdivision consists of a mixture of cell types (Cant and Morest, 1979a). Although Osen did not make a major point of it, she did note that her small spherical cell area contained other cell types, especially along the periphery. She classified most of these cells as small cells. The posterodorsal part (APD) might appear to be a dorsal extension of the anterior subdivision, since it contains mostly spherical bushy cells; however, it is bordered by a large group of other cell types (to be discussed below; Cant & Morest, 1979a).

The globular cell area of Osen corresponds, more or less, to the posterior division of AVCN (AVCN-P) of Brawer and associates, who further subdivided the posterior division into dorsal and ventral parts (PD and PV, respectively), the ventral part corresponding to the region of the entering nerve root. The proportion of various cell types appears to differ in PD and PV (Tolbert & Morest, 1982a). The posterior division of AVCN is also included in Osen's multipolar cell area, which overlaps with the globular cell area but also extends caudally into the PVCN. As will be considered in detail later, multipolar cell types occur throughout the ventral cochlear nucleus and, except for the fact that rostral PVCN seems to contain only this type in Nissl-stained material, there appears to be no compelling reason to distinguish a multipolar cell area per se.

It is PVCN that provides the greatest difference between the two schemes. Osen considered PVCN to be divisible into two major parts. The caudal pole of the nucleus was called the octopus cell area (OCA) after the predominant cell type found there. The anterior part of PVCN was included in the multipolar cell area. Brawer and co-workers, on the other hand, were able to define seven areas in PVCN, four of which (posterior, ventral, dorsal, and central) were in the caudal region of the nucleus and probably correspond to Osen's octopus cell area. Two of the most rostral parts – the anterior and anterodorsal subdivisions – probably correspond to the caudal part of Osen's multipolar cell area (Brawer et al., 1974). The seventh subdivison – the lateral part of the PVCN – may include part of Osen's peripheral cap of small cells, although this subdivision also contains many fairly large stellate cells (lateral nucleus of Lorente de Nó, 1933a; Brawer et al., 1974).

The last of Osen's cell areas – the peripheral cap of small cells – is, in Nissl-stained sections, a poorly delimited area along the lateral aspect of the ventral cochlear nucleus. Because larger cells are often mixed in with the small cells along the margins of the nucleus, Brawer and colleagues (1974) did not define a separate area in Nissl sections. However, a region apparently equivalent in location and extent to Osen's small cell cap can be easily distinguished in Golgi- or myelin-stained preparations, because the main branches of the auditory nerve do not enter it and thinly myelinated axons interconnecting DCN and AVCN run through it (Cant & Morest, 1978; unpublished observations). The small cell cap lies along the dorsolateral edges of the anterior and posterior division of AVCN, continues caudally dorsal to the cochlear nerve root, and lies along the ventrolateral edges of PVCN. It is located just medial to the granule cell layer throughout its extent.

The utility of dividing the cochlear nuclear complex into smaller parts has been confirmed by the findings that the subdivisions receive different arrangements of inputs from cochlear and noncochlear sources (Brawer & Morest, 1975; Cant & Gaston, 1982; Cant & Morest, 1978; Kane, 1976; Lorente de Nó, 1933a, 1976, 1981; Osen & Roth, 1969; Rasmussen, 1967), that they form distinct projections (Warr, 1966, 1969, 1972, 1982), and that they contain different types of physiologically defined single units (e.g., Bourk, 1976, Godfrey et al., 1975a,b). Within most of the subdivisions, however, more than one cell type can be identified, and the connections and physiology of each of these may differ as well. Therefore, although the parcellation into regions provides a first step toward an understanding of the neuronal organization of the cochlear nucleus, it is at the level of cell types that a basic understanding must be sought.

CELL TYPES IN THE COCHLEAR NUCLEAR COMPLEX

Study of the cochlear nucleus reveals obvious differences in neuronal populations both within and among the subdivisions. As a working hypothesis, we assume that morphologically different types of neurons are functionally different. Ways of testing this hypothesis are to study other differences among the neurons, such as differences in their synaptic organization and efferent connections, and to provide sufficiently detailed descriptions of the distribution and organization of the neurons to allow correlations of physiological (see Young, chapter 12) and neurochemical data with the anatomical findings. If neuronal types defined in these studies could be correlated with the morphological types, the hypothesis that the structural differences underlie functional differences would be strengthened.

The first two detailed studies of cell types in the cochlear nucleus of the cat (Osen, 1969a, and Brawer et al., 1974, cited above) agree in many respects, and correspondence among some of their respective cell types can be readily demonstrated. However, in other instances, confusions arise when one tries to relate the two schemes. Since one or the other or both of these classification schemes for the cochlear nucleus of the cat have been applied in most recent studies of other species (e.g., Caspary, 1972; Disterhoft, Perkins, & Evans, 1980; Jones, 1979; Konigsmark, 1973; Martin, 1981; Moore & Osen, 1979; Moskowitz & Liu, 1972; Perry & Webster, 1981; Webster, 1971; Webster & Trune, 1982; Zook & Casseday, 1982), we shall discuss in detail some of the more important agreements and differences between the two schemes and, with some new data, suggest a more complete synthesis.

It is possible to relate the cell types defined by Osen (1969a) most clearly to those defined by Brawer and associates (1974) for those cells whose distribution is limited to a small part of the nucleus. The appearance of these neurons in Nissl and Golgi preparations is discussed in the following paragraphs; then we deal with the populations of neurons whose distribution is more widespread and for which correspondences are less clear.

Cell Types That Have a Limited Distribution Within the Cochlear Nuclear Complex

Six cell types are recognized in both systems of classification and can be uniquely defined on the basis of morphology in Golgi and Nissl preparations and location within the cochlear nucleus. They are the spherical bushy cells, the globular bushy cells, and the octopus cells of the ventral cochlear nucleus, the fusiform cells and the giant cells of the DCN, and the granule cells, which are associated with both nuclei.

Spherical bushy cells. Osen used the term, "spherical," to name the most prominent cell type in the rostral part of AVCN. The name describes a shape, of course, and, in fact, many of these cells are round in section; however, the shapes seen in sections alone do not provide a criterion sufficient for defining a homogeneous cell population in AVCN. We have suggested a simple criterion to specify a unique cell population in AVCN-A that can be correlated with types defined in other ways, namely the presence of a layer of Nissl substance apposed to the nuclear envelope (Cant & Morest, 1979a). This definition agrees very well with Osen's initial description of both large and small spherical cells. By this criterion, there are other cell types present in the posterior subdivision (Cant & Morest, 1979a – to be discussed in a later section). In any case, when "spherical" is used to name a population of cells, it cannot refer to the shape of each cell per se, since the shapes of the individual cells are variable (Cant & Morest, 1979a).

In the cat, it is possible to equate the spherical cell population almost completely, if not exclusively, with the bushy cell population of AVCN-A (Cant & Morest, 1979a). Since bushy cells occur throughout the AVCN (Brawer et al., 1974), we propose that these cells in the anterior division be called *spherical bushy cells* to distinguish them from the *globular bushy cells* (discussed below).

The spherical bushy cells, in Golgi impregnations, are characterized by tufts of dendritic processes that arise from one or a few short, thin proximal dendrites (Figure 11-1A; Brawer et al., 1974; Cant & Morest, 1979a). The soma of the cell is often studded with spines but the dendrites are relatively smooth. Adendritic bushy cells, present in young kittens (Brawer et al., 1974), are not frequently observed in adult cats (Cant & Morest, 1979a). The distribution within the ventral cochlear nucleus of cells identified as spherical bushy cells is shown in Figure 11-5.

Globular bushy cells. Globular cells occur in AVCN-P and, to a certain extent, in the anterior part of PVCN (Osen, 1969a; Tolbert & Morest, 1982a). They are large, pale cells with an eccentrically located nucleus and a fine granular appearance in Nissl-stained preparations (Osen, 1969a). In a study of AVCN in the vicinity of the cochlear nerve root, Tolbert and Morest (1982a) provided evidence that the globular cells of Nissl stains correspond to the bushy cells of AVCN-P as seen in Golgi preparations, although they caution that the morphology of the bushy cells is heterogeneous and that the correspondence may not be absolute. Definite resolution of this issue awaits further study, but, since it seems clear that most globular cells do have the bushy dendrites, we propose to refer to them as globular bushy cells to distinguish them from the spherical bushy cells common more rostrally.

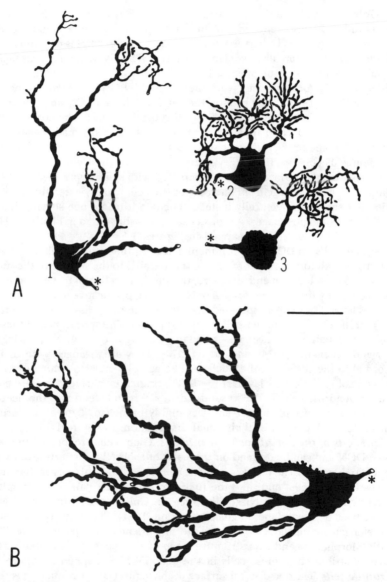

Figure 11-1. (A.) *Neuronal types in the anterior division of the anteroventral cochlear nucleus.* Both medium-sized stellate cells (1) and spherical bushy cells (2 and 3) are present in the posterior part of the anterior division. Only spherical bushy cells are common in the anterior part of the anterior division. (B.) Typical octopus cell in the caudal part of the posteroventral cochlear nucleus. (∗) Initial segment of axon. Adult cat, Golgi–Kopsch method. Bar = 50 μm.

In Golgi material, many bushy cells in AVCN-P resemble those in AVCN-A; others, with less highly branched tufts of longer appendages, are found exclusively in the posterior division (Tolbert & Morest, 1982a). Two examples of globular bushy cells found in AVCN-P are illustrated in Figure 11-2. The distribution of cells identified as globular bushy cells is mapped in Figure 11-5.

Octopus cells. Octopus cells were first named by Osen (1969a) and described in detail by Kane (1973). They occupy the caudal pole of PVCN and, for the most part, are segregated from the rest of the cell types in PVCN. The correspondence between the Golgi and Nissl appearance of these cells is easily made because of the characteristic shape of the cell body and the fact that the central part of the caudal cochlear nucleus contains this cell type almost exclusively. Octopus cells are large neurons. The somatic surface is heavily encrusted with spiny appendages and several very large dendrites emerge from one pole of the cell, usually extending in a dorsal direction but sometimes ventrally instead. The dendrites branch several times and end in little tufts of appendages. A typical example is illustrated in Figure 11-1B. The distribution of octopus cells is mapped in Figure 11-5.

Fusiform cells. In DCN one prominent cell type, the fusiform cell (or pyramidal cell, Osen, 1969a), forms a layer of cell bodies parallel to the surface of the nucleus. In addition to their location and large size, the fusiform cells can be defined in Nissl-stained sections by their unique pattern of Nissl substance relative to the other smaller cells in this layer. They appear speckled, with large clumps of Nissl substance scattered throughout the otherwise rather pale perikaryoplasm. The appearance of these cells in Golgi impregnations has been described in detail by Lorente de Nó (1933a, 1981), Brawer and colleagues (1974), and Kane (1974). They are arranged with their long axis normal to the surface of the nucleus. The apical dendrites, which extend into the superficial or molecular layer of the DCN, branch extensively and are covered with short dendritic spines. The basal dendrites, which extend into the deep layer of the nucleus, are usually longer and less highly branched. Typical fusiform cells are illustrated in Figure 11-3; their usual distribution, in Figure 11-5.

Giant cells of the dorsal cochlear nucleus. Giant cells are located in the deep layers of DCN and can be defined on the basis of their Nissl pattern, even without reference to their size. The nucleus in these cells is considerably larger than in other cell types (Osen, 1969a) and, like the fusiform cells, their pale perikaryoplasm is speckled by large chunks of Nissl substance. In Golgi material five types of giant cells have been defined (Kane, Puglisi, & Gordon, 1981). These five types – elongate bipolar, elongate multipolar, globular, radiate, and oriented multipolar – have different dendritic morphology and fine structure. One of the types is illustrated in Figure 11-3. The distribution of these cells in the deep DCN is mapped in Figure 11-5.

Granule cells. The dorsolateral surface of the ventral cochlear nucleus is covered by a thin layer of extremely small neurons known as granule cells. This layer, the external granular layer, widens posteriorly and is continuous with a tongue of granule cells that partially separates the ventral from the dorsal cochlear nucleus. In addition to the granular layer, granule cells are found throughout the layer formed by the fusiform cells and also in the molecular and deep layers of DCN. Granule cells may

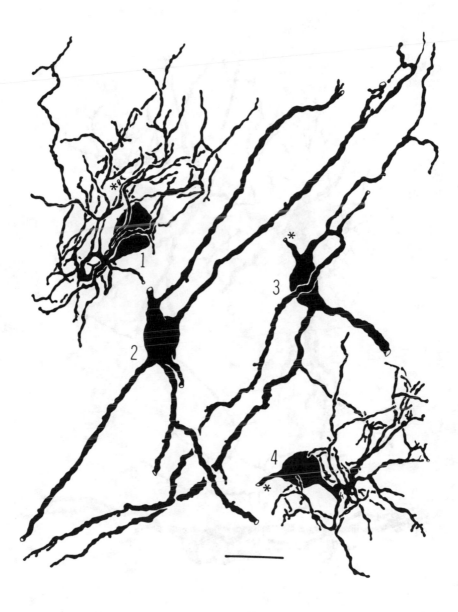

Figure 11-2. *Neuronal types in the posterior division of the anteroventral cochlear nucleus.* Globular bushy cells (1 and 4) and large stellate or elongate cells (2 and 3) are intermingled throughout this part of the nucleus. (∗) Initial segment of axon. Adult cat, Golgi–Kopsch method. Bar = 50 μm.

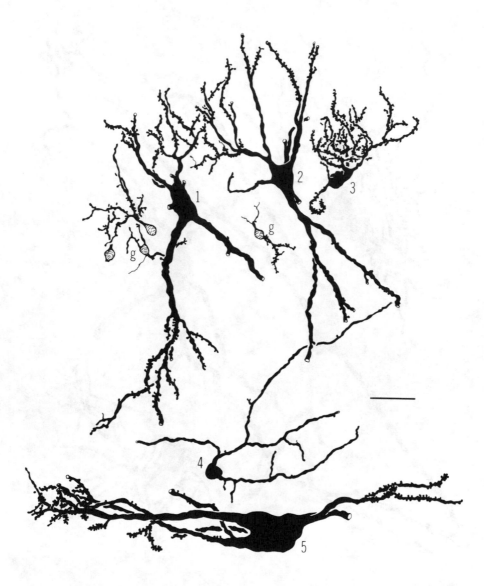

Figure 11-3. *Neuronal types in the dorsal cochlear nucleus.* Fusiform cells (1 and 2) and granule cells (g) form a densely packed layer of cell bodies. Small cells include cartwheel cells (3) and small stellate cells (4). Giant cells (5) occupy the deep layer. Adult cat, Golgi–Kopsch method. Bar = 50 μm.

also be found in other parts of the ventral cochlear nucleus. These tiny cells have been studied by Mugnaini and associates (1980a,b). They resemble, but are not identical to, the granule cells of the cerebellum. Their very small size relative to all other neurons makes them easily distinguishable in Nissl or Golgi material. In all probability, they are glutamatergic or aspartatergic neurons (Oliver, Potashner, Jones, & Morest, 1983; see also Wenthold & Martin, chapter 10, this volume). Examples of this cell type are illustrated in Figure 11-3. The distribution of individual granule cells was not mapped in the study illustrated in Figures 11-5 to 11-7; however, the regions of densest aggregations are indicated.

Cell Types That Have a Widespread Distribution Throughout the Cochlear Nuclear Complex

Many cells in the cochlear nuclear complex do not fit into the categories discussed above. Osen (1969a) called these neurons small cells, multipolar cells, and giant cells, but noted that clear-cut distinctions among these types could not be made, since there appears to be a continuum in cell size from small to giant and much variability in Nissl-staining characteristics. These cells presumably correspond to the cells in the ventral cochlear nucleus referred to as small cells, stellate cells, elongate cells, and giant cells on the basis of their morphology in Golgi material and to some or all of the several types characteristic of the rostral PVCN, for example, clavate cells, antenni-form cells, shrub cells, and bushy multipolar cells (Brawer et al., 1974). Although attempts have been made to correlate the types seen in Nissl and Golgi material, they have not been entirely satisfactory, since, unlike the neuronal types discussed in the previous section, these cell types are not uniquely definable on the basis of their Nissl pattern alone. Moreover, even though size has been used to classify the cells, in general, it is still not clear from one study to the next if comparable populations of cells have been defined. For simplicity, in the following discussion, all of these cells will be referred to as multipolar cells to distinguish them from those neurons discussed in the previous section. The term is fairly descriptive of the appearance in Nissl-stained material of most of these cells, from the smallest to the very largest, although some do appear to be more fusiform or bipolar in shape.

Measurements. There is some indication that multipolar cells of various sizes may be distributed differentially throughout the cochlear nuclear complex (Osen, 1969a), but no quantitative data have been available. We tried to see if classes among the multipolar cells could be more clearly specified, using not only their Nissl-staining patterns but also quantitative information about their size relative to their locations. We therefore made measurements of the cross-sectional area of all multipolar neurons in nine evenly spaced horizontal sections through the cochlear nuclear complex. The locations of all neurons in the nine sections were mapped onto drawings of the sections at a magnification of approximately 100 ×. Then every neuron with an intact nucleus was examined under oil immersion. Those cells that could be classified as one of the types discussed in the previous section were identified (e.g., Figure 11-5), and the profiles of all remaining neurons – the multipolar cells – were drawn and their areas measured with a digital planimeter. The data were organized and analyzed with the use of a computer program available through the Duke University Computing Center (Statistical Analysis System, SAS Institute, Inc.).

Results of the measurements are summarized in Figure 11-4 and the locations of neurons of various sizes in three of the nine sections are illustrated in Figures 11-6 and 11-7. Note that in these figures the cells are divided into four arbitrary size categories for the purposes of illustration. Typical examples of cells within each size group are shown in Figure 11-8. The rationale for suggesting that there are at least four size groups is discussed below, but, unfortunately, it has not proved feasible to define neuronal types on the basis of size alone. The histograms clearly show overlap in cell sizes.

Comparisons of various parts of the nucleus show some marked differences in the sizes of the multipolar cells in different regions (Figure 11-4). On this basis, three main areas stand out. The DCN contains, for the most part, cells of the smallest size group. The AVCN-A and the small cell cap contain small cells and also numerous medium-sized cells. The AVCN-P and anterior PVCN, meeting at the entrance of the cochlear nerve root, contain both small and medium-sized cells and also a population of large cells found only rarely in other parts of the nucleus. Each of these areas is discussed, in turn, in the following paragraphs.

Dorsal cochlear nucleus. As expected, the multipolar neurons in DCN are quite small. In the Nissl preparations, almost all of these cells have the appearance of typical small cells with a highly infolded nuclear envelope and a scant perikaryon so that the nuclear envelope rests very close to the external membrane of the cell (Figure 11-8). Some of the larger neurons of this group have a markedly different appearance: the nuclear envelope is rounder and the perikaryon is considerably plumper. It is clear, however, from the histogram in Figure 11-4 that it is not possible to distinguish two types based on size alone, and, while the Nissl appearance at the two extremes is quite clear, there are many cases in which it would be difficult to place a neuron into one group or another. Thus, while a hint exists that this is not a completely homogeneous population of small cells, we have no good basis at present for definitively subdividing the group in Nissl-stained material.

In Golgi material, on the other hand, several morphologically distinct types of small cells are obvious. Lorente de Nó (1933a) and Brawer and associates (1974) defined at least three types. One of these – the cartwheel neuron – appears to be found only in the superficial layer. The cartwheel cells (Figure 11-3, *3*) have several short dendrites which, after branching, curve back toward the cell soma. The dendrites are typically covered with spines. The other two types of small cells – small stellate and small elongate neurons – are found throughout the dorsal cochlear nucleus (Brawer et al., 1974). A small stellate cell is illustrated in Figure 11-3 *(4)*. Both of these small cell types have long thin dendrites that bear a few appendages along their course. The small elongate cells may have a slightly larger and more elongated soma than the small stellate cells. One or more of these cell types could correspond to the small cells referred to as "golgi cells" by Mugnaini and associates (1980a), or it may be that the golgi cell is a fourth type of cell that is not readily impregnated in adult

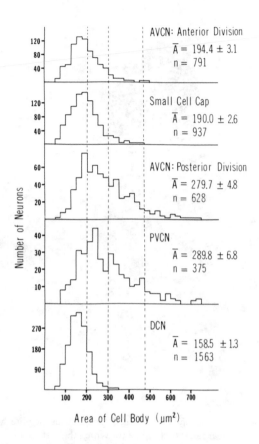

Figure 11-4. *Histograms that illustrate the distribution of cell areas (in micrometers squared) in five parts of the cochlear nuclear complex.* Nine evenly spaced horizontal sections through the cochlear nucleus were traced at a magnification of 100 × and the location of every neuron with an intact nucleus, mapped. Each neuron was then examined under oil immersion (63 × Neofluar lens, N.A. 1.25). Cells in the following categories were identified as described in the text: spherical bushy cells, globular bushy cells, octopus cells, fusiform cells, giant cells of the dorsal cochlear nucleus, and granule cells. The locations of these cells (except the granule cells) were plotted, as shown in Figure 11-5. All of the remaining cells – the multipolar cells – were drawn, and their areas were measured with a digital planimeter. The data were organized by subdivisions and the histograms were generated by a computer program. The dashed lines on the figure show the cut-off points arbitrarily selected for illustration of the distribution of cell sizes shown in Figures 11-6 and 11-7. A, average area ±SEM; n, total number of neurons measured. The mean for DCN is significantly less than those for the anterior division of AVCN and for the small cell cap. The latter means are, in turn, significantly less than those for the posterior division of AVCN and for PVCN.

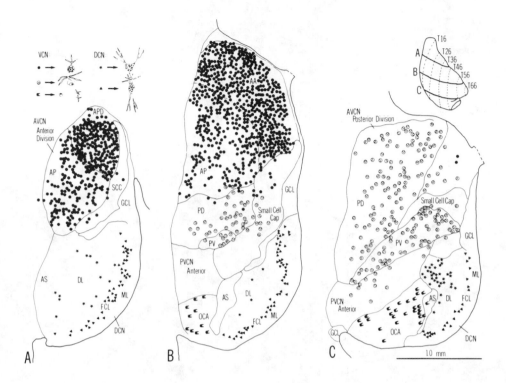

Figure 11-5. *Distribution of qualitatively definable cell types.* Three of nine horizontal sections
through the cochlear nuclear complex for which the distributions of cell types were
plotted (see Figure 11-4 and text). Rostral is toward the top of the figure; lateral,
to the right. The approximate locations of these three sections are indicated in the
inset drawing of the complex. On the inset, the numbers and dashed lines indicate
the location of transverse sections in the block model atlas of Kiang and associates
(1975), T16 being the most rostral. Symbols for cell types: (•), spherical bushy cells;
(⊙), globular bushy cells; (⊂), octopus cells; (▲), fusiform cells; (★), giant cells of
the dorsal cochlear nucleus. Abbreviations for this and the next two figures: AVCN,
anteroventral cochlear nucleus; APD, posterodorsal part of the anterior division
of AVCN, AP, posterior part of the anterior division of AVCN; AA, anterior part
of the anterior division of AVCN; SCC, small cell cap: GCL, granule cell layer; PD,
dorsal part of the posterior division of AVCN; PV, ventral part of the posterior division of AVCN; DCN, dorsal cochlear nucleus; ML, molecular layer of DCN; FCL,
fusiform cell layer of DCN; DL, deep layers of DCN; AS, acoustic striae; PVCN,
posteroventral cochlear nucleus; OCA, octopus cell area.

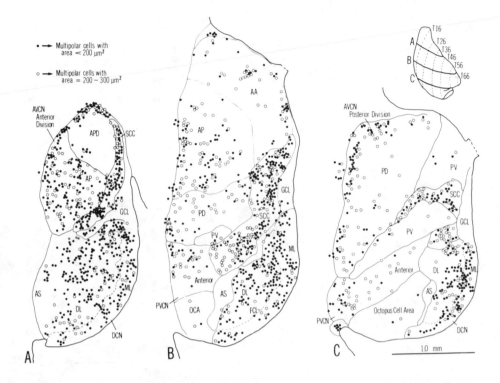

Figure 11-6. *Distribution of small and medium-sized multipolar cells.* Horizontal sections through the cochlear nuclear complex are as shown in Figure 11-5. Symbols: (•), multipolar cells with area less than 200 μm^2; (o), multipolar cells with area 200–300 μm^2.

animals. The difficulty in establishing a correspondence between small cell types in Nissl and Golgi material renders study of each cell type with the electron microscope more difficult.

   Anterior division of AVCN and the small cell cap. Although the small cell population of DCN appears to be morphologically heterogeneous, the range of cell sizes is relatively restricted (Figure 11-4). If we arbitrarily define cells in this size range as "small cells," how do cell sizes in other parts of the cochlear nucleus compare? The AVCN-A and the small cell cap, when compared to each other, have almost identical multipolar cell populations in terms of their size (Figure 11-4) and Nissl-staining patterns (Figure 11-8). The mean area of the cells in AVCN-A is not significantly different, statistically, from that of the cells in the small cell cap. However, the mean areas in these two regions are significantly greater than that of the cells in the DCN. Therefore, it seems reasonable to suggest that these regions contain populations of neurons not appropriately referred to as small cells, if the small cell

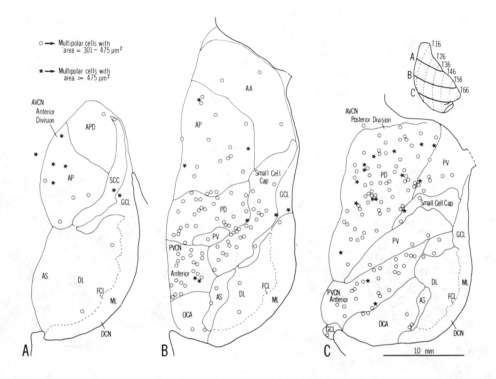

Figure 11-7. *Distribution of large and giant multipolar cells.* Horizontal sections through the cochlear nuclear complex are as shown in Figure 11-5. Symbols: (o), multipolar cells with area 301–475 μm²; (★), multipolar cells with area greater than 475 μm².

of DCN is taken as the standard. On the other hand, since the population on the whole is significantly smaller than that found in the more caudal parts of the ventral cochlear nucleus (Figure 11-4, discussed below), we shall refer to the larger multipolar cells in AVCN-A and the small cell cap as medium-sized cells. It has previously been shown that the larger of the multipolar (or "ovoid") neurons in the anterior division overlap in size to a certain extent with the spherical cells (when average diameter of the neuron is used as an index of size; Cant & Morest, 1979a). Although Nissl-staining patterns of the smallest and largest multipolar cells are clearly different (Cant & Morest, 1979a; Figure 11-8), the intermediate types are difficult to classify on the basis of Nissl pattern and/or size, since there is considerable overlap. Furthermore, the distributions of cells of particular sizes within the anterior division are not sufficiently different to permit a classification of two (or more) populations, although the smallest cells do tend to be concentrated along the extreme margins of the nucleus (Figure 11-6). Additional criteria, such as information about the synaptic organization

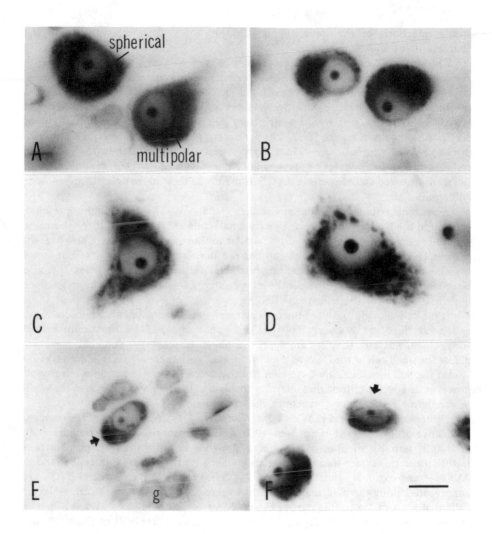

Figure 11-8. *Examples of multipolar cells of various sizes in the cochlear nuclear complex.* (A) A medium-sized multipolar cell and a spherical cell in the anterior division of the anteroventral cochlear nucleus. (B) Medium-sized multipolar cells in the small cell cap. (C) Large multipolar cell in the posterior division of the anteroventral cochlear nucleus. (D) Giant cell in the region of the cochlear nerve root. (E) Small cell (arrow) in the dorsal cochlear nucleus surrounded by granule cells. (F) Small cell (arrow) in the small cell cap. Cresyl violet stain; Bar = 10 μm.

and connections of the neurons, may aid in more definitely specifying the characteristics of each group.

The small and medium-sized multipolar cells of AVCN-A have been shown to correspond to the small and stellate cell types of Golgi preparations (Cant & Morest, 1979a). The distinction between small and stellate cells in Golgi preparations has been mainly on the basis of size. In Nissl preparations, a distinction between size groups in the histograms would be arbitrary (Figure 11-4). A typical stellate cell of AVCN-A is shown in Figure 11-1A. These neurons have long, relatively smooth dendrites, some of which may end in a fairly complex tuft of appendages. The small cells are similar in appearance to the small stellate cells of the DCN and differ from the medium-sized stellate cells in AVCN-A mainly in their more delicate appearance and smaller size.

A neuronal population essentially similar to that of AVCN-A is found in the small cell cap in the Nissl preparations. Typical small cells are prominent throughout the cap, but many medium-sized neurons, similar to those in AVCN-A, are also present (Figure 11-8). Since the small cell cap has not been studied in any detail, it is not possible to make suggestions regarding further classifications of cell types. It would be of interest to determine whether the morphology of the cells in Golgi impregnations is similar to that of the cells of AVCN-A.

It is likely that almost all of the cells referred to here as small and medium-sized cells were classified by Osen (1969a) as small cells since, in the total population of the cochlear nucleus, they are among the smallest. However, as stated above, if we define the small cell of the DCN as the typical small cell, there are cells in both AVCN-A and the small cell cap that are significantly larger. It is not possible at present, however, to specify criteria that unambiguously assign any given neuron to the small or medium-sized category, except at the extremes.

Posterior division of AVCN and anterior part of PVCN. The part of the cochlear nuclear complex referred to by Osen (1970) as the central region also contains small cells and, perhaps, medium-sized cells, although overlap in the histograms makes it difficult to be certain that the population of medium-sized stellate cells found in AVCN-A also extends caudally. The smaller cells in AVCN-P and rostral PVCN are congregated along the margins and are thus segregated in large part from the larger cells that are unique to this part of the cochlear nucleus (Figures 11-6, 11-7). The large cells, which undoubtedly correspond to the multipolar cells of Osen (1969a), are found in the interior of the nucleus where they are intermingled with the globular cells (Figures 11-5, 11-6, 11-7). Tolbert and Morest (1982a) demonstrated that the large multipolar cells probably correspond to the stellate and elongate cells in that region. Small cells and small stellate cells were observed in AVCN-P also and, therefore, in both Golgi and Nissl preparations, there appears to be a continuum in size from the small cells to the large multipolar cells. Clarification of exactly how many cell types are present awaits further study. For example, the critical distinction between stellate cells and elongate cells has not been established (Tolbert & Morest, 1982a). Stellate and elongate cells of AVCN-P are illustrated in Figure 11-2 *(2, 3)*. Although they resemble the stellate cells of AVCN-A in some respects, many of the stellate and elongate cells in AVCN-P are considerably larger. In general, the cell bodies give rise to relatively smooth dendrites that branch only a few times and may extend for considerable distances (Tolbert & Morest, 1982a).

The correspondence of the multipolar cells with cell types defined in the rostral PVCN in Golgi preparations is still not completely clear. This part of the cochlear nucleus of the cat has not been studied in the same detail as AVCN and is an important area for future investigation.

There are a very few large, or giant, neurons in AVCN-P and anterior PVCN that are also found more anteriorly. Both Osen (1969a) and Brawer and associates (1974) recognized giant neurons as a distinct group. Not only are they considerably larger than the other neurons present, their nucleus is also relatively very large (Osen, 1969a), so that these cells stand out even in a qualitative survey of the ventral cochlear nucleus. The giant cells are found in every part of the ventral cochlear nucleus, although there may be a concentration of them in the dorsal region of the cochlear nerve root (Figure 11-7). Very large cells, distributed sparsely throughout the ventral cochlear nucleus, project to the cochlear nucleus of the opposite side (Cant & Gaston, 1982; see below), suggesting that the giant cells may actually represent a separate functional class.

One's confidence in classifications of cell types developed and refined as discussed above is considerably strengthened when differences in other features reasonably considered to be relevant to the function of the cells can be correlated with the cell types. As detailed in the following sections, major areas of investigation along these lines have been in studies of differences in afferent input to and synaptic organization of the neurons in the cochlear nucleus and in studies of the efferent projections of particular cell types.

AFFERENT INPUT TO THE COCHLEAR NUCLEAR COMPLEX: LIGHT MICROSCOPIC STUDIES

Cochlear Fibers

The structure and organization of the central axonal processes of spiral ganglion cells have been described in rapid Golgi preparations (Brawer & Morest, 1975; Feldman & Harrison, 1969; Held, 1893; Koelliker, 1896; Lorente de Nó, 1933a,b; 1976; 1981; Ramón y Cajal, 1909), and in experimental studies (Cohen, Brawer, & Morest, 1972; Jones & Casseday, 1979a; Lewy & Kobrak, 1936; Osen, 1970; Powell & Cowan, 1962; Sando, 1965; van Noort, 1969). The cochlear nerve projects to all parts of the cochlear nucleus except for certain parts of the external granule cell layer. It projects most heavily to the ventral cochlear nucleus but contributes only a fraction of the endings in DCN (Rasmussen, 1957). The cochlear nerve fibers enter the ventral cochlear nucleus, dividing it into anterior and posterior parts. Most, but not necessarily all, of the fibers bifurcate in the entrance zone into ascending and descending branches (Figures 11-9, 11-10). As a rule, the descending branches of the cochlear nerve root

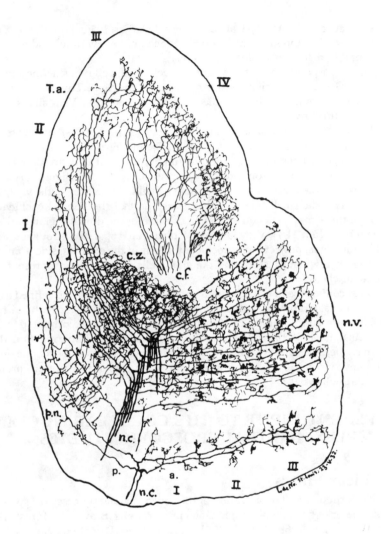

Figure 11-9. *Parasagittal section through the cochlear nucleus of a 4-day-old cat.* Cochlear nerve
fibers (n.c.) bifurcate into anterior (a) and posterior (p) branches. The anterior
branches cross through three regions (I, II, III) of the anteroventral cochlear nucleus
(n.v.). The posterior branches cross through the posteroventral cochlear nucleus
(p.n.), where they form collaterals, to end in the dorsal cochlear nucleus (T.a.).
Abbreviations: a.f., association fibers connecting the dorsal and ventral nuclei; c.f.,
centrifugal fibers ending in the cortex of the T.a.; c.z., confluence zone. Rapid Golgi
method. From Lorente de Nó, 1981.

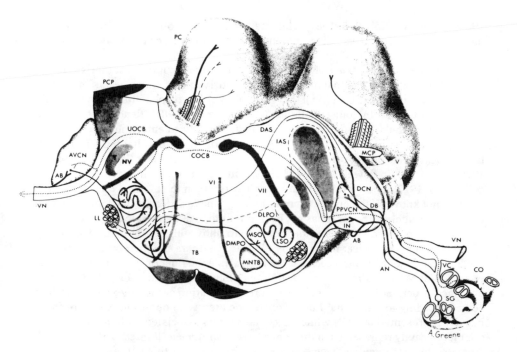

Figure 11-10. *Wiring diagram of some of the principal connections of the bulbar auditory nuclei.*
Although the cochlear nerve is represented as a single channel, in fact it contains
at least two populations of spiral ganglion cells innervating inner and outer hair
cells separately (Dunn, 1975; Dunn & Morest, 1975; Ginzberg & Morest, 1983;
Perkins & Morest, 1975). AB, ascending branch of cochlear nerve; AN, cochlear
nerve; AVCN, anteroventral cochlear nucleus; CO, cochlea; COCB, crossed olivocochlear bundle; CP, cerebral peduncle; DAS, dorsal acoustic stria; DB, descending
branch of cochlear nerve; DCN, dorsal cochlear nucleus; IAS, intermediate acoustic
stria; IN, posteroventral part of AVCN; LL, lateral lemniscus; LSO, lateral superior
olive; MCP, middle cerebellar peduncle; MNTB, medial trapezoid nucleus; MSO,
medial superior olive; PC, inferior colliculus; PCP, inferior cerebellar peduncle;
PPVCN, posteroventral cochlear nucleus; SG, spiral ganglion; TB, trapezoid body;
TNV, descending trigeminal tract and nucleus; UOCB, uncrossed olivocochlear
bundle; VC, vestibulocochlear anastomosis; VN, vestibular nerve; V, trigeminal
nerve root; VI, abducens nerve root and nucleus; VII, facial nerve foot.

are a little thinner than the ascending branches, although the latter are usually shorter.
Some of the root fibers may not form ascending branches or only very short ones
ending near the point of bifurcation. As the ascending fibers course through AVCN,
they give rise to numerous collateral branches that end in small end-bulbs or boutons
in the posterior division and as very large end-bulbs in the anterior division. The
ascending branch of an individual fiber may form branches and terminals in all subdivisions of AVCN or in only one or two (Brawer & Morest, 1975; Feldman & Harrison,

1969; Lorente de Nó, 1976, 1981). The small cell cap is probably not entered by the main segments of the ascending branches but appears rather to receive collaterals from them (Osen, 1970).

The descending branches of the cochlear nerve fibers course posteriorly through PVCN, forming branches that arborize into extensive pericellular nests. The lateral part (in particular, the small cell cap – see above) is not penetrated by the main branches but rather by long collaterals (Lorente de Nó, 1981). Reaching the caudal pole of the nucleus, cochlear nerve fibers turn dorsally to enter the deep layers of DCN where they arborize extensively. Most authors maintain that the terminals of the cochlear fibers do not penetrate beyond the fusiform cell layer (Jones & Casseday, 1979a; Osen, 1970; Powell & Cowan, 1962; van Noort, 1969); however, Cohen and colleagues (1972) report a few primary cochlear fibers in the molecular layer as well.

It is not known if the outer and inner hair cells have different connections within the cochlear nucleus. So far it has not been possible to demonstrate such differences qualitatively; however, there is evidence for quantitative differences in the distribution of fine and coarse cochlear nerve axons. The largest fibers and their branches project predominantly to the ventral cochlear nucleus, while the finer ones favor DCN (Cohen et al., 1972; Morest, 1981; Morest & Bohne, 1983; Rasmussen, 1960). There is also evidence, albeit indirect, for a differential representation of the inner and outer hair cells, according to which the finer axons associated with outer hair cells are more heavily represented in DCN while the coarser fibers associated with inner hair cells are more heavily represented in the ventral cochlear nucleus (Morest & Bohne, 1983). (See also the arguments advanced by Kim, chapter 7, in this volume.)

Golgi studies suggest that the distribution of individual cochlear nerve fibers within the cochlear nuclear complex is orderly (Figure 11-9), and the results of experimental studies confirm this (Osen, 1970; Powell & Cowan, 1962; Sando, 1965). Fibers arising from spiral ganglion cells in the apical turn of the cochlea are situated ventrolaterally in both the ventral and dorsal nuclei and those arising in the basal cochlea are situated dorsomedially (Rasmussen, Gacek, McCrane, & Baker, 1960; Sando, 1965). Whether the organization of the collateral branches in the small cell cap is also cochleotopic is not known.

The systematic arrangement of the cochlear axons within the cochlear nucleus forms the anatomical basis for the observation that neurons in the ventral parts of the ventral and dorsal nuclei respond most readily to low-frequency tonal stimulation, whereas those in the dorsal parts respond to high-frequency stimulation (Bourk, 1976; Bourk et al., 1981; Godfrey et al., 1975a,b; Rose, 1960; Rose et al., 1959). At some points in the nucleus, there appear to be deviations from this systematic order, especially in the region of the cochlear nerve root itself (Bourk et al., 1981). The tonotopic organization of DCN and PVCN is still known only in outline, but a detailed map of the tonotopic organization of the AVCN is available (Bourk et al., 1981). The AVCN appears to be arranged in isofrequency laminae in which the fibers from a restricted part of the cochlea are presumed to terminate. Each lamina extends through the entire AVCN in a plane approximately perpendicular to the boundaries of the major divisions of that nucleus. Likewise, van Noort (1969) and Osen (1970) have demonstrated that axons arising from a limited region of the cochlea form sheets of fibers in the cochlear nucleus that slope in a ventromedial direction.

Since fibers from restricted parts of the cochlea project throughout the cochlear nuclear complex, each of the three major divisions of the complex would be expected to contain neurons responsive to the entire relevant tonal spectrum (Rose, 1960; Rose et al., 1959). There is actually only one tonotopic map in the cochlear nucleus formed by the cochlear nerve fibers. On the other hand, there appear to be several different maps with respect to the various groups of neurons sampling the cochlear input. The traverse of the ascending and descending branches across the boundaries of several subdivisions in AVCN and PVCN, respectively, could result in a complete representation of the entire frequency range within each subdivision. In AVCN, at least, this appears to be the case. Both the anterior and posterior divisions of AVCN contain units responsive to all frequencies tested (Bourk et al., 1981). In the AVCN-A, the posterior part (AP) also contains representation of all frequencies, but the anterior (AA) and posterodorsal (APD) parts do not, unless they are considered together (Bourk et al., 1981). Therefore, although the anatomical arrangement of the ascending fibers results in an apparently continuous mapping throughout AVCN, functionally, this arrangement could be considered to result in a number of parallel tonotopic maps with respect to the second-order neurons.

It would be interesting to know if tonotopic maps could be generated by recordings from particular unit types. Within many of the tonotopically organized subdivisions of the ventral cochlear nucleus, there are several cell types, which could be organized differently with respect to the auditory nerve fibers. For example, in AVCN-P, the smaller multipolar cells are found mainly along the margins of the nucleus and so would seem to lie in a different relationship to the cochlear nerve fibers than do the globular and larger multipolar cells. There are deviations from a systematic tonotopic organization in the region of the bifurcations of the cochlear nerve fibers (Bourk et al., 1981). It is possible that the deviant neurons form a separate class of cells intermingled with cell types that are organized tonotopically.

The organization of the auditory nerve fibers within the small cell cap is not known. Recordings in this region reveal progressively changing best frequencies, but in a direction opposite from that of the adjacent parts of the nucleus (Bourk, 1976; Rose, 1960; Rose et al., 1959). Therefore, it might be expected that the collateral input to the small cell cap is organized in an orderly way, although it seems to differ from the basic plan of the rest of the complex.

Noncochlear Fibers

Noncochlear inputs to neurons of the cochlear nuclear complex have been described in rapid Golgi preparations (Cant & Morest, 1978; Feldman & Harrison, 1969; Held, 1893; Lorente de Nó, 1933a, 1976, 1981). Experimental studies have revealed that the main sources of these inputs are the superior olivary complex, the contralateral cochlear nucleus, the nuclei of the lateral lemniscus, and the inferior colliculus (Adams & Warr, 1976; Cant & Gaston, 1982; Conlee & Kane, 1982; Elverland, 1977; Kane, 1976, 1977a,b; Kane & Finn, 1977; Osen & Roth, 1969; Rasmussen,

1960, 1967; Spangler, Henkel, & Cant, 1983; van Noort, 1969). In addition, there are intrinsic fibers interconnecting various parts of the nucleus (Cant & Morest, 1978; Lorente de Nó, 1933a, 1976, 1981; Oliver, 1984; Oliver, Potashner, Jones, & Morest, 1983). The best known are the reciprocal connections between the external granular layer and the molecular layer of DCN, the projections from DCN to AVCN, which probably arise, in part, from the corn cells, and those from AVCN to DCN, which probably arise, in part, from recurrent collaterals of stellate cells.

Projections to the cochlear nucleus from the superior olivary complex arise in all periolivary areas but not from the medial or lateral superior olivary nuclei (Elverland, 1977; Spangler et al., 1983). The heaviest projections arise in the ipsilateral lateral nucleus of the trapezoid body and in both the ipsilateral and contralateral ventral nuclei of the trapezoid body. Inputs from the superior olivary complex are distributed throughout the cochlear nuclear complex (Elverland, 1977; Kane, 1976; Spangler et al., 1983), although the input is not equally dense in all areas. Osen and Roth (1969) present histochemical evidence that acetylcholinesterase-positive axons, arising in the superior olivary complex and traveling with the olivocochlear bundle, project to the granular cell layer.

Projections from the contralateral cochlear nucleus arise from large cells scattered throughout the complex (Cant & Gaston, 1982). Their major sites of termination are the anterior division of AVCN, PVCN, and the superficial layers of DCN, but sparse input is found throughout the cochlear nucleus.

There are a few neurons in the ventrocaudal part of the ventral nucleus of the lateral lemniscus that project to the cochlear nucleus (Adams & Warr, 1976; Spangler et al., 1983). The dorsal nucleus of the lateral lemniscus sends projections to PVCN and DCN of both sides (Conlee & Kane, 1982; Kane & Conlee, 1979; Kane & Finn, 1977). The entire PVCN receives a relatively sparse input (Kane & Conlee, 1979). The projection to the dorsal cochlear nucleus appears to be confined to the fusiform cell layer and deep layers (Conlee & Kane, 1982).

The well-known projections to DCN from the inferior colliculus (Lorente de Nó, 1933a; Rasmussen, 1960, 1964; van Noort, 1969) were described in some detail by Conlee and Kane (1982). They concluded that there is a topographic arrangement of projections from the inferior colliculus to the layers of DCN. All the projections are bilateral. There is also a sparse bilateral projection from the inferior colliculus to PVCN, but a projection to AVCN has not been described.

SYNAPTIC ORGANIZATION OF SPECIFIC NEURONAL TYPES IN THE COCHLEAR NUCLEAR COMPLEX: ELECTRON MICROSCOPIC STUDIES

Anterior Division of the Anteroventral Cochlear Nucleus

Spherical bushy cells. Neurons in AVCN-A of cats and other species have been the subject of several electron microscopic studies (Cant & Morest, 1979b; Gentschev

& Sotelo, 1973; Ibata & Pappas, 1976; Lenn & Reese, 1966; McDonald & Rasmussen, 1971; Schwartz & Gulley, 1978; Sotelo, Gentschev, & Zamora, 1976). It is likely that most of the cells described in these studies were the spherical bushy cells, although exact correlations with cell types defined in the light microscope were not always made. To be sure that their sample was restricted to the spherical bushy cells, Cant and Morest (1979b) identified the cell types in the electron microscope based on their location and appearance in the light microscope. Because part of AVCN-A contains only this cell type, they could describe the synaptic organization of both the cell soma and dendrites.

At least 70% (usually more) of the somatic surface of the bushy cells is contacted by synaptic terminals (Cant, 1981), including the end-bulbs of Held, which attain their largest size in this part of the nucleus. Each end-bulb forms multiple small synaptic contacts with the somatic surface. The fine structure of the cochlear endings is similar throughout the cochlear nuclear complex (Cant & Morest, 1979b; Kane, 1973, 1974; Lenn & Reese, 1966; Tolbert & Morest, 1982b), although, as is obvious from Golgi studies, the size of the terminals varies greatly. Synaptic terminals arising from cochlear axons contain large, round synaptic vesicles rather loosely scattered about in the ending (Figure 11-11). The synaptic contact is short, and usually the postsynaptic surfaces and the associated densities arch slightly toward the terminal. In the anterior division of AVCN, at least, it appears that all terminals of this type disappear after cochlear ablation (Cant & Morest, 1979b). The proximal dendrites and their bushy appendages are also contacted by inputs from the cochlea, either processes of the end-bulb or boutons arising from collateral branches. Much of the surfaces of the soma and proximal dendrites also form synapses with terminals that survive cochlear ablation. These noncochlear terminals can be distinguished from the cochlear inputs by the distinctly smaller size of their synaptic vesicles (Figure 11-11; Cant & Morest, 1979b; Ibata & Pappas, 1976; Lenn & Reese, 1966; McDonald & Rasmussen, 1971; Schwartz & Gulley, 1978). Cant & Morest (1979b) identified at least three groups based on the shape of the synaptic vesicles, finding terminals with flattened, pleomorphic, or, rarely, small spherical vesicles. The sources of the individual noncochlear terminal types have not been demonstrated, but the possibilities include other parts of the cochlear nucleus, the contralateral cochlear nucleus, a number of periolivary cell groups, and the ventral nucleus of the lateral lemniscus.

The bushy dendritic appendages characteristic of spherical bushy cells appear to be contacted by relatively few terminals (Cant & Morest, 1979b), so that the physiological responses of this cell type should primarily reflect the organization of inputs on the somatic surface and the proximal dendrite(s).

Stellate cells. Cant (1981) concluded that the larger multipolar, or stellate, cells in AVCN-A are represented by two groups of cells in the electron microscope. The cells of the first group – the type I stellate cells – must receive most of their synaptic inputs on their dendrites, since usually less than 30% of their somatic surface receives synaptic contacts. These few contacts on the somatic surface and the many contacts on the proximal dendrites are similar to those on the bushy cells, including cochlear endings with their characteristic large, spherical vesicles as well as inputs from other sources (Figure 11-11). The cochlear endings are never as large as end-bulbs, so they probably correspond to the boutons that arise from cochlear nerve fibers. Whether the noncochlear sources of input to the type I stellate cells are the same as for the bushy cells remains to be determined, but the fine structure of the noncochlear terminals is similar (Figure 11-11).

The neurons in the second group of stellate cells – the type II stellate cells – are apposed by endings covering at least 70% of the cell surface. Dense clusters of terminals also form synapses with the dendrites as far as they can be followed from the soma. Thus activity in these neurons reflects the interplay of the inputs to both the dendrites and the soma. Like the other cell types in AVCN-A, these neurons receive both cochlear and noncochlear inputs, although the fine structure of one of the noncochlear inputs is different from that of any of those on the other cell types (Cant, 1981). It does not appear that type II stellate cells receive their cochlear input from end-bulbs, although definitive studies with serial sections are not available.

Small cells. The smallest cells in the anterior division, like those in the rest of the ventral cochlear nucleus, have not been studied in any detail in the electron microscope. The typical small cell with scant, pale perikaryoplasm and a highly infolded nucleus is present, especially around the margins of this region. Further study with the electron microscope should shed light on the cytological distinctions among the small cells and stellate cells.

Posterior Division of the Anteroventral Cochlear Nucleus

Globular bushy cells. The fine structure of globular bushy cells has been described by Tolbert and Morest (1982b), who identified them in electron micrographs by comparing their characteristic features in the light and electron microscopes. Globular cells are distinguished from other cell types by the relatively abundant free polyribosomes throughout the perikaryon and by the absence of complex arrays of granular endoplasmic reticulum. An average of 83% of the somatic and proximal dendritic surface is apposed by synaptic terminals, which appear to be of the same types identified in AVCN-A (Figure 11-11). The small end-bulbs described in this region in Golgi material appear in the electron microscope as large endings with large, spherical vesicles that form multiple synaptic contacts. Therefore, the fine structure of these cochlear afferent terminals is the same as that seen in the anterior division and in other parts of the nucleus (see below). About 40% of the terminals contacting the globular bushy cell soma and proximal dendrites have smaller vesicles and, since they remain unchanged after cochlear ablation, appear to be of noncochlear origin. These noncochlear terminals are of at least two morphological types (Figure 11-11). The distal dendritic appendages of the globular cells have not been described, and the nature of their input is not known.

Stellate and elongate cells. At least some of the stellate cells in AVCN-P are considerably larger than those in AVCN-A. Tolbert & Morest (1982b) demonstrated that these large cells correspond to the multipolar cells described by Osen (1969a).

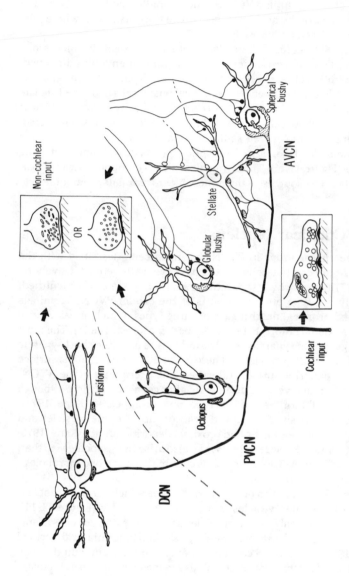

Figure 11-11. *Schematic illustration of the afferent connections and synaptic organization of several cell types in the anteroventral (AVCN), posteroventral (PVCN), and dorsal (DCN) cochlear nuclei.* Cochlear fibers bifurcate and the branches form terminals throughout the nucleus. Cochlear terminals (stippled) contact spherical bushy cells, globular bushy cells, and stellate cells in AVCN, octopus cells in PVCN, and fusiform cells in DCN. Cochlear terminals vary in size but generally contain large round synaptic vesicles and make multiple, short, asymmetric contacts with the postsynaptic surface (lower inset). Terminals of noncochlear fibers (filled or clear boutons on the cell bodies and dendrites) usually contain highly flattened synaptic vesicles (top terminal in upper inset) or small pleiomorphic vesicles (bottom terminal in upper inset). Both types form nearly symmetric contacts with the postsynaptic surfaces. A rarer type of noncochlear terminal contains small, round vesicles and makes asymmetric contacts (not illustrated).

Although they have not been described in detail, smaller stellate cells, perhaps like those in AVCN-A, are also present in AVCN-P. These smaller stellate cells tend to congregate along the margins of the nucleus, especially in the dorsal part, where they mingle with the true small cells (Figures 11-6, 11-7).

Tolbert & Morest (1982b) defined the stellate cells in the electron microscope on the basis of their very large and prominent stacks of granular endoplasmic reticulum. The synaptic organization of these cells is quite different from that of the globular cells, the differences paralleling those between spherical bushy cells and type I stellate cells in AVCN-A (Cant, 1981; Cant & Morest, 1979b). Specifically, less than 15% of the somatic surface of the stellate cells is apposed by synaptic terminals. The axosomatic terminals that are present, as well as the more abundant terminals forming synapses with the proximal dendrites, are of the same types as those found contacting the globular bushy cells (Figure 11-11). The terminals with large, round vesicles apparently arise in the cochlea. The sources of the noncochlear terminals are not known.

Posteroventral Cochlear Nucleus

Octopus cells. The only neurons in PVCN that have been described with the electron microscope are the octopus cells, which have been studied extensively by Kane (1973, 1974b, 1977a; also Schwartz & Kane, 1977). They are easily identified, since they are the only cell type present in parts of the caudal PVCN. Terminals contacting the soma and proximal dendrite are of three types, which are similar to those seen in the AVCN (Cant & Morest, 1979b; Tolbert & Morest, 1982b). The most numerous type has large, round synaptic vesicles and makes multiple short synaptic contacts with the octopus cell (Figure 11-11). These cover 50% of the somatic surface and 70% of the proximal dendritic surface. Like the similar terminals in the AVCN, these terminals with large, round vesicles degenerate after cochlear ablation, although at 4 days after surgery not all terminals of this type have disappeared (Kane, 1973). A second type of terminal has small, round to oval, or pleomorphic, vesicles and contacts approximately 15% of the somatic and proximal dendritic surface. Kane (1973) presents evidence that some of these terminals may also arise in the cochlea, so that, unlike the cells so far studied in AVCN, the octopus cells may receive two morphologically different types of inputs from the cochlea.

One type of axosomatic terminal on octopus cells, a type which survives cochlear ablation, contains small, flattened vesicles and is relatively sparse (Figure 11-11). Another type of terminal, found only on the distal dendrites of the octopus cells (Kane, 1977a), contains small, spherical vesicles. These are similar to terminals described by Cant and Morest (1979b, their SV-S category) that terminate mainly on the dendrites of spherical bushy cells. After very large lesions are made in the superior olivary complex, degeneration in the ipsilateral octopus cell area is mainly confined to the terminals on the distal dendrites, whereas in the contralateral octopus cell area, the somatic terminals with small, flattened vesicles appear to undergo degenerative changes (Kane, 1977a). The exact sources of these terminals are not known, but some areas that appear to have a major input to the octopus cell area are the contralateral cochlear nucleus (Cant & Gaston, 1982) and the ipsilateral posterior periolivary nucleus (Spangler et al., 1983).

Dorsal Cochlear Nucleus

Fusiform cells (Figure 11-12). The fine structure of fusiform cells, which can be easily identified in the electron microscope because of their location in a distinct layer and their relatively large size, has been described by Kane (1974a,b, 1977b; Kane & Habib, 1978). Synaptic terminals cover the somatic surface and the proximal portions of the apical and basal dendrites. At least eight types of synaptic terminals have been distinguished in the fusiform cell layer (Kane, 1977b), but not all of them are known to contact fusiform cells.

The cochlear input to the fusiform cells is morphologically similar to that in the rest of the cochlear nuclear complex (Figure 11-11), the terminals being characterized by large, round synaptic vesicles and forming multiple short synaptic complexes with the soma and proximal dendrites (Kane, 1974a). Three types of terminals with flattened vesicles make up the noncochlear input to the soma and proximal dendrites (Kane, 1974a, 1977b). After very large lesions of the contralateral superior olivary complex or of the contralateral inferior colliculus, some of these terminals with flattened vesicles degenerate (Kane, 1977b), indicating that some of the noncochlear input to the fusiform cells is from these sources. No differences between the types of terminals on the proximal portions of the apical and basal dendrites have been reported, although light microscopic studies would suggest that their sources of input are different (e.g., Jones & Casseday, 1979b).

Rapid Golgi studies of the three types of small cells in DCN led to the conclusion that axons of all three types might form contacts with fusiform cells (Kane, 1974a; Lorente de Nó, 1933a), but the terminals have not been identified in the electron microscope.

Small cells. The fine structure of the small cells of DCN has been studied by Kane (1974a,b, 1977b) and by Mugnaini and associates (1980b). In general, types of small cells have not been distinguished in the electron microscope, although Mugnaini and co-workers (1980b) have used the term "golgi cells" for small neurons that are intermingled with the granule cells in the molecular layer. They are easily distinguished from granule cells but have not been clearly distinguished from the types of small cells described by Brawer and associates (1974). These neurons have the typical lobulated nucleus of the small cells, and the somatic surface is highly irregular with bulges and depressions, which are the sites of contacts with very large endings presumably belonging to mossy fibers (Mugnaini et al., 1980b). These endings (type Ia of Kane, 1974a) contain small, round vesicles and form multiple synaptic contacts with the cell soma and dendrites.

The small cell dendrites described by Mugnaini and colleagues (1980b) participate in synaptic glomeruli. Their dendrites surround a central large terminal and are also associated with peripherally located boutons with pleomorphic vesicles. A similar, but somewhat different account has been given for the fusiform cell layer (Kane, 1974a,b). The source of the mossy fiber terminals is not known, although Kane (1974b) suggests, on the basis of degeneration studies, that some type 1a fibers reaching the fusiform cell layer are of cochlear origin. Kane (1974a,b) has presented evidence that small cells receive input from the cochlea and also that they receive inputs from the superior olivary complex (Kane, 1977b), although the exact source is unknown.

Giant cells. Only one study of the synaptic organization of the giant cells of DCN is available (Kane et al., 1981). These authors described five types of giant cells and noted some differences in the arrangement of synaptic inputs on the surface of each type. The proximal dendrites of all five kinds of giant cell are contacted by synaptic inputs. The distal dendrites were not studied. The elongate multipolar cells and radiate cells receive many somatic inputs as well. Although the sources of the inputs were not established, Kane and associates (1981) noted that one type of terminal resembles the cochlear inputs to the fusiform cells. This type, with large, round synaptic vesicles, forms contacts with all types of giant cells, but light microscopic observations of axons degenerating after cochlear ablation give the impression that the pattern of distribution of cochlear inputs is different on each type (Kane et al., 1981).

Granule cells. Some aspects of the fine structure of granule cells have been described by Kane (1974a) in the fusiform cell layer and by Mugnaini and associates (1980b) in the molecular layer. The soma and proximal portion of the dendrite receive a few synapses and the boutons contacting them may have either round or pleomorphic vesicles. At some distance from the cell soma the dendrites enter the complex synaptic structures known as glomeruli, so called because of their resemblance to similar structures in the cerebellum. In the center of the glomerulus, a large terminal with round synaptic vesicles makes contacts with the dendrites of many granule cells. Smaller boutons with pleomorphic vesicles make contacts with the granule cell dendrites in the periphery of the glomerulus. The sources of the inputs to the glomeruli are not known, but the small peripheral terminals might arise from the axons of small cells that are intermingled with the granule cells. There may be several sources of mossy fibers, including collaterals of the olivocochlear bundle.

Other Parts of the Cochlear Nuclear Complex

No electron microscopic studies are yet available of the small cell cap of the ventral cochlear nucleus (Osen, 1969a). It would be of interest to compare the synaptic organization of the cells in this region with that of the stellate and small cells of AVCN-A since, based on the measurements presented in an earlier section and on their Nissl-staining patterns, these cell populations are indistinguishable. However, some differences might be expected, as the different locations of the cells would expose them to different synaptic inputs.

Another region that has not yet been studied in any detail is the anterior part of PVCN which contains several cell types that are unique to this part of the ventral cochlear nucleus (Brawer et al., 1974).

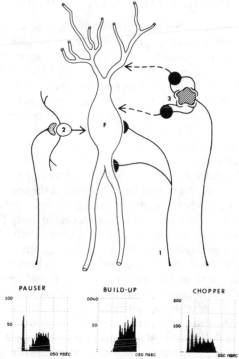

Figure 11-12. *Schematic of some of the principal inputs to the fusiform cells (F) in the dorsal cochlear nucleus.* The fusiform cells receive direct projections from cochlear nerve fibers (1) and an even larger input from interneurons, including small cells (2), some of which are thought to be inhibitory and GABAergic, and granule cells (3), which are thought to be excitatory and glutamatergic. Small cells (2) receive direct projections from cochlear nerve fibers, including axosomatic synapses (stippled ending), and noncochlear sources. Granule cells also receive direct cochlear projections by way of axosomatic and axodendritic synapses. The latter include those of mossy fibers (hatched ending in the fusiform cell layer). However, most of the inputs to the interneurons are noncochlear in origin, including many, if not most, mossy fibers. Typical time-patterns of unit activity following acoustic stimulation recorded in the fusiform cell layer are shown in the poststimulus time histograms, representing number of spikes as a function of time after stimulus onset (short tone bursts at characteristic frequency). Pauser and build-up patterns can be attributed to fusiform cells, the chopper pattern, to small cells, fusiform cells, or even artifactual causes (Godfrey et al., 1975b; Kane 1974a; Rhode et al., 1983a). The initial peak of activity in the pauser pattern could result from the direct excitatory input of cochlear nerve fibers to certain fusiform cells (1), followed with an inhibition generated by small cells (2), which in due course could succumb to the more diffuse and slowly developing excitatory activity elaborated by the granule cells (3). Build-up units would differ primarily in lacking enough direct excitation by auditory nerve fibers to overcome the prevailing inhibition by noncochlear inputs. From Kane, 1974a.

EFFERENT PROJECTIONS OF SPECIFIC CELL TYPES

A series of studies by Warr (1966, 1969, 1972) and by van Noort (1969) established the general patterns of efferent projections from the subdivisions of the cochlear nucleus of the cat, and a detailed review has recently appeared (Warr, 1982). A brief summary is given in Figures 11-10, 11-13, and 11-14. AVCN-A projects to the ipsilateral lateral superior olivary nucleus and anterior part of the lateral nucleus of the trapezoid body. It further projects to the medial superior olivary nucleus, the dorsal and ventral nuclei of the lateral lemniscus, and the central nucleus of the inferior colliculus of both sides (Warr, 1966; van Noort, 1969). In contrast, PVCN projects to the ipsilateral and contralateral periolivary nuclei and to the contralateral ventral nucleus of the lateral lemniscus and central nucleus of the inferior colliculus (Warr, 1969). When lesions of PVCN are made sufficiently large that they encroach on the region of the nerve root, degeneration is also seen in the contralateral medial nucleus of the trapezoid body, where the degenerating fibers terminate in the large calyces of Held, and in the ventral nucleus of the trapezoid body (Warr, 1972). In almost all cases, more than one cell type would have been involved in the lesions, so that it is not possible to obtain information about projections of specific cell types from these experiments. More recent studies, using techniques based on the axonal transport of horseradish peroxidase to label individual cells, have provided some information about projections of certain of the cell types, although in no case have all of the projections of a single cell type been catalogued with certainty.

Spherical bushy cells. Indirect evidence from a number of laboratories has led to the conclusion that the spherical bushy cells project topographically to the ipsilateral lateral superior olivary nucleus and to both medial superior olivary nuclei (Harrison & Warr, 1962; Osen 1969b; Stotler, 1953; van Noort, 1969, Warr, 1966). Small injections of horseradish peroxidase into these nuclei confirm the suggestion that the spherical bushy cells are a main source of their input (Cant & Casseday, unpublished results). Osen (1969b) suggested that the spherical cells formed two populations with the rostrally located "large spherical" cells projecting to the two medial superior olivary nuclei and the more caudal "small spherical" cells projecting to the lateral superior olivary nucleus. However, it is now clear that spherical cells in both the anterior and posterior parts of AVCN-A project to both the medial and lateral superior olivary nuclei (Cant & Casseday, unpublished results, Tolbert et al., 1982; Warr, 1982), although it is not known whether a given neuron projects to both targets.

For the most part, there is no evidence that the spherical bushy cells project to the inferior colliculus (Adams, 1979; Cant, 1982; Roth, Aitkin, Andersen, & Merzenich, 1978), although Adams does report at least one bushy cell labeled after very large injections of horseradish peroxidase into the inferior colliculus. Cells in the rostral AVCN project heavily into the contralateral ventral nucleus of the lateral lemniscus (Glendenning, Brunso-Bechtold, Thompson, & Masterson, 1981; Warr, 1966), but it is not known whether this projection arises in the spherical bushy cells and/or in other cell types.

Globular bushy cells. It has long been suspected that the globular cells of the posterior AVCN are the source of the calyces of Held that form synapses with the principal cells of the contralateral medial nucleus of the trapezoid body (e.g., Harrison & Irving, 1966a,b). Tolbert, Morest, and Yurgelun-Todd (1982) demonstrated this projection by injecting horseradish peroxidase into the medial nucleus of the trapezoid body and observing the subsequent labeling of globular bushy cells. The axons of the fibers that form the calyces also send collateral branches into the dorsomedial periolivary nucleus (Morest, 1968) – so this nucleus also receives inputs from the globular bushy cells.

Other targets of the globular bushy cells, if they exist, are unknown. Roth and associates (1978) report that many globular cells are labeled after horseradish peroxidase injections into the central nucleus of the inferior colliculus, but Adams (1979) reports that few if any globular cells are labeled. This question deserves further study.

Small, medium-sized, and large multipolar cells of the ventral cochlear nucleus. After injections of horseradish peroxidase into the inferior colliculus, neurons throughout the contralateral ventral cochlear nucleus are labeled, as are a few neurons in the ipsilateral ventral cochlear nucleus (Adams, 1979; Roth et al., 1978). In Adams' study, in which some of the labeled cells and their dendrites were heavily filled with reaction product, most of the labeled cells could be identified as stellate or small cells. Both Roth and colleagues and Adams report a tendency for the labeled cells in the AVCN to be arranged in "columns" with intervening rows of unlabeled cells (see also Cant, 1982). A similar tendency is apparent in the distribution of the multipolar cells in the AVCN, as shown in Figures 11-6 and 11-7. For example, in the posterior part of the anterior division (AP), the multipolar cells often occur in groups separated by clusters of spherical bushy cells.

The medium-sized stellate cells of AVCN-A that project to the inferior colliculus correspond to the type I stellate cells defined in electron microscopic studies (Cant, 1981, 1982). The type II stellate cells do not appear to project to the inferior colliculus and their targets are unknown. Smaller cells in the AVCN may also project to the inferior colliculus (Adams, 1979; Cant, 1982). It has not been explicitly stated that cells in the small cell cap project to the inferior colliculus, although it appears from the published figures that some of them probably do (see Adams, 1979).

Stellate cells of the ventral cochlear nucleus are also sometimes labeled after horseradish peroxidase injections in the superior olivary complex (Tolbert et al., 1982), but it is possible that their axons are only passing through the region. The recurrent collaterals of the stellate cells in AVCN-P can be filled retrogradely with horseradish peroxidase following injections in either the trapezoid body (Tolbert et al., 1982) or DCN (Oliver et al., 1983). Thus the stellate cells of AVCN-P contribute to the ventro-tubercular tract of Lorente de Nó (1981).

Octopus cells. Indirect evidence suggests that the main targets of the octopus cells are in the ipsilateral and contralateral periolivary regions (Adams & Warr, 1976; Osen, 1969b; van Noort, 1969; Warr, 1969). The target periolivary nuclei include the posterior periolivary cell group, which has a substantial input back into PVCN (Spangler et al., 1983), and the dorsomedial, dorsolateral, and anterolateral periolivary cell groups. There are conflicting reports as to whether the octopus cells also project to the inferior colliculus (Adams, 1979; Roth et al., 1978).

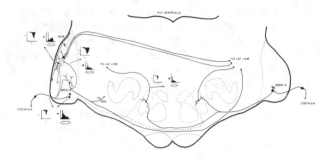

Figure 11-13. *Circuits of cell types and their proposed relation to signal processing in the bulbar auditory pathways: Medial superior olive (MSO) and dorsal cochlear nucleus (DCN).* In AVCN-A (anterior division of the anteroventral cochlear nucleus) each spherical bushy cell receives very large excitatory, axosomatic synaptic endings from one or sometimes two cochlear nerve fibers. The synaptic organization of the spherical bushy cells faithfully preserves both the sharp tuning of individual cochlear nerve fibers, as shown by a typical tuning curve of threshold versus frequency (T vs. F), and the time-pattern of response (primary-like pattern), as shown by a typical peristimulus time histogram (No. of spikes vs. time stimulus envelope) of unit spiking activity as a function of time associated with stimulation by short tone bursts at characteristic frequency. An individual spherical bushy cell projects bilaterally to MSO, synapsing on the homolateral dendrites of the disc-shaped principal cells. The dotted line tracing this projection suggests that a single axon may establish this connection by way of a collateral, although this has not been established for the cat, as it has for the chicken (Jhaveri & Morest, 1982; Young & Rubel, 1983). In MSO this synaptic arrangement would be suitable for binaural interactions dependent on timing differences, while the tuning characteristics and time-pattern of response are being preserved through its projections to the inferior colliculus. The stellate cell of AVCN-A and AVCN-P (posterior division of the anteroventral cochlear nucleus) forms a parallel pathway with that of the spherical bushy cell – MSO principal cell projection, while itself projecting directly to the inferior colliculus. The synaptic organization provides for a transformation of the time-pattern of response from primarylike in the auditory input to the chopper pattern, while preserving fairly well the tuning characteristics of the cochlear nerve. In AVCN-P recurrent collaterals of the stellate axon project to DCN. In DCN, the fusiform cells and giant cells establish parallel pathways projecting directly to the contralateral inferior colliculus, after receiving collateral inputs from the cochlear nerve fibers and the AVCN. The synaptic organization of the fusiform cells, as well as some of the giant cells, can introduce striking transformations in the auditory response properties. The tuning curves tend to be broader and more irregular than those of the primary afferents and the response areas typically are modified by inhibitory zones, while the time patterns of response can produce pauser or build-up or chopper patterns (see Figure 11-12). Granule cells with parallel fibers provide for local circuits, along with small cells, such as the corn cell, which also is thought to project to AVCN. LAT. LEM., lateral lemniscus; SOC, superior olivary complex.

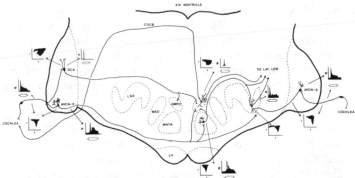

Figure 11-14. *Circuits of cell types and their proposed relation to signal processing in the bulbar auditory pathways: Lateral superior olive (LSO) and crossed olivocochlear bundle (COCB).* In AVCN-P (posterior division of the anteroventral cochlear nucleus), globular bushy cells receive multiple, presumably excitatory synapses from cochlear nerve fibers belonging to spiral ganglion cells innervating hair cells in the cochlea. Although the synaptic organization of the globular bushy cell preserves the sharp tuning of the auditory nerve, as shown by a typical tuning curve (T vs. F), it introduces a slight modification of the time-pattern of response (pri-notch pattern), as shown by typical peristimulus time histograms (No. vs. time stimulus envelope). An individual globular bushy cell projects to the contralateral MNTB (medial nucleus of the trapezoid body) by way of a large excitatory axosomatic calyx that synapses on one, and only one, principal type of neuron – a synaptic arrangement that faithfully preserves the tuning characteristics and time-pattern of response generated by globular bushy cells. Collaterals of the bushy cell axons also project to some, if not all, of the same types of neurons in the contralateral DMPO (dorsomedial periolivary nucleus) that contribute to the COCB. Since some DMPO neurons also project into the lateral lemniscus (TO LAT. LEM.), it remains to be proved that the bushy cell collaterals synapse on the very same cells that project back to the cochlea – where the precise relations of this circuit of cell types to inner and outer hair cells and their respective sensory neurons also remain to be determined. The principal neurons of MNTB also project to DMPO by way of an inhibitory pathway to LSO, a site of intensity-dependent binaural interactions, no doubt involving ipsilateral excitatory projections from spherical bushy cells in AVCN-A (anterior division of AVCN). Of interest would be the mechanism by which the sharply tuned pri-notch input from MNTB and the sharply tuned primary-like input from AVCN-A converge to generate sharply tuned chopper patterns in LSO. These pathways could be construed as parts of a recurrent circuit hypothesized to relate intensity coding to a lateralization function (Tolbert et al., 1982). In OCA (octopus cell area) the octopus cells establish a parallel pathway with the preceding ones, all of which eventually overlap in the DMPO. The synaptic organization of the octopus cell differs from that of the bushy cell and presumably introduces a dramatic signal transformation, reflected by a greatly broadened tuning curve and an onset type of time-pattern. These physiological features are also seen in some of the units in the DMPO, but comparable electrophysiological recordings of COCB neurons are not available.

Giant cells of the ventral cochlear nucleus. Whether or not the giant cells of the ventral cochlear nucleus are among the multipolar cells labeled after injections of horseradish peroxidase into the inferior colliculus has not been established. The giant cells appear to project to the contralateral cochlear nucleus (Cant & Gaston, 1982), since the labeled cells scattered in the contralateral nucleus after horseradish peroxidase injections are relatively very large and their distribution is quite similar to that seen for giant cells (e.g., Figure 11-7).

Fusiform cells of the dorsal cochlear nucleus. The fusiform cells project via the dorsal acoustic stria to the central nucleus of the inferior colliculus (Adams, 1979; Adams & Warr, 1976; Brunso-Bechtold, Thompson, & Masterson, 1981; Osen, 1972; Roth et al., 1978). The projection is mainly contralateral and is topographically organized. There is evidence that the projection is mainly to the medial and central parts of the central nucleus (Brunso-Bechtold et al., 1981; Oliver, 1984). No other target for these neurons has been conclusively demonstrated, but recurrent collaterals exist within DCN (Kane, 1974a; Osen & Morest, unpublished; Rhode, Oertel, & Smith, 1983a). There may be sparse projections from DCN to the nuclei of the lateral lemniscus (Glendenning et al., 1981), but the cell types of origin have not been identified.

Small cells of the dorsal cochlear nucleus. Adams (1979) reports that a few of the small cells in the superficial layers of DCN project to the inferior colliculus. Small cells also send axons to the AVCN (e.g., corn cells of Lorente de Nó, 1933a, 1981, and Brawer et al., 1974), where at least some of them end as baskets around cells of the posterior division (Cant & Morest, 1978). Within DCN itself, small cells appear to form synaptic contacts with fusiform cells (Kane, 1974a) and possibly also with other small cells and granule cells (Mugnaini et al., 1980b).

Giant cells of the dorsal cochlear nucleus. The giant cells project to the inferior colliculus (Adams, 1979; Osen, 1972; Winkler, 1921). Some of them also project to the contralateral cochlear nucleus (Cant & Gaston, 1982). This latter projection may arise from the vertical giant cells (Kane et al., 1981). Other targets of the giant cells, if they exist, have not been definitely demonstrated.

Granule cells. The granule cells, found throughout the cochlear nuclear complex, appear to send axons from the external granular cell layer and deeper layers of DCN into the molecular layer, where they form parallel fibers presumably ending on the apical dendrites of fusiform cells and possibly also other cell types (Brawer et al., 1974; Mugnaini et al., 1980a). Granule cells also form connections in the deeper layers of DCN by way of parallel fibers (Kane, 1974a).

SIGNAL CODING IN THE COCHLEAR NUCLEUS

By signal coding we mean the systematic representation in the CNS of acoustic stimuli. This can be defined in terms of the electrical response patterns of individual neurons to acoustic stimuli. So far it has been possible to describe the response areas, thresholds, latencies, and time-patterns of electrical activity of single units following simple acoustic stimuli in a systematic way in the cochlear nerve and the cochlear nucleus. Unit responses to complex acoustic stimuli can also be characterized (see Sachs, chap. 8), but we shall not attempt to relate the structural basis for these phenomena. Following simple acoustic stimuli, cochlear nerve fibers respond in predictable ways, generally with a sharp tuning curve and a characteristic time-pattern as seen in the peristimulus time histogram. While these response properties have been well characterized for most cochlear nerve fibers, namely, the larger myelinated ones (1–6 μm in diameter in the cat; Arneson & Osen, 1978), it is not yet clear if the smaller axons, including myelinated and unmyelinated ones less than 1μm in diameter, have been fairly represented. This is a question of some theoretical importance, since there is evidence that the smaller axons are more closely linked to the outer hair cells, while the larger ones innervate predominately the inner hair cells. Among the larger ones, three varieties have been described: (1) the giant fibers from the apical turn (Ginzberg & Morest, 1983; Perkins & Morest, 1975; Spoendlin, 1972) and the radial fibers ending on the (2) inner or (3) outer aspects of the inner hair cells (Liberman, 1980). Thus at least two input channels to the cochlear nucleus can be defined anatomically, but we are not certain how the signal coding properties of these channels differ. Be that as it may, it is still useful to ask how the signal codes so far demonstrated in the cochlear nerve are processed in the cochlear nucleus.

The signal transmission properties of the cochlear nucleus are such that the discharge patterns established by the cochlear nerve fibers will be preserved across the synaptic interruptions that occur in the cochlear nucleus, or they will be transformed. Provided that the signal transformations occur in a predictable pattern, one may correlate the transmission properties of the cochlear nucleus with the specific locations and structures in which they occur. There are consistent locations in a number of cases that correlate with certain types of unit responses in particular locations in the cochlear nucleus and, in a few instances, with specific kinds of structures. The plausibility of this approach is suggested by referring the results of electrophysiological experiments to the cytoarchitecture of the cochlear nucleus and its connections. This can be illustrated with a standard wiring diagram for the caudal levels of the brain stem auditory system in the cat (Figure 11-10). Information from the cochlea can be transmitted directly by the cochlear nerve to every subdivision of the cochlear nucleus. Because many of the cochlear nerve fibers entering the cochlear nucleus bifurcate into branches of nearly equal diameter, the same pattern of activity can be conveyed to each of the major divisions in response to a simple stimulus. Hence there is an opportunity in the cochlear nucleus to determine what roles the different types of neurons and their patterns of synaptic organization may play in signal preservation or transformation by comparing their response types to identical stimuli.

A comparison of some of the characteristic tuning curves of units recorded in the cochlear nerve and in various subdivisions of the cochlear nucleus is shown in Figures 11-13 and 11-14 (see also Kiang, Morest, Godfrey, Guinan, & Kane, 1973; Tsuchitani, 1978). The available findings indicate that many units in the ventral cochlear nucleus have tuning curves as sharp as those in the cochlear nerve, including most units in AVCN-A and certain ones in AVCN-P. On the other hand, some units typically exhibit broader tuning curves and very irregular response areas, for example, in DCN and in the octopus cell area. Thus, in parts of the cochlear nucleus, this aspect of the signal code is consistently preserved, while in others it is predictably altered.

One can also illustrate consistent differences in the time-pattern of response for units in the cochlear nucleas. This temporal aspect of signal coding can be respresented by peristimulus time histograms, which assume a consistent configuration for units typically recorded in the cochlear nerve (Figures 11-13 and 11-14; see also Kiang et al., 1973; Tsuchitani, 1978). This pattern is faithfully preserved in AVCN-A by the same units which have sharp tuning curves. Since they appear to preserve different aspects of the signal input from the cochlear nerve fibers, these units have been classified as primarylike. A similar case can be made for some of the units recorded in AVCN-P; however, in many of these units a small dip or notch may appear in the histogram at a relatively short latency. The latency of the notch may correspond to the absolute refractory period of this so-called "pri-notch" type of unit. In other units there can be a dramatic transformation of the time-pattern of response transmitted by the cochlear nerve. For example, the units with broad tuning curves in the octopus cell area of PVCN typically respond maximally at the minimum latency, with little or no activity at longer latencies ("onset" type). Still other typical time-patterns have been described within the cochlear nucleus, for example, "choppers," "pausers," and "build-up" responses and their subclasses. Some of these tend to appear more frequently in one region than another (e.g., pausers in DCN), while others may have a broad distribution within the cochlear nucleus (e.g., certain kinds of choppers) (see Young, chap. 12).

It is possible to extend this approach to the more central levels of the auditory pathways. For example, primarylike units can be demonstrated in the medial superior olivary nucleus, to which cells in AVCN-A with similar properties presumably project. Likewise, the cells representing pri-notch units in AVCN-P are thought to project to the medial nucleus of the trapezoid body, where a similar response type has been demonstrated. In this way one could presumably follow the wiring diagram of the auditory pathways while describing the response types from level to level. However, a wiring diagram is unlikely to provide an accurate picture of signal transmission in the central auditory system. The reason for this is that the wiring diagram as such simply does not exist as a structural organization in the auditory pathways. Being merely a mnemonic device, such a diagram does not truly represent the pattern of connections between the individual neurons. But it is the individual neurons that process information. Ultimately, then, one would require a map of their individual connections in order to define signal transmission during auditory information processing. Moreover, information of this type is necessary to begin a study of the synaptic mechanisms responsible for signal transmission.

To identify the mechanisms that account for signal preservation or transformation, it is necessary to develop an appropriate morphological analysis at the cellular level. Since it is not yet feasible to identify individual cells in vertebrate brains, the morphological analysis must depend on the definition of types of cells and axonal endings, which can be compared as a class between different brains with respect to their structural and functional properties. Perhaps the best known of the structural bases for signal coding in the cochlear nucleus relate to the primarylike response type of AVCN-A, the pri-notch cell type of AVCN-P, the onset type of the octopus cell area, and the build-up and pauser types of DCN.

In AVCN-A many of the ascending branches of the cochlear nerve fibers form large endings, the end-bulbs of Held, which synapse on the cell bodies of a specific type of neuron, the spherical bushy cells. Since only one, usually, or sometimes two or three fibers synapse on individual bushy cells, these neurons are able to maintain the tonotopic sequence with as much precision as the cochlear nerve itself (Figure 11-13). Since the end-bulbs and the cell body of bushy cells are distinctive structures, which can be identified unambiguously in thin sections, their fine structure has been clearly analyzed (Figure 11-11). Forming large, clear spherical vesicles, a widened synaptic cleft, and pronounced asymmetric membrane densities, the end-bulb junctions resemble other excitatory synapses in the CNS. In fact, electrophysiological studies correlated with the known morphology and connections of the bushy cells have confirmed that the end-bulbs function as powerful excitatory synapses with a high degree of synaptic security. In anesthetized preparations the input–output transmission ratio is approximately unity, which result is reasonable since each end-bulb forms a large number of synaptic complexes with a target cell. These properties could account for the observation that the primarylike units in AVCN-A preserve the time-pattern of response transmitted by cochlear nerve fibers with high fidelity. In other words, these neurons would be especially effective in preserving the temporal patterns of ongoing low-frequency cochlear signals, including phase-locked ones (Rose et al., 1974), which occur in this part of the cochlear nucleus. On the other hand, differences in stimulus onset times could vary slightly in individual units. This circumstance would render the bushy cells of AVCN-A especially useful for setting up effective binaural interactions based on ongoing time differences in the medial superior olive, to which they project (Figures 11-10, 11-13).

In AVCN-P the cochlear nerve fibers near their bifurcations also form end-bulbs qualitatively similar to those described in AVCN-A, but they are smaller, on the average, and do not attain the size of the biggest end-bulbs more rostrally (Figure 11-11). It is likely that a few more cochlear fibers form end-bulbs on a single globular bushy cell, although not enough to compromise the sharpness of tuning. In view of the similarity of the synaptic organization of the globular bushy cell in AVCN-P to that of the spherical bushy cell in AVCN-A, one would expect to encounter some similarities in the response properties of these two types of neurons. For example, both types should have sharp tuning curves and similar time-patterns of response. However, a notch could be expected in the peristimulus time histogram of the globular bushy cell, if enough cochlear nerve fibers converged on this neuron with excitatory synapses so as to ensure consistent firing at the minimum latency. Thus it is very likely that the globular bushy cells correspond to pri-notch unit types. There is strong evidence that these neurons project by way of very large fibers to the medial nucleus of the trapezoid body, there to form the enormous calyces of Held, the large excitatory axosomatic synaptic endings on the principal cell type. These latter neurons, like the spherical bushy cells and the end-bulbs of Held in AVCN-A, provide for a faithful preservation of the globular bushy cell input from AVCN-P, even to the point of reproducing the pri-notch pattern (Figure 11-14).

The functions of the principal neurons of the trapezoid nucleus are probably multiple, since they project to one of the origins of the crossed olivocochlear bundle in the dorsomedial periolivary nucleus and to the lateral superior olive, perhaps to introduce, directly or indirectly, an inhibitory input to the binaural interactions that occur there (Figure 11-14). Some of these interactions may depend on binaural intensity differences. The synaptic organization of the cochlear nerve–globular bushy cell–trapezoid body principal cell–lateral superior olive circuit could contribute to such a function. Since the projection of the principal cell of the medial trapezoid nucleus to the dorsomedial periolivary nucleus is a collateral of the inhibitory pathway to the lateral superior olive, it could also be inhibitory to these periolivary neurons. At the same time, the projection of the globular bushy cells to the dorsomedial periolivary nucleus by way of collaterals from the excitatory calyciferous axons might be expected to provide excitatory input to these periolivary neurons. Thus neurons in the dorsomedial periolivary nucleus could monitor the input–output function of the principal cells of the medial trapezoid nucleus with reference to a balance between these excitatory and inhibitory pathways. Such a balance would be subject to modification by the projections of small axons from the cochlear nucleus to the peridendritic plexus of the principal cells in the medial trapezoid nucleus and by the projection from PVCN to the dorsomedial periolivary nucleus. The latter projection may involve octopus cells and the crossed olivocochlear neurons, although other pathways arise in the dorsomedial periolivary nucleus to the inferior or superior colliculi. The arrangement of end-bulbs on the globular bushy cell would presumably enhance the dynamic range of the pri-notch units compared to that of primarylike units in AVCN-A, while the calycine endings in the medial trapezoid nucleus would tend to preserve the globular bushy cell output with high fidelity.

In PVCN-OCA the descending cochlear nerve fibers produce a large number of synaptic endings, which virtually encrust the bodies and dendritic trunks of the octopus cells. On some octopus cells there may be so many endings that they collect in stacks or irregular layers, while the numerous somatic appendages typical of these cells reach out to contact endings in the second or third row, as it were. These large synaptic endings have the same cytological features as the excitatory synapses of the end-bulbs in AVCN-A (Figure 11-11) and the calyces in the medial trapezoid nucleus. Many such endings are formed, *en passant,* by each cochlear nerve fiber, especially the large ones, and many thick individual fibers converge on individual octopus cells. Although the descending branches of the cochlear nerve fibers generally maintain the sequential arrangement characteristic of the tonotopic organization elsewhere (Figure 11-9), the dendritic trunks of individual octopus cells extend at right angles across large sectors of the afferent fiber spectrum. This arrangement could provide the basis for the broad tuning curves characteristic of units in this region. In fact, some of the cochlear fibers with large endings, turning out of the fiber laminae, wander along the dendrites making synapses *de passage,* and these could contribute to the irregular shapes of the tuning curves often observed in the octopus cell area of PVCN.

The basis for the onset response of octopus cells can only be surmised at present. Presumably some powerful inhibitory input arrives shortly after the onset of a typical response and is sustained for the duration of the stimulus, as long as its parameters do not change. This hypothesis is consistent with the available evidence (Rhode et al., 1983b) but requires further evaluation. The source of such an inhibition is unknown, but it could be generated by the smaller fibers that form nests of small synaptic endings on the cell body and dendritic trunks. The cytological features of these endings (Figure 11-11), with small pleiomorphic vesicles, narrowed synaptic cleft, and nearly symmetrical membrane densities, resemble those of other putative inhibitory synapses, for example, those of the inhibitory interneurons of the cerebellar cortex. In the case of the octopus cell these endings could come from interneurons within PVCN or they might come directly from the cochlear nerve itself or possibly even from collaterals of some of the thicker cochlear nerve fibers with large endings (Kane, 1973, 1976). Whatever its source, the inhibitory input would have to be large, precisely timed, with a short time constant, and closely linked to the initial excitation. This would presumably require synchronization of many small axons entering the synaptic nests. For these reasons, it would be tempting to hypothesize an inhibitory input from the cochlea itself or at least from interneurons very near the octopus cells. Another property of the octopus cells that contributes to the effectiveness of the onset response is the constancy of the first spike at the minimum latency. This response property no doubt results from the overwhelming array of large excitatory cochlear endings, which cover some 50–70% of the perikaryal surface. Because the dendrites are often oriented in the vertical plane in one direction or another – usually dorsally, but sometimes ventrally – the sequential arrangement of the tonotopically arranged cochlear axons could provide a structural basis for directional sensitivity to sweeping frequencies, on the assumption that the cochlear inputs from these fibers are excitatory and that the spike generator resides in the initial segment of the octopus cell axon (Morest et al., 1973). And indeed some units with directional sensitivity have been demonstrated in the OCA, but these are not common (Godfrey et al., 1975a,b; Rhode et al., 1983b). Moreover, it is not clear that the individual afferents are uniformly related to these cells in the postulated sequence.

The functional significance of the octopus cells is unclear, although they are thought to project bilaterally to portions of the periolivary complex (Figures 11-10, 11-14). Consequently, these cells could be involved in the regulation of the olivocochlear pathways or in binaural interactions, perhaps related to binaural differences of onset times. Whether octopus cells could play a role in detection of onset times or of complex stimuli, such as sweeping frequencies or vocal inflections, is an interesting matter for speculation. Suffice it to say that the synaptic organization of octopus cells is one that would facilitate responses to changing stimuli.

In DCN the descending fibers of the cochlear nerve and their branches are finer than in the ventral cochlear nucleus and include both medium-sized and fine axons. While these axons still conform to the tonotopic map in terms of their sequential arrangement within DCN, their terminations are organized according to an entirely different principle than in the ventral cochlear nucleus. Although one may still analyze these with reference to the different cell types, it is necessary to relate the synaptic organization to the cortical structure of DCN. The cortical structure consists of four morphologically distinct layers of the neuropil, which are crossed to varying extents by the dendrites of the fusiform and giant cells and which are interconnected by a local circuit of small neurons and granule cells. The incoming cochlear nerve axons synapse on most, if not all, of these cell types, but not uniformly. Most of the cochlear nerve synapses occur in the deep layers and the deeper zone of the fusiform cell layer, where the fusiform cell bodies are. The fusiform cells have their elongated dendrites extended in planes that are parallel to the cochlear nerve fiber branches, thus helping to preserve the tuning of the cochlear inputs.

The basal dendrites and somata of the fusiform cells are thought to receive the bulk of the cochlear nerve endings on these neurons (Figure 11-12). Many, if not all, of the cochlear endings have cytological features resembling those of the excitatory synapses in AVCN, where, no doubt, collaterals of some of the same axons project (Figure 11-11). The apical dendrites clearly receive most of their input from the small endings of noncochlear axons, including parallel fibers of granule cells and axons of small cells, although there probably is not a clear segregation of inputs. Many of these endings have morphological characteristics consistent with those of inhibitory interneurons of the cerebellar cortex. Other small endings resemble those of the excitatory cerebellar parallel fibers. This suggests the hypothesis that some of the small neurons of DCN may function in a local circuit as inhibitory neurons which receive excitatory input from the cochlea in parallel with the fusiform cells but which elaborate an inhibition of the fusiform cell responses. In this way a wave of inhibition could produce the early suppression of activity which characterizes the pauser and build-up units that have been correlated with the fusiform cells (Figures 11-12, 11-13). Since there is an enormous number of granule cells impinging on individual fusiform cells, including basal as well as apical dendrites, these interneurons could generate an extensive wave of excitation, although this would require a period of time to build up. However, as stimulus-driven excitatory input continued to impinge on the granule cell population, the firing of the fusiform cells could increase to a significant level, as observed in the build-up and pauser units (Figure 11-12).

Given the cortical structure of DCN, the presence of granule cells whose dendrites synapse with mossy fibers in glomerular structures and whose axons form parallel fibers synapsing on dendrites and stellate interneurons, one could consider an analogy with the cerebellar cortex, as Lorente de Nó (1981) and some others have (e.g., Cohen, 1972; Mugnaini et al, 1980a). However, the analogy is defective, since there appears to be no counterpart to the Purkinje cell in DCN, the fusiform cell having basal dendrites and a very different synaptic organization. Likewise the cartwheel cell, while having a certain superficial resemblance to the Purkinje cell because of its many dendritic appendages, is a much smaller cell with a very different dendritic arrangement. Granule cells and glomeruli occur in all layers of DCN. There is no counterpart of the giant cells, cartwheel cells, or corn cells in the cerebellar cortex. It is not clear which neurons, if any, are equivalent to the large Golgi type II cells of the cerebellum, although Mugnaini and associates (1980b) have proposed a candidate. So far the principal similarity seems to be the existence of granule cells, which appear to be excitatory interneurons that use glutamate or aspartate as a transmitter (Oliver et al., 1981, 1983). (See Wenthold & Martin, chapter 10.)

Neither are the DCN circuits analogous to those of the cerebellar cortex. The excitatory input from the climbing fiber is not common to both granule and Purkinje cells. Although cerebellar granule cells may also use L-glutamate as an excitatory transmitter at synapses with Purkinje cells, the latter receive excitatory inputs from two separate sources, climbing and parallel fibers. The mossy fiber input is to the granule cell, which in turn projects to the Purkinje cell. Moreover, the climbing fiber and granule cell synapses have a different arrangement on the Purkinje cell than do the cochlear and parallel fiber synapses on the fusiform cells of DCN.

In any case, in DCN it appears that excitatory as well as inhibitory local circuits could play a role in determining the response properties of fusiform cells (Evans & Nelson, 1973a,b; Godfrey et al., 1975b; Kane, 1974a; Rhode et al., 1983a; Voigt & Young, 1980; Young, 1980). Since these circuits are not well studied, speculations on this basis about the functional significance of the patterns of synaptic organization in the cat would be premature and vague. Certainly one could hope to explain some of the complexity of the response areas of the fusiform cells in terms of the modifications introduced by interneurons, such as the small cells (Young, chapter 12). Other recent studies suggest a particularly strong input to DCN from the outer hair cells of the cochlea (Morest, 1981; Morest & Bohne, 1983). We do not have enough detailed information on the synaptic organization of the intrinsic neurons or of the extrinsic noncochlear input of DCN to permit testable hypotheses like those proposed for certain types of neurons in the ventral cochlear nucleus. The predominant physiological response types in the ventral cochlear nucleus tend to provide a secure representation of simple acoustic stimuli that are readily defined in terms of frequency, intensity, and phase (Kiang, et al., 1973; Morest et al., 1973; Rhode et al., 1983a) and a predominance of inner hair cell input (Morest & Bohne, 1983). The synaptic organization of DCN seems to introduce another type of acoustic analysis, heavily influenced by its many interneurons and noncochlear inputs (Young & Brownell, 1976). Thus, ongoing activity in the central auditory system may dominate the function of DCN and its physiological relationships to the hair cells, especially to the outer hair cells (Morest & Bohne, 1983; see Kim, chapter 7).

CONCLUDING REMARKS

Several points in the preceding review seem worth emphasizing. Among these is the finding that most of the subdivisions of the cochlear nucleus contain several different types of neurons. While nearly pure populations of neurons occur in certain regions, such as the central zone of the octopus cell area and the rostral extreme of the ventral cochlear nucleus, most parts of the nucleus contain two or more populations. One cannot subdivide the cochlear nucleus on the basis of cell size alone or of some other simple criterion such as perikaryal shape in thin sections. Principal neurons, such as spherical cells, are not always meaningfully distinguished by size, nor are varieties of smaller cells. Consequently, we have argued for a definition of neuronal types based on multiple criteria, which emphasize the spatial arrangements of axons and dendrites in the neuropil and the fine structure of their synapses. Cell types and subdivisions thus defined can be related to specific synaptic connections with other kinds of neurons in particular locations. In this way we define specific circuits of cell types. It is these circuits that can be most meaningfully correlated with the response properties of unit types that are characterized physiologically. Ultimately this approach should provide the structural basis for explaining information processing in the central auditory pathways, not only in terms of their input–output functions but in terms of the synaptic mechanisms operating in the central circuits. When viewed in this light, the morphology of central auditory neurons will not be limited to a static configuration but can be used to define functional models.

Of the problems that remain for defining the relations of structure to signal coding in the cochlear nucleus, perhaps the most serious are those of the intrinsic organization of indigenous neurons and of the synaptic organization of the distal dendrites of the different cell types. This information is necessary to explain the role of the descending auditory pathways, as well as the local circuits in the cochlear nucleus, in the modifications imposed on signal processing by the central nervous system. In solving these, it will be necessary to make use of labeling methods of individual cells identified as to type in both the light and electron microscopes. This approach is tedious and time consuming but feasible.

Definitions of cell types and of boundaries of subdivisions are continually subject to change and refinement. As newer data are gathered, the older definitions are improved and made more explicit. Already, with recent studies of its individual parts, our understanding of the cochlear nucleus has advanced beyond the first detailed descriptions of its overall organization. As it is to be expected that this evolution will continue, the goal of this chapter is to make present conceptions of the cochlear nucleus sufficiently clear that workers not directly involved in studies of its structural organization will be able to follow and to profit from new insights.

REFERENCES

Adams, J.C. (1979). Ascending projections to the inferior colliculus. *Journal of Comparative Neurology, 182,* 519–538.

Adams, J.C., & Warr, W.B. (1976). Origins of axons in the cat's acoustic striae determined by injection of horseradish peroxidase into severed tracts. *Journal of Comparative Neurology, 170,* 107–122.

Arneson, A.R., & Osen, K.K. (1978). The cochlear nerve in the cat: Topography, cochleotopy, and fiber spectrum, *Journal of Comparative Neurology, 178,* 661–678.

Bourk, T.R. (1976). *Electrical responses of neural units in the anteroventral cochlear nucleus of the cat.* Unpublished doctoral dissertation, Massachusetts Institute of Technology.

Bourk, T.R., Mielcarz, J.M., & Norris, B.E. (1981). Tonotopic organization of the anteroventral cochlear nucleus of the cat. *Hearing Research, 4,* 215-241.

Brawer, J.R., & Morest, D.K. (1975). Relations between auditory nerve endings and cell types in the cat's anteroventral cochlear nucleus seen with the Golgi method and Nomarski optics. *Journal of Comparative Neurology, 160,* 491-506.

Brawer, J.R., Morest, D.K., & Kane, E. (1974). The neuronal architecture of the cochlear nucleus of the cat. *Journal of Comparative Neurology, 155,* 251-300.

Britt, R.H. (1976). Intracellular study of synaptic events related to phase-locking responses of cat cochlear nucleus cells to low frequency tones. *Brain Research, 112,* 313-327.

Britt, R.H., & Starr, A. (1976a). Synaptic events and discharge patterns of cochlear nucleus cells. I. Steady-frequency tone bursts. *Journal of Neurophysiology, 39,* 162-178.

Britt, R.H., & Starr, A. (1976b). Synaptic event and discharge patterns of cochlear nucleus cells. II. Frequency-modulated tones. *Journal of Neurophysiology, 39,* 179-194.

Brugge, J.F., Javel, E., & Kitzes, L.M. (1978). Signs of functional maturation of peripheral auditory system in discharge patterns of neurons in anteroventral cochlear nucleus of kittens. *Journal of Neurophysiology, 41,* 1557-1579.

Brugge, J.F., Kitzes, L.M., & Javel, E. (1981). Postnatal development of frequency and intensity sensitivity of neurons in the anteroventral cochlear nucleus of kittens. *Hearing Research, 5,* 217-229.

Brunso-Bechtold, J.K., Thompson, G.C., & Masterson, R.B. (1981). HRP study of the organization of auditory afferents ascending to central nucleus of inferior colliculus in cats. *Journal of Comparative Neurology, 197,* 705-722.

Cant, N.B. (1981). The fine structure of two types of stellate cells in the anterior division of the anteroventral cochlear nucleus of the cat. *Neuroscience, 6,* 2643-2655.

Cant, N.B. (1982). Identification of cell types in the anteroventral cochlear nucleus that project to the inferior colliculus. *Neuroscience Letters, 32,* 241-246.

Cant, N.B., & Gaston, K.C. (1982). Pathways connecting the right and left cochlear nuclei. *Journal of Comparative Neurology, 212,* 313-326.

Cant, N.B., & Morest, D.K. (1978). Axons from non-cochlear sources in the anteroventral cochlear nucleus of the cat. A study with the rapid Golgi method. *Neuroscience, 3,* 1003-1029.

Cant, N.B., & Morest, D.K. (1979a). Organization of the neurons in the anterior division of the anteroventral cochlear nucleus of the cat. Light-microscopic observations. *Neuroscience, 4,* 1909-1923.

Cant, N.B. & Morest, D.K. (1979b). The bushy cells in the anteroventral cochlear nucleus of the cat. A study with the electron microscope, *Neuroscience, 4,* 1925-1945.

Caspary, D. (1972). Classification of subpopulations of neurons in the cochlear nuclei of the kangaroo rat. *Experimental Neurology, 37,* 131-151.

Cohen, E.S. (1972). *Synaptic organization of the caudal cochlear nucleus of the cat: A light and electron microscopical study.* Unpublished doctoral dissertation, Harvard University.

Cohen, E.S., Brawer, J.R., & Morest, D.K. (1972). Projections of the cochlea to the dorsal cochlear nucleus in the cat. *Experimental Neurology, 35,* 470-479.

Conlee, J.W., & Kane, E.S. (1982). Descending projections from the inferior colliculus to the dorsal cochlear nucleus in the cat: An autoradiographic study. *Neuroscience, 1,* 161-178.

Disterhoft, J.F., Perkins, R.E., & Evans, S. (1980). Neuronal morphology of the rabbit cochlear nucleus. *Journal of Comparative Neurology, 192,* 687-702.

Dunn, R.A. (1975). *A comparison of Golgi-impregnated innervation patterns and fine structural morphology in the cochlea of the cat.* Unpublished doctoral dissertation, Harvard University.

Dunn, R.A., & Morest, D.K. (1975). Receptor synapses without synaptic ribbons in the cochlea of the cat. *Proceedings of the National Academy of Sciences, USA, 72,* 3599-3603.

Elverland, H.H. (1977). Descending connections between the superior olivary and cochlear nuclear complexes in the cat studied by autoradiographic and horseradish peroxidase methods. *Experimental Brain Research, 27,* 397–412.

Evans, E.F., & Nelson, P.G. (1973a). The responses of single neurons in the cochlear nucleus of the cat as a function of their location and the anesthetic state. *Experimental Brain Research, 17,* 402–427.

Evans, E.F., & Nelson, P.G. (1973b). On the functional relationship between the dorsal and ventral divisions of the cochlear nucleus of the cat. *Experimental Brain Research, 17,* 428–442.

Feldman, M.L., & Harrison, J.M. (1969). The projection of the acoustic nerve to the ventral cochlear nucleus of the rat. A Golgi study. *Journal of Comparative Neurology, 137,* 267–294.

Fuse, G. (1913). Das Ganglion ventrale und das Tuberculum acusticum beim einigen Sauglingen und beim Menschen. *Arbeiten aus dem Hirnanatomischen Institut in Zuerich, 7,* 1–210.

Gentschev, T., & Sotelo, C. (1973). Degenerative patterns in the ventral cochlear nucleus of the rat after primary deafferentation. An ultrastructural study. *Brain Research, 62,* 37–60.

Gibson, M.M., Hind, J.E., Kitzes, L.M., & Rose, J.E. (1977). Estimation of traveling wave parameters from the response properties of cat AVCN neurons. In E.F. Evans & J.P. Wilson (Eds.), *Psychophysics and physiology of hearing.* London: Academic Press.

Ginzberg, R.D., & Morest, D.K. (1983). A study of cochlear innervation in the young cat with the Golgi method. *Hearing Research, 10,* 227–246.

Gisbergen, J.A.M. van, Grashuis, J.L., Johannesma, P.I.M., & Vendrik, A.J.H. (1975). Spectral and temporal characteristics of activation and suppression of units in the cochlear nucleus of the anesthetized cat. *Experimental Brain Research, 23,* 367–386.

Glendenning, K.K., Brunso-Bechtold, J.K., Thompson, G.C., & Masterson, R.B. (1981). Ascending auditory afferents to the nuclei of the lateral lemniscus. *Journal of Comparative Neurology, 197,* 673–703.

Godfrey, D.A., Kiang, N.Y.S., & Norris, B.E. (1975a). Single unit activity in the posteroventral cochlear nucleus of the cat. *Journal of Comparative Neurology, 162,* 247–268.

Godfrey, D.A., Kiang, N.Y.S., & Norris, B.E. (1975b). Single unit activity in the dorsal cochlear nucleus of the cat. *Journal of Comparative Neurology, 162,* 269–284.

Goldberg, J.M., & Brownell, W.E. (1973). Discharge characteristics of neurons in anteroventral and dorsal cochlear nuclei of cat. *Brain Research, 64,* 35–54.

Goldberg, J.M., & Greenwood, D.D. (1966). Response of neurons of the dorsal and posteroventral cochlear nuclei of the cat to acoustic stimuli of long duration. *Journal of Neurophysiology, 29,* 72–93.

Greenwood, D.D., & Goldberg, J.M. (1970). Response of neurons in the cochlear nuclei to variations in noise bandwidth and to tone–noise combinations. *Journal of the Acoustical Society of America, 47,* 1022–1040.

Greenwood, D.D., & Maruyama, N. (1965). Excitatory and inhibitory response areas of auditory neurons in the cochlear nucleus. *Journal of Neurophysiology, 28,* 863–892.

Greenwood, D.D., Merzenich, M.M., & Roth, G.L. (1976). Some preliminary observations on the interrelations between two-tone suppression and combination tone driving in the anteroventral cochlear nucleus of the cat. *Journal of the Acoustical Society of America, 59,* 607–633.

Harrison, J.M., & Irving, R. (1965). The anterior ventral cochlear nucleus. *Journal of Comparative Neurology, 124,* 15–42.

Harrison, J.M., & Irving, R. (1966a). Ascending connections of the anterior ventral cochlear nucleus in the rat. *Journal of Comparative Neurology, 126,* 51–64.

Harrison, J.M. & Irving, R. (1966b). The organization of the posterior ventral cochlear nucleus in the rat. *Journal of Comparative Neurology, 126,* 391–402.

Harrison, J.M., & Warr, W.B. (1962). A study of the cochlear nuclei and ascending auditory pathways of the medulla. *Journal of Comparative Neurology, 119*, 341–379.

Held, H. (1891). Die centralen Bahnen des Nervus acusticus bei der Katze. *Archives für Anatomie und Physiologie Anatomische Abteilung, 15*, 271–291.

Held, H. (1893). Die centrale Gehörleitung. *Archives für Anatomie and Physiologie Anatomische Abteilung*, 201–248.

Ibata, Y., & Pappas, G.D. (1976). The fine structure of synapses in relation to the large spherical neurons in the anterior ventral cochlear (sic) of the cat. *Journal of Neurocytology, 5*, 395–406.

Jhaveri, S., & Morest, D.K. (1982). Neuronal architecture in nucleus magnocellularis of the chicken auditory system with observations on nucleus laminaris: A light and electron microscope study. *Neuroscience, 7*, 809–836.

Jones, D.R. (1979). *Auditory pathways in the brainstem of the tree shrew, Tupaia glis.* Unpublished doctoral dissertation, Duke University.

Jones, D.R., & Casseday, J.H. (1979a). Projections of auditory nerve in the cat as seen by antero-grade transport methods. *Neuroscience, 4*, 1299–1313.

Jones, D.R., & Casseday, J.H. (1979b). Projections to laminae in dorsal cochlear nucleus in the tree shrew, *Tupaia glis*. *Brain Research, 160*, 131–133.

Kane, E.S.C. (1973). Octopus cells in the cochlear nucleus of the cat: Heterotypic synapses upon homeotypic neurons. *International Journal of Neuroscience, 5*, 251–279.

Kane, E.S. (1974a). Synaptic organization in the dorsal cochlear nucleus of the cat: A light and electron microscopic study. *Journal of Comparative Neurology, 155*, 301–330.

Kane, E.S. (1974b). Patterns of degeneration in the caudal cochlear nucleus of the cat after cochlear ablation. *Anatomical Record, 179*, 67–92.

Kane, E.S. (1976). Descending projections to specific regions of cat cochlear nucleus: A light microscopic study. *Experimental Neurology, 52*, 372–388.

Kane, E.S. (1977a). Descending inputs to the octopus cell area of the cat cochlear nucleus: An electron microscopic study. *Journal of Comparative Neurology, 173*, 337–354.

Kane, E.S., (1977b). Descending inputs to the cat dorsal cochlear nucleus: An electron microscopic study. *Journal of Neurocytology, 6*, 583–605.

Kane, E.S., & Conlee, J.W. (1979). Descending inputs to the caudal cochlear nucleus of the cat: Degeneration and autoradiographic studies. *Journal of Comparative Neurology, 4*, 759–783.

Kane, E.S., & Finn, R.C. (1977). Descending and intrinsic inputs to dorsal cochlear nucleus of cats: A horseradish peroxidase study. *Neuroscience, 2*, 897–912.

Kane, E.S., & Habib, C.P. (1978). Development of the dorsal cochlear nucleus of the cat: An electron microscope study. *The American Journal of Anatomy, 153*, 321–343.

Kane, E.S., Puglisi, S.G., & Gordon, B.S. (1981). Neuronal types in the deep dorsal cochlear nucleus of the cat. I. Giant neurons. *Journal of Comparative Neurology, 198*, 483–513.

Kiang, N.Y.S., Godfrey, D.A., Norris, B.E., & Moxon, S.E. (1975). A block model of the cat cochlear nucleus. *Journal of Comparative Neurology, 162*, 221–246.

Kiang, N.Y.S., Morest, D.K., Godfrey, D.A., Guinan, J.J., & Kane, E.S. (1973). Stimulus coding at caudal levels of the cat's auditory system. I. Response characteristics of single units. In A.R. Møller (Ed.), *Basic mechanisms in hearing.* New York: Academic Press.

Kiang, N.Y.S., Pfeiffer, R.R., Warr, W.B., & Backus, A.S.N. (1965). Stimulus coding in the cochlear nucleus. *Annals of Otology, Rhinology and Laryngology, 74*, 463–485.

Koelliker, A. (1896). *Handbuch der Gewebelehre des Menschem Bd. 2.* Leipzig: Wilhelm Engelman.

Koerber, K.C., Pfeiffer, W.B., Warr, W.B., & Kiang, N.Y.S. (1966). Spontaneous spike discharges from single units in the cochlear nucleus after destruction of the cochlea. *Experimental Neurology, 16*, 119–130.

Konigsmark, B.W. (1973). Cellular organization of the cochlear nuclei in man. *Journal of Neuropathology and Experimental Neurology, 32,* 153–154.

Lenn, T.R., & Reese, T.S. (1966). The fine structure of nerve endings in the nucleus of the trapezoid body and the ventral cochlear nucleus. *American Journal of Anatomy, 118,* 375–390.

Lewy, F.H., & Kobrak, H. (1936). The neural projection of the cochlear spiral on the primary acoustic centers. *Archives of Neurological Psychiatry, 35,* 839–852.

Liberman, M.C. (1980). Morphological differences among radial afferent fibers in the cat cochlea: An electron-microscopic study of serial sections. *Hearing Research, 3,* 45–63.

Lorente de Nó, R. (1933a). Anatomy of the eighth nerve. III. General plans of structure of the primary cochlear nuclei. *Laryngoscope, 43,* 327–350.

Lorente de Nó, R., (1933b). Anatomy of the eighth nerve: The central projection of the nerve endings of the internal ear. *Laryngoscope, 43,* 1–38.

Lorente de Nó, R. (1976). Some unresolved problems concerning the cochlear nerve. *Annals of Otology, Rhinology, and Laryngology, 85 (Supplement 34),* 1–28.

Lorente de Nó, R. (1981). *The primary acoustic nuclei.* New York: Raven Press.

Martin, M.R. (1981). Morphology of the cochlear nucleus of the normal and reeler mutant mouse. *Journal of Comparative Neurology, 197,* 141–152.

McDonald, D.M., & Rasmussen, G.L. (1971). Ultrastructural characteristics of synaptic endings in the cochlear nucleus having acetylcholinesterase activity. *Brain Research, 28,* 1–18.

Moore, J.K., & Osen, K.K. (1979). The cochlear nuclei in man. *American Journal of Anatomy, 154,* 393–418.

Morest, D.K., (1968). The collateral system of the medial nucleus of the trapezoid body of the cat, its neuronal architecture and relation to the olivo-cochlear bundle. *Brain Research, 9,* 288–311.

Morest, D.K. (1981). Degeneration in the brain following exposure to noise. In R.P. Hamernik, D. Henderson, & R. Salvi, (Eds.), *New perspectives on noise-induced hearing loss.* New York: Raven Press.

Morest, D.K., & Bohne, B.A. (1983). Noise-induced degeneration in the brain and representation of inner and outer hair cells. *Hearing Research, 9,* 145–151.

Morest, D.K., Kiang, N.Y.S., Kane, E.C., Guinan, J.J., & Godfrey, D.A. (1973). Stimulus coding at caudal levels of the cat's auditory nervous system. II. Patterns of synaptic organization. In A.R. Møller (Ed.), *Basic mechanisms in hearing.* New York: Academic Press.

Moskowitz, N., & Liu, J.-C. (1972). Central projections of the squirrel monkey. *Journal of Comparative Neurology, 144,* 335–344.

Mugnaini, E., Warr, W.B., & Osen, K.K. (1980a). Distribution and light microscopic features of granule cells in the cochlear nuclei of cat, rat, and mouse. *Journal of Comparative Neurology, 191,* 581–606.

Mugnaini, E., Osen, K.K., Dahl, A.-L., Friedrich, V.L., & Korte, G. (1980b). Fine structure of granule cells and related interneurons (termed Golgi cells) in the cochlear nuclear complex of cat, rat, and mouse. *Journal of Neurocytology, 9,* 537–570.

Oliver, D.L. (1984). Dorsal cochlear nucleus projections to the inferior colliculus in the cat. A light and electron microscopic study. *Journal of Comparative Neurology, 224,* 155–172.

Oliver, D.L., Jones, D.R., Potashner, S.J., & Morest, D.K. (1981). Evidence for selective uptake, release, and axonal transport of D-aspartate in the auditory system and cerebellum of cat and guinea pig. *Anatomical Record,* 186A.

Oliver, D.L., Potashner, S.J., Jones, D.T., & Morest, D.K. (1983). Selective labelling of spiral ganglion and granule cells with D-aspartate in the auditory system of cat and guinea pig. *Journal of Neuroscience, 3,* 455–472.

Osen, K.K. (1969a). Cytoarchitecture of the cochlear nuclei in the cat. *Journal of Comparative Neurology, 136,* 453–484.

Osen, K.K. (1969b). The intrinsic organization of the cochlear nuclei in the cat. *Acta Oto-laryngology, 67,* 352–359.

Osen, K.K. (1970). Course and termination of the primary afferents in the cochlear nuclei of the cat: An experimental anatomical study. *Archives Italiennes de Biologie (Pisa), 108,* 21–51.

Osen, K.K. (1972). Projection of the cochlear nuclei on the inferior colliculus in the cat. *Journal of Comparative Neurology, 144,* 355–372.

Osen, K.K., & Roth, K. (1969). Histochemical localization of cholinesterases in the cochlear nuclei of the cat with notes on the origin of acetylcholinesterase-positive afferents and the superior olive. *Brain Research, 16,* 165–185.

Perkins, R.E., & Morest, D.K. (1975). A study of cochlear innervation patterns in cats and rats with the Golgi method and Nomarski optics. *Journal of Comparative Neurology, 163,* 129–158.

Perry, D.R., & Webster, W.R. (1981). Neuronal organization of the rabbit cochlear nucleus: Some anatomical and electrophysiological observations. *Journal of Comparative Neurology, 197,* 623–638.

Pfeiffer, R.R. (1966a). AVCN: Waveforms of extracellularly recorded spike potentials. *Science, 154,* 667–668.

Pfeiffer, R.R. (1966b). Classification of response patterns of spike discharges for units in the cochlear nucleus: Tone-burst stimulation. *Experimental Brain Research, 1,* 220–235.

Pfeiffer, R.R., & Kiang, N.Y.S. (1965). Spike discharge patterns of spontaneous and continuously stimulated activity in the cochlear nucleus of anesthetized cats. *Biophysics Journal, 5,* 301–316.

Pirsig, W. (1968). Regionen, Zelltypen und Synapsen im ventralen Nucleus cochlearis des Meerschweinchens. *Archiv für Klinische und Experimentelle Ohren-, Nasen-, und Kehlkopfheilkunde (Berlin), 192,* 333–350.

Powell, T.P.S., & Cowan, W.W. (1962). An experimental study of the projection of the cochlea. *Journal of Anatomy, 96,* 269–284.

Powell, T.P.S., & Erulkar, S.D. (1962). Transneuronal cell degeneration in the auditory relay nuclei of the cat. *Journal of Anatomy (London) 96,* 249–268.

Ramón y Cajal, S. (1909). *Histologie du système nerveux de l'homme et des vertébrés* (1952 reprint). Madrid: Instituto Ramón y Cajal.

Rasmussen, G.L. (1957). Selective silver impregnation of synaptic endings. In W.F. Windle (Ed.), *New research techniques of neuroanatomy.* Springfield: Thomas.

Rasmussen, G.L. (1960). Efferent fibers of the cochlear nerve and cochlear nucleus. In G.L. Rasmussen & W. Windle (Eds.), *Neural mechanisms of the auditory and vestibular systems.* Springfield: Thomas.

Rasmussen, G.L. (1964). Anatomic relationships of the ascending and descending auditory systems. In W.S. Fields & B.R. Alford (Eds.), *Neurological aspects of auditory and vestibular disorders.* Springfield: Thomas.

Rasmussen: G.L. (1967). Efferent connections of the cochlear nucleus. In A.B. Graham (Ed.), *Sensorineural hearing processes and disorders.* Boston: Little, Brown.

Rasmussen, G.L., Gacek, R.R., McCrane, E.P., & Baker, C.C. (1960). Model of cochlear nucleus (cat) displaying its afferent and efferent connections. *Anatomical Record, 136,* 344.

Rhode, W.S., Oertel, D., & Smith, P.H. (1983a). Physiological response properties of cells labeled intracellularly with horseradish peroxidase in cat ventral cochlear nucleus. *Journal of Comparative Neurology, 213,* 448–463.

Rhode, W.S., Smith, P.H., & Oertel, D. (1983b). Physiological response properties of cells labeled intracellularly with horseradish peroxidase in cat dorsal cochlear nucleus. *Journal of Comparative Neurology, 213,* 426–447.

Romand, R. (1979). Intracellular recording of 'chopper responses' in the cochlear nucleus of the cat. *Hearing Research, 1,* 95–99.

Rose, J.E. (1960). Organization of frequency sensitive neurons in the cochlear nuclear complex of the cat. In G.L. Rasmusen & W.F. Windle (Eds.), *Neural mechanisms of the auditory and vestibular systems.* Springfield: Thomas.

Rose, J.E., Galambos, R., & Hughes, J.R. (1959). Microelectrode studies of the cochlear nuclei of the cat. *Bulletin of Johns Hopkins Hospital, 104,* 211–251.

Rose, J.E., Kitzes, L.M., Gibson, M.M., & Hind, J.E. (1974). Observations on phase-sensitive neurons of anteroventral cochlear nucleus of the cat: Nonlinearity of cochlear output. *Journal of Neurophysiology, 37,* 218–253.

Roth, G.L., Aitkin, L.M., Andersen, R.A., & Merzenich, M.M. (1978). Some features of the spatial organization of the central nucleus of the inferior colliculus of the cat. *Journal of Comparative Neurology, 182,* 661–680.

Sala, L. (1893). Ueber den Ursprang des Nervus acusticus. *Archiv für Mikroskopische Anatomie, 42,* 18–52.

Sando, I. (1965). The anatomical interrelationships of the cochlear nerve fibers. *Acta Oto-laryngologica, 59,* 417–436.

Schwartz, A.M., & Gulley, R.L., (1978). Non-primary afferents to the principal cells of the rostral anteroventral cochlear nucleus of the guinea pig. *American Journal of Anatomy, 153,* 489–508.

Schwartz, A.M., & Kane, E.S. (1977). Development of the octopus cell area in the cat ventral cochlear nucleus. *The American Journal of Anatomy, 148,* 1–18.

Sotelo, C., Gentschev, T., & Zamora, A.J. (1976), Gap junctions in ventral cochlear nucleus of the rat. A possible new example of electronic junctions in the mammalian central nervous system. *Neuroscience, 1,* 5–7.

Spangler, K.M., Henkel, C.K., & Cant, N.B. (1983). Descending projections from the superior olivary complex to the cochlear nucleus of the cat. *Neuroscience Abstracts, 9,* 766.

Spoendlin, H. (1972). Innervation densities of the cochlea. *Acta Otolaryngologica, 73,* 235–248.

Stotler, W.A. (1953). An experimental study of the cells and connections of the superior olivary complex of the cat. *Journal of Comparative Neurology, 98,* 401–431.

Tolbert, L.P., & Morest, D.K. (1982a). The neuronal architecture of the anteroventral cochlear nucleus of the cat in the region of the cochlear nerve root: Electron microscopy. *Neuroscience, 7,* 3053–3068.

Tolbert, L.P., & Morest, D.K. (1982b). The neuronal architecture of the anteroventral cochlear nucleus of the cat in the region of the cochlear nerve root: Golgi and Nissl methods. *Neuroscience, 7,* 3013–3030.

Tolbert, L.P., Morest, D.K., & Yurgelun-Todd, D.A. (1982). The neuronal architecture of the anteroventral cochlear nucleus of the cat in the region of the cochlear nerve root: Horseradish peroxidase labelling of identified cell types. *Neuroscience, 7,* 3031–3052.

Tsuchitani, C. (1978). Lower auditory brain stem structures of the cat. In R.R. Naunton & C. Fernandez. (Eds.), *Evoked electrical activity in the auditory nervous system.* New York: Academic Press.

van Gehuchten, A. (1902). Recherches sur la voie acoustique centrale (voie acoustique bulbo-mesencephalique). *Le Nevraxe, 4,* 251–300.

van Gehuchten, A. (1906). Recherches sur la termination centrale des nerfs sensibles peripheriques. VI. Le nerf cochleaire. *Le Nevraxe, 8,* 125–146.

van Noort, J. (1969). The anatomical basis for frequency analysis in the cochlear nucleus complex. *Psychiatria, Neurologia, Neurochirurgia, 72,* 109–114.

Voight, H.F., & Young, E.D. (1980). Evidence of inhibitory interactions between neurons in dorsal cochlear nucleus. *Journal of Neurophysiology, 44,* 76–96.

Warr, W.B. (1966). Fiber degeneration following lesions in the anterior ventral cochlear nucleus of the cat. *Experimental Neurology, 14,* 453–474.

Warr, W.B. (1969). Fiber degeneration following lesions in the posteroventral cochlear nucleus of the cat. *Experimental Neurology, 23,* 140–155.

Warr, W.B. (1972). Fiber degeneration following lesions in the multipolar and globular cell areas in the ventral cochlear nucleus of the cat. *Brain Research, 40,* 247–270.

Warr, W.B. (1982). Parallel ascending pathways from the cochlear nucleus: Neuroanatomical evidence of functional specialization. *Contributions to Sensory Physiology, 7,* 1–38.

Webster, D.B. (1971). Projection of the cochlea to cochlear nuclei in Merriam's kangaroo rat. *Journal of Comparative Neurology, 143,* 323–340.

Webster, D.B., & Trune, D.R. (1982). Cochlear nuclear complex of mice. *The American Journal of Anatomy, 163,* 103–130.

Winkler, C. (1921). *Anatomie du systeme nerveux. Ile partie l'appareil nerveux du n. trigeminus et celiui du n. octavus.* Bohn: Haalem.

Young, E.D. (1980). Identification of response properties of ascending axons from dorsal cochlear nucleus. *Brain Research, 200,* 23–37.

Young, E.D., & Brownell, W.E. (1976). Responses to tones and noise of single cells in dorsal cochlear nucleus of unanesthetized cats. *Journal of Neurophysiology, 39,* 282–300.

Young, E.D., & Voigt, H.F. (1982). Response properties of type II and type III units in dorsal cochlear nucleus. *Hearing Research, 6,* 153–169.

Young, S.R., & Rubel, E.W. (1983). Frequency specific projections of individual neurons in chick brain stem auditory nuclei. *Journal of Neuroscience, 3,* 1373–1378.

Zook, J.M., & Casseday, J.H. (1982). Cytoarchitecture of auditory system in lower brainstem of the mustache bat, *Pteronotus parnellii. Journal of Comparative Neurology, 207,* 1–13.

Chapter 12

Response Characteristics of Neurons of the Cochlear Nuclei[1]

Eric D. Young

The ultimate goal of research on the nervous system is gaining an understanding of relationships between brain mechanisms and mental function. In the case of sensory systems, this general goal can be broken into three parts: generating a description of the patterns of activity of sensory neurons, working out the form of the internal representation of the sensory environment in those patterns, and formulating testable hypotheses about the relationships between the neuronal patterns and perception. There are many lines of investigation which must be followed to achieve these goals. In the process of working out the patterns of activity of sensory neurons, it seems especially productive at present to attempt to describe the morphological characteristics of neurons in the relevant sensory nuclei, the patterns of connectivity among the neurons of different morphological classes, and the response properties of the neurons of each morphological class. This descriptive information, once obtained, will serve as a framework for the more difficult goals mentioned above. The immediate goal, in other words, is to generate a neural circuit diagram for the system to serve as the basis for analysis of information processing by the system.

The cochlear nuclei (CN) serve as a good example of the usefulness of this approach. The morphological cell types making up the CN have been defined reasonably well, as have many (but not all) aspects of their connectivity (see the review by Cant & Morest in chap. 11 of this volume). At the same time, studies of single neurons in the CN with microelectrode techniques have revealed a number of identifiable patterns of response to sound. Both the morphological and physiological analyses make it clear that the CN consists of a complex of subsystems. Each subsystem has its own structure, connections, and response characteristics. Each subsystem receives a complete representation of the cochlear frequency map; that is, auditory nerve fibers from the whole length of the cochlea terminate within the regions occupied by each subsystem (Lorente de Nó, 1933; Osen, 1970) and the tonotopic maps in the CN cut across the boundaries between subdivisions (Bourk, Mielcarz, & Norris, 1981; Rose, Galambos, & Hughes, 1960). The major subsystems are reviewed schematically in Figure 12-1. The differences between these subsystems are significant enough to

[1]The preparation of this chapter was supported by NIH Grants 5 RO1 NS12524 and 5 KO4 NS00381.

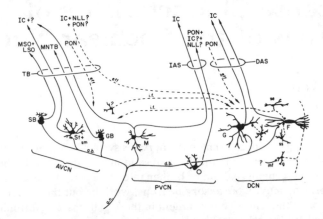

Figure 12-1. Schematic summary of major subsystems of cochlear nuclei (CN). Synaptic terminals in CN come from auditory nerve (a.n.) fibers (Lorente de Nó, 1933; Ramón y Cajal, 1909); from efferent axons of higher auditory centers (eff; Adams & Warr, 1976; Cant & Morest, 1978; Elverland, 1977; Kane & Finn, 1977; Lorente de Nó, 1933); from intrinsic axons of interneurons, mainly in DCN, and from intranuclear association fibers (i.f.) connecting CN subdivisions (Lorente de Nó, 1933, 1981). Major cell types and their connections are shown in a roughly sagittal view of CN (Brawer et al., 1974; Osen, 1969); SB – spherical bushy cells receive large calyces of Held on their somata from small numbers of a.n. fibers and have limited dendritic trees (Cant and Morest, 1979b; Ramón y Cajal, 1909). SB axons travel through trapezoid body (TB) to principal nuclei of superior olivary complex (van Noort, 1969; Warr, 1966). GB – globular bushy cells have synaptic inputs similar to SB; their axons are the largest in the TB and terminate in the medial nucleus of the trapezoid body (Tolbert & Morest, 1982a,b; Tolbert et al., 1982). St – stellate neurons have long dendritic trees upon which a.n. and other inputs make bouton terminals. Some have no terminals on soma, others have somatic input (Cant, 1981; Cant & Morest, 1979a). sm – Small stellate neurons. M – multipolar neurons have stellate or elongate morphology and receive bouton terminals on dendritic trees only (Tolbert & Morest, 1979a,b; Tolbert et al., 1982). Axons of St, sm, and M cells travel through TB (or intermediate acoustic stria [IAS] for M cells) to inferior colliculus (Adams, 1979). O – octopus cells of caudal PVCN (octopus cell area, OCA) receive massive input from a.n. on somata and proximal dendritic trees (Kane, 1973); destinations of axons are poorly understood, but include periolivary nuclei of superior olivary complex (van Noort, 1969; Warr, 1969). F – fusiform cells, one type of principal cell in DCN. F cells have large apical and basal dendritic trees which receive inputs from many sources, including a.n., via three routes: directly on their somata and dendrites, indirectly through small cell interneurons (se, ss), and through granule cell (g)/parallel fiber system (Kane, 1974a; Lorente de Nó, 1981; Mugnaini et al., 1980; Osen & Mugnaini, 1981). G – giant cell, large cells which are the other DCN principal cell type (Kane et al., 1981). The nature of synaptic inputs to G is poorly understood. F and G axons project through dorsal acoustic stria (DAS) to inferior colliculus (Adams, 1979). Abbreviations: a.b. – ascending branch of a.n. fiber; a.n. – auditory nerve; AVCN – anteroventral division of CN; BF – best frequency; CN – cochlear nuclei; DAS – dorsal acoustic stria; d.b. – descending branch of a.n. fiber; DCN – Dorsal division of CN; IC – inferior colliculus; LSO – lateral nucleus of superior olive; mf – mossy fiber terminal on granule cell; MNTB – medial nucleus of trapezoid body; MSO – medial nucleus of superior olive; NLL – nuclei of lateral lemniscus; OCA – octopus cell area of PVCN; PON – periolivary nuclei; PVCN – posteroventral division of CN; TB – trapezoid body; VCN – ventral cochlear nucleus (AVCN + PVCN).

support the working hypothesis that they are different neural systems which are performing distinct functions within the overall organization of the auditory system.

This chapter reviews current knowledge about the response properties of neurons in the CN. The emphasis is on schemes for organizing the diversity of response characteristics found in the CN and on showing how these schemes can be related to the morphologically defined neural subsystems. The focus is purposefully narrow, concentrating on the mammalian CN. This narrow focus allows detailed consideration of the large body of work on this system in the limited space available.

PHYSIOLOGICAL RESPONSE TYPES

A fruitful approach to the problem of analyzing the characteristics of a diverse group of neurons such as those making up the CN is to attempt to define an inclusive set of unit[2] types which can be used as a classification scheme around which to organize the analysis. Each unit type is defined by a group of response properties; ideally, the unit types are distinguished from each other by clear criteria so that identification of a particular unit as belonging to one type or another can be done with a few simple tests. Perhaps the most important goal of this sort of analysis is finding unit types that can be associated with particular morphological cell types. This association allows, for example, the response characteristics of projection cells to be differentiated from those of interneurons and serves as a basis for the study of information processing by the system.

Two approaches have been taken to the definition of response types in the CN, one based on response maps (Evans & Nelson, 1973a) and the second based on the temporal patterns of units' responses to best frequency (BF) stimuli (Pfeiffer, 1966a). These are discussed separately below.

Unit Types Based on Response Maps

A response map is a description of the sensory receptive field of an auditory neuron. In the form used here, it is a map of the distribution of excitatory and inhibitory[3] responses at various stimulus frequencies and sound levels. Figure 12-2 shows an example of a response map for a unit in the DCN of a decerebrate cat (Young & Brownell, 1976). The small plot at lower left in this figure is the response map. Shaded regions show the frequencies (abscissa) and sound levels (ordinate) at which tones produced excitatory responses; the unshaded regions enclosed by dotted lines show the frequency–sound level combinations that produced inhibitory responses.

---

[2]The term "unit" is used to refer to the activity of a neuron as recorded with a microelectrode. It is distinguished from "cell" or "neuron," which refer to the anatomical entity from which the recording is made.

[3]The terms "excitatory" and "inhibitory" must be interpreted with caution. Strictly speaking, these terms refer to postsynaptic effects of EPSPs and IPSPs, that is, to direct excitation or inhibition of the cell. With extracellular recording, it is only possible to detect increases or decreases in action potential discharge rate. Rate changes, particularly rate decreases, are not necessarily produced by direct excitation or inhibition occurring in the cell under study. Unfortunately there are no convenient alternative terms. In this paper, excitation and inhibition are used, in most cases, to refer to rate increases or decreases. Usually this usage will be made clear by attaching a word like "responses" to indicate that the response obtained from the neuron is like a response produced by direct excitation, or inhibition.

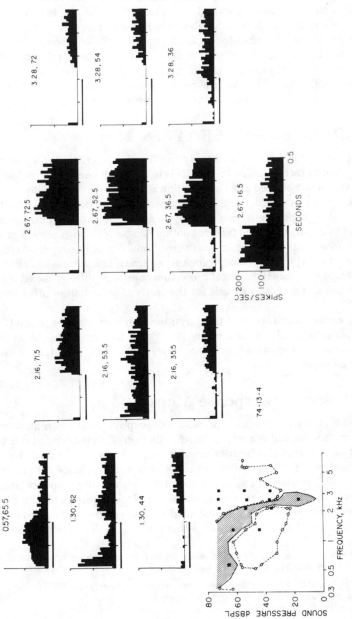

Figure 12-2. Response map of a DCN type IV unit (lower left) and PST histograms of responses of the same unit to tone bursts at various frequencies and sound levels. In the response map, shaded regions are excitatory responses (20% increase in discharge rate over spontaneous rate) and unshaded regions surrounded by dashed lines are inhibitory responses (20% decrease in rate below spontaneous). Dots on response map show frequency/sound level combinations at which PST histograms were taken. Numbers on PST histograms are frequency (kilohertz) and sound level (decibels SPL) at which the histogram was made. Heavy bar beneath PST histogram abscissa shows duration of stimulus. (From Young & Brownell, 1976; used with permission)

The remainder of Figure 12-2 shows PST histograms[4] of this unit's responses at particular frequency–sound level combinations (indicated on the response map by dots).

Figure 12-2 illustrates the point that a response map is an overall summary of a unit's responses which leaves out many details. For example, inspection of the PST histograms in Figure 12-2 shows that the inhibitory responses at 2.67 kHz (third column from the left) contain a number of features not observable in the inhibitory responses at higher or lower frequencies. The inhibitory responses at 3.28 kHz (fourth column) or 1.3 kHz (first column) consist only of a simple suppression of discharge rate during the stimulus, whereas the inhibitory responses at 2.67 kHz are followed by a strong afterdischarge, a large increase in discharge rate after the stimulus is turned off. The difference in these inhibitory responses is not reflected in the response map. A similar comment can be made about the excitatory response regions. Although response maps can be extended to show more features by plotting measures of other aspects of responses (such as afterdischarges), analysis of response maps in the CN has not been carried beyond the basic discrimination of excitatory and inhibitory responses. Fortunately, the presence or absence and the distribution of inhibitory response areas has proven to be useful in differentiating unit types in the CN.

Classification of units in the CN on the basis of response maps was first done by Evans and Nelson (1973a). Variants of their scheme have been applied by others, not only in the cat (van Gisbergen, Grashuis, Johannesma, & Vendrick, 1975a; Young & Brownell, 1976) but also in the rabbit (Hui & Disterhoft, 1980) and redwing blackbird (Sachs & Sinnott, 1978). Response map classification depends on differences in the prevalence of inhibitory responses. Because inhibitory responses are suppressed by anesthesia (Evans & Nelson, 1973a; Young & Brownell, 1976), response map classification is most useful in unanesthetized animals. Indeed, some of the response map types are not observed in anesthetized animals.

Five response map types are distinguished, denoted types I through V. These are defined below and in Figure 12-3. These definitions of response types are slightly different from those originally used by Evans and Nelson (1973a) and are more similar to the definitions used by Young and Voigt (1982) and Gibson (1983). Figure 12-3 shows schematic response maps for the unit types as well as examples of the behavior of their discharge rate in response to BF tones and broadband noise (rate versus level functions).

Type I units have strictly excitatory response maps (Figure 12-3). Auditory nerve fibers are type I and the excitatory response regions of type I units in the CN resemble the tuning curves of auditory nerve fibers. Type I units generally have monotonically increasing rate versus level functions and respond to broadband noise. Type I units do not display inhibitory responses to sound; that is, there is no single tone stimulus that will produce a net reduction in a type I unit's spontaneous activity during the stimulus.[5] The reductions of discharge rate that are observed following stimuli are

---

[4]A PST histogram is a plot of discharge rate (spikes/second) versus time. It is constructed by presenting a stimulus repeatedly (20 times in the case of Figure 12-2) and counting the number of spikes which occur at various times during and after the stimulus. For the histograms in Figure 12-2, the time axis is divided into 10-MS bins for the counting. In Figure 12-4 the time axis is divided into 0.25-ms bins.

[5]Auditory-nerve fibers and type I CN units show two-tone suppression (Sachs & Kiang, 1968), which is similar to inhibition in that stimulus energy at frequencies above and below the excitatory response area can suppress rate responses to other stimuli. There is no suppression of spontaneous discharge rate by this mechanism, however, and this feature distinguishes two-tone suppression from true inhibition.

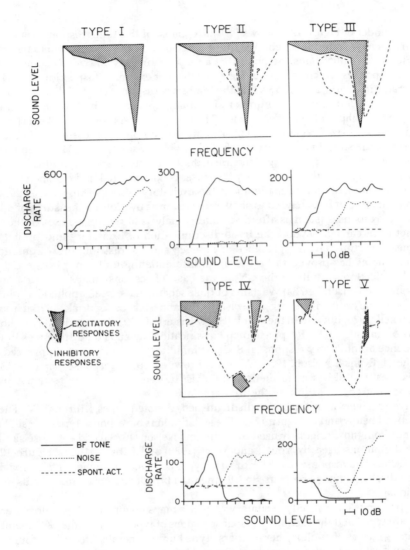

Figure 12-3. Examples of response maps (top) and rate versus sound level functions (bottom) for the five response map types. Types are labeled above each response map. Response maps are schematic, showing the general layout of response maps for each type. Question marks indicate variable or unknown features. Excitatory response (increase in discharge rate) regions are shaded; inhibitory response (decrease in discharge rate) regions are unshaded, enclosed in dashed lines. Rate versus level functions are actual examples of average discharge rate during 200-ms BF tone bursts (solid lines) or noise bursts (dotted lines), plotted as a function of the sound pressure level of the stimulus. Horizontal dashed lines show spontaneous rate.

not considered to be inhibitory responses. Poststimulus rate reductions are likely to be secondary to similar poststimulus rate reductions in auditory nerve fibers, that is, to peripheral adaptation (van Gisbergen et al., 1975a).

Type II units have excitatory response regions qualitatively similar to those of type I units. Type II units are distinguished by their lack of spontaneous activity and their lack of response to broadband stimuli. As is shown in the example in Figure 12-3, type II units respond to tones with high discharge rates, up to 400 spikes/s (Young & Voigt, 1982) but give little or no response to broadband noise. For the purposes of definition, it is convenient to consider a unit to be type II if its spontaneous rate is less than 2.5 spikes/s and if the ratio of its maximum BF tone response rate to its maximum noise response rate is greater than 2.8 (Gibson, 1983). Since type II units are not spontaneously active, it is not possible to determine directly whether they have inhibitory response areas. However, the fact that they do not respond to broadband stimuli while they do respond strongly to tonal stimuli suggests that they have very effective inhibitory input at frequencies above and below their excitatory response area. Inhibitory inputs are also suggested by the fact that their excitatory response areas are slightly narrower than those of auditory nerve fibers and that the thresholds of their low-frequency excitatory tails are 10 to 20 dB higher than those of auditory nerve fibers (Young & Voigt, 1982).

Type III units have excitatory response regions like those of type I and II units, but also have inhibitory regions at frequencies above or below their excitatory area (inhibitory sidebands). Type III units respond to noise at rates comparable to their response rates to BF tones.

Type IV units (Figures 12-2 and 12-3) give excitatory responses to BF tones near threshold; at higher levels, usually within 20 to 40 dB of threshold, the response to BF tones becomes inhibitory. As a consequence, the response maps of type IV units are predominantly inhibitory. The only consistently observed excitatory area is the small one near BF threshold. Other excitatory areas are usually present, but their location and configuration varies from unit to unit. Type IV units have characteristic rate–level functions for BF tones which are highly nonmonotonic (Figure 12-3). Type IV units respond strongly to broadband noise; indeed, over half of them give higher response rates to broadband noise than to BF tones (Young & Brownell, 1976).

Type V units are those which give only inhibitory responses to BF tones. They differ from type IV units by lacking the excitatory area near BF threshold (Figure 12-3).

In practice it is necessary to add a marginal response type to the list above, type I/III. These units respond to noise so they are not type II. However, they lack spontaneous activity, so it is not possible to test for the presence of inhibitory sidebands and thereby to distinguish between types I and III. Inhibitory sidebands can be detected in units without spontaneous activity by application of excitant amino acids to produce spontaneous activity (Martin & Dickson, 1983); this technique has not been generally applied.

The response map classification scheme is most useful if its unit types can be related to morphological cell types. In the case of the DCN, a relationship has been established by the use of antidromic stimulation, as is summarized in the first two columns of Table 12-1 (Young, 1980). Most of the type IV units tested could be stimulated from the efferent fiber tract of the DCN, the dorsal acoustic stria (DAS), implying that type IV responses are recorded from the principal cells of the DCN (fusiform cells and giant cells, labeled F and G in Figure 12-1). Almost no type II units could be antidromically activated from the DAS, suggesting that type II responses are recorded from a DCN interneuron. Furthermore, type II units were activated occasionally from the region of the VCN through which run association fibers (labeled i.f. in Figure 12-1) connecting AVCN and DCN (column 2 of Table 12-1). One source of these association fibers in the DCN is a variety of small cell interneuron called the corn cell or vertical cell by Lorente de Nó (1981); probably the small elongate cell of Brawer, Morest, & Kane, 1974). Corn cell axons send a collateral to the AVCN before entering the DCN neuropil (designated se in Figure 12-1). Antidromic stimulation results for type III DCN units are mixed and it is likely on this and other grounds (Gibson, 1983; Voigt & Young, 1980) that type III units are recorded from more than one DCN cell type.

The right half of Table 12-1 shows the distribution of the response map types among the subdivisions of the CN. Note that there are considerable differences in the prevalence of various unit types in different regions of the CN. The AVCN contains mostly type I or type I/III units; the PVCN contains more type III units than the AVCN; and the DCN contains mostly types II through IV. Type II units are found almost exclusively in the deep DCN, which finding is consistent with the location of corn cells (Lorente de Nó, 1981). Type IV units predominate in the fusiform cell layer of the DCN, in the vicinity of the cell bodies of the fusiform cells and are also found in the deep DCN, where giant cells are located.

The prevalence of inhibitory responses increases progressively from rostral to caudal in the CN. The responses of most units in the AVCN resemble those of auditory nerve fibers in that they do not show inhibitory responses, whereas almost all units in the DCN do. This fact has been noted in anesthetized preparations as well (Gisbergen et al., 1975a; Goldberg & Brownell, 1973). Thus there are significant differences among the response maps of units in the subdivisions of the CN, with a general increase in complexity as the recording site moves from AVCN to DCN.

Unit Types Based on PST Histograms

The second approach to classification of CN response patterns was developed by Kiang and Pfeiffer (Kiang, Pfeiffer, Warr, & Backus, 1965b; Pfeiffer, 1966a). This scheme classifies units according to the shape of PST histograms of their responses to brief BF tone bursts. In subsequent investigations (Bourk, 1976; Godfrey, Kiang, & Norris, 1975a,b; Kiang, Morest, Godfrey, Guinan, & Kane, 1973), PST histogram shape has been found to predict a number of other properties, as is required of a useful classification scheme. This approach has been applied to the CN of cat (Gisbergen et al., 1975a), chinchilla (Mast, 1970a), rabbit (Hui & Disterhoft, 1980;

TABLE 12-1

Locations from which units in the DCN can be antidromically stimulated (left two columns) and distribution of the response map types among various subdivisions of the cochlear nucleus (right five columns)

Response map type	Units in DCN antidromically activated from[a]		% of units[b] of each type found in			
	DAS	VCN	DCN^c_{FCL}	DCN^c_{Deep}	PVCN	AVCN
I			•	•	X	XX
I/III					XX	XX
II	1/30	6/32	•	XX	•	•
III	4/16	1/11	X	X	XX	X
IV	34/43	0/22	XXXX	XX		
V			•	•		

[a]From Young (1980). Units in DCN only; no units in remainder of CN were tested. Given as number antidromically driven/number tested. VCN stimulus site is in dorsal, posterior VCN, near the location of association fibers connecting DCN and AVCN.

[b]Scale: no symbol, < 1%; (•) = 1–15%; (X) = 16–30%; (XX) = 31–45%; (XXX) = 46–60%; (XXXX) = 61–76%; (XXXXX) = > 75%. Percentages express fraction of units in each column. DCN data are from Young and Voigt (1982; 86 units in FCL, 108 units in deep layer). VCN data are from Gibson (1983; 41 units in AVCN, 26 units in PVCN).

[c]DCN_{FCL} = fusiform and molecular cell layers of the DCN; DCN_{Deep} = deep layer of the DCN.

Perry & Webster, 1981), kangaroo rat (Caspary, 1972) and gerbil (Frisina, Chamberlain, Brachman, & Smith, 1982).

Figure 12-4 illustrates the basic response types of this scheme; a few types which are encountered infrequently have been left out of this figure. The PST histograms illustrated in Figure 12-4 have been redrawn from examples provided by Godfrey and associates (1975a,b) and Bourk (1976).

Primarylike responses (top row) are characterized by a high rate of discharge at stimulus onset followed by a gradual decline to a more or less steady response through the remainder of the stimulus. The left-hand example in the top row of Figure 12-4 is characteristic of auditory nerve fibers as well as CN neurons, which is the reason for the name primarylike.

Onset responses are shown in the second row of Figure 12-4. They are characterized by a single spike or a brief burst of spikes at stimulus onset with little or no discharge during the remainder of the stimulus burst.

Chopper responses are illustrated in the third row of Figure 12-4. They are characterized by fluctuations in response rate that are synchronized with stimulus onset. The peaks and valleys in the chopper PST histograms are not produced by phase locking to individual cycles of the stimulus tone. Instead, they reflect the tendency of these cells to discharge action potentials at regularly spaced intervals.

Pausers give an onset spike, followed by a pause of significant duration (at least 5 ms), followed by a gradual resumption of activity. Buildup responses are like pause responses except that the onset spike is missing. The *onset-S* pattern is characterized by an onset burst followed by a gradual decline in activity through the rest of the stimulus burst; the decline in response rate is more rapid than in primarylike units and less rapid than in other onset units. An additional response type not illustrated in Figure 12-4 is similar to type V described previously, in that it shows only reduction of spontaneous activity in response to BF tone stimuli (Gisbergen et al., 1975a; Godfrey et al., 1975b).

The PST histogram shapes in Figure 12-4 illustrate the range of response types encountered in the CN. In fact, the histograms in each row are typical of subtypes of the major response types (i.e., two subtypes of primarylike units, three of onset units, and so forth); these subtypes are listed in the caption to Figure 12-4. Bourk (1976) and Godfrey and colleagues (1975a,b) have shown that, to varying degrees, each of these subtypes has a constellation of properties consistently associated with it. Thus the subtypes can be considered to be different unit types, each with its own set of characteristics.

A problem for the classification based on PST histograms is that units frequently show more than one PST histogram shape. For example, as the stimulus level is increased, a unit may show a primarylike response, then a pauser response, and then a chopper response (an example is provided in Figure 2 of Godfrey et al., 1975a). The problem is worse if stimulus frequency is moved away from BF. Therefore, it is not possible, in general, to characterize a unit's responses in terms of one type of PST histogram. Rather, the PST histogram response type that seems most typical of a unit is chosen, and then the unit's other properties are examined. The ultimate unit type is defined in terms of a constellation of properties, only one of which is its most typical PST histogram type. Unit types have been given the names of their most typical PST response type, and one must be careful to remember the distinction between unit types and PST histograms in considering this literature (e.g., a pauser unit can give a chopper PST histogram under certain circumstances).

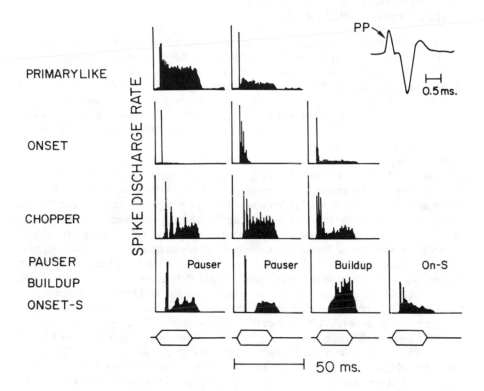

Figure 12-4. Examples of various types of PST histograms recorded in the CN of anesthetized cat. Computed from 25-ms BF tone bursts with envelope rise times of 2.5 ms, repeated once every 100 ms. Primarylike responses (top row) are identical to the responses of auditory nerve fibers (first example) or show a brief pause in firing (second example, called pri-notch). Onset responses (second row) vary in the degree of steady-state response they show. The example first from left is On-I (Godfrey et al., 1975a,b); the second is On-A (Bourk); the third is On-L (Godfrey et al., 1975a,b) or On-P (Bourk, 1976). Chopper units (third row) differ in the rate of chopping and the duration over which coherent chopping is observed. The examples are Chop-L (long interval), Chop-S (sustained) and Chop-T (transient), respectively, from left to right (Bourk, 1976). Pauser and buildup units (bottom row) show a long latency steady-state response which may be accompanied by an onset spike (pausers). Bourk called units similar to On-S *On-G*. The inset at upper right shows the shape of triphasic waveforms containing prepotentials (PP) that are observed in the AVCN. Histograms are redrawn from Godfrey and associates (1975a,b) and Bourk (1976).

Correspondence of Response Types and Morphological Cell Types

Bourk (1976) used an additional property of his recordings to classify units in the AVCN. Many units in the AVCN have triphasic action potentials, which consist of two components: a positive potential (PP) followed by a diphasic action potential of the usual configuration (Pfeiffer, 1966b). An example of one of these triphasic action potentials is shown at top right in Figure 12-4. Prepotentials are observed in regions containing large synaptic terminals such as the end-bulbs of Held on bushy cells in the AVCN (SB and GB in Figure 12-1; Brawer & Morest, 1975; Feldman & Harrison, 1969; Lenn & Reese, 1966; Pfeiffer, 1966b; Ramon y Cajal, 1909; and similar end-bulbs on the principal cells of the medial nucleus of the trapezoid body (MNTB; Li & Guinan, 1971; Morest, 1968). The prepotential is thought to be the action potential discharge of the large presynaptic terminal. Li and Guinan (1971) analyzed this synapse by recording from cells in the MNTB where the incoming axons that form end-bulbs can be orthodromically stimulated from the TB and the axons of the postsynaptic MNTB cells can be antidromically stimulated from the lateral superior olive (LSO). Orthodromic stimulation from the TB gives the full triphasic action potential, whereas antidromic stimulation from the LSO gives only the second, diphasic component, the presumed postsynaptic discharge. Based on this and other evidence, Li and Guinan concluded that the prepotential was recorded from the end-bulb and the diphasic spike from the postsynaptic cell. It seems safe to draw a similar conclusion for triphasic action potentials in the AVCN, that is, to conclude that AVCN prepotential units are recorded from bushy cells (Bourk, 1976). The distinction between prepotential and nonprepotential units is a third classification scheme for units in the VCN. Bourk (1976) found that virtually all AVCN units with prepotentials were primarylike and vice versa (but see Martin & Adams, 1979, who reported some nonprimarylike units with prepotentials). On this basis, he suggested that primarylike units are recorded from bushy cells. It follows that nonprimarylike response types in the VCN are recorded from stellate cells (labeled St in Figure 12-1). Stellate cells differ from bushy cells by having long dendritic trees upon which they receive bouton terminals from auditory nerve fibers; end-bulbs are not observed on stellate cells (Cant, 1981; Cant & Morest, 1979a; Tolbert & Morest, 1982a,b).

The best evidence for correspondence of primarylike responses and bushy cells and of nonprimarylike responses and stellate cells is provided by results of intercellular dye injection experiments.[6] Rhode, Oertel, and Smith (1983b) marked 16 stellate cells in the AVCN and PVCN with horseradish peroxidase (HRP); 14 of these cells were choppers and 2 of them gave onset responses. Two bushy cells were marked, both of which gave primarylike responses. A third cell with morphology similar to that of a bushy cell was also marked; its responses were primarylike, except that its response latency was rather long for a primarylike response. This cell was smaller than most bushy cells and may have been a small cell. Although the conclusion will stand on firmer ground when a larger number of marked cells is available, the HRP

---

[6]In these experiments, a microelectrode is used to record from a cell and then, in fortunate cases, the cell is injected with a solution of horseradish peroxidase (HRP) from the microelectrode. The enzyme spreads throughout the cell and the cell can be visualized later by using the enzyme to catalyze a reaction, leaving an opaque precipitate.

marking experiments provide direct evidence that primarylike responses are recorded from bushy cells and nonprimarylike responses are recorded from stellate cells.

The correspondence between bushy cells and primarylike responses and between stellate and nonprimarylike responses can be extrapolated to the globular bushy cells and multipolar cells (which have stellate morphology) of the caudal AVCN and PVCN. Because they have the shortest latencies of antidromic activation from the TB, Bourk (1976) concluded that the primarylike-notch unit type (see caption to Figure 12-4) was recorded from globular bushy cells. These cells are the source of the largest axons in the trapezoid body (Tolbert, Morest, & Yurgelun-Todd, 1982; van Noort, 1969).

The distribution of PST histogram response types among the subdivisions of the CN is summarized in Table 12-2. The subdivisions of the AVCN for the data listed in the right-hand five columns of this table are those introduced by Brawer and associates (1974). The data in Table 12-2 show that there are significant differences in the distribution of primarylike (prepotential) and nonprimarylike response types in the various subregions of the AVCN. The distribution of primarylike and nonprimarylike units corresponds well with the distribution of bushy and stellate cells in the various subdivisions of the VCN (Brawer et al., 1974; Cant & Morest, 1979a).

The octopus cell area (OCA) is a region in the posterior part of the PVCN containing only one cell type, the octopus cell (Kane, 1973; Osen, 1969). Almost all of the responses recorded in the OCA by Godfrey and associates (1975a) were onset responses (third column of Table 12-2). Rhode and colleagues (1983b) filled one octopus cell with HRP and it showed an onset response pattern. Thus, it seems likely that octopus cells give onset responses in the anesthetized preparation. In unanesthetized, decerebrate cats, Ritz and Brownell (1982) also found onset responses to predominate in the OCA (32/49 cells), but the response characteristics of these onset cells were quite different from those of Godfrey and co-workers (1975a). The problems raised by Ritz and Brownell's results will be discussed in more detail below.

The predominant response type in the DCN of anesthetized animals is the pauser/buildup type (first two columns of Table 12-2; Godfrey et al., 1975b). There is evidence that these responses are recorded from the principal cells of the DCN. First, three pauser units could be antidromically stimulated from the DAS (Kiang et al., 1973) and five DCN pauser units could be antidromically stimulated from the central nucleus of the inferior colliculus (Bourk, 1976). Second, Rhode, Smith, and Oertel (1983a) filled 26 DCN pauser or buildup cells with HRP; 24 of them were fusiform cells, one of the two types of DCN principal cell. The response type of giant cells, the other DCN principal cell type, is unclear; Rhode, Smith and Oertel (1980) reported that giant cells did not respond to sound, perhaps because of the barbiturate anesthesia.

Units with response characteristics like those of type IV units in unanesthetized preparations are not often encountered in anesthetized preparations (but see Gisbergen et al., 1975a). It seems clear that, in the presence of anesthesia, type IV units give pauser or buildup responses. This correspondence has been demonstrated directly by administering an anesthetic dose of sodium pentobarbital to decerebrate cats during

TABLE 12-2

Location of various PST histogram types

	DCN		PVCN		AVCN				
	FCL	Deep	OCA	Other	PV	PD	AP	APD	AA
Primarylike (prepotential)		•	•	•	XXXX	X	XXX	XXXXX	XXXXX
Onset		•	XXXX	X	•	X	X		•
Chopper	•	X	•	XXXX	XX	XXX	XX	X	•
On-S		X							
Pauser-buildup	XXXXX	XXX	•	•			•		
Other		•	•				•	•	

Notes. Each column shows how the units encountered in one region of the cochlear nucleus are distributed among various types. Data are from Godfrey and associates, 1975a,b and Bourk, 1976. Scale: no symbol, <1%; (•) = 1–15%; (X) = 16–30%; (XX) = 31–45%; (XXX) = 46–60%; (XXXX) = 61–75%; (XXXXX) = >75%. Percentages express fraction of units in each column. For the AVCN, all units with prepotentials (Bourk's PP1 and PP2 categories) were counted as primarylike. Abbreviations: FCL DCN fusiform cell layer; Deep, deep region of DCN; OCA otopus cell area; PV, PD regions of posterior division of AVCN (Brawer et al., 1974); AP, APD, AA regions of anterior AVCN. Numbers of units in columns are 118, 224, 52, 48, 50, 115, 203, 37, 297, respectively, from left to right.

the study of type IV units and showing that the units' inhibitory responses at BF are converted to excitatory pauser responses (Evans & Nelson, 1973a; Young & Brownell, 1976). Another piece of evidence consistent with the correspondence of type IV and pauser/buildup units is the fact that both types can be antidromically stimulated from the DAS and IC (Table 12-1 and the paragraph above).

A final interesting point about the distribution of response types in the DCN is that onset-S responses are found primarily in the deep layer of the DCN (Table 12-2). Their distribution thus resembles that of type II units in the decerebrate preparation (Table 12-1). These two unit types share other properties (Godfrey, 1971; Godfrey et al., 1975b; Young & Voigt, 1982). They are the only units in the CN that do not respond well to broad- band stimuli such as clicks or noise bursts; they are not spontaneously active; and they have rather characteristic gradually nonmonotonic rate–level functions (Figure 3 and Figure 6 of Godfrey et al., 1975b). These similarities make it likely that they are recorded from the same morphological cell type. As was discussed above, evidence from antidromic stimulation studies suggests that these responses are recorded from small cell interneurons in the DCN (Young, 1980).

RESPONSE PROPERTIES IN THE VCN

Differences Between Primarylike and Nonprimarylike Units in VCN

Table 12-1 shows that the response maps of neurons in the CN diverge progressively from those of auditory nerve fibers (i.e., type I) as the recording site moves from the AVCN to the DCN; the most striking change is that more inhibitory responses are observed in caudal areas. Table 12-2 contains a similar result, in that the prevalence of nonprimarylike response types increases from rostral to caudal. The general correlation in the location of primarylike and type I responses (i.e., most common in rostral AVCN) raises the question of whether there is a general correspondence of type I and primarylike units and of type III and nonprimarylike units. Sufficient evidence to answer this question is not available, but there is some evidence to support such a correspondence. Inhibitory sidebands have not been observed in the rostral AVCN (Goldberg & Brownell, 1973) or in units with prepotentials (Bourk, 1976; Gibson, unpublished observation). Inhibitory sidebands were observed in all nonprepotential units studied by Martin and Dickson (1983). There is, however, a conflicting observation; Brownell (1975) observed inhibitory sidebands in the large-diameter axons of the trapezoid body; these axons come from globular bushy cells in the posterior AVCN and PVCN (Tolbert, Morest, & Yurgelun-Todd (1982) and give a variety of types of primarylike response (primarylike-notch; Bourk, 1976). Final resolution of this question must await further study.

The nonprimarylike response types differ from primarylike units (and auditory nerve fibers) in a number of ways other than the shape of their PST histograms. Table 12-3 summarizes some of these differences.

Nonprimarylike response types generally have longer response latencies (column 2) and show weaker phase locking to the stimulus (columns 3 and 4). The results summarized in Table 12-3 were obtained by direct observation of responses to tones or clicks. van Gisbergen, Grashuis, Johannesma, & Vendrick (1975b) obtained similar results by computing the cross correlation between a noise stimulus and the spike train it evoked. The amplitudes of these cross correlation functions were smaller for nonprimarylike units, which finding is consistent with weaker phase locking to the stimulus.

An additional difference between primarylike and nonprimarylike units is in response regularity. While a simple quantitative comparison of regularity cannot be made because of differences in the way in which regularity has been studied, the results can be summarized as follows. Auditory nerve fibers and primarylike units discharge in a very irregular fashion (Bourk, 1976; Goldberg & Brownell, 1973; Kiang,

Watanabe, Thomas, & Clark, 1965a; Pfeiffer & Kiang, 1965). Irregular means that the time interval between successive spikes varies over a wide range of values in a random fashion; in fact, a Poisson point process serves as a reasonable approximation to primary auditory spike trains, except for refractoriness (Kiang et al., 1965a). Nonprimarylike units have more regular discharge; the most regular unit types are choppers and pausers in the DCN (Bourk, 1976; Gisbergen et al., 1975c; Godfrey et al., 1975a,b; Goldberg & Brownell, 1973; Pfeiffer & Kiang, 1965). The effects of regular discharge show up most clearly in the chopper PST response pattern. Chopping is basically a reflection of an even spacing between action potentials in a unit's responses. When responses to several stimulus bursts are averaged together to compute a PST histogram, the spikes tend to occur at the same times in all bursts, producing a series of peaks and valleys in the histogram. In contrast, for an irregular primarylike unit, spikes occur at random times following stimulus onset, resulting in a smooth histogram which reflects only average discharge rate.

Primarylike Responses and Bushy Cells

It is interesting to consider the differences in response properties of primarylike and nonprimarylike units in terms of differences in their synaptic organizations. The clearest contrast is between bushy cells, presumed to be primarylike, and stellate cells, presumed to be nonprimarylike. The bushy cells receive a few very large end-bulb terminals on their somata, whereas the stellate cells receive a large number of small bouton inputs on their dendritic trees and in some cases also on their somata (Brawer & Morest, 1975; Cant, 1981; Cant & Morest, 1979b; Feldman & Harrison, 1969; Tolbert & Morest, 1982a,b). The two types of terminals, although different in form, come from the same auditory nerve fibers (Brawer & Morest, 1975; Feldman & Harrison, 1969; Lorente de Nó, 1933, 1981), so the patterns of activity at the inputs of bushy and stellate cells are the same. They differ only in the number of auditory nerve fibers contacting each cell and in the form and distribution of the inputs on their surfaces.

The effect of placement of synaptic inputs on the soma or at varying distances from the soma on the dendritic tree can be understood from the theory of dendritic electrotonus (Jack, Noble, & Tsien, 1975; Rall, 1977). Generally, the synaptic potentials observed in the soma are low-pass filtered versions of the potentials generated at the synaptic site. As the synaptic site moves away from the soma along the dendritic tree, the potentials observed in the soma change by having slower rise times, longer durations, and smaller amplitudes. Thus, on electrotonic grounds alone, postsynaptic potentials in bushy cells should be large with rapid rise times and those in stellate cells should be smaller, with slower rise times. The results of intracellular recording in the CN are generally consistent with these predictions (Rhode et al., 1983b; Romand, 1978, 1979) and are summarized in Figure 12-5.

The first column of Figure 12-5 shows five examples of intracellular recordings in primarylike units. These results are typical of primarylike neurons (Romand, 1978)

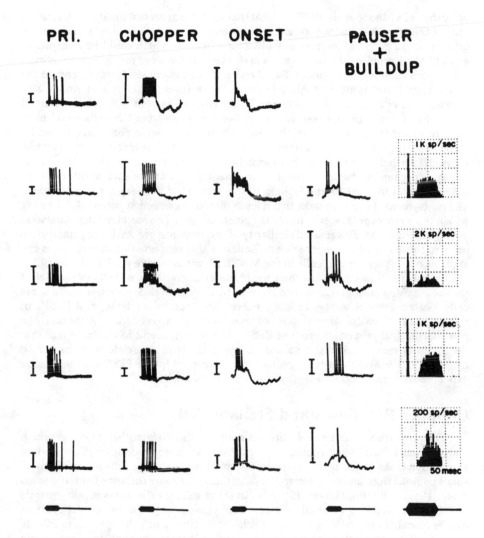

Figure 12-5. Examples of intracellular recordings of responses to BF tone bursts. Each column
shows examples from four or five different units of one PST histogram type (labeled
at top). For pauser/buildup group only, PST histograms of responses are also shown
(right-hand column). Vertical scale marks 10 mV in all cases. Tone bursts, shown
at bottom of each column, were 25 ms in duration. In primarylike column, top
3 records are from primarylike and bottom two from primarylike-notch units. Top
3 onset units were On-A or On-I; fourth unit is On-L; bottom unit is On-S. All
pauser/buildup units are from the DCN. (Redrawn with permission from Romand,
1979.)

or bushy cells (Rhode et al., 1983b) in that there is little or no sustained depolarization during the stimulus. Instead, membrane potential rises very rapidly and develops into an action potential without any obvious inflection which could be interpreted as an EPSP. A problem of interpretation in this case is that these recordings sometimes come from auditory nerve fibers. Based on their click latencies, Romand concluded that a significant number of his recordings were from CN cells and Rhode and colleagues (1983b) reported similar results for two bushy cells which were stained with HRP. Even in those cases, however, the responses from CN cells could have been recorded from the axons of the cells, where the synaptic potentials cannot be seen. Thus, there is some uncertainty about the intracellular potentials of primarylike units. Nevertheless, the data at present favor the idea that bushy (primarylike) neurons, because of the large size of their synaptic inputs from each auditory nerve fiber, respond in a one-to-one fashion to the arrrival of primary action potentials. The postsynaptic EPSP is so large that it leads directly to an action potential, following which the membrane is reset to its resting potential, giving no sustained depolarization during the stimulus. The general similarity of the response properties of primarylike units to those of auditory nerve fibers (Bourk, 1976) supports this idea, as does the analysis of the prepotential cells in the MNTB discussed above (Li & Guinan, 1971).

Oertel (1982) has analyzed the membrane characteristics of cells in the CN of the mouse using intracellular recording in an in vitro brain slide preparation. In some cells located anterior to the auditory nerve, she found very large, fast EPSPs in response to electrical stimulation of the auditory nerve root. Although the pharmacological properties of these EPSPs do not correspond to current ideas that the auditory nerve transmitter substance is glutamate or aspartate (see chapter 10 by Wenthold & Martin in this volume), they are the type of EPSP which is to be expected from the model of bushy cells discussed above.

Chopper Responses and Stellate Cells

The properties of stellate cells are consistent with a different situation, in which many small inputs must summate to produce an action potential. This sort of summation is suggested by the synaptic morphology of stellate cells in which many small boutons from auditory nerve fibers terminate at some distance from the soma (Cant, 1981; Tolbert & Morest, 1982a,b). In some stellate cells, no synaptic contacts are observed on the soma at all. The electrophysiological properties of stellate cells can be examined by looking at intracellular recordings from chopper units (Rhode et al., 1983b). The electrophysiological properties of some chopper units are shown in the second column of Figure 12-5. In the majority of chopper units, Romand (1978, 1979) observed relatively large, steady depolarizations during the stimulus.

One of the significant differences between chopper units and auditory nerve fibers is the regularity of their discharge. Gisbergen and associates (1975c) considered two possible ways in which the irregular discharges of auditory nerve fibers could be turned into regular discharges in CN cells. One explanation presumes that a large number of separate synaptic events must summate in order to lead to a discharge. The inputs are summated in the membrane capacitance of the postsynaptic neuron;

when the membrane potential reaches threshold, a spike occurs and the membrane potential is reset to its resting value. Molnar and Pfeiffer (1968) had previously shown that, under these circumstances, superposition of a large number of irregular spike trains could lead to a regular output. The regularity of the output in this situation derives from the fact that the neuron must accumulate the discharges of many inputs to reach threshold (see Goldberg & Brownell, 1973, and Nilsson, 1975, for slightly different formulations of this point). Notice that this explanation focuses on the integration of input events preceding a spike discharge in the postsynaptic cell.

The alternative hypothesis considered by Gisbergen and colleagues (1975c) is that, following a spike discharge, the postsynaptic neuron is refractory for a long period of time. Even though the summated input process may be sufficient to significantly depolarize the cell, it does not produce an action potential until recovery from the preceding one is complete (Goldberg, Adrian, & Smith, 1964). Regularity in this instance derives from the properties of the recovery process. This explanation focuses on events following spike discharge.

Gisbergen and associates (1975c) reasoned that these two models could be differentiated by considering the first spike in response to a stimulus; this spike is not preceded by another spike, and therefore could be affected by prespike integration of inputs, but not by postspike refractoriness. Gisbergen and colleagues showed that there is a correlation between regularity of discharge and the latency of the first spike evoked by a stimulus. This is to be expected if the behavior of regularly discharging units is controlled by the integration time required for input events to summate to threshold, but is not expected from the refractoriness model.

Examination of the intracellular potentials of chopper units is partly consistent with the idea of integration time as the controlling factor in chopper units' discharge. Romand (1979, figure 2) has shown an example of a chopper unit in which the rise time of click-evoked EPSPs in the cell is rather slow (more than 1 ms). However, the integration time hypothesis seems to require a resetting of membrane potential to rest following a spike, followed by a period of integration back up to threshold (Molnar & Pfeiffer, 1968). This does not appear to occur, because chopper units display a steady depolarization during the stimulus (Figure 12-5). It may be, as suggested by Rhode and co-workers (1983b), that both mechanisms operate; integration effects produce long first spike latencies in these cells, but some membrane property similar to a recovery process produces the perstimulatory regularity.

The synaptic morphology of stellate cells can be used to explain another aspect of the response properties of choppers, their relatively weak phase locking (Table 12-3). A large number of auditory nerve fiber inputs at some distance from the spike initiation site should lead to severe low-pass filtering of EPSPs by dendritic electrotonus. This filtering should damp out phase-locked variations in postsynaptic potentials as they propagate to the spike trigger zone.

Onset Responses

Units showing onset responses are found throughout the CN (Bourk, 1976; Godfrey et al., 1975a,b), usually mixed with other response types. The exception is the caudal PVCN, where onset responses predominate in anesthetized animals (Table 12-2). Onset responses in the OCA are thought to be recorded from octopus cells, the predominate cell type of this region (Kane, 1973; Osen, 1969). The discussion that follows applies to onset cell types other than the onset-S and onset-G types, which appear to be different from other onset types.

The properties of units giving onset responses are similar to those of primarylike units in many features, the PST histograms being the most significant exception. The response latencies of onset cells are short and onset cells phase lock to reasonably high frequencies (Table 12-3). The onset units of the OCA are typical in these regards. Octopus cells share with bushy cells the property of having massive synaptic input from the auditory nerve on their somata. They differ from bushy cells in that octopus cells receive a large number of bouton terminals from many auditory nerve fibers (Kane, 1973) as opposed to a large number of synaptic contacts gathered up into a few large terminals from a small number of auditory nerve fibers. Nevertheless, it is likely that the similarity of latency and phase-locking data for these two cell types derives from the similar arrangement of auditory nerve input on their somata.

A number of suggestions have been offered to explain the onset character of octopus cell responses. Kane (1973) found that there were two morphologically different types of synaptic contact made by auditory nerve fibers on octopus cells; she suggested that one might be inhibitory, so that the octopus cell would be excited and then immediately inhibited by a volley of auditory nerve activity. However, intracellular recordings from onset cells, including the one octopus cell identified by Rhode and associates, (1983b; also Britt & Starr, 1976a; Romand, 1978), have usually found large steady depolarizations in these cells during stimulation (third column of Figure 12–5). In the one case in Figure 12–5 with a hyperpolarization, the hyperpolarization was attributed by Romand (1978) to spike afterpotentials. Such steady depolarization is clearly inconsistent with the involvement of inhibition in producing transient responses in these cells.

Ritz and Brownell (1982) found onset responses to predominate in the OCA of unanesthetized, decerebrate cats. However, their onset units had several properties that are significantly different from those of onset units in anesthetized animals. Most of their onset units were spontaneously active and many had inhibitory sidebands. One group of units (called *onset-in*) were invariably spontaneously active and displayed inhibitory responses essentially identical to those of type IV units in the DCN (12/32 onset units localized histologically to the OCA). The responses to BF tones of onset-in units were excitatory near threshold, but became inhibitory at higher levels. The inhibitory response consisted of an onset burst of spikes, followed by cessation of discharge for the duration of the tone burst, followed by an offset burst of spikes after the stimulus, a typical pattern for DCN type IV neurons (Young & Brownell, 1976).

It is not clear that Ritz and Brownell's onset-in units were recorded from the same type of cell as the OCA onset units of Godfrey and associates (1975a). In two cases where onset-in units were studied before and after administration of barbiturate anesthesia, the response properties of the cells in the anesthetized state were more like

TABLE 12-3

Some properties of various response types in anesthetized cats

	% with spont. act[b]	Click latency[c] (ms.)	Avg. vector strength at 1.5 kHz[d,e]	Freq. at which VS = 0.2[e](kHz)	Other properties
Primarylike[a]	93	0–1	0.73	4	
Onset	0	0–1.2	≃0.63	≃3	Slightly broader tuning curves than other types; strong response to clicks
Chopper	63	1–4.5	0.1	1.2	
On-S	0	1–4	–	–	Give weak response to broadband stimuli (8/12 did not respond to noise bursts, 15/26 did not respond to clicks; Godfrey, 1971)
Pauser/buildup	84	1–6	0.09	–	

[a]AVCN prepotential units (PP1 and PP2 of Bourk, 1976).

[b]Spont. > 2.5/s for PVCN and DCN are data of Godfrey and colleagues (1975a,b); spont. > 1/s for AVCN are data of Bourk (1976).

[c]Latency relative to average auditory nerve fiber value, units with BFs > 2 kHz only; clicks are 20–40 dB above threshold (Godfrey et al., 1975a,b; Bourk, 1976).

[d]Data for primarylike, onset, and chopper units from AVCN only (Bourk, 1976); onset values are based on very few units; the value in pauser/buildup row is for DCN cells of all types encountered (Goldberg & Brownell, 1973; 73% of their units had pauser/builtup patterns).

[e]Vector strength (VS) is a measure of the strength of phase locking (Goldberg & Brownell, 1973). It is computed by plotting a vector of unit length for each spike in the record; the angle between the vector and the x axis is equal to the phase of the sinusoidal stimulus at which the spike occurred. Vector strength equals the length of the vectorial sum of these unit vectors divided by the number of spikes. Perfect phase locking gives a vector strength of 1; no phase locking at all gives a vector strength near 0.

those of choppers than onset units. Nevertheless, the possibility that octopus cells might show inhibitory responses raises the difficult question of how these responses might arise. Given the general finding of depolarizing intracellular potentials in onset units, and the paucity of synaptic input to octopus cells from sources other than auditory nerve fibers (Kane, 1973), it seems unlikely that synaptic inhibition could be involved.

Ritz and Brownell (1982) suggested that the apparently inhibitory responses might result from depolarization block, a blockage of action potential discharge caused by inactivation of sodium channels by sustained depolarization. This mechanism is thought to account for the stoppage of spike discharge that occurs when large doses of excitant amino acids are applied to certain cells, including prepotential cells in the AVCN (Martin & Adams, 1979). Depolarization block usually produces onset responses, because at least one spike is produced at the onset of depolarization before the block is asserted. Regardless of whether Ritz and Brownell's onset-in units were recorded from octopus cells, depolarization block is an attractive explanation for the properties of onset cells. Depolarization block is consistent with the large intracellular depolarizations in onset units during stimulation (Britt & Starr, 1976a; Romand, 1978; Rhode et al., 1983b) and the small size of extracellularly recorded action potentials in the OCA (Godfrey et al., 1975a). However, a problem for the depolarization block hypothesis is that excitant amino acids (glutamate and aspartate) do not produce depolarization block in onset units of the PVCN (Caspary, Havey, & Faingold, 1981); rather, they produce a general increase in excitability of these cells. At the present time, the physiology of onset cells in general and octopus cells in particular is incompletely understood.

RESPONSE PROPERTIES IN THE DCN

The DCN has the most complex morphology of the subdivisions of the CN. It contains a variety of morphological cell types and a quite complex neuropil (Kane, 1974a; Osen & Mugnaini, 1981; Lorente de Nó, 1981). It is the only subdivision of the CN which has been shown to have significant numbers of interneurons. At least three different pathways exist for transfer of activity between the inputs to the DCN and its principal cells (Figure 12-1). These include direct synaptic terminals on the principal cells, and indirect pathway via small cell interneurons (labeled se and ss in Figure 12-1), and a mossy fiber/granule cell system (labeled mf, g in Figure 12-1) similar to that of the cerebellum (Kane, 1974a,b; Lorente de Nó, 1981; Mugnaini, Warr, & Osen, 1980; Osen & Mugnaini, 1981). The DCN also receives a large efferent input from parts of the superior olivary complex and the inferior colliculus (Adams & Warr, 1976; Elverland, 1977; Jones & Casseday, 1979; Kane & Finn, 1977; Rasmussen, 1964) and is less dependent on its auditory nerve input than are other regions of the CN (Bird, Gulley, Wenthold, & Fex, 1978; Koerber, Pfeiffer, Warr, & Kiang, 1966; Rasmussen, 1964). The efferent input to the DCN explains the prominence of responses to contralateral ear stimuli in DCN neurons (Mast, 1970b, 1973; Young & Brownell, 1976).

The most striking feature of the response characteristics of cells in the DCN is the prevalence of anesthesia-sensitive inhibitory responses (type IV and type V; Evans & Nelson, 1973a; Young & Brownell, 1976). These responses are recorded from the principal neurons of the DCN (fusiform and giant cells; Young, 1980). Evans and Nelson (1973b) showed that predominantly inhibitory responses were observed in the DCN in preparations in which the efferent input to the DCN from higher auditory centers had been surgically removed by making a knife cut medial to the nucleus. This implies that a significant fraction of the inhibition was generated within the CN.

There is evidence to support the existence of at least two different sources of inhibitory influence on DCN principal cells. Evans and Nelson (1973b) showed that powerful and long-lasting inhibition of spontaneous activity of DCN units could be produced by single shock stimuli in the AVCN, especially the part of the AVCN through which the association fibers connecting the DCN and AVCN run (Lorente de Nó, 1933). This inhibitory effect was observed in preparations in which the auditory nerve had been sectioned 2 weeks previously and allowed to degenerate. Evans and Nelson concluded that the association fibers from cells in the AVCN were a major source of inhibitory input to cells in the DCN.

The second potential source of inhibitory input to DCN principal cells is from small cell interneurons in the DCN (Voigt & Young, 1980; Young & Brownell, 1976). As was mentioned above, the results of antidromic stimulation imply that type IV units are recorded from DCN principal cells (fusiform and giant cells, F and G in Figure 12-1), whereas type II responses are recorded from DCN interneurons (Young, 1980). Young and Brownell (1976) pointed out that the responses of these two unit types are reciprocal: type IV units are active when type II units are silent and vice versa. For example, type IV units are spontaneously active whereas type II units are not (Young & Voigt, 1982). Figure 12-6 illustrates results from a type II and a type IV unit recorded simultaneously with two electrodes in the same DCN (Young & Voigt, 1981). Note that in parts A and B of Figure 12-6 the excitatory area of the type II unit overlaps the inhibitory response area of the type IV unit. The arrows at the top of the figure point to the best frequencies (BFs) of the two units to aid in alignment. Figure 12-6C shows rate versus level functions for the two units responding to tone bursts at the BF of the type II unit. The type II unit begins to discharge at about the level at which the type IV unit's rate begins to decline. In fact, type II units consistently have thresholds which are 10 dB or so higher than those of type IV units with similar BFs in the same preparation (Young & Brownell, 1976).

Figure 12-6D shows more direct evidence for an inhibitory contact between these two units. This figure shows a cross correlogram (Moore, Segundo, Perkel, & Levitan, 1970; Perkel, Gerstein, & Moore, 1967) of the simultaneously recorded spike trains of the two units whose response maps are plotted above. The cross correlogram shows the average discharge rate of the type IV unit in relation to spikes in the type II unit. Note that there is a drop in type IV average firing rate just after type II spikes (i.e., just to the right of the origin). Such an "inhibitory trough" was found in the cross correlograms of 11/14 type II/type IV neuron pairs isolated on the same electrode (Voigt & Young, 1980) and in 20/55 pairs isolated with two electrodes (Voigt & Young,

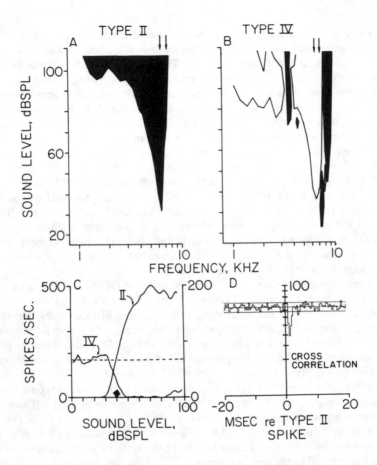

Figure 12-6. (A) Response map of type II unit from DCN. (B) Response map of type IV unit from DCN. These two units were isolated in the same nucleus using two electrodes and studied simultaneously. BFs of the units are slightly different, shown by arrows at the top of the response maps. (C) Plots of discharge rate versus sound level for 200-ms tone bursts at BF of type II unit. Black diamond shows sound level at which steady tone was presented to evoke activity in both units from which the cross correlogram in (D) was computed. (D) Cross correlogram of activity of the two units during presentation of steady tone at BF of type II unit, 40 dB SPL. Generated by constructing histograms of type IV discharge rate versus time, centered on each type II spike. These were superimposed to estimate average rate in type IV unit as a function of time before and after spikes in type II unit. Type II spikes all occur at time 0 on abscissa; plot shows type IV rate in vicinity of type II spikes. Square root of rate was plotted for statistical reasons (Voigt & Young, 1980). Horizontal lines show ±2 standard deviation confidence limits on individual bins in cross correlogram, assuming long delay mean value (from Young & Voigt, 1981).

unpublished data). An inhibitory trough must be found in the cross correlograms of units connected by a monosynaptic inhibitory connection (Moore et al., 1970). The consistent occurrence of inhibitory troughs in DCN type II and type IV units' cross correlograms supports the idea that type II units are inhibitory interneurons terminating on type IV units.

The reciprocal nature of the responses of type II and type IV units persists in the presence of anesthesia, if it is accepted that type II units correspond to onset-S units and type IV units correspond to pausers or buildup units. The decay of activity in onset-S units corresponds qualitatively to the inverse of the buildup of activity in pausers or buildup units (see Figure 12–4). It is attractive to explain the transition from profound inhibition to pausing in type IV units when anesthesia is given by a corresponding weakening of discharge in type II inhibitory interneurons. Type II units in the DCN of unanesthetized preparations give strong excitatory responses in which high rates of discharge are maintained throughout the duration of a 200-ms stimulus (unpublished observation), whereas onset-S units in anesthetized preparations give rapidly adapting responses (Figure 12–4).

Another piece of evidence to support the idea of local inhibitory interneurons comes from an analysis of field potentials in the DCN. Manis and Brownell (1983) inferred the distribution of current sources and sinks in the DCN following electrical stimulation of the auditory nerve. They interpreted their results as reflecting the postsynaptic currents from three sources of synaptic input to fusiform cells: the first is a direct monosynaptic excitatory input from the auditory nerve, the second is a longer latency excitatory input of unknown origin, and the third is a disynaptic inhibitory input, at a depth corresponding to fusiform cell somata, where many DCN interneurons form synaptic terminals (Lorente de Nó, 1981).

It is important to point out that neither the cross-correlation evidence nor the field potential analysis proves the existence of local inhibitory circuits. In either case, there are alternate interpretations of the data, discussed in the original papers (Manis & Brownell, 1983; Voigt & Young, 1980). Nevertheless, the weight of evidence supports the idea that DCN principal cells receive powerful inhibitory connections from local circuits. These inhibitory inputs must be superimposed on excitatory inputs with the same frequency selectivity, because the inhibitory responses at BF become excitatory when anesthesia is given (Evans & Nelson, 1973a; Young & Brownell, 1976).

A problem for our understanding of the DCN is that there is currently no information about the mossy fiber/granule cell/parallel fiber circuit in the DCN. It seems likely that granule cells form excitatory connections on fusiform cells, by analogy with the cerebellum where granule cells have an excitatory effect on Purkinje cells (Llinas, 1981). However, there is no evidence, at present, concerning the effects of granule cell activity in the DCN.

An attractive feature of the local inhibitory interneuron model of the DCN is that the response properties of the presumed inhibitory interneuron, the type II unit, explain some of the unusual features of the response properties of type IV units. One of these features is the strong responses to broad band noise that type IV units generally give (Figure 12–3), despite their predominantly inhibitory responses to tones.

Figure 12-7 shows an analysis of the noise response of a type IV unit. Figure 12-7B shows rate versus level functions for responses to bandpass noise of three different bandwidths: 0.5, 1.0, and 2.0 kHz. These noise bands were centered arithmetically on the unit's BF. Their extent in frequency is indicated by the horizontal bars labeled 0.5, 1.0, and 2.0 on the unit's response map in Figure 12-7A. Note that as the bandwidth of the noise is widened, the response rate at moderate and high sound levels (above − 70 dB) increases; that is, the rate versus level function for 2.0-kHz noise lies above the functions for 1.0 and 0.5 kHz. This increase in discharge rate implies that the frequency components added to the noise as the bandwidth was widened should have an excitatory effect on the unit when presented alone. The data in Figure 12-7C show that this is not so. When pairs of noise bands covering the frequencies between the 0.5 and 1.0 kHz bands or the frequencies between the 1.0 and 2.0 kHz bands (the two pairs of bars labeled 0.5–1.0 and 1.0–2.0 on the response map) were presented alone, their effect was in the inhibitory direction over a wide range of sound levels (approximately − 80 to − 45 dB. Yet it was over precisely this range of sound levels that energy in these marginal frequency regions, when added to the 0.5-kHz band of noise to widen it to 1.0 kHz or to the 1.0-kHz band to widen it to 2.0 kHz, produced an excitatory effect on the unit (Figure 12-7B). The frequency components in the marginal noise bands had an inhibitory effect when presented alone (Figure 12-7C), but an excitatory effect when presented together with frequency components nearer the unit's BF (Figure 12-7B).

The properties of the type II interneuron can be invoked to explain the behavior shown in Figure 12-7. Type II units have no spontaneous activity and do not respond to broadband stimuli. For the purposes of this discussion, assume that type II units are prevented from responding to broadband stimuli by powerful inhibitory sidebands. Therefore, as noise bands are widened (0.5 to 1.0 to 2.0 kHz), the type II units' responses grow weaker, reducing the inhibitory drive on the type IV unit and increasing its discharge rate (disinhibition, Figure 12-7B). When the frequency components in the marginal bands (0.5–1.0 or 1.0–2.0 kHz) are presented alone, however, the type II units are strongly inhibited. Because type II units are not spontaneously active, their discharge rate cannot decrease; they simply do not respond at all to the marginal noise bands, and no change in the input to the type IV unit from type II units occurs when the marginal noise bands are turned on. This explains how the marginal noise bands can act to increase discharge rate in one case by disinhibition, but be prevented from having the same effect when presented alone, because they cannot inhibit the response of the type II units to rates below zero. It does not explain the inhibitory effect on the type IV unit of the marginal noise bands presented by themselves (Figure 12-7C). This inhibitory effect must be explained as a direct, but rather weak, inhibition by these frequency components of the type IV unit through other inhibitory inputs (inhibitory sidebands). Ordinarily, the effects of the type II units on the type IV unit are much stronger than the effects of these inhibitory sidebands, so their inhibitory effects are not clearly observed.

Intracellular recordings in DCN principal cells have only been made in anesthetized animals, so intracellular potentials must be compared to the pauser and buildup

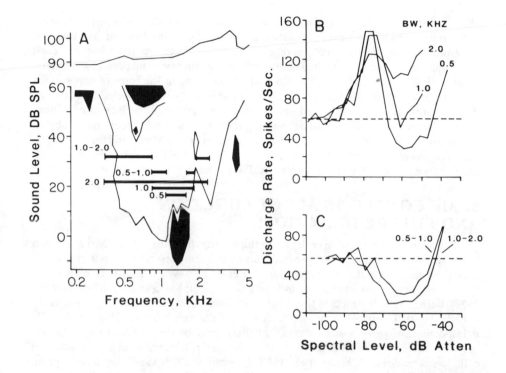

Figure 12-7. (A) Response map of DCN type IV unit with acoustic calibration (above), on same
frequency axis. Calibration shows spectrum of broadband noise at cat's eardrum.
Horizontal bars on response map show bandwidths of noisebands used to study
this unit. (B) Discharge rate versus spectrum level for three noisebands centered
at unit's BF. Bandwidths are given next to plots and correspond to continuous bars
(0.5, 1.0, 2.0) on the response map in (A) (C). Discharge rate versus spectrum level
for pairs of marginal noise bands. These are bands of noise added to the 0.5-kHz
band to make a 1.0-kHz band (0.5–1.0) and bands of noise added to the 1.0-kHz
band to make a 2.0-kHz band (1.0–2.0).

responses observed in anesthetized animals. The fourth column from the left in Figure
12-5 illustrates some examples from Romand (1978); corresponding PST histograms
are shown in the last column. These are typical of many intracellular recordings in
pauser/buildup units in that, with BF stimuli, a hyperpolarization suggestive of inhibitory input is not observed at the time of the pause in spike discharge (Britt & Starr,
1976a; Gerstein, Butler, & Erulkar, 1968; Rhode et al., 1983a; Starr & Britt, 1970).
According to the model for type IV responses discussed above, this pause should
be a remnant of the inhibitory response observed in unanesthetized preparations and
so should be consistently associated with hyperpolarization. Fortunately, hyperpolarizations corresponding to pauses in firing have been observed in some cases (e.g.,

Starr & Britt, 1970, Figure 1; Rhode et al., 1983a; Figures 2C,D); hyperpolarization is commonly observed during stimulation at frequencies away from BF and immediately after the end of BF stimuli. There is evidence that these hyperpolarizations result from inhibitory synaptic input to fusiform cells in the form of reductions of membrane noise during hyperpolarization (Rhode et al., 1983a) and in the form of suppression by acoustic stimuli of discharges evoked by depolarizing currents injected into the cells (Starr & Britt, 1970). Gerstein and associates (1968) explained the lack of consistent hyperpolarizations to BF stimuli as resulting from the electrode recording site being remote from the site of spike generation and inhibitory input. This is still the best explanation of this phenomenon; the problem awaits further study, especially in unanesthetized animals where the effects of any inhibitory input should be more evident.

SOME COMMENTS ABOUT FUNCTION AND FUTURE DIRECTIONS

There are many questions relating to the wiring diagram of the CN that remain to be answered. Although the general plan of the auditory nerve input to the CN is known, recent results have raised some interesting new questions. There are two types of auditory nerve ganglion cells (type I and type II; Kiang et al., 1982; Spoendlin, 1978); both of which project to the CN (Leake-Jones & Snyder, 1982; Ruggero, Santi, & Rich, 1982). The question of how the axons of the two types terminate in the CN is important, in view of suggestions that there may be differences in distribution between the two (Morest & Bohne, 1983). Similarly, a subclass of type I ganglion cells has been defined (Kiang et al., 1982; Liberman, 1978, 1980) that has different physiological and morphological characteristics from the majority of type I ganglion cells. It is important to know whether there are differences in the distributions of axons of these two groups (Rouillier, Schreiber, Fekete, & Ryugo, 1983).

Many sources of efferents to the CN from higher auditory structures are known, and much remains to be learned about the distribution of these potentially important feedback pathways within the CN and about their effects on the response properties of CN cells. The distribution of outputs of the CN in higher nuclei, particularly the inferior colliculus, is known only in general. The problem of interpretation of the response characteristics of CN neurons would be greatly facilitated by knowing, in detail, the termination patterns of the different cell types and the relationships of these patterns to those of other sources of input. The inferior colliculus promises to be fertile ground for this sort of analysis, since all ascending auditory pathways terminate there and there is evidence that these terminal fields are not uniformly distributed (Oliver & Morest, 1979; Roth, Aitkin, Andersen, & Merzenich, 1978; Semple & Aitkin, 1979).

The question of the analysis of specific subsystems of the CN has formed the core of this chapter. The properties of the subsystems of the CN are significantly different, suggesting different functional roles for these subsystems within the auditory system. Although it is simplistic to think that well-defined separate functions can be found for each bit of neural tissue in a system which is as tightly integrated with ascending and descending connections as is the auditory system, it is useful to consider how the transformation of the representation of the acoustic environment which occurs in each CN subsystem might serve to aid the overall system in solving the perceptual problems which it faces. At present, this can be done only to a limited extent.

The bushy cells of the AVCN are clearly specialized to provide precise information about the stimuli in the two ears to the cells of the principal nuclei of the superior olivary complex (SOC) for the purposes of sound localization. Sound localization depends on precise comparison of the arrival time and intensity of the stimuli in the two ears. The cells of the SOC receive roughly equal innervation from the CN of the two sides and many cells in the SOC are sensitive to interaural stimulus parameters in a fashion appropriate to sound localization (see review by Brugge & Geisler, 1978). A number of behavioral studies have shown that lesions of the TB or of the AVCN disrupt sound localization in animals (e.g., Casseday & Neff, 1975; Casseday & Smoak, 1981; Jenkins & Masterton, 1982; Thompson & Masterton, 1978). The simple synaptic structure of bushy cells and the general similarity of their response characteristics to those of auditory nerve fibers can be understood as specializations for transmitting precise information about auditory nerve firing patterns. An intriguing question left unanswered by the theory that bushy cells are a relay from auditory nerve to SOC is the role of the other inputs known to terminate on bushy cells as boutons (Cant & Morest, 1978, 1979b; Schwartz & Gulley, 1978).

The contributions of the other subsystems of the CN to sound localization are unclear. Cells in both DCN and VCN respond to stimuli in the contralateral ear (Dunker, Grubel, & Pfalz, 1964; Klinke, Boerger, & Gruber, 1969; Mast, 1970b, 1973; Pfalz, 1962; Young & Brownell, 1976), but these inputs are much weaker than ipsilateral inputs. Since sound localization seems to require precise comparison of roughly equal representations of the activity in the two ears, it seems unlikely that the contralateral responses of CN neurons contribute directly to sound localization. However, there is some evidence to support the idea that the principal cells of the DCN play a role in modulating sound localization in the inferior colliculus. Semple and Aitkin (1980) examined the properties of cells in the IC whose activity could be affected with short latency by stimulation of the DAS. The cells most commonly affected by DAS stimulation had binaural response properties similar to those of neurons in the LSO, suggesting a convergence of inputs from the DCN and the LSO on these cells. Furthermore, Bengry, Silverman, and Clopton (1977) reported that the binaural response properties of IC units were modified by sectioning the DAS and IAS.

Besides its role in relaying information to the SOC for sound localization, the VCN has been implicated as a necessary link in other brainstem auditory reflexes. Borg (1973) showed that lesions of the TB raised the threshold of or weakened the middle ear muscle reflex, whereas lesions of the DCN or DAS and IAS did not. Davis, Gendelman, Tischler, and Gendelman (1982) have shown that lesions in the VCN greatly reduce the acoustic startle reflex, whereas lesions of the DCN have no effect.

Some recent evidence indicates that the CN may play a role in detection of stimuli in noisy environments. Human and animal observers are able to detect and discriminate auditory stimuli over a very wide intensity range and in the presence of high levels of background noise (Costalupes, 1983; Dye & Hafter, 1980; Moore & Raab, 1975; Viemeister, 1974). Behavioral performance stays reasonably constant over this wide range of sound levels despite the fact that auditory nerve fibers have limited dynamic ranges (Sachs & Abbas, 1974). That is, auditory nerve fibers are able to signal changes in stimulus level with changes in rate over only a limited range of sound levels (similar to the rate–level function of the type I unit in Figure 12-3). Because of this limited dynamic range, the representation of acoustic stimuli in auditory nerve discharge patterns is degraded by, for example, high levels of background noise (e.g., Costalupes, Gibson, & Young, 1984; Gibson, 1983; Palmer & Evans, 1982; Sachs, Voigt, & Young, 1983). The noise saturates the rate response of the fibers; that is, the fibers are driven at their maximum rate by the noise and are no longer sensitive to changes in the level of a stimulus present with the noise.

Saturation is partly ameliorated, in the case of a BF tone in the presence of continuous broadband background noise, by a shift in the dynamic range of auditory nerve fibers (Costalupes et al., 1984). That is, the noise causes a shift to higher sound levels of the range of sound levels over which the fiber is sensitive to changes in stimulus level. These dynamic range shifts extend the range over which auditory nerve fibers can respond to the BF tone stimulus, but they do not prevent ultimate saturation of the fibers by the noise. In the CN, the situation is different in subtle ways (Gibson, 1983). The dynamic range shifts of CN units are only slightly larger than those of auditory nerve fibers. However, many CN units are not saturated by the noise and thereby retain good responsiveness at high noise levels. Type II units, for example, do not respond to the background noise at all.

Palmer and Evans (1982) studied a different situation, the responses of auditory nerve fibers and CN units to BF tones in the presence of bandstop noise, with the stop band centered on BF. Although bandstop noise is not as realistic a model for everyday background noise situations as is broadband noise, it did allow Palmer and Evans to demonstrate a difference between auditory nerve fibers and CN units. Most auditory nerve fibers were unable to signal changes in level of the tone with changes in rate at high noise levels because of saturation of their responses by the noise. The only fibers to retain significant responsiveness to the tone at high noise levels were low-spontaneous-rate fibers, which usually have wide dynamic ranges (Liberman, 1978; Sachs & Abbas, 1974). In the CN, especially the DCN, a larger percentage of units avoided saturation by the noise and retained good sensitivity to the BF tones by shifting their dynamic ranges to higher test levels in the presence of the noise. The difference in auditory nerve fiber results between Costalupes and colleagues (1984) and Palmer and Evans (1982) derives mainly from the effects of the frequency components of the noise close to BF, which were missing in Palmer and Evans' bandstop noise background. Frequencies close to BF have the strongest dynamic range shifting effect in auditory nerve fibers (Costalupes et al., 1984; Javel, 1981). The differences between Palmer and Evans' auditory nerve and CN unit behavior probably resulted from the effects of sideband inhibition in the CN which augmented the effect of peripheral dynamic range shift. This led Palmer and Evans to suggest that the inhibitory processes in the DCN are designed to broaden the dynamic range of the system.

Further evidence of a role for the CN in signal detection in noise was provided by Pickles (1976; Pickles & Comis, 1973), who investigated the critical band phenomenon in cats. The critical band is a measure of the frequency resolving power of the auditory system; it expresses the range of frequencies over which stimuli will interact in various psychophysical tests (Scharf, 1970). Cats show critical band behavior similar to that seen in humans (Costalupes, 1983; Pickles, 1975). Pickles (1976) implanted a cannula over the CN and showed that when atropine solutions were applied to the CN, cats' critical bandwidths became enormously wider, or the critical bandwidth mechanism was abolished. He interpreted this result as a reflection of the blockade of cholinergic efferent pathways from the superior olive to the CN (Comis & Davies, 1969; Comis & Whitfield, 1968; Osen & Roth, 1969). Regardless of the mechanism, the fact that a complex behavioral measure like the critical band could be affected by pharmacological modification of the CN suggests a critical role for the CN in detection of signals in noise.

The results in Figure 12-7 illustrate the point that the responses of CN neurons to complex stimuli may sometimes not be straightforward extensions of their responses to tones. Similar results have been reported in other situations, such as responses to frequency- and amplitude-modulated tones (Britt & Starr, 1976b; Erulkar, Gerstein, & Butler, 1966; Fernald & Gerstein, 1972; Møller, 1977; Nelson & Evans, 1971). In many situations, of course, the responses to complex stimuli may be predicted from a summation of the pure-tone responses of the unit (Greenwood & Goldberg, 1970; Langner, Bonke, & Scheich, 1981; Sachs & O'Connell, 1983). The results of this sort of analysis apparently depend on the unit under study and the stimulus.

Responses to complex stimuli have only begun to be studied in the auditory system (for reviews of this area, see Pickles, 1982, and Møller, 1983). The importance of this sort of analysis is clear, since the natural stimuli with which the auditory system deals in real-life situations are all complex and time varying. Studies of responses to carefully chosen complex stimuli which relate the responses to specific physiological or anatomical unit types will be essential to the analysis of auditory information processing.

There are many facets of the response properties of CN units that remain to be worked out. The problem of associating response types with cell types, which is the crucial underpinning for the analysis of information processing in the CN, can now be approached using the powerful technique of intracellular staining of physiologically identified neurons. This technique promises to clarify the questions remaining in this area. Once the CN wiring diagram is worked out, it will allow an intelligent approach to such problems as responses to complex, natural stimuli and the response properties of CN cells in conscious, intact animals. It is in the intact preparation that our ultimate understanding of information processing in the CN will be gained. The next few years should bring great progress in the analysis of the function of the CN in hearing.

REFERENCES

Adams, J.C. (1979). Ascending projections to the inferior colliculus. *Journal of Comparative Neurology, 183,* 519–538.

Adams, J.C., & Warr, W.B. (1976). Origins of axons in the cat's acoustic striae determined by injection of horseradish peroxidase into severed tracts. *Journal of Comparative Neurology, 170,* 107–121.

Bengry, M.F., Silverman, M.S., & Clopton, B.M. (1977). Effects of lesioning the dorsal and intermediate acoustic striae on binaural interaction at the inferior colliculus. *Experimental Brain Research, 28,* 211–219.

Bird, S.J., Gulley, R.L., Wenthold, R.J., & Fex, J. (1978). Kainic acid injections result in degeneration of cochlear nucleus cells innervated by the auditory nerve. *Science, 202,* 1087–1089.

Borg, E. (1973). On the neuronal organization of the acoustic middle ear reflex. A physiological and anatomical study. *Brain Research, 49,* 101–123.

Bourk, T.R. (1976). *Electrical responses of neural units in the anteroventral cochlear nucleus of the cat.* Doctoral dissertation, Massachusetts Institute of Technology, Cambridge.

Bourk, T.R., Mielcarz, J.P., & Norris, B.E. (1981). Tonotopic organization of the anteroventral cochlear nucleus of the cat. *Hearing Research, 4,* 215–241.

Brawer, J.R., & Morest, D.K. (1975). Relations between auditory nerve endings and cell types in the cat's anteroventral cochlear nucleus seen with the Golgi method and Nomarski optics. *Journal of Comparative Neurology, 160,* 491–506.

Brawer, J.R., Morest, D.K., & Kane, E.S. (1974). The neuronal architecture of the cochlear nucleus of the cat. *Journal of Comparative Neurology, 155,* 251–300.

Britt, R., & Starr, A. (1976a). Synaptic events and discharge patterns of cochlear nucleus cells. I. Steady frequency tone bursts. *Journal of Neurophysiology, 39,* 162–178.

Britt, R., & Starr, A. (1976b). Synaptic events and discharge patterns of cochlear nucleus cells. II. Frequency-modulated tones. *Journal of Neurophysiology, 39,* 179–194.

Brownell, W.E. (1975). Organization of the cat trapezoid body and the discharge characteristics of its fibers. *Brain Research, 94,* 413–433.

Brugge, J.F., & Geisler, C.D. (1978). Auditory mechanisms of the lower brainstem. *Annual Review of Neuroscience, 1,* 363–394.

Cant, N.B. (1981). The fine structure of two types of stellate cells in the anterior division of the anteroventral cochlear nucleus of the cat. *Neuroscience, 6,* 2643–2655.

Cant, N.B., & Morest, D.K. (1978). Axons from noncochlear sources in the anteroventral cochlear nucleus of the cat. A study with the rapid Golgi method. *Neuroscience, 3,* 1003–1029.

Cant, N.B., & Morest, D.K. (1979a). Organization of the neurons in the anterior division of the anteroventral cochlear nucleus of the cat: Light microscopic observations. *Neuroscience, 4,* 1909–1923.

Cant, N.B., & Morest, D.K. (1979b). The bushy cells in the anteroventral cochlear nucleus of the cat. A study with the electron microscope. *Neuroscience, 4,* 1925–1945.

Caspary, D. (1972). Classification of subpopulations of neurons in the cochlear nuclei of the kangaroo rat. *Experimental Neurology, 37,* 131–151.

Caspary, D.M., Havey, D.C., & Faingold, C.L. (1981). Glutamate and aspartate: Alteration of thresholds and response patterns of auditory neurons. *Hearing Research, 4,* 325–333.

Casseday, J.H., & Neff, W.D. (1975). Auditory localization: Role of auditory pathways in brain stem of the cat. *Journal of Neurophysiology, 38,* 842–858.

Casseday, J.H., & Smoak, H.A. (1981). Effects of unilateral ablation of anteroventral cochlear nucleus on localization of sound in space. In J. Syka & L. Aitkin (Eds.), *Neuronal mechanisms of hearing* (pp. 277-282). New York: Plenum.

Comis, S.D., & Davies, W.E. (1969). Acetylcholine as a transmitter in the cat auditory system. *Journal of Neurochemistry, 16,* 423-429.

Comis, S.D., & Whitfield, I.C. (1968). Influence of centrifugal pathways on unit activity in the cochlear nucleus. *Journal of Neurophysiology, 31,* 62-68.

Costalupes, J.A. (1983). Broadband masking noise and behavioral pure tone threshold in cats. *Journal of the Acoustical Society of America, 74,* 758-764.

Costalupes, J.A., Young, E.D., & Gibson, D.J. (1984). Effects of continuous noise backgrounds on rate response of auditory-nerve fibers in cat. *Journal of Neurophysiology, 51,* 1326-1344.

Davis, M., Gendelman, D.S., Tischler, M.D., & Gendelman, P.M. (1982). A primary acoustic startle circuit: Lesion and stimulation studies. *Journal of Neuroscience, 2,* 791-805.

Dunker, F., Grubel, G., & Pfalz, R. (1964). Influence of spontaneously active, deafferented single units of the cat's cochlear nucleus by contralateral stimulation. *Pflugers Archiv, 278,* 610-623.

Dye, R.H., Jr., & Hafter, E.R. (1980). Just-noticeable differences of frequency for masked tones. *Journal of the Acoustical Society of America, 67,* 1746-1753.

Elverland, H.H. (1977). Descending connections between the superior olivary and cochlear nuclear complexes in the cat studied by autoradiographic and horseradish peroxidase methods. *Experimental Brain Research, 27,* 397-412.

Erulkar, S.D., Gerstein, G.L., & Butler, R.A. (1966). Transmembrane potentials from cat cochlear nucleus in response to pure and frequency-modulated (FM) tonal stimuli. *Federation Proceedings, 25,* 463.

Evans, E.F., & Nelson, P.G. (1973a). The responses of single neurones in the cochlear nucleus of the cat as a function of their location and the anaesthetic state. *Experimental Brain Research, 17,* 402-427.

Evans, E.F., & Nelson, P.G. (1973b). On the functional relationship between the dorsal and ventral divisions of the cochlear nucleus of the cat. *Experimental Brain Research, 17,* 428-442.

Feldman, M.L., & Harrison, J.M. (1969). Projections of acoustic nerve to ventral cochlear nucleus of rat. A Golgi study. *Journal of Comparative Neurology, 137,* 267-295.

Fernald, R.D., & Gerstein, G.L. (1972). Response of cat cochlear nucleus neurons to frequency and amplitude modulated tones. *Brain Research, 45.* 417-435.

Frisina, R.D., Chamberlain, S.C., Brachman, M.L., & Smith, R.L. (1982). Anatomy and physiology of the gerbil cochlear nucleus: An improved surgical approach for microelectrode studies. *Hearing Research, 6,* 259-275.

Gerstein, G.L., Butler, R.A., & Erulkar, S.D. (1968). Excitation and inhibition in cochlear nucleus. I. Tone-burst stimulation. *Journal of Neurophysiology, 31,* 526-536.

Gibson, D.J. (1983). *Similar dynamic range adjustments in the auditory nerve and cochlear nuclei of the decerebrate cat.* PhD dissertation, Johns Hopkins University, Baltimore.

Godfrey, D.A. (1971). *Localization of single units in the cochlear nucleus of the cat: An attempt to correlate neuronal structure and function.* Doctoral thesis, Harvard University.

Godfrey, D.A., Kiang, N.Y.S., & Norris, B.E. (1975a). Single unit activity in the posteroventral cochlear nucleus of the cat. *Journal of Comparative Neurology, 162,* 247-268.

Godfrey, D.A., Kiang, N.Y.S., & Norris, B.E. (1975b). Single unit activity in the dorsal cochlear nucleus of the cat. *Journal of Comparative Neurology, 162,* 269-284.

Goldberg, J.M., Adrian, H.O., & Smith, F.D. (1964). Response of neurons of the superior olivary complex of the cat to acoustic stimuli of long duration. *Journal of Neurophysiology, 27,* 706-749.

Goldberg, J.M., & Brownell, W. E. (1973). Discharge characteristics of neurons in the anteroventral and dorsal cochlear nuclei of cat. *Brain Research, 64.* 35–54.

Greenwood, D.D., & Goldberg, J.M. (1970). Response of neurons in the cochlear nuclei to variations in noise bandwidths and to tone-noise combinations. *Journal of the Acoustical Society of America, 47,* 1022–1040.

Hui, G.S., & Disterhoft, J.F. (1980). Cochlear nucleus unit responses to pure tones in the unanesthetized rabbit. *Experimental Neurology, 69,* 576–588.

Jack, J.J.B., Noble, D., & Tsien, R.W. (1975). *Electric current flow in excitable cells.* Oxford: Clarendon Press.

Javel, E. (1981). Suppression of auditory nerve responses. I. Temporal analysis, intensity effects and suppression contours. *Journal of the Acoustical Society of America, 69,* 1735–1745.

Jenkins, W.M., & Masterton, R.B. (1982). Sound localization: Effects of unilateral lesions in central auditory system. *Journal of Neurophysiology, 47,* 987–1016.

Jones, D.R., & Casseday, J.H. (1979). Projections to laminae in dorsal cochlear nucleus in the tree shrew, Tupaia glis. *Brain Research, 160,* 131–133.

Kane, E.C. (1973). Octopus cells in the cochlear nucleus of the cat: heterotypic synapses upon homeotypic neurons. *International Journal of Neuroscience, 5,* 251–279.

Kane, E.C. (1974a). Synaptic organization in the dorsal cochlear nucleus of the cat: A light and electron microscopic study. *Journal of Comparative Neurology, 155,* 301–330.

Kane, E.C. (1974b). Patterns of degeneration in the caudal cochlear nucleus of the cat after cochlear ablation. *Anatomical Record, 179,* 67–92.

Kane, E.S., & Finn, R.C. (1977). Descending and intrinsic inputs to dorsal cochlear nucleus of cats: A horseradish peroxidase study. *Neuroscience, 2,* 897–912.

Kane, E.S., Puglisi, S.G., & Gordon, B.S. (1981). Neuronal types in the deep dorsal cochlear nucleus of the cat: I. Giant neurons. *Journal of Comparative Neurology, 198,* 483–513.

Kiang, N.Y.S., Watanabe, T., Thomas, E.C., & Clark, L.F. (1965a). *Discharge patterns of single fibers in the cat's auditory nerve.* Research monograph 35. Cambridge: MIT Press.

Kiang, N.Y.S., Pfeiffer, R.R., Warr, W.B., & Backus, A.S.N. (1965b). Stimulus coding in the cochlear nucleus. *Annals of Otology, Rhinology and Laryngology, 74,* 463–485.

Kiang, N.Y.S., Morest, D.K., Godfrey, D.A., Guinan, J.J., & Kane, E.C. (1973). Stimulus coding at caudal levels of the cat's auditory nervous system. I. Response characteristics of single units. In A.R. Moller (Ed.), *Basic mechanisms in hearing.* New York: Academic Press.

Kiang, N.Y.S., Rho, J.M., Northrup, C.C., Liberman. M.C., & Ryugo, D.K. (1982). Hair-cell innervation by spiral ganglion cells in adult cats. *Science, 217,* 175–177.

Klinke, R., Boerger, G., & Gruber, J. (1969). Studies on the functional significance of efferent innervation in the auditory system: Afferent neuronal activity as influenced by contralaterally-applied sound. *Pfluegers Archiv, 306,* 165–175.

Koerber, K.C., Pfeiffer, R.R., Warr, W.B., & Kiang, N.Y.S. (1966). Spontaneous spike discharges from single units in the cochlear nucleus after destruction of the cochlea. *Experimental Neurology, 16,* 119–130.

Langner, G., Bonke, D., & Scheich, H. (1981). Selectivity of auditory neurons for vowels and consonants in the forebrain of the mynah bird. In J. Syka & L. Aitkin (Eds.), *Neuronal mechanisms of hearing.* New York: Plenum.

Leake-Jones, P.A., & Snyder, R.L. (1982). Uptake and transport of horseradish peroxidase by cochlear spiral ganglion neurons. *Hearing Research, 8,* 199–223.

Lenn, N.J., & Reese, T.S. (1966). Fine structure of nerve endings in the nucleus of the trapezoid body and the ventral cochlear nucleus. *American Journal of Anatomy, 118,* 375–390.

Li, R. Y-S., & Guinan, J.J. (1971). Antidromic and orthodromic stimulation of neurons receiving calyces of Held. *MIT Research Laboratory of Electronics, Quarterly Progress Report, 100,* 227–234.

Liberman, M.C. (1978). Auditory-nerve response from cats raised in a low-noise chamber. *Journal of the Acoustical Society of America, 63,* 442–455.

Liberman, M.C. (1980). Morphological differences among radial afferent fibers in the cat cochlea: An electron-microscopic study of serial sections. *Hearing Research, 3,* 45–63.

Llinas, R.R. (1981). Electrophysiology of the cerebellar networks. In V.B. Brooks (Ed.), *Handbook of physiology* (Vol. II), *Neurophysiology.* Baltimore: Waverly Press.

Lorente de No, R. (1933). Anatomy of the eighth nerve. III. General plan of structure of the primary cochlear nuclei. *Laryngoscope, 43,* 327–350.

Lorente de No, R. (1981). *The primary acoustic nuclei.* New York: Raven Press.

Manis, P.B., & Brownell, W.E. (1983). Synaptic organization of eighth nerve afferents to the cat dorsal cochlear nucleus. *Journal of Neurophysiology, 50,* 1156–1181.

Martin, M.R., & Adams, J.C. (1979). Effects of DL α-aminoadipate on synaptically and chemically evoked excitation of anteroventral cochlear nucleus neurons of the cat. *Neuroscience, 4,* 1097–1105.

Martin, M.R., & Dickson, J.W. (1983). Lateral inhibition in the anteroventral cochlear nucleus of the cat: A microiontophoretic study. *Hearing Research, 9,* 35–45.

Mast, T.E. (1970a). Study of single units of the cochlear nucleus of the chinchilla. *Journal of the Acoustical Society of America, 48,* 505–512.

Mast, T.E. (1970b). Binaural interaction and contralateral inhibition in dorsal cochlear nucleus of the chinchilla. *Journal of Neurophysiology, 33,* 108–115.

Mast, T.E. (1973). Dorsal cochlear nucleus of the chinchilla: Excitation by contralateral sound. *Brain Research, 62,* 61–70.

McDonald, D.M., & Rasmussen, G.L. (1971). Ultrastructural characteristics of synaptic endings in the cochlear nucleus having acetylcholinesterase activity. *Brain Research, 28,* 1–18.

Moller, A.R. (1977). Coding of time-varying sounds in the cochlear nucleus. *Audiology, 17,* 446–468.

Moller, A. (1983). *Auditory physiology.* New York: Academic Press.

Molnar, C.E., & Pfeiffer, R.R. (1968). Interpretation of spontaneous spike discharge patterns of cochlear nucleus neurons. *Proceedings of the IEEE, 56,* 993–1002

Moore, B.C.J., & Raab, D.H. (1975). Intensity discrimination for noise bursts in the presence of a continuous bandstop background: Effects of level, width of the bandstop, and duration. *Journal of the Acoustical Society of America, 57,* 400–405.

Moore, G.P., Segundo, J.P., Perkel, D.H., & Levitan, H. (1970). Statistical signs of synaptic interaction in neurons. *Biophysics Journal, 10,* 876–900.

Morest, D.K. (1968). The collateral system of the medical nucleus of the trapezoid body of the cat, its neuronal architecture and relation to the olivo-cochlear bundle. *Brain Research, 9,* 288–311.

Morest, D.K., & Bohne, B.A. (1983). Noise-induced degeneration in the brain and representation of inner and outer hair cells. *Hearing Research, 9,* 145–151.

Mugnaini, E., Warr, W.B., & Osen, K.K. (1980). Distribution and light microscopic features of granule cells in the cochlear nuclei of cat, rat, and mouse. *Journal of Comparative Neurology, 191,* 581–606.

Nelson, P.G., & Evans, E.F. (1971). Relationship between dorsal and ventral cochlear nuclei. In M.B. Sachs (Ed.) *Physiology of the auditory system.* Baltimore: National Educational Consultants.

Nilsson, H.G. (1975). Model of discharge patterns of units in the cochlear nucleus in response to steady state and time-varying sounds. *Biol. Cybernetics, 20,* 113–119.

Oertel, D. (1982). Intracellular responses of cells in mouse cochlear nucleus to electrical stimulation of the auditory nerve *in vitro. Neuroscience Abstracts, 8,* 149.

Oliver, D.L., & Morest, D.K. (1979). Cochlear nucleus projections to the inferior colliculus of the cat studied with light and electron microscopic autoradiography. *Neuroscience Abstracts, 5,* 27.

Osen, K.K. (1969). Cytoarchitecture of the cochlear nuclei in the cat. *Journal of Comparative Neurology, 136,* 453–484.

Osen, K.K. (1970). Course and termination of the primary afferents in the cochlear nuclei of the cat. An experimental anatomical study. *Archives Italienne de Biologie, 108,* 21–51.

Osen, K.K., & Mugnaini, E. (1981). Neuronal circuits in the dorsal cochlear nucleus. In J. Syka & L. Aitkin (Eds.) *Neuronal mechanisms of hearing.* New York: Plenum.

Osen, K.K., & Roth, K. (1969). Histochemical localization of cholinesterases in the cochlear nuclei of the cat, with notes on the origin of acetylcholinesterase-positive afferents and the superior olive. *Brain Research, 16,* 165–185.

Palmer, A.R., & Evans, E.F. (1982). Intensity coding in the auditory periphery of the cat: Responses of cochlear nerve and cochlear nucleus neurons to signals in the presence of bandstop masking noise. *Hearing Research, 7,* 305–323.

Perkel, D.H., Gerstein, G.L., & Moore, G.P. (1967). Neuronal spike trains and stochastic point processes. II. Simultaneous spike trains. *Biophysics Journal, 7,* 419–440.

Perry, D.R., & Webster, W.R. (1981). Neuronal organization of the rabbit cochlear nucleus: Some anatomical and electrophysiological observations. *Journal of Comparative Neurology, 197,* 623–638.

Pfalz, R.K.J. (1962). Centrifugal inhibition of afferent secondary neurons in the cochlear nucleus. *Journal of the Acoustical Society of America, 34,* 1472–1474.

Pfeiffer, R.R. (1966a). Classification of response patterns of spike discharges for units in the cochlear nucleus: Tone burst stimulation. *Experimental Brain Research, 1,* 220–235.

Pfeiffer, R.R. (1966b). Anteroventral cochlear nucleus: Wave forms of extracellularly recorded spike potentials. *Science, 134,* 667–668.

Pfeiffer, R.R., & Kiang, N.Y.S. (1965). Spike discharge patterns of spontaneous and continuously stimulated activity in the cochlear nucleus of anesthetized cats. *Biophysical Journal, 5,* 301–316.

Pickles, J.O. (1975). Normal cortical bands in the cat. *Acta Otolaryngology, 80,* 245–254.

Pickles, J.O. (1976). Role of centrifugal pathways to cochlear nucleus in determination of critical bandwidth. *Journal of Neurophysiology, 39,* 394–400.

Pickles, J.O. (1982). *An introduction to the physiology of hearing.* New York: Academic Press.

Pickles, J.O., & Comis, S.D. (1973). Role of centrifugal pathways to cochlear nucleus in detection of signals in noise. *Journal of Neurophysiology, 36,* 1131–1137.

Rall, W. (1977). Core conductor theory and cable properties of neurons. In E.R. Kandel (Ed.), *Handbook of physiology* (Vol. I), *Cellular biology of neurons.* Baltimore: Waverly Press.

Ramon y Cajal, S. (1909). *Histologie du systeme nerveaux de l'homme et des vertebres.* Paris: Maloine.

Rasmussen, G.L. (1964). Anatomical relationships of ascending and descending auditory system. In W. Fields & B.R. Alford (Eds.) *Neurological aspects of auditory and vestibular disorders.* Springfield: Thomas.

Rhode, W.S., Smith, P., & Oertel, D. (1980). Intracellular recording and staining in cat cochlear nucleus. *Neuroscience Abstracts, 6,* 554.

Rhode, W.S., Smith, P.H., & Oertel, D. (1983a). Physiological response properties of cells labeled intracellularly with horseradish peroxidase in cat dorsal cochlear nucleus. *Journal of Comparative Neurology, 213,* 426–447.

Rhode, W.S., Oertel, D., & Smith, P.H. (1983b). Physiological response properties of cells labeled intracellularly with horseradish peroxidase in the cat ventral cochlear nucleus. *Journal of Comparative Neurology, 213,* 448–463.

Ritz, L.A., & Brownell, W.E. (1982). Single unit analysis of the posteroventral cochlear nucleus of the decerebrate cat. *Neuroscience, 7,* 1995–2010.

Romand, R. (1978). Survey of intracellular recording in the cochlear nucleus of the cat. *Brain Research, 148,* 43–65.

Romand, R. (1979). Intracellular recording of 'chopper responses' in the cochlear nucleus of the cat. *Hearing Research, 1,* 95–99.

Rose, J.E., Galambos, R., & Hughes, J. (1960). Organization of frequency sensitive neurons in the cochlear nuclear complex of the cat. In G.L. Rasmussen & W.F. Windle (Eds.), *Neuronal mechanisms of the auditory and vestibular systems.* Springfield: Thomas.

Roth, G.L., Aitkin, L.M., Andersen, R.A., & Merzenich, M.M. (1978). Some features of the spatial organization of the central nucleus of the inferior colliculus of the cat. *Journal of Comparative Neurology, 182,* 661–680.

Rouillier, E.M., Schreiber, C., Fekete, D.M., & Ryugo, D.K. (1983). Morphology of auditory nerve fiber innervation of the cat cochlear nucleus in relation to spontaneous rate activity. *Abstracts of the 13th Meeting of the Society for Neuroscience,* 495.

Ruggero, M.A., Santi, P.A., & Rich, N.C. (1982). Type II cochlear ganglion cells in the chinchilla. *Hearing Research, 8,* 339–356.

Sachs, M.B., & Abbas, P.J. (1974). Rate versus level functions for auditory-nerve fibers in cats: Tone burst stimuli. *Journal of the Acoustical Society of America, 56,* 1835–1847.

Sachs, M.B., & Kiang, N.Y.S. (1968). Two-tone inhibition in auditory-nerve fibers. *Journal of the Acoustical Society of America, 43,* 1120–1128.

Sachs, M.B., & O'Connell, N.A. (1983). Frequency analysis in the central nervous systems of non-mammalian vertebrates. In B. Lewis (Ed.) *Bioacoustics.* London: Academic Press.

Sachs, M.B., & Sinnott, J.M. (1978). Responses to tones of single cells in nucleus magnocellularis and nucleus angularis of the redwing blackbird (Agelaius phoniceus). *Journal of Comparative Physiology, 126,* 347–361.

Sachs, M.B., Voigt, H.F., & Young, E.D. (1983). Auditory nerve representation of vowels in background noise. *Journal of Neurophysiology, 50,* 27–45.

Scharf, B. (1970). Critical bands. In J.V. Tobias (Ed.), *Foundations of modern auditory theory.* New York: Academic Press.

Schwartz, A.M., & Gulley, R.L. (1978). Non-primary afferents to the principal cells of the rostral anteroventral cochlear nucleus of the guinea pig. *American Journal of Anatomy, 153,* 489–508.

Semple, M.N., & Aitkin, L.M. (1979). Representation of sound frequency and laterality by units in central nucleus of cat inferior colliculus. *Journal of Neurophysiology, 42,* 1626–1639.

Semple, M.N., & Aitkin, L.M. (1980). Physiology of pathway from dorsal cochlear nucleus to inferior colliculus revealed by electrical and auditory stimulation. *Experimental Brain Research, 41,* 19–28.

Spoendlin, H. (1978). The afferent innervation of the cochlea. In R.F. Naunton & C. Fernandez (Eds.) *Evoked electrical activity in the auditory nervous system.* New York: Academic Press.

Starr, A., & Britt, R. (1970). Intracellular recordings from cat cochlear nucleus during tone stimulation. *Journal of Neurophysiology, 33,* 137–147.

Thompson, G.C., & Masterton, R.B. (1978). Brain stem auditory pathways involved in reflexive head orientation to sound. *Journal of Neurophysiology, 41,* 1183–1202.

Tolbert, L.P., & Morest, D.K. (1982a). The neuronal architecture of the anteroventral cochlear nucleus of the cat in the region of the cochlear nerve root: Electron microscopy. *Neuroscience, 7,* 3053–3067.

Tolbert, L.P., & Morest, D.K. (1982b). The neuronal architecture of the anteroventral cochlear nucleus of the cat in the region of the cochlear nerve root: Golgi and Nissl methods. *Neuroscience, 7,* 3013–3030.

Tolbert, L.P., Morest, D.K., & Yurgelun-Todd, D.A. (1982). The neuronal architecture of the anteroventral cochlear nucleus of the cat in the region of the cochlear nerve root: Horseradish peroxidase labelling of identified cell types. *Neuroscience, 7,* 3031–3052.

van Gisbergen, J.A.M., Grashuis, J.L., Johannesma, P.I.M., & Vendrick, A.J.H. (1975a). Spectral and temporal characteristics of activation and suppression of units in the cochlear nuclei of the anesthetized cat. *Experimental Brain Research, 23,* 367–386.

van Gisbergen, J.A.M., Grashuis, J.L., Johannesma, P.I.M., & Vendrick, A.J.H. (1975b). Neurons in the cochlear nucleus investigated with tone and noise stimuli, *Experimental Brain Research, 23,* 387–406.

van Gisbergen, J.A.M., Grashuis, J.L., Johannesma, P.I.M., & Vendrick, A.J.H. (1975c). Statistical analysis and interpretation of the initial response of cochlear nucleus neurons to tone bursts. *Experimental Brain Research, 23,* 407–423.

van Noort, J. (1969). *The structure and connections of the inferior colliculus.* The Netherlands: van Gorcum.

Viemeister, N.F. (1974). Intensity discrimination of noise in the presence of band reject noise. *Journal of the Acoustical Society of America, 56,* 1594–1600.

Voigt, H.F. & Young, E.D. (1980). Evidence of inhibitory interactions between neurons in dorsal cochlear nucleus. *Journal of Neurophysiology, 44,* 76–96.

Warr, W.B. (1966). Fiber degeneration following lesions of the anterior-ventral cochlear nucleus of the cat. *Experimental Neurology, 14,* 453–474.

Warr, W.B. (1969). Fiber degeneration following lesions in the posteroventral cochlear nucleus of the cat. *Experimental Neurology, 23,* 140–155.

Young, E.D. (1980). Identification of response properties of ascending axons from dorsal cochlear nucleus. *Brain Research, 200,* 23–37.

Young, E.D., & Brownell, W.E. (1976). Responses to tones and noise of single cells in dorsal cochlear nucleus of unanesthetized cats. *Journal of Neurophysiology, 39,* 282–300.

Young, E.D., & Voigt, H.F. (1981). The internal organization of the dorsal cochlear nucleus. In J. Syka (Ed.), *Neuronal mechanisms of hearing.* New York: Plenum.

Young, E.D., & Voigt, H.F. (1982). Response properties of type II and type III units in the dorsal cochlear nucleus. *Hearing Research, 6,* 153–169.

Chapter 13

Asymmetries in Evoked Potentials

C.I. Berlin

L.J. Hood

P. Allen

INTRODUCTION

In the opening chapter of this book, Stebbins, Coombs, and Prosen discuss hemispheric or lateral asymmetries in many species. Recently it has even been suggested that "no animal species, no matter how humble, lacks cerebral dominance" (Geschwind, cited in Marx, 1983). The corollaries suggest that studies of human brain asymmetry, almost exclusively related to temporal lobes and "language function," may also be subcortical and need to be reexamined.

The orthodox work from which much of today's thinking developed cites the well-known anatomic and functional asymmetries in the human cortex (Celesia, 1976; Geschwind & Levitsky, 1968). Many writers (e.g., Kimura, 1973, summarized in Berlin & McNeil, 1976; Berlin, Lowe-Bell, Cullen, Thompson, & Loovis, 1973; Cullen, Thompson, Hughes, Berlin, & Samson, 1974; Porter & Hughes, 1983; Sidtis, 1982) have suggested that dichotic listening asymmetries are the least invasive ways of studying cerebral dominance for speech. We were not alone in suggesting some years ago that these asymmetries may not be restricted to cortical hemispheric specialization, but may have *subcortical underpinnings* (Berlin, 1977; Riklan & Cooper, 1977). Eidelberg and Galaburda (1982) and Ferraro and Minckler (1977) are among those who have recently shown *anatomic* asymmetries in the rostral brainstem. A number of other workers have suggested that there may be subcortical *physiological* auditory brainstem response asymmetries in the dorsal brainstem area (Chiappa, Gladstone & Young, 1979; Decker & Howe, 1981). There are also well-documented auditory *perceptual* asymmetries that have been in the literature for many years (examples include Bakker, 1968; Deutsch, 1974; Efron & Yund, 1974; Morais & Darwin, 1974; Murphy & Venables, 1971).

Few human body structures are perfectly symmetrical, and therefore it is reasonable to assume that there should be structural and physiological asymmetries in the *lower* brainstem. Yet we have built entire theories of cortical hemispheric specialization on the notion that only the hemispheres are asymmetrical and the rest of the brain is not. In this work, we studied asymmetries electrophysiologically (rather than with dichotic listening) at both subcortical and cortical levels using monaural versus binaural stimulation to elicit various forms of evoked potentials. We uncovered a number of provocative and interesting new observations. The data to follow show that (1) There are distinct right–left ear differences in almost every evoked potential we studied. (2) The binaural interaction component (that is, the residual obtained by subtracting monaurally elicited evoked potentials from binaurally elicited evoked potentials) is asymmetrical only so far as individual ears show asymmetry. (3) In some, but not all, of the evoked potentials there is a difference between the responses acquired from the C_z–A_1 and C_z–A_2 derivations even during simultaneous binaural stimulation. (4) In some evoked potentials, there appear to be differences in evoked potentials which vary with handedness.

In this chapter we address three types of evoked potentials – the early (auditory brainstem) response (0 to 10 ms), the middle latency response (10 to 75 ms), and the N_1–P_2 complex of the late response (75 to 200 ms).

THE EXTRACTION OF EVOKED POTENTIAL ASYMMETRIES

We discuss the stimulus and filtering characteristics of the early (auditory brainstem) response, middle latency response, and late response in their respective sections. However, in extracting and analyzing the data in all three of the potentials, we have followed a uniform pattern. Stimuli were always 100-μs pulses presented via TDH-39 or Koss HV/X earphones at 75 dB HLN. Evoked potential data were acquired in a four-electrode, two-channel array. That is, the "hot" electrode was always at the vertex (C_z), the respective references were on the mesial surface of the ear lobes (A_1 and A_2), while the ground was placed at the nasion.

Because all of these experiments were concerned with uncovering asymmetries in the auditory system, it was necessary to eliminate contributions of the electronics or the acoustics to the respective asymmetries. Care was taken to match the phase, frequency response, and intensity of the right and left earphones, and to match the frequency responses of each channel of the preamplifiers and postamplifiers. Each subject was studied under the following conditions:

1. *Standard condition:* red earphone on right ear, channel 1 electronics from the C_z–A_2 montage;
2. *Earphones reversed:* red earphone on left ear, but electronics set up as in condition 1;
3. *Electronics reversed:* earphones as in condition 1, but channel 1 electronics now handles output from the C_z–A_1 montage;
4. *Earphones and electronics reversed:* red earphone on left ear, electronics as in condition 3.

Each of these conditions was repeated on four separate occasions with a serial order change. In this way studies by statistical time series analysis enabled us to parcel out those factors due to physiologic asymmetries and those secondary to asymmetries in the equipment.

Stimuli were presented monaurally to the right ear, monaurally to the left ear, or to both ears simultaneously. During monaural stimulation we acquired both ipsilateral and contralateral recordings. Thus the following data were acquired from each experimental run:

1. RIP = Right ear stimulated, ipsilateral recording;
2. RCO = Right ear stimulated, contralateral recording;
3. LIP = Left ear stimulated, ipsilateral recording;
4. LCO = Left ear stimulated, contralateral recording;
5. SRT = Sum of all right ear stimulations, made up of RIP + RCO;
6. SLT = Sum of all left ear stimulations, made up of LIP + LCO;
7. BRT = Binaural stimulation recorded from the C_z-A_2 montage;
8. BLT = Binaural stimulation recorded from the C_z-A_1 montage;
9. SBIN = Sum of binaural stimulation, or (BRT + BLT).

From these data we acquired a number of derived potentials. The differences between all traces were acquired by linear subtraction; that is, there was no normalization of any of the data that went into the subtractions. All waveforms were acquired with equal numbers of stimulations and identical amplification settings. The *derived* responses were as follows.

1. BIC = The binaural interaction component = SBIN − (SRT + SLT);
2. BIC_R = The contribution of the right side to the binaural interaction component = $\dfrac{SBIN - SLT}{2}$;
3. BIC_L = The contribution of the left side to the binaural interaction component = $\dfrac{SBIN - SRT}{2}$;
4. SRT − SLT = Ear asymmetries (that is the difference between monaural results);
5. BRT − BLT = Binaural stimulation asymmetries;
6. BIC_R − BIC_L = Binaural interaction component asymmetries.

Each response was amplified 100,000 times through a combination of Grass P15 preamplifiers and custom-built postamplifiers. Responses were digitized on a Nicolet 1072 Signal Averager. The ASCII representation of the averaged waveforms was transmitted to a Perkin–Elmer 8/32 computer for storage and processing. An analysis protocol enabled us to add the waveforms acquired from all subjects under similar conditions and to statistically study the time series of grouped as well as individual waveforms.

The primary method of statistical analysis used was a time series analysis of variance (ANOVA) which incorporated the evoked potential waveform as one of the variables with each point in the waveform treated as a level of the time series variable. This application of ANOVA principles (developed by L.F. Hughes of our laboratory) enabled us to evaluate the waveforms on a point-by-point basis for similarity with baseline responses.

In summary, we were able to study (sometimes in the same subjects) the early (auditory brainstem) response, middle latency response, and late response asymmetries and binaural interactions. The results are presented in individual sections for each of the three potentials.

THE POTENTIALS

The Early Latency (Auditory Brainstem) Response

Data collection. Click stimuli were presented at a rate of 11 to 17 pulses per second. The auditory brainstem responses were acquired using bandpass filters of 100 to 3000 Hz. The digitizing rate was at 20 µs per point and two channels were acquired simultaneously. The multiplexing system alternated between channels giving an interpoint interval of 40 ms for this potential. Counterbalancing of earphones and electronics channels was completed as described earlier.

Results. Figures 13-1 and 13-2 show that, as a group, our subjects have a binaural interaction (BIC) at approximately 6 ms. Some subjects have a reliable binaural interaction; that is, under repeated measures and repeated conditions over 4 days the subjects show identical binaural interaction and virtually identical asymmetries. Other subjects show reliable auditory brainstem responses, but no binaural interaction. The early response of virtually all subjects shows asymmetry when both ears are stimulated simultaneously (BRT – BLT; see Figure 13-1 and Allen, Berlin, & Parrish, 1982.).

Discussion. These experiments have been repeated three times, twice in New Orleans and once in England (Lobaugh, Parker, Thornton, & Berlin, 1980). Although the earphone and electronics rotations were not performed in all the other experiments, we obtained basically the same results; that is, there is a right–left asymmetry and a binaural-right versus binaural-left asymmetry as well as a binaural interaction asymmetry. Note first that the sum of the monaural responses is about 20% larger (only at Wave V) than the sum of the binaural responses. Note also the slight slope differences that suggest the BIC is a "background potential" present only during binaural stimulation. The binaural interaction asymmetry, however, is secondary almost totally to the individual asymmetry between the ears.

This asymmetry is the one proposed by Decker and Howe (1981). They proposed that the binaural interaction (BIC) was inherently asymmetrical based on whether or not one noted the contribution of the right ear or the left ear to that binaural interaction. Their argument was as follows:

When one adds the responses from the two monaural conditions together, and subtracts the resultant waveform from the binaural response, the asymmetry is obscured. They felt that the sums of the right ear should be subtracted from the binaural response first, *followed* by subtraction of the sums of the left ears. When they did that, they uncovered what was clearly an asymmetry in the contribution of right versus left ears to the binaural interaction.

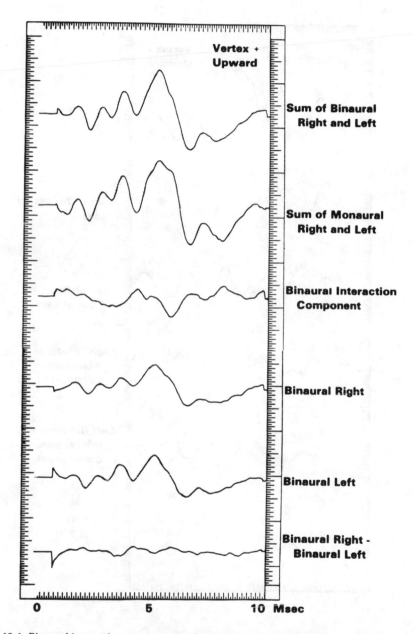

Figure 13-1. Binaural interaction component and right–left asymmetry for responses to binaural stimulation for the early (auditory brainstem) response. Data represent an average of 16 subjects.

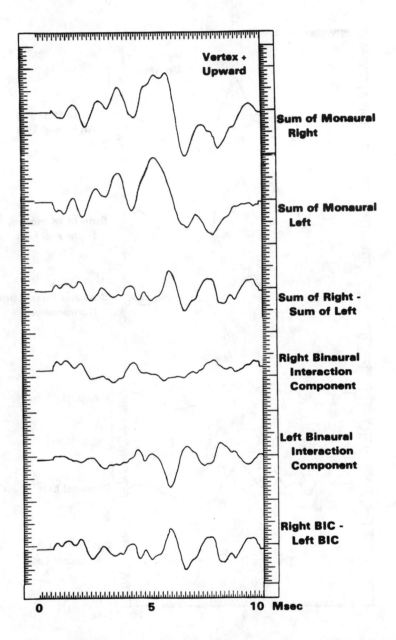

Figure 13-2. Right–left asymmetry for responses to monaural stimulation and binaural interaction asymmetry for the early (auditory brainstem) response for 16 subjects.

We have duplicated Decker and Howe's work and also have found an asymmetry; however, we know that virtually all of the asymmetry is contributed to by the individual asymmetries acquired during the right and left ear monaural stimulation. Figures 13-1 and 13-2 show this clearly. In the upper portion of Figure 13-1, we see the binaural interaction acquired by our method of summing the two monaural traces and subtracting those from the binaural. The individual right and left binaural interactions acquired by Decker and Howe's method and the difference of these are shown in the lower portion of Figure 13-2. Finally we show the result of subtracting the left ear brainstem response (SLT) from the right ear brainstem response (SRT) (Figure 13-2, upper portion); we find that the resultant curve is identical in virtually all respects to the binaural interaction asymmetries generated by Decker and Howe's method.

This finding can be predicted algebraically as follows:

If $\dfrac{SBIN}{2} - SLT = BIC_R$ and $\dfrac{SBIN}{2} - SRT = BIC_L,$

then $BIC_R - BIC_L = \left(\dfrac{SBIN}{2} - SLT\right) - \left(\dfrac{SBIN}{2} - SRT\right) = SRT - SLT$

We also observed that some subjects had a binaural interaction component while others did not. Our preliminary observations suggest that this "binaural interaction" to simultaneous signals may be secondary to temporal order judgment asymmetries; some subjects who consistently showed large and reliable binaural interaction components also had large asymmetry in their temporal order judgment abilities when asked to tell which ear was stimulated first in a two-item forced choice paradigm. Contrastively, subjects with no temporal order bias in favor of one ear or the other also failed to show consistent binaural interaction components in their evoked potentials.

Our most interesting finding on the theoretical level was the BRT–BLT asymmetry, which suggested a second through fourth-order neuron asymmetry unrelated to peripheral ear differences.

The Middle Latencies

Dobie and Norton (1980) showed that binaural interaction also occurred in the middle latency response. The interaction component was evident in the 20- to 40-ms latency range that encompasses Wave P_a. The following section confirms that observation and shows that the binaural interaction is larger, more stable, and easier to extract in the middle latencies than in the auditory brainstem response. Additional data also describe asymmetries in right–left comparisons of middle latency responses.

Data collection. Dobie and Norton (1980) used linked earlobe electrodes for the reference sites and reported large postauricular muscle artifacts in some of their subjects. We elected to use a two-channel recording system with reference electrodes on the mesial surface of the earlobe. The stimuli, which again were 100-μs pulses, were presented at a rate of 3.3 per second. The digitizing rate was 400 μs per point and thus the resolution using two-channel multiplexing was equal to 800 μs. The total time window was 204.8 ms and 512 sweeps were acquired per condition. All other data collection and manipulation were the same as in the auditory brainstem response section.

Bandpass filters on the Grass P15 preamplifiers were set at 10–100 Hz with a slope of 6 dB per octave. Comparison of responses obtained with these filter settings to responses obtained with no filtering showed that, for adult normal-hearing subjects, use of these filter settings did not alter the averaged responses, the asymmetry, or the interaction derivations.

Stimuli were presented monaurally to the right ear, monaurally to the left ear, and binaurally at 75 dB HLN. Subjects remained awake for all test sequences, but were allowed to read during recording.

Each individual sweep was recorded on an FM recorder. The averaged data acquired through the Nicolet 1072 Signal Averager were transmitted to the main laboratory computer for disk storage and statistical analyses.

Results. Hood, Berlin, and Hughes (1983a) investigated binaural interaction in the middle latency response, right–left asymmetries to monaural and binaural stimulation, binaural interaction asymmetries, and the replicability of these interactions and asymmetries in right-handed subjects.

The primary components identified in our data for responses to both monaural and binaural stimulation were Waves P_0, P_a, and P_b. These peaks occurred in the latency region between 10 and 70 ms poststimulus.

To obtain the binaural interaction component (BIC), the responses to left- and right-ear stimulation were added, then the sum of the two monaural stimulation conditions was subtracted from the sum of the binaural responses. Figure 13-3 shows that there is a large, statistically significant binaural interaction component in the middle latency response between 20 and 40 ms latency.

Asymmetries were obtained by subtracting left from right responses for the monaural condition, binaural condition, and for the right and left components of the binaural interaction. For the monaural comparisons the ipsilateral and contralateral responses were added together to yield the summed right and left ear responses (SRT and SLT, respectively).

Those right–left asymmetries, that compare responses to monaural stimulation of each ear were quite marked and statistically significant. This SRT–SLT asymmetry, shown in Figure 13-4, indicates that the asymmetry is primarily in the latency region of 30 to 60 ms.

Figure 13-4 shows that the right and left portions of the binaural interaction need not be symmetrical, a finding which is consistent with the report of Decker and Howe (1981) for the auditory brainstem response. When the asymmetries between these two components are closely examined and compared to the monaural right–left differences, it is clear that the binaural interaction asymmetry is again accounted for by the monaural differences (Figure 13-4).

Only minimal right–left asymmetry was observed in responses to binaural stimulation and statistical analysis showed that these differences were not significant in the middle latency response, in contrast to the findings for the auditory brainstem response.

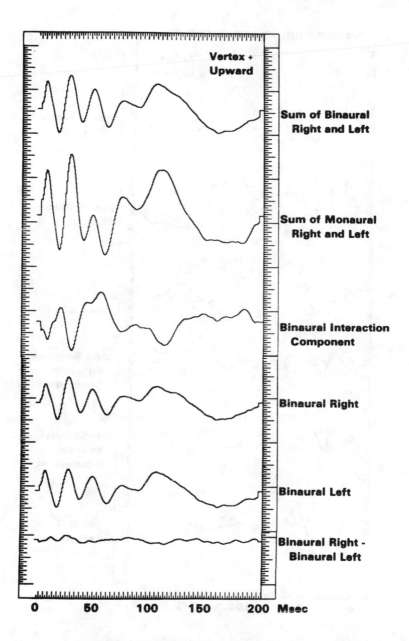

Figure 13-3. Binaural interaction component and right–left asymmetry for responses to binaural stimulation for the middle latency response. Data represent an average of six subjects.

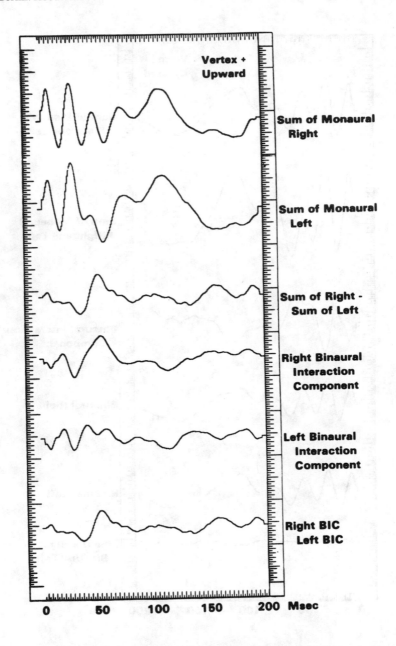

Figure 13-4. Right–left asymmetry for responses to monaural stimulation and binaural interaction asymmetry for the middle latency response for six subjects.

Discussion. The presence of a binaural interaction component in the middle latency response is in agreement with the results of Dobie and Norton (1980). In contrast to their report, however, our findings indicated good replicability of the binaural interaction and no observable interference of the postauricular muscle artifact. The binaural interaction component seems to be related more to an *amplitude* difference between the monaural and binaural tracings than a slope or latency difference, as is observed in the auditory brainstem response. This is particularly evident in the latency region of Wave P_a.

In the middle latency response the increase in amplitude with binaural stimulation over that observed with monaural stimulation was less than for the ABR. Therefore, when the sum of monaural responses is compared to the binaural responses, amplitude differences may be a greater source in the binaural interaction observed in the middle latency response than in the auditory brainstem response. To examine the influence of amplitude, we divided the summed monaural responses by 2. When the summed monaural response is divided by 2 and then subtracted from the binaural response, the "W" configuration remains. This is consistent with the presence of a latency difference as well in the components entering into the binaural interaction.

As observed in the ABR data, the BIC_R and BIC_L differences or the binaural interaction asymmetry can be accounted for by monaural asymmetries (SRT–SLT). The fact that the binaural interaction right–left asymmetries and the monaural right–left asymmetries are alike is not surprising, given that the binaural right–left differences are minimal and the primary asymmetry is observed in the responses to monaural stimuli.

Since the stimuli were broad band clicks, the two most likely sources of this and the related monaural asymmetries are (1) resonance peak differences in ear canal and middle ear structures and (2) true asymmetries in the neural generators for these potentials. At present, we have no data on peripheral resonance peaks; however, evidence for a neural source for the asymmetry comes from the finding that asymmetries are less evident in the latency region of Wave P_0 than in the later components of the middle latency response. This argument is similar to that used in support of the neural source for the binaural interaction in the auditory brainstem response.

Subjects showed greater individual variability in monaural asymmetries than in the binaural interaction component both in the amplitude of the asymmetry and in replicability.

The same asymmetries and interactions were examined in left-handed listeners (Hood, Martin & Berlin, 1983b). Right–left asymmetries and binaural interaction were similar in both right- and left-handed subjects. However, measures of absolute latency of Waves P_0, P_a, and P_b showed a marked latency difference between groups in Wave P_b with longer latencies in left-handed subjects by an average of 7 to 8 ms (Figure 13-5). This difference between groups in Wave P_b latency was highly significant, while latency differences observed for Waves P_0 and P_a were 0.6 and 1.6 ms, respectively.

Test–retest replicability of latencies in our subjects was 1.6 to 2 ms in the middle latency response which suggests that the observed differences in P_b latency between right- and left-handed groups could not be attributed to intertest variability.

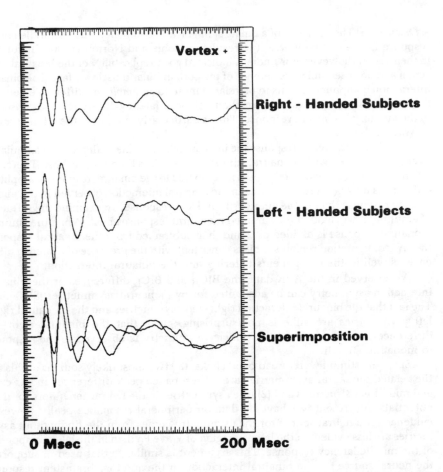

Figure 13-5. Middle latency response for right-handed subjects (top trace) and left-handed subjects (middle trace) and superimposition of both traces.

The Late Potentials

Binaural interaction and lateral asymmetries were also examined in the N_1–P_2 complex of the late potentials. The following section describes data which show that a large binaural interaction component can be observed in the late potentials while right–left asymmetries are less apparent than in the auditory brainstem response and the middle latency response.

Data collection. Stimuli were presented monaurally to the right ear, monaurally to the left ear, and binaurally at 75 dB HLN. The stimuli, 100-μs pulses, were presented at a rate of 1.1 per second.

A two-channel recording system was used as in data collection for the earlier evoked potentials, and bandpass filters were set at 0.1–10 Hz with a slope of 6 dB per octave. The digitizing rate was 1000 μs per point and thus the resolution using two-channel multiplexing was equal to 2000 μs. The total time window was 512.0 μs and 128 sweeps were acquired per condition.

Subjects remained awake for all test sequences and counted the number of stimuli for each test run. All other data collection and manipulation were the same as in the auditory brainstem response and middle latency response sections.

Each individual sweep was recorded on an FM recorder. The averaged data acquired through the Nicolet 1072 Signal Averager were transmitted to the main laboratory computer for disk storage and statistical analyses.

Results. Figures 13–6 and 13–7 show the data we acquired (Hood et al., 1983b). The main peaks in our data were at 80 μs for N_1 and 150 μs for P_2. The binaural interaction, which was quite easy to acquire, was seen in all subjects as a large vertex negative component at approximately 150 μs.

Monaural asymmetries were greater than binaural asymmetries as in the middle latency response. The asymmetry between the right binaural interaction and the left binaural interaction again is the same as that asymmetry observed for the monaural right–left comparison.

Discussion. These data show that less asymmetry is present in evoked potential recordings for the late potentials than for the early and middle potentials. One explanation for this finding probably relates to the numerous interconnections between the right and left hemispheres at cortical versus subcortical levels. Surface recordings of responses at the cortical level are more apt to reflect responses which are distributed equally between the hemispheres. In addition, the fact that asymmetries are clearly present in the middle latency response suggests that the middle latencies derive their activity from different neural units than do the late responses.

When the binaural interaction is derived after dividing the summed monaural response by 2, the amplitude of the binaural interaction component is markedly reduced and actually reverses direction in some subjects. This suggests that, unlike the middle latency or ABR binaural interaction, the monaural–binaural differences may be almost entirely due to amplitude differences as a result of summing waveforms. The amplitude differences between responses to monaural and binaural stimulation were minimal in our data. Thus, the process of summing monaural responses resulted in a greater monaural amplitude as compared to the binaural than for the ABR or MLR.

Similar asymmetries and interactions were observed for right- and left-handed subjects in the late potentials. In addition, no significant differences in absolute latencies of N_1 or P_2 have been reported (Hood et al., 1983b).

Overall Discussion

The 1983 Harvard Conference "Biological Foundations of Cerebral Dominance" (Marx, 1983) highlighted a number of newly uncovered anatomic and behavioral brain

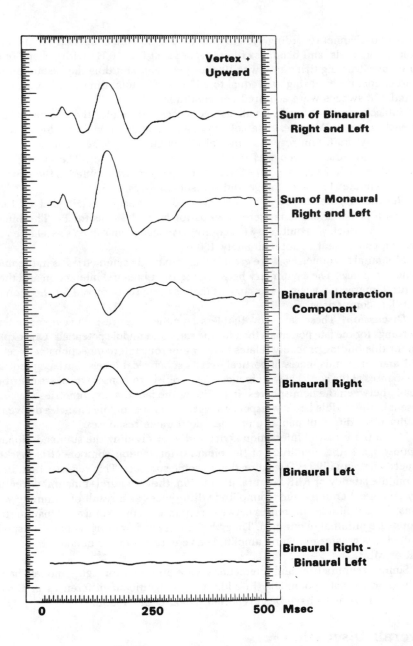

Figure 13-6. Binaural interaction component and right–left asymmetry for responses to binaural stimulation for the late response. Data represent an average of six subjects.

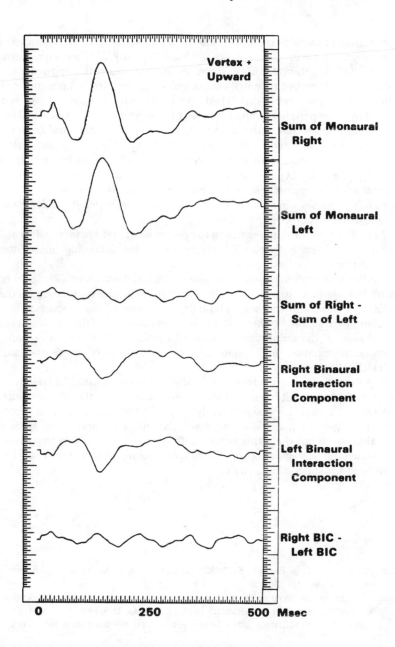

Figure 13-7. Right-left asymmetry for responses to monaural stimulation and binaural interaction asymmetry for the late response for six subjects.

asymmetries in human, bird, ape, and even rat. Some of these asymmetries seem to be subject to hormonal influences. Although many of these asymmetries seem to be related to cerebral cortex, some are in fact subcortically mediated. In this investigation of evoked potentials supposedly deriving from different levels of the auditory system we found that (1) Almost every evoked potential we studied was affected by some peripheral right versus left ear asymmetry. (2) A binaural interaction component (the residual activity after the subtraction of monaural from binaurally elicited responses) found in all potentials was asymmetrical physiologically only insofar as the responses from the ears were peripherally asymmetrical. (3) There was a C_z-A_2 versus C_z-A_1 asymmetry in the (early) auditory brainstem response to binaural clicks at approximately the third- and fourth- order neuron levels. (4) *In the middle responses wave P_b latency averaged 7 ms later in left-handed subjects* than in right-handed subjects.

In addition to the data regarding the presence of and characteristics of binaural interaction and evoked potential asymmetries, the following observations have emerged from these studies:

Auditory brainstem responses to binaural stimuli are on an average at least 60% greater in amplitude than responses recorded to monaural stimulation. In the middle latency response and the late potentials, the sums of the responses to binaural stimulation are actually somewhat *smaller* than the sums of the monaural responses. This change in the amplitude increase of responses to binaural as compared to monaural stimulation may relate to Zwislocki's theory of central summation (Zwislocki, 1971).

The second observation involves the differences in the middle latency responses between right- and left-handed subjects. We have found that the absolute latency of Wave P_b of the MLR is significantly longer in left-handed subjects. Both earlier responses (P_0 and P_a) and later responses (N_1 and P_2) (more likely to derive from cortical area) do not show this latency difference. This suggests that there may be independent physiological indices which correlate with hand preference, but are not manifested in late cortical activity.

REFERENCES

Allen, P., Berlin, C.I., & Parrish, K. (1982). Asymmetries in the binaural auditory brainstem response. *Asha, 24,* 770.

Bakker, D. (1968). Ear asymmetry with monaural stimulation. *Psychonomic Science, 12,* 62.

Berlin, C.I. (1977). Hemispheric asymmetry in auditory tasks. In S. Harnad, R. Doty, L. Goldstein, J. Jaynes, & G. Krauthamer (Eds.), *Lateralization in the nervous system.* New York: Academic Press.

Berlin, C.I., Lowe-Bell, S.S., Cullen, J.K., Thompson, C.L., & Loovis, C.F. (1973). Dichotic speech perception: An interpretation of right-ear advantage and temporal offset effects. *Journal of the Acoustical Society of America, 53,* 699–709.

Berlin, C.I., & McNeil, M.R. (1976). Dichotic listening. In N. Lass (Ed.), *Contemporary issues in experimental phonetics,* New York: Academic Press.

Celesia, G.G. (1976). Organization of auditory cortical areas in man. *Brain, 99,* 403–414.

Chiappa, K.H., Gladstone, K.J., & Young, R.R. (1979). Brainstem auditory evoked responses: Studies of waveform variations in 50 human subjects. *Archives of Neurology, 36,* 81–87.

Cullen, J.K., Jr., Thompson, C.L., Hughes, L.F., Berlin, C.I., & Samson, D.S. (1974). The effects of varied acoustic parameters on performance in dichotic speech perception tasks. *Brain and Language, 1,* 307–322.

Decker, T.N., & Howe, S.W. (1981). Auditory tract asymmetry in brainstem electrical responses during binaural stimulation. *Journal of the Acoustical Society of America, 69,* 1084–1090.

Deutsch, D. (1974). An auditory illusion. *Nature (London), 251,* 307–309.

Dobie, R.A., & Norton, S.J. (1980). Binaural interaction in human auditory evoked potentials. *Electroencephalography and Clinical Neurophysiology, 49,* 303–313.

Efron, R., & Yund, E.W. (1974). Dichotic competition of simultaneous tone bursts of different frequency. I. Dissociation of pitch from lateralization and loudness. *Neuropsychologia, 12,* 249–256.

Eidelberg, D., & Galaburda, A.M. (1982). Symmetry and asymmetry in the human posterior thalamus. *Archives of Neurology, 39,* 325–332.

Ferraro, J.A., & Minckler, J. (1977). The human lateral lemniscus and its nuclei. The human auditory pathways: A quantitative study. *Brain and Language, 4,* 277–294.

Geschwind, N., & Levitsky, W. (1968). Human brain: Left–right asymmetries in temporal speech region. *Science, 161,* 186–187.

Hood, L.J., Berlin, C.I., & Hughes, L.F. (1983a). Binaural interaction in the middle latency response. *Journal of the Acoustical Society of America, 73,* S79.

Hood, L.J., Martin, D.A., & Berlin, C.I. (1983b). Auditory evoked potential asymmetries in right- and left-handed listeners. *Journal of the Acoustical Society of America, 74,* S40.

Kimura, D. (1973). The asymmetry of the human brain. *Scientific American, 227,* 70–78.

Lobaugh, P., Parker, D., Thornton, A.R.D., & Berlin, C.I. (1980). Binaural interaction asymmetries in human ABR's. *Journal of the Acoustical Society of America, 68,* S20.

Marx, J.L. (1983). The two sides of the brain. *Science, 220,* 488–490.

Morais, J., & Darwin, C.J. (1974). Ear differences for same–different reaction times to monaurally presented speech. *Brain and Language, 1,* 383–390.

Murphy, E.H., & Venables, P.H. (1971). The effects of caffeine citrate and white noise on ear asymmetry in the detection of two clicks. *Neuropsychologia, 9,* 27–32.

Porter, R.J., Jr., & Hughes, L.F. (1983). Dichotic listening to CV's: Method, interpretation and application. In J.B. Hellige (Ed.), *Cerebral hemisphere asymmetry: Method, theory and application.* Praeger Scientific Publishers, University of Southern California Press.

Riklan, M., & Cooper, I.S. (1977). Thalamic lateralization of psychological functions: Psychometric studies. In S. Harnad, R. Doty, L. Goldstein, J. Jaynes, & G. Krauthamer (Eds.), *Lateralization in the nervous system.* New York: Academic Press.

Sidtis, J.J. (1982). Predicting brain organization from dichotic listening performance: Cortical and subcortical functional asymmetries contribute to perceptual asymmetries. *Brain and Language, 17,* 287–300.

Zwislocki, J.J. (1971). Central masking and neural activity in the cochlear nucleus. *Audiology, 10,* 48–59.

AUTHOR INDEX

A

Abbas, P.J., 263, 276, 354, 452
Achor, L.J., 349, 356
Adams, J.C., 161, 168, 170, 247, 347, 348, 352, 359, 393, 394, 402, 403, 406, 434, 444
Ades, H.W., 36
Adrian, H.O., 441
Agelfors, E., 318
Agranoff, B.W., 160
Ahrron, W., 24
Aitkin, L.M., 402, 403, 406, 450, 451
Albe, F., 217, 225, 234
Albers, R.W., 160
Allanson, J.T., 354
Allegra, L.A., 327, 330
Allen, J.B., 219
Allen, P., 464
Altman, D.W., 252
Altman, P.L., 97
Altschuler, R.A., 162, 164, 165, 166, 172, 173, 186, 342, 345, 350, 356, 358
Andersen, R.A., 402, 403, 406, 450
Anderson, D.J., 26, 263, 266
Anderson, S.D., 251
Änggard, L., 118
Anlezark, G., 349
Anniko, M., 200, 201
Ansberry, M., 37
Anson, B.J., 110, 118
Anson, J., 169
Aran, J.-M., 133, 252
Ardell, L.A., 309
Arenberg, I.K., 201
Arlien-Soberg, P., 349
Armitage, S.E., 130
Arneson, A.R., 407
Arthur, R.M., 263, 270
Ary, M., 142
Ascher, P., 161
Ashby, P., 349
Axelrod, F.S., 229

B

Babitz, L., 361
Bachelard, H.S., 358
Backus, A.S.N., 372, 430
Baker, C.C., 392
Bakker, D., 461
Baldwin, B.A., 130

Banerjee, S.D., 61
Banfai, P., 311, 316
Barelli, A.E., 216
Baru, A.V., 5
Bast, T.H., 118
Bantini, C., 188
Batkin, S., 37
Baylis, J.R., 19
Beaton, R.D., 3
Beaudet, A., 342, 346
Beecher, M.D., 2, 5, 9, 13, 14, 31
Békésy, G. von, 216, 218, 225, 249
Belford, G.R., 141
Bench, J., 130
Benes, F.M., 144
Bengry, M.F., 451
Benoit, J.A.A., 61, 102
Bergstrom, L., 309, 324
Berlin, C.I., 319, 461, 464, 468, 471, 473
Berliner, K.I., 310
Bernardin, C.P., 270
Bernfield, M.R., 61
Bhargava, V.K., 356
Bilger, R.C., 312
Bird, S.J., 444
Biscoe, T.J., 168, 346
Bjorkroth, B., 310, 328
Black, F.O., 328
Black, R.C., 309
Blakeslee, E.A., 29
Bladon, R.A.W., 280
Blamey, P.J., 319
Bledsoe, S.C., Jr., 164, 166, 167, 168, 170, 171, 172
Blumstein, S.E., 283
Bobbin, R.P., 159, 161, 162, 163, 164, 165, 166, 167, 168, 169, 170, 171, 172
Bock, G.R., 37, 111, 112, 133
Boerger, G., 451
Bogert, B.P., 301
Bohne, B.A., 29, 30, 31, 36, 248, 251, 326, 392, 413, 450
Boisvert, P., 29
Bonazolli, R., 51, 102
Bonke, B.A., 188
Bonke, D., 453
Bonke, H., 188
Bone, R.C., 30, 31, 32, 200
Bonnevie, K., 89, 102
Borg, E., 451
Born, D.E., 136
Bornstein, J.C., 349
Bosher, S.K., 109, 201
Bourgois, M., 309

Bourk, T.R., 347, 372, 375, 392, 393, 423, 430, 431, 432, 434, 435, 437, 438, 440, 441
Bowery, N.G., 167
Boyle, A.J.F., 215, 218, 225, 235
Brachman, M.L., 36, 263, 283, 290, 431
Brachmann, D.E., 310, 315, 326, 327
Bradford, H.F., 169
Brady, J.V., 31
Brawer, J.R., 343, 347, 371, 372, 373, 374, 375, 376, 378, 381, 382, 389, 391, 392, 399, 400, 406, 430, 434, 435, 438
Bredberg, G., 115, 118, 225, 235
Brehingstall, G., 111
Britt, R., 372, 442, 444, 449, 450, 453
Brocaar, M.P., 24
Brodal, A., 247
Brooks, D., 111
Brown, C.H., 1, 2, 14
Brown, J.C., 351
Brown, M.C., 214, 253
Brownell, W.E., 251, 372, 413, 425, 427, 429, 430, 435, 436, 437, 438, 442, 444, 445, 447, 451
Brugge, J.F., 37, 120, 148, 263, 266, 270, 372
Bruggencate, G. Ten, 353
Brummer, S.B., 310, 330
Bruns, V., 17
Brunso-Bechtold, J.K., 402, 406
Bryant, G., 165, 168, 173
Buchwald, J.S., 349
Bullock, T.H., 3
Burda, H., 22
Burdick, C.K., 5, 6, 29
Burgio, P.A., 200, 201
Burian, K., 311
Burkhalter, A., 342
Burns, E.M., 318
Butikofer, R., 323
Butler, R.A., 449, 450, 453

C

Caceres, A., 144
Caesar, G., 164, 167
Calas, A., 169
Cameron, R., 200, 201
Camp, R.T., Jr., 6, 29
Canlon, B., 199
Cant, N.B., 119, 373, 374, 375, 376, 388, 389, 393, 394, 395, 396, 398, 399, 402, 403, 406, 434, 435, 438, 440, 451
Canzek, V., 345
Capranica, R.R., 217, 229, 230
Carlborg, B., 169
Carlier, E., 110, 115, 133
Carter, J.A., 169
Caspary, D.M., 348, 354, 355, 356, 375, 431, 444

Casseday, J.H., 37, 375, 389, 392, 399, 402, 444
Cataland, S., 172
Celesia, G.G., 461
Chamberlain, S.C., 431
Champagnat, J., 353
Cheatham, M.A., 251
Cheney, D.L., 3
Cheng, S.-S., 141
Cheung, H.C., 249
Chiappa, K.H., 461
Chihal, D.M., 166, 167, 168, 170, 172
Chikamori, Y., 356
Chistovich, L.A., 302
Chole, R.A., 133
Chuang, H.H., 52, 102
Chung, D.Y., 36
Churchill, J.A., 162
Clark, C.S., 31
Clark, G.M., 32, 309, 310, 312, 319
Clark, L.F., 438
Clark, L.S., 22
Clark, W.W., 30, 31, 251
Clarke, G.P., 311
Clements, M., 37, 111
Clopton, B.M., 37, 148, 310, 313, 314, 319, 324, 329, 451
Cody, A.R., 221, 225, 235
Cohen, E.S., 389, 392, 412
Cohen, G.M., 118, 122
Cohen, R.H., 61
Colavita, F.B., 36
Colburn, H.S., 303
Coleman, J.R., 145
Coleman, J.W., 115
Coles, R.B., 111, 120, 122, 123, 136
Collins, G.G.S., 169
Collins, J.F., 349
Collins, M.J., 309
Coloumbre, A.J., 92
Comegys, T.H., 169, 201
Comis, S.D., 162, 163, 167, 172, 249, 347, 352, 354, 355, 356, 453
Conlee, J.W., 134, 145, 148, 393, 394
Conley, E., 51, 102
Constantine-Paton, M., 148
Contreras, N.E., 358
Coombs, S., 17, 22, 24, 25, 26, 30
Cooper, I.S., 461
Cooper, W.E., 317
Corey, D.P., 252
Cornsweet, T.N., 19
Costalupes, J.A., 452, 453
Cotanche, D.A., 118, 119
Cotman, C.W., 169
Cowan, W.M., 133, 140
Cowan, W.W., 389, 392
Cox, D.W.G., 169
Crane, H.D., 248

Cranford, J.L., 36
Crawford, A.C., 234, 252
Crossland, W.J., 140
Croucher, M.J., 349
Cuenod, M., 342, 346
Cullen, J.K., 461
Curtis, D.R., 170, 346, 349, 353, 354, 359, 360
Cutting, J.E., 298

D

Dahl, A.-L., 381, 399, 400, 406, 412
Dahlstrom, A., 360
Dallos, P., 32, 33, 130, 224, 248, 251, 252
D'Amico-Martel, A., 73, 102
Dancer, A., 217, 225, 235
Danto, J., 37
Darwin, C.J., 461
Davies, J., 168, 346, 349
Davies, W.E., 353, 453
Davis, H., 249, 254
Davis, M., 451
Dawkins, R., 3
Deatherage, B.H., 254
DeBoer, E., 219, 249, 299
Decker, T.N., 461, 464, 468
Deitch, J.S., 144
Delgutte, B., 263, 288, 291, 292, 293, 297, 299, 303
DeMott, J.E., 169
Denavit-Saubie, M., 353
Densert, B., 169
Densert, O., 169
Deol, M.S., 71, 97, 99, 102
Derlacki, E.L., 32
De Rosier, D.J., 119, 232, 251
Desmedt, J.E., 162, 164, 165, 166
Desmond, M.E., 92
deSouza, E., 141
DesRasiers, M.H., 195
Detwiller, S.R., 52, 102
Deutsch, D., 461
Devigne, C., 37, 115
Dewson, J.H. III, 5, 303
Dichter, M., 182
Dickson, J.W., 358, 429, 437
Dietrich, W.D., 142
Diggs, J., 140
Disterhoft, J.F., 375, 427, 430
Djupesland, G., 110
Dobelle, W.H., 310
Dobie, R.A., 326, 327, 330, 467, 471
Donaldson, J.A., 110
Dooling, R.J., 16, 19, 22
Doran, R., 162
Douek, E., 311
Dowell, R.C., 319

Dragsten, P.R., 217
Drenckhahn, D., 249
Drescher, D.G., 165, 166, 168, 170, 172, 173
Drescher, M.J., 165, 166, 168, 170, 172, 173
Duckert, L.G., 329, 330
Duggan, A.W., 353
Dunker, F., 451
Durham, D., 141, 142
Duvall, A.J., 31
Duvall, F., 310
Dye, R.H., Jr., 452

E

Easter, S.S., 120
Eckenstein, F., 162
Eddington, D.K., 310, 311, 315, 319, 322
Edgerton, B.J., 310
Edstrom, L., 204
Edwards, J.S., 140
Efron, R., 461
Egelman, E.H., 119, 232
Ehret, G., 16, 17, 22, 31, 120, 140
Eidelberg, D., 461
Eisenberg, L.S., 310
Eldredge, D.H., 31, 241, 254
Eldredge, N., 16
Elliott, D.N., 29
Elverland, H.H., 393, 394, 444
Engstrom, H., 241
Erulkar, S.D., 139, 372, 449, 450, 453
Evans, E.F., 15, 172, 218, 225, 233, 248, 249, 263, 270, 276, 318, 321, 372, 413, 425, 427, 436, 445, 447, 452, 453
Evans, R.H., 167, 168, 346
Evans, S., 375
Eybalin, M., 169, 171

F

Faingold, C.L., 348, 444
Fant, C.G.M., 273
Farbman, A.I., 77
Farley, G.R., 247, 359, 360
Fass, B., 140
Fay, R.R., 5, 16, 19, 22, 24, 26, 30
Fee, W.E., Jr., 133
Feitosa, A.G., 32
Fekete, D.M., 450
Feldman, M.L., 389, 391, 393, 434, 438
Felix, D., 353
Feng, A.S., 37, 134, 145, 148, 247
Fermin, C.F., 118, 122
Fernald, R.D., 453
Ferraro, J.A., 461
Fettiplace, R., 234, 252

Fex, J., 161, 162, 164, 165, 166, 168, 172, 173, 186, 247, 342, 344, 345, 358, 444
Fex, R.L., 182, 183
Finn, R.C., 393, 394, 444
Fischler, H., 216
Fisher, S.K., 353
Flamnino, F., 37
Flock, A., 164, 200, 223, 224, 231, 232, 249, 251
Flock, B., 231
Fong, M., 310
Foote, S.L., 361
Foulke, E., 309
Fourcin, A.J., 311, 315, 327
Francis, A.A., 168
Frankenhaeuser, B., 323, 324
Franks, A., 349
Freedman, R., 361
Frei, E.H., 216
Friedrich, V.L., 381, 399, 400, 406, 412
Frishkopf, L.S., 229
Frisina, R.D., 431
Fromme, H.D., 182, 183
Frush, D.P., 133
Fujimoto, S., 119, 356
Fuse, G., 371, 372
Fuxe, K., 356, 360

G

Gacek, R.R., 392
Galaburda, A.M., 461
Galambos, R., 3, 372, 392, 393, 423
Galley, N., 247
Gannon, R.P., 254
Garfinkle, T.J., 110, 231
Gaston, K.C., 375, 389, 393, 394, 399, 406
Gates, G.R., 111, 120, 122, 123, 136
Geisler, C.D., 215, 221, 263, 270, 283, 288, 303
Gendelman, D.S., 451
Gendelman, P.M., 451
Gentschev, T., 394, 395
Gerstein, G.L., 445, 449, 450, 453
Geschwind, N., 461
Gessert, C.F., 254
Gheewala, T.R., 310
Gibson, D.J., 427, 429, 430, 452
Gibson, M.M., 270, 372
Gifford, M.L., 253
Gilula, N.B., 113
Ginzberg, R.D., 113, 407
Giraudi, D.M., 19, 30
Gisbergen, J.A.M. van, 372, 427, 429, 430, 432, 435, 437, 438, 440, 441
Gladstone, K.J., 461
Glass, I., 310, 313, 319, 323, 324
Gleason, H.A., 273
Glendenning, K.K., 402, 406

Globus, A., 133, 140
Glorig, A., 32
Godfrey, D.A., 169, 351, 353, 372, 375, 392, 401, 407, 408, 411, 413, 430, 431, 432, 435, 436, 437, 438, 441, 444
Gold, T., 249
Goldberg, J.M., 372, 430, 437, 438, 441, 453
Goldstein, J.L., 263, 268, 299, 301, 303, 324
Goldstein, M.H., Jr., 229
Gondra, M., 165
Goodman, R.R., 356
Goodwin, P., 188, 206
Gorda, M.P., 359
Gordon, B.S., 378, 400, 406
Gottlieb, G., 37, 120, 134, 148
Gould, S.J., 16
Gourevitch, G., 16
Grashuis, J.L., 372, 427, 429, 430, 432, 435, 437, 438, 440, 441
Gray, L., 111, 120, 134, 136, 144, 146, 148
Green, S., 3, 9, 11, 12
Greenberg, J., 188, 201
Greenwood, D.D., 320, 372, 453
Grimwade, J., 130
Grobstein, C., 61, 102
Grubel, G., 451
Gruber, J., 451
Grynderup, V., 349
Guerry, T.L., 133
Guillery, R.W., 133, 140
Guinan, J.J., Jr., 183, 241, 247, 253, 407, 408, 411, 413, 430, 434, 435, 440
Gulley, R.L., 166, 182, 183, 395, 444, 451
Gunderson, T., 215
Guth, P.S., 159, 161, 162, 164, 165, 166, 168, 173, 352
Guttman, R., 323

H

Haas, H.L., 353
Habib, C.P., 399
Hachmeister, L., 323
Hackett, J.T., 119, 122, 134, 142
Hafft, L.P., 61
Hafter, E.R., 452
Haldeman, S., 346
Hall, E.K., 86
Hall, J.G., 346
Hall, L., 26
Hall, M., 273
Halperin, H.R., 319
Hamberger, A., 169
Hamernik, D., 19
Hamernik, R.P., 22, 29, 30, 31, 263
Handy, I.C., 359
Hans, J., 31

Hansson, E., 345
Harmison, G.G., 342, 345
Harris, D.M., 32, 33, 130, 248, 251
Harrison, J.M., 343, 372, 389, 391, 393, 402, 403, 434, 438
Harrison, R.G., 50, 52, 86, 89, 102
Harrison, R.V., 248
Harrison, W.H., 32
Hartman, B.K., 355
Hartman, W., 22
Hashimoto, T., 263
Havey, D.C., 348, 355, 444
Hawkins, A.D., 16
Hawkins, J.E., Jr., 1, 29, 30, 31, 33, 133, 248
Hay, E.D., 61
Hayabuchi, I., 119
Headley, P.M., 346
Healy, M.J.R., 301
Heffner, H., 36
Heinz, J.M., 293
Heinz, R.D., 16, 22, 31
Held, H., 371, 389, 393
Helfenstein, W.M., 215
Helmerich, L.F., 310
Helmholtz, H.L.F. von, 264
Henderson, D., 19, 22, 29, 30, 31
Hendricks, D.M., 89
Hendriksen, O., 349
Henkel, C.K., 394, 399, 403
Henry, K.R., 133
Herkenham, M., 356
Herndon, M.K., 310
Hertwig, P., 89, 97, 102
Heywood, P., 77
Hilding, D., 115
Hill, B.C., 216
Hill, D.R., 167
Hill, R.G., 354
Hillman, P., 215
Hillyard, V., 32
Himelfarb, M.Z., 111
Hind, J.E., 263, 266, 270, 372
Hinojosa, R., 309, 324
Hirokawa, N., 118, 122, 249
Hochmair, E.S., 311, 313, 315, 316, 318, 322
Hochmair-Desoyer, I.J., 311, 313, 315, 316, 318, 321, 322, 327
Hoffman, D.W., 172, 186
Hokfelt, T., 356
Holton, T., 231, 232
Holtzer, H., 61, 102
Hood, L.J., 468, 471, 473
Horten, R., 349
Hortmann, G., 311
Hoshino, T., 247, 255
Hosli, L., 353
Houde, R.A., 309
House, W.F., 32, 310, 326

Howe, S.W., 461, 464, 468
Howlett, B., 351
Howse, P.E., 19
Huang, C.M., 349
Hubbard, A.E., 234, 251, 263
Hudson, A.L., 167
Hudspeth, A.J., 231, 252
Huffman, R.D., 346
Hughes, J.R., 372, 392, 393, 423
Hughes, L.F., 461, 468
Hui, G.S., 427, 430
Hungerbuhler, J.P., 188, 201
Hunt, K., 168
Hunt, S., 352
Hunter-Duvar, I., 29, 200, 201
Huxley, A.F., 323, 324
Hynson, K., 29, 30

I

Ibata, Y., 395
Irvine, D.R.F., 111, 120
Irving, R., 343, 372, 403
Iverson, L.L., 182

J

Jack, J.J.B., 438
Jackson, H., 110, 119, 122, 134, 136, 142
Jacobs, J., 217
Jacobson, A.G., 92
Jacobson, R., 273
Jansson, E., 203
Jarrett, L.S., 51, 102
Jaskoll, T.F., 110
Jasser, A., 162
Javel, E., 37, 120, 263, 359, 372, 452
Jenison, G.L., 164, 165, 166, 167, 168, 169, 170
Jenkins, W.M., 36, 451
Jerger, J.F., 111, 319
Jerger, S., 111
Jhaveri, S., 119, 134
Johannesma, P.I.M., 372, 427, 429, 430, 432, 435, 437, 438, 440, 441
Johns, M.E., 133
Johnson, D.H., 268, 270, 293, 297
Johnson, G.A., 217
Johnsson, L.-G., 1, 29, 30, 31, 133, 248, 326, 328
Johnston, G.A.R., 346, 353, 354
Johnstone, B.M., 17, 162, 163, 213, 214, 215, 216, 218, 221, 222, 225, 235, 248, 249, 250
Johnstone, J.R., 214, 235, 248
Jones, D.R., 343, 346, 375, 389, 392, 399, 413, 444
Jones, D.T., 381, 394
Jun, S., 22

K

Kaan, H.W., 86, 102
Kakaurda, O., 195
Kaltenbach, J.A., 110, 111, 123
Kane, E., 372, 373, 374
Kane, E.C., 140, 407, 408, 430, 435, 442, 444
Kane, E.S., 186, 343, 375, 376, 378, 381, 382,
    389, 393, 394, 395, 398, 399, 400, 406, 411,
    413
Karduck, A., 255
Karlstedt, J., 345
Kasamatsu, T., 142
Katsuki, Y., 165, 170, 172
Katayama, Y., 263
Katz, D.D., 97
Katzman, R.K., 160
Kauer, J.S., 361
Kaufmann, R., 206
Kay, R., 15
Keister, T.E., 5
Keith, R.W., 111
Keithley, E.M., 318
Keller, 249
Kelliher, E.M., 310
Kelly, J.B., 37, 111
Kelly, J.P., 227
Kemp, D.T., 249, 251
Kennedy, C., 195
Kerr, A.G., 309
Kerr, L.M., 111, 134, 146, 148
Kessler, D.K., 324
Khanna, S.M., 213, 214, 215, 216, 217, 218, 221,
    225, 226, 227, 235, 249
Kiang, N.Y.S., 22, 25, 134, 241, 247, 248, 263,
    276, 284, 299, 310, 318, 319, 343, 352, 372,
    375, 392, 407, 408, 411, 413, 430, 431, 432,
    435, 436, 437, 438, 441, 442, 444, 450
Killackey, H.P., 140, 141, 247
Kim, D.O., 233, 234, 248, 249, 250, 251, 252,
    253, 263, 264, 248, 270
Kimm, J., 326
Kimura, D., 461
Kitzes, L.M., 37, 120, 140, 247, 270, 343, 372
Klinke, R., 159, 162, 165, 166, 167, 172, 182,
    183, 233, 247, 255, 451
Kliauga, P., 215
Knight, P.L., 264
Kobayashi, R.M., 359
Kobrak, H., 389
Koelliker, A., 371, 389
Koerber, K.C., 134, 352, 372, 444
Kohllöffel, L.U.E., 217, 218, 225, 235
Koizumi, K., 359, 360
Konigsmark, B.W., 375
Konishi, M., 22
Konishi, T., 161, 162, 163
Konkle, D.F., 111

Korte, G., 381, 399, 400, 406, 412
Kraus, H., 182, 185
Krebs, J.R., 3
Krnjevic, K., 182, 186, 352, 353, 354, 355
Kromer, L.F., 355
Kronester-Frei, A., 247
Kubik, S., 311
Kuhar, M.J., 352, 353
Kuhl, P.K., 6, 7, 8, 309
Kuriyama, K., 164

L

Lam, D.M.K., 164
Landolt, I., 200, 201
Langner, G., 453
Laplante, S., 188
Lawrence, P.D., 323
Leake, P.A., 142
Leake-Jones, P.A., 247, 309, 328, 329, 330, 450
Le Douarin, N.M., 71
Leng, G., 162, 163, 167, 172
Lenn, N.J., 434
Lenn, T.R., 395
Lenoir, M., 110, 115, 133
Leonard, D.G.B., 213, 214, 215, 217, 218, 221,
    225, 226, 227, 249
LePage, E.L., 214, 216, 249, 252
Lessac, M.S., 148
Levi-Montalcini, R., 110, 134, 136
Levine, R.A., 247, 248
Levitan, H., 445, 447
Levitsky, W., 461
Levitt, H., 309
Levitt, P., 355
Levy, O., 86
Lewis, M.S., 352
Lewis, W.H., 71
Lewy, F.H., 389
Li, C.W., 55, 68, 76, 86, 97, 102, 113
Li, R.Y-S., 434, 440
Liberman, A.M., 5
Liberman, M.C., 241, 247, 248, 256, 263, 276,
    318, 343, 407, 450, 452
Liff, H., 229
Lim, D.J., 172, 231, 247, 255
Lindblom, B., 280
Ling, A., Jr., 215, 231, 232
Linthicum, F.H., Jr., 326
Lipes, R., 219
Lippe, W.R., 109, 123, 126, 134, 140
Littlefield, W.M., 268
Liu, J.-C., 375
Ljungdahl, A., 356
Llinas, R.R., 447
Lobaugh, P., 464
Lockberg, 217

Lodge, D., 167, 349
Loeb, G.E., 303, 310, 314, 319
Loftus-Hill, J.J., 217
Long, G., 17, 22
Lonsbury-Martin, B.L., 36
Loovis, C.F., 461
Lorente de Nó, R., 343, 372, 374, 375, 378, 382,
    389, 392, 393, 394, 399, 403, 406, 412, 423,
    430, 438, 444, 445, 447
Lowe-Bell, S.S., 461
Lowry, O.H., 142
Lowy, W.A., 161
Lubinska, V.V., 302
Lukas, S.E., 31
Lynch, J.C., 5

M

Macartney, J.C., 249
Maderson, P.F.A., 110
Magnaini, E., 381
Malamed, B., 165
Malik, R., 170
Manis, P.B., 447
Manley, G.A., 3, 17, 225
Mannberg, 249
Marion, M., 309, 324
Marler, P., 3
Marshall, A.T., 199
Marshall, K.C., 346
Martin, D.A., 471, 473
Martin, G.K., 36
Martin, M.R., 165, 168, 170, 343, 346, 347, 348,
    349, 351, 352, 354, 358, 361, 375, 429, 434,
    437, 444
Martinez-Hernanez, A., 350
Marty, R., 118, 130
Maruyama, N., 372
Marx, J.L., 461, 473
Mast, T.E., 430, 444, 451
Masta, R.I., 253
Masterton, R.B., 37, 402, 406, 451
Mathews, R.G., 319, 322
Matschinsky, F.M., 169, 206
Matsuoka, I., 356
Matthews, D., 15
Matthews, J.W., 233, 234
Matthews, M.R., 144
Mauldin, L., 111
May, G.A., 310
McCrane, E.P., 392
McCullock, R.M., 346
McDonald, D.M., 351, 395
McFadden, D., 30
McGee, T., 32, 33
McGinn, M.D., 133
McHardy, J., 310

McKean, C.M., 356
McLennan, H., 167, 346, 353
McLennan, J., 160
McLoughlin, C.B., 61
McNeil, M.R., 461
McPhee, J., 68
Medina, J.E., 165, 166, 168, 170, 172, 173
Meier, S., 61, 99
Melamed, B., 168, 173
Meldrum, B.S., 349, 354
Melen, R.D., 310
Mermelstein, P., 302
Merzenich, M.M., 264, 303, 309, 310, 311, 314,
    315, 322, 328, 330, 343, 372, 402, 403, 406,
    450
Mesulam, M.-M., 182
Meyer, M.R., 140
Michelson, R.P., 216, 310, 311
Mielcarz, J.M., 372, 392, 393, 423
Miller, J.D., 5, 6, 8, 31
Miller, J.M., 3, 31, 310, 326, 328, 329, 330, 331
Miller, L.C., 119, 122, 123, 129
Miller, M.I., 283, 284, 288, 291, 301
Mills, J.H., 31
Minckler, J., 461
Mladejovsky, M.G., 310
Model, P.G., 51, 102
Moffat, A.J.M., 229, 230
Mogi, G., 172
Møller, A.R., 216, 453
Molnar, C.E., 233, 234, 248, 263, 268, 441
Monaco, P., 164, 165, 166
Monaghan, P., 172
Moody, D.B., 1, 2, 5, 9, 13, 14, 29, 30, 31, 32,
    33, 248
Moore, B.C.J., 26, 130, 311, 452
Moore, D.R., 111, 120
Moore, G.P., 445, 447
Moore, J.K., 343, 375
Moore, M., 355, 359
Moore, R.Y., 355
Morais, J., 461
Morest, D.K., 119, 134, 247, 343, 346, 347, 351,
    353, 372, 373, 374, 375, 376, 378, 381, 382,
    388, 389, 391, 392, 393, 394, 395, 396, 398,
    399, 400, 402, 403, 406, 407, 408, 411, 413,
    430, 434, 435, 436, 437, 438, 440, 450, 451
Morgan, D.N., 166, 167, 170, 172
Morgenstern, K., 206
Morley, B.J., 359
Morrison, D., 343
Morse, D.B., 5
Mosinger, J.L., 345
Moskowitz, N., 375
Mountain, D.C., 234, 251, 253
Moxon, E.C., 247, 248, 263, 299, 310, 319
Mozo, B.T., 6, 29
Mueller-Preuss, P., 3

Mugnaini, E., 382, 399, 400, 406, 412, 444
Muir, D., 111
Muller, C., 310
Mulroy, M.J., 119, 232, 251, 252
Muraski, A.A., 31, 231
Murato, K., 263
Muria-Garcia, F., 102
Murphy, E.H., 461
Murray, E., 231

N

Nábêlek, I.V., 31
Nachlas, M.M., 141
Nadol, J.B., Jr., 309, 324
Narins, P.M., 229
Neely, S.T., 249, 250, 252
Neff, W.D., 37, 451
Neises, G.R., 342
Neiswander, P., 217, 225
Nelson, D.A., 5
Nelson, P.G., 372, 413, 425, 427, 436, 445, 447, 453
Neuweiler, G., 17
Newman, J.D., 3
Nielsen, D.W., 23, 29
Nienhuys, T.G.W., 32
Nilsson, H.G., 441
Noble, D., 438
Noden, D.M., 73, 99, 102, 110, 113
Nokes, M.A., 216
Nordeen, K.W., 140, 247
Nordemar, H., 200, 201
Norenberg, M.D., 350
Norris, B.E., 372, 375, 392, 393, 411, 413, 423, 430, 431, 432, 435, 436, 437, 438, 441, 442, 444
Norris, C.H., 159, 161, 162, 165, 168, 173
Northrup, C.C., 241, 343, 450
Norton, S.J., 467, 471
Nuttall, A.L., 214, 253

O

Oakes, D.J., 168
Oberholtzer, M., 36
O'Connell, N.A., 453
O'Connor, P., 145
O'Connor, T.A., 3, 36, 148
O'Dorisio, T.M., 172
Oertel, W., 165, 166, 167, 172, 182, 372, 406, 411, 413, 434, 435, 438, 440, 441, 442, 444, 449, 450
Oliver, A.P., 361
Oliver, D.L., 343, 346, 381, 394, 403, 406, 413, 450

O'Loughlin, B.J., 26
Oppenheim, A.V., 301
Orawski, A., 24
O'Reilly, B.F., 309, 329
Orr, M.F., 61, 113
Orsulakova, A., 206
Osborne, M.P., 172
Osen, K.K., 247, 343, 351, 372, 373, 375, 376, 378, 381, 382, 388, 389, 392, 393, 394, 396, 399, 400, 402, 403, 406, 407, 412, 423, 435, 442, 444, 452
Ostapoff, E.M., 111, 134, 146, 148
Otte, J., 309, 324
Owens, E., 309, 324
Özdamer, Ö., 32, 33

P

Padden, D.M., 6, 7
Palmer, A.R., 263, 452
Pappas, G.D., 395
Parakkal, M.H., 162, 165, 166, 345, 358
Parker, D., 464
Parkin, J.L., 310
Parks, T.N., 110, 119, 126, 134, 136, 144, 145, 148
Parrish, K., 464
Partsch, C.J., 89
Passow, B., 22
Patlak, C.S., 195
Paton, J.A., 217
Patrick, J.F., 309, 312
Patricoski, M., 26
Patterson, J.H., 6, 29
Patuzzi, R., 213, 214, 215, 218, 221, 222, 225, 249, 250
Pause, M., 255
Peake, W.R., 215
Peake, W.T., 231, 232, 254
Pedley, T., 349
Peduzzi, J.D., 140
Peet, M.J., 170, 349
Peggemonti, L., 359
Perkel, D.H., 445, 447
Perkins, R.E., 375, 407
Perry, D.R., 375, 431
Perry, J., 30, 31
Pert, C.B., 356
Peters, R., 3
Petersen, M.R., 1, 2, 9, 13, 31, 32, 248
Pettigrew, J.D., 142
Pettigrew, K.D., 195
Pettit, C.R., 310
Pfalz, R., 354, 451
Pfeiffer, R.R., 134, 248, 263, 264, 347, 352, 372, 425, 430, 434, 438, 441, 444

Pfingst, B.E., 3, 36, 309, 310, 313, 316, 321, 322, 324, 326, 330
Pickles, J.O., 25, 219, 245, 355, 356, 453
Pirsig, W., 354, 355, 372
Plattsmier, H.S., 30
Plomp, P., 319
Pohl, P., 8
Popelav, J., 30
Popelka, G.R., 111
Popper, A.N., 16, 22, 24, 25
Porter, R.J., Jr., 461
Potashner, S.J., 343, 346, 349, 381, 394, 403, 413
Pourcho, R.G., 182
Powell, T.P.S., 139, 144, 372, 389, 392
Pribram, K.H., 5
Price, G.R., 133
Probett, G.A., 169
Prosen, C.A., 31, 32, 33, 248
Puglisi, S.G., 378, 400, 406
Puil, E., 348, 353
Pujol, R., 37, 110, 115, 118, 130, 133, 169

Q

R

Raab, D.H., 36, 452
Rabiner, L.R., 301
Rall, W., 438
Ramón y Cajal, S., 343, 371, 372, 389, 434
Ramon-Moliner, E., 359
Rang, H.P., 161
Rarey, K.E., 171
Rasmussen, G.L., 303, 351, 372, 375, 389, 392, 393, 394, 395, 444
Reale, R.A., 263, 270, 303
Rebillard, G., 111, 120
Rebillard, M., 118
Reagan, J., 71, 102
Reese, T.S., 395, 434
Regan, D., 15
Reid, M., 310
Reivich, M., 188, 195, 201
Relkin, E.M., 110, 111, 112, 123, 251
Retzius, G., 115, 118
Reubi, J.C., 342
Rho, J.M., 241, 343, 450
Rhode, W.S., 214, 215, 218, 221, 222, 225, 235, 249, 372, 406, 411, 413, 434, 435, 438, 440, 441, 442, 444, 449, 450
Rich, N.C., 247, 450
Richrath, W., 182, 183
Richter, H.G., 255
Riklan, M., 461

Riley, D.A., 142
Risberg, A., 318
Ritz, L.A., 442, 435, 444
Robertson, D., 162, 163, 216, 225, 233, 235, 248
Robles, L., 215, 221, 235
Rodenburg, M., 24
Rogowski, B.A., 134, 145, 148
Romand, R., 118, 120, 372, 438, 440, 441, 442, 444, 449
Roomans, G.M., 203
Rose, J.E., 113, 263, 264, 266, 270, 372, 392, 393, 423
Rosenthal, M.H., 136
Rosenzweig, M., 36
Rosner, B.S., 298
Rosowski, J.J., 110
Ross, M.D., 171, 200
Roth, G.L., 264, 372, 402, 403, 406, 450
Roth, K., 351, 375, 393, 394, 453
Rouillier, E.M., 450
Rubel, E.W., 37, 109, 111, 113, 115, 119, 120, 122, 123, 126, 133, 134, 136, 140, 141, 142, 144, 146, 148
Ruben, R.J., 37, 55, 68, 71, 76, 77, 81, 86, 89, 97, 99, 113, 114, 118
Rubenstein, M., 215, 216
Rubin, R.P., 342
Ruggero, M.A., 247, 343, 450
Rugh, R., 63
Russell, I.J., 163, 164, 166, 170, 223, 224, 225, 252
Rustioni, A., 342, 346
Ryals, B.M., 109, 115, 123, 126, 133, 136
Ryan, A., 30, 31, 32, 33, 130, 166, 169, 183, 186, 188, 200, 206, 248
Ryugo, D.K., 241, 343, 450

S

Sachs, M.B., 3, 16, 22, 263, 268, 270, 273, 283, 284, 288, 291, 296, 301, 302, 303, 320, 354, 427, 452, 453
Saidel, W.N., 22
Sala, L., 371
Salvi, R.J., 19, 22, 29, 30, 32
Samson, D.S., 461
Sandanaga, M., 354
Sando, I., 264, 389, 392
Sanes, D.H., 148
Santi, D.A., 343
Santi, P.A., 247, 450
Santos-Sacchi, J., 224
Sasa, M., 356
Sasaki, C.T., 361
Saunders, J.C., 17, 29, 30, 37, 110, 111, 112, 119, 120, 122, 123, 133, 136, 188, 201, 231, 232

Savaki, H.E., 172
Schacht, J., 199
Schafer, R.W., 301
Schalk, T.B., 263, 276, 280
Scharf, B., 453
Schechter, H., 215
Schechter, N., 359
Scheich, H., 188, 453
Schindler, D.N., 311
Schindler, R.A., 310, 311, 313, 328, 343
Schmeidt, R.T., 263
Schmidt, J., 352, 359
Schmiedt, R.A., 247, 252
Schnerson, A., 115
Schnitzler, H.-U., 17, 22
Schon, F., 182
Schreiber, C., 450
Schubert, E.D., 216, 310, 324
Schuknecht, H.F., 32, 162, 309
Schwab, J., 217, 225, 235
Schwartz, A.M., 395, 398, 451
Schwartz, I.R., 166, 169, 353
Schwitzer, L., 119
Scott, G.E., 113
Searcy, M.H., 19
Segal, P., 111
Segundo, J.P., 445, 447
Seifter, E.J., 37, 111, 112, 133
Seikin, R.L., 302
Seligman, A.M., 141
Sellick, P.M., 213, 214, 215, 218, 221, 222, 223, 224, 225, 249, 250, 252
Sellstrom, A., 345
Selters, W.A., 315
Semple, M.N., 450, 451
Serafin, J.V., 2, 29, 30
Serviere, J., 188
Sewell, W., 168, 173
Sewell, W.F., 159
Seyfarth, R.M., 3
Shambaugh, G.E., Jr., 32
Shamma, S.A., 310
Shannon, R.V., 310, 315, 322, 326
Shanon, E., 111
Sharp, F.R., 186, 188, 206
Shaw, E.A.G., 110, 111
Shea, C.A., 55, 68, 76, 86, 89, 113
Shen, J.J., 32
Sherrick, C., 235
Shiff, W., 309
Shinohara, M., 195
Shiosaka, S., 356
Shnerson, A., 37
Shofner, W.P., 37
Sidtis, J.J., 461
Siebert, W.M., 219, 301, 303
Siegel, G.J., 160
Siegel, J.H., 248, 251, 253, 263

Sikkeland, T., 215
Silverman, M., 330
Silverman, N.S., 37, 148, 313, 314, 451
Simada, Z., 359, 360
Simmonds, M.A., 354
Simmons, D.D., 247
Simmons, F.B., 303, 310, 311, 327, 328, 330
Sinex, D.G., 283, 288
Sinnott, J.M., 3, 5, 8, 10, 16, 22, 427
Sitler, R., 31
Sitler, R.W., 22
Sjostrand, F.S., 241
Skärsteen, O., 215
Slapnick, S.M., 113
Slepian, J.Z., 163
Slettemoen, G.A., 217, 225
Smigielski, P., 217, 225, 235
Smith, C.A., 254, 255
Smith, C.B., 171
Smith, D.E., 133
Smith, D.I., 214
Smith, D.J., 142
Smith, F.D., 441
Smith, L., 327, 330
Smith, P.H., 372, 406, 411, 413, 434, 435, 438, 440, 441, 442, 444, 449, 450
Smith, R.L., 36, 263, 283, 290, 431
Smith, S., 319
Smith, Z.D.J., 119, 122, 123, 129, 134, 136, 142, 144, 146, 148
Smoak, H.A., 451
Smoorenburg, G.F., 319
Snowdon, C.T., 5
Snyder, R.L., 247, 450
Snyder, S.H., 356
Sobkowicz, H.M., 113
Sohmer, H.S., 254
Sokolich, W.G., 263
Sokoloff, L., 195
Solomon, R.L., 148
Soma, M., 310
Sondhi, M.M., 219
Sonn, M., 310
Sonnhof, U., 353
Sosamma, J.B., 169
Sotelo, C., 395
Spangler, K.N., 394, 399, 403
Sparks, D.W., 309
Spelman, F., 309, 310
Spelman, F.A., 313, 314
Spemann, H., 86
Spira, D., 216
Spoendlin, H., 186, 241, 247, 343, 407, 450
Srulovicz, P., 301, 303
Starr, A., 327, 349, 356, 372, 442, 444, 449, 450, 453
Stebbins, W.C., 1, 2, 5, 9, 13, 14, 16, 29, 30, 31, 32, 33, 37, 248, 252

Steele, C.R., 219
Stevens, K.N., 283, 293, 317, 318
Steward, O., 134, 136, 140, 144
Stiglbrunner, H.K., 318
Stotler, W.A., 402
Straughan, D.W., 354
Stream, K.S., 111
Stream, R.W., 111
Streeter, G.L., 86
Streit, P., 342
Strelioff, D., 223, 231
Strevens, P., 293
Suga, N., 3, 15, 263
Sulik, K.K., 118, 119
Sutton, D., 313, 326, 328, 329, 330
Swanson, L.W., 355
Syka, J., 30

T

Taber, L.S., 219
Tachibana, M., 159, 164, 168, 173, 356
Takaori, S., 356
Takasaka, T., 255
Tanaka, Y., 165, 172
Taniguchi, L., 263
Tansley, B., 15
Taylor, K.J., 214, 218, 225
Tebecis, A.K., 353, 360
Tees, R.C., 37, 148
Telleen, C.C., 309
Terhardt, E., 299
Thalmann, I., 171, 206
Thalmann, R., 169, 171, 172, 201, 206
Thielemeir, M.A., 310
Theiler, K., 63
Thomas, E.C., 438
Thomas, F.C., 22
Thompson, C.L., 461
Thompson, G.C., 402, 406, 451
Thompson, M.H., 165, 167, 172
Thornhill, R.A., 172
Thornton, A.R.D., 464
Tilney, L.G., 29, 30, 37, 119, 231, 232, 249
Tischler, M.D., 451
Todd, J.R., 77
Toerien, M.J., 89
Tolbert, L.P., 347, 374, 376, 378, 388, 389, 395,
    396, 398, 402, 403, 434, 435, 437, 438, 440
Toner,J., 130
Tong, Y.C., 310, 312, 315, 319, 322
Tonndorf, J., 216
Torda, C., 360
Tousimis, A.J., 199
Trune, D.R., 140, 375
Tsien, R.W., 438
Tsou, K.-C., 141

Tsuchitani, C., 407, 408
Tukey, J.W., 301
Turner, C.W., 29
Turner, M.J., 310, 330
Turner, R.G., 231

U

Uhl, G.R., 356

V

Valverde, F., 144
Van de Water, T.R., 51, 55, 68, 71, 76, 77, 81,
    86, 89, 92, 97, 99, 102, 110, 113
Van Dyke, R.H., 52, 102
van Gehuchten, A., 371
van Noort, J., 372, 389, 392, 394, 402, 403, 435
Venables, P.H., 461
Vendrick, A.J.H., 372, 427, 429, 430, 432, 435,
    438, 440, 441
Verschuure, J.V., 24
Vertes, D., 31
Viemeister, N.F., 19, 24, 318, 452
Vince, M.A., 130
Vinnikov, Y.A., 161
Vivion, M.C., 309, 330
Vogten, L.L.M., 24
Voigt, H.F., 291, 296, 303, 372, 413, 427, 429,
    430, 436, 445, 447, 452
Voldrich, L., 22
von During, M., 255
Vurek, L.S., 310

W

Wada, T., 115, 118
Waddington, C.H., 52, 99, 102
Walcott, W.W., 216
Walker, D., 130
Walker, J.R., 111
Walker, M.G., 310
Walsh, J.K., 22
Walsh, S.M., 309, 310, 329
Walzl, E.M., 130
Wamsley, J.K., 352, 353, 358, 359
Wang, C.-Y., 251, 252
Wann, J.R., 140
Ward, W.D., 29, 31
Warr, W.B., 134, 183, 241, 247, 303, 343, 352,
    372, 375, 381, 382, 393, 394, 402, 403, 406,
    412, 430, 444
Warren, R.L., 109, 201
Watanabe, T., 22, 354, 359, 360, 438
Watkins, J.C., 167, 168, 346, 347

Webb, W.W., 217
Webster, D.B., 37, 134, 140, 144, 148, 343, 375
Webster, M., 37, 134 140, 144, 148, 343
Webster, W.R., 188, 375, 431
Weiss, T.F., 231, 232, 251, 252, 254, 263
Welt, C., 142
Wenthold, R., 164, 165, 166, 182, 183, 342, 345, 351, 353, 359, 444
Wenzel, R.P., 133
Werman, R., 160, 161
Wersall, J., 343
Wessells, N.K., 61
Wever, E.G., 227
Wexler, K.F., 319
Wheal, H.V., 346
White, D.G., 349
White, M.W., 303, 310, 314, 315, 330
White, R.L., 310, 311
Whitfield, I.C., 15, 347, 352, 354, 356, 453
Wickman, M.G., 200
Wiederhold, M.L., 172, 253
Wiedmer, B., 309
Wightman, F.L., 299
Wilkenson, R., 19
Willott, J.F., 140
Wilson, J.P., 214, 216, 218, 225, 235, 248, 249
Winberg, S., 167
Winbery, S.L., 164
Winkler, C., 371, 406
Wood, C., 130
Wollberg, Z., 3
Woodford, C., 22
Woolf, N.K., 3, 32, 130, 186, 188, 206
Woolsey, C.N., 130
Woolsey, T.A., 140, 142
Wong-Riley, M.T.T., 142
Worden, F.G., 3
Wright, A., 231
Wroblewski, R., 200, 201, 203
Wustrow, F., 311

X, Y

Yamamoto, K., 119
Yates, G.K., 215, 218, 225, 235
Ylikoski, J., 32
Yntema, C.L., 49, 50, 52, 55, 71, 99, 102, 113
Yoshizuka, M., 119
Yost, W.A., 303
Young, E.D., 263, 268, 270, 273, 281, 283, 291, 296, 303, 320, 372, 413, 425, 427, 429, 430, 436, 437, 442, 444, 445, 447, 451, 452
Young, R.R., 461
Young, S.R., 119, 126
Young, W.S., 352
Yund, E.W. 461
Yurgelun-Todd, D.A., 402, 403, 435, 437

Z

Zamora, A.J., 395
Zarbin, M.A., 353, 359
Zeisberg, B., 311
Zieglgansberger, W., 348
Zimmerman, D.McG., 170
Zoloth, S.R., 2, 9, 13, 19
Zook, J.M., 375
Zurek, P.M., 251
Zweig, G., 219
Zwicker, E., 24
Zwilling, E., 52, 99
Zwislocki, J.J., 110, 219, 263, 476

SUBJECT INDEX

Page numbers in *italics* refer to illustrations: (t) indicates tables.

A

Acetylcholine, afferent as transmitter, of cochlea, 161
  of lateral line organ, 163
  as efferent transmitter, of cochlea, 161–163
  of lateral line organ, 163–164
  as neurotransmitter, of cochlear nucleus, 351–352
  of inferior colliculus, 359–360
  of medial geniculate nucleus, 360
Acousticolateralis systems, monoamines as transmitters in, 171–172
ALSR. See *Rate, synchronized, average localized.*
Amino acids, as neurotransmitters, of inferior colliculus, 359
  of medial geniculate nucleus, 360
  cochlear uptake of, as indicator of transmitter function, 182–186
  excitatory, as afferent transmitter, of cochlea, 167–169
    as afferent transmitter, of lateral line organ, 170–171
    as efferent transmitter, of cochlea, 170
    as efferent transmitter, of lateral line organ, 171
  inhibitory, as neurotransmitters of cochlear nucleus, 353–355
γ-Aminobutyrate, as afferent transmitter, of cochlea, 164–166
  of lateral line organ, 166
  as efferent transmitter, of cochlea, 166
  of lateral line organ, 166–167
Amphibians, papilla of, nerve fiber tuning in, 229–230, *230*
Amplitude spectrum, of /ɛ/, 265
ANAS. See *Auditory nerve stimulating substance.*
Angular nucleus. See *Nucleus angularis.*

Audiograms, from various fish, *18*
Auditory cortex, neurotransmitters of, 360
Auditory form, and function, comparative analysis of, 16–38
Auditory nerve, anatomy of, 343–344
  biochemistry of, 344–346
  characteristic frequency of fibers, *264, 265*
  neurotransmitters of, 341–362
  pharmacology of, 346–349
  speech encoding in, 263–304
  synapse of, model of, *350*
Auditory nerve activating substance, as afferent neurotransmitter of cochlea, 173
Auditory nuclei, bulbar, principal connections of, *391*
Auditory system, bulbar, cell circuits and their relationships to signal processing, *404, 405*
  central, neurotransmitters of, 341–362
  development of, extrinsic influences on, 132–149
  recent advances in understanding of, 109–149
  functional activity of, autoradiography and, 186–199
  uptake of deoxyglucose in, 186-199
Autoradiography, for determining functional activity in auditory system, 186–199

B

Basilar membrane, electrical responses of, and susceptibility to trauma, 223–225
  measurement of, 213–217
  techniques of, 215–217
  mechanical response of, measured by laser interferometer, 217–218
  response of, in guinea pig, *250*
  sharp tuning response of, and susceptibility to trauma, 218–220
  tuning curve of, 218, *219*
    effect of trauma on, 221
    versus hair cell curve, 225, *226*
    versus neural tuning curve, 221, *222*

tuning of, and condition of outer hair
cells, histological correlation
between, 225–229
tuning response of, nonlinearity of,
221–223, *223*
Basal papilla. See *Cochlea.*
Biological signals, comparative perception
of, 3–16
Brain stem, functional roles of inner- and
outer-hair-cell subsystems in, 241–258
Brain stem evoked potentials, asymmetries
in, 461–476
extraction of, 462–464
auditory brain stem response, 464–467,
465, 466
early latency, 464–467, *465, 466*
for chick hatchlings, *147*
middle latencies, 467–472, *469, 470*
late potentials, 472–473, *474, 475*
Bundle, olivocochlear, crossed, effect of on
otoacoustic signal, *254*
Bushy cells, globular, 376–378, *379, 384*
efferent projections of, 402–403
synaptic organization of, 396, *397*
spherical, 376, *377, 384*
efferent projections of, 402
synaptic organization of, 394–395, *397*

C

Capacitive probe, for measuring basilar
membrane, 216
Cartwheel cells, *380*
Catecholamines, as neurotransmitters, of
cochlear nucleus, 355–356
of inferior colliculus, 360
of medial geniculate nucleus, 360
Cells. See also *Neurons.*
bushy, globular, 376–378, *379, 384*
efferent projections of, 402–403
synaptic organization of, 396, *397*
spherical, 376, *377, 384*
efferent projections of, 402
synaptic organization of, 394–395, *397*
cartwheel, *380*
fusiform, 378, *380, 384*

of dorsal cochlear nucleus, efferent
projections of, 406
synaptic organization of, *397, 399, 401*
giant, 378, *380, 384*
efferent projections of, 406
synaptic organization of, *397,* 400
granule, 378–381, *380*
efferent projections of, 406
synaptic organization of, *397,* 400
in cochlear nucleus, measurements of,
381–382, *383*
multipolar, of ventral cochlear nucleus,
efferent projections of, 403
octopus, *377,* 378, *384*
efferent projections of, 403
synaptic organization of, *397,* 398–399
small, of dorsal cochlear nucleus, efferent
projections of, 406
stellate, *377*
synaptic organization of, 395–396, *397*
types of, and cochlear nucleus response
types, 434–437
efferent projections of, 402–406
in cochlear nuclear complex, 375–389
distribution of by area, *383*
Central nervous system, role of in
development of auditory system,
134–149
Cepstrum, pitch, computed from spectrum
of /da/, *302*
Characteristic frequency, of auditory nerve
fibers, 264, *265*
versus normalized rate, for /ɛ/, *291*
versus normalized rate for low
spontaneous rate units, *280*
Chemical elements, variation in across stria
vascularis and spiral ligament, *208*
Cochlea. See also *Cochlear nucleus.*
energy dispersive X-ray analysis of, effect
of noise exposure on, 206–210, *209*
functional roles of inner- and outer-hair-
cell subsystems in, 241–258
implants of, 309–332. See also *Cochlear
implants.*
inner- and outer-hair-cell subsystems of,
comparisons of, 256–258, 257(t)
evidence for, 247–255, *250,254*
hypotheses for, 243–247, *246*

interpretation of observations, 255–258
ion distribution in, energy dispersive X-
    ray analysis for, 199–210
    of cochlear tissues, 203–206, 205,
        207–209
    of fluid spaces, 201–203, *202–205*
neurotransmitters of, 159–163, 164–166,
    167–170, 172–173
opening of, sources of trauma in,
    213–215
physiological parameters of, anatomical
    measures of, 181–210
positions of outer hair cells or spiral
    ganglion cells in, *116*
removal of, and effect on development of
    auditory system, 134–142, *138, 139,
    141, 143*
sharp tuning response of, reversible loss
    of, 233–234
trauma to, from measurement techniques,
    215–217
    from opening, 213–215
uptake of amino acids by, as indicator of
    transmitter function, 182–186
uptake of deoxyglucose by, 192–199
Cochlear implants, candidate selection for,
    324–327
    clinical approaches for, 310–312
    current approaches, 312
    intra- versus extracochlear, 315–317
    mechanisms of function, 322–324
    morbidity of, 327–331
    physiological considerations for, 318–321
    processor strategies for, 317–324
    psychophysical considerations for,
        321–322
    single- versus multichannel, 312–315
    speech models for, 317–318
Cochlear nerve, 389–393, *390, 391*
    afferent input to, 398–394
    anatomy of, 371–375
    anteroventral, anterior division of,
        synaptic organization of, 394–396,
        397
        cell types of, 385–389
        posterior division of, synaptic
            organization of, 396–398, *397*

cell types in, 375–389
    distribution of by area, *383*
    of limited distribution, 376–381, *377,
        379, 380*
    of widespread distribution, 381–389
    synaptic organization of, 394–401
dorsal, cell circuits and relationships to
    signal processing in, *404*
    cell types of, 382–385
    response properties in, 444–450
    synaptic organization of, *397, 399–400*
neurons of, physiological response types
    of, 425–437
response characteristics of, 423–453
neurotransmitters of, 343–351, *350*
noncochlear fibers in, 393–394
posteroventral, synaptic organizations of,
    397, 398–399
signal coding in, *404, 405,* 406–413
stimulus coding in, structural basis for,
    371–414
subdivisions of, 371–375
subsystems of, schematic summary of,
    424
ventral, chopper responses and stellate
    cells, 440–441
    onset responses of, 441–444
    primarylike versus nonprimarylike
        units, 437–438
    response properties of, 437–444
Colliculus, inferior, neurotransmitters of,
    359–360
Conductive elements, of ear, development
    of, 110–112
Congenital malformations, of mammalian
    inner ear, mechanisms of, 97–99, *98,
    100*
Consonants, fricative. See *Fricative
    consonants.*
    stop. See *Stop consonants.*
Corti, organ of. See *Organ of Corti.*
Crossed olivocochlear bundle. See
    Olivocochlear bundle, crossed.
Cytochochleogram, of guinea pig treated
    with kanamycin, *34*

D

Deafferentation, partial, effect of on development of auditory system, 142–144, *145, 146*

Deoxyglucose, uptake of, in auditory system, 186–199

Discriminability functions, for various mammalian species, *23*

Duct, endolymphatic. See *Endolymphatic duct.*

E

Ear. See also *Auditory system; External ear; Inner ear; Middle ear.*

development of. See *Auditory system, development of; Inner ear, mammalian, developmental mechanisms of.*

mechanics of, effect of inner ear damage on, 234–235

EDXA. See *Energy dispersive X-ray analysis.*

Electrical responses, of basilar membrane and hair cells, and susceptibility to trauma, 223–225

Endolymph, residue of, energy dispersive X-ray analysis of, *203*

Endolymphatic duct, ablation experiments on, 92, *93–95*

anlage of, role of in development of mammalian inner ear, 89–97, *93–96*

cannulation experiments on, 92–97, *96*

Energy dispersive X-ray analysis, of cochlear ion distribution, 199–210, *203–205, 207–209*

Environmental influences, effect of on development of the auditory system, 144–149

Epitheliomesenchymal interactions, in development of inner ear, 61–76, *64, 66, 67, 69, 70, 72, 73*

External ear, development of conducting elements of, 110–112

F

Fate map, of abnormal otocyst, 89, *90*

of normal otocyst, 86–89, *87, 88, 90*

Fate mapping, in development of mammalian ear, 86–89, *87, 88, 90,* 91(t)

Frequency, characteristic, of auditory nerve fibers, 264, *265*

ranges of to which animals respond, 120, *122(t)*

Fricative consonants, poststimulus histograms for /ma/ and /ba/, *294*

power spectra of, *295*

representation of, in speech encoding, 293–298

steady-state discharge rate versus characteristic frequency, *296*

Fusiform cells, 378, *380, 384*

of dorsal cochlear nucleus, efferent projections of, 406

synaptic organization of, *397, 399, 401*

G

GABA. See *γ-Aminobutyrate.*

Ganglion, statoacoustic. See *Statoacoustic ganglion.*

Giant cells, of dorsal cochlear nucleus, 378, *380, 384*

efferent projections of, 406

synaptic organization of, *397, 400*

Granule cells, 378–381, *380*

efferent projections of, 406

synaptic organization of, *397, 400*

H

Hair cell(s), electrical responses of, and susceptibility to trauma, 223–225

in amphibian papilla, *228*

in basilar papilla, *229*

inner and outer, numbers of, and associated afferent neurons, 243(t)

inner and outer subsystems of,
    comparisons of, 256–258, 257(t)
functional roles of, 241–258
    evidence for, 247–255, 250, 254
    in cochlea and brain stem, 241–258
    working hypotheses for, 243–247, 246
    interpretation of observations, 255–258
maximum loss of, following exposure to
    high-intensity pure tones, 129
mechanical tuning of, and function of
    inner ear, 213–235
number of, as function of position along
    chick cochlea, 128
outer, condition of, and correlation with
    basilar membrane tuning, 225–229
    energy dispersive X-ray analysis of, 205
    exposed to noise, energy dispersive
        X-ray analysis of, 209
    tuning curve of, versus basilar membrane
        curve, 225, 226
    tuning of, basis of, 231–232
    tuning response of, nonlinearity of,
        221–223, 223
Hearing capabilities, comparative analysis
    of, 16–38
Histograms, interspike interval, 266
    of dynamic ranges for CF tones, 280
    period, 266, 267
    poststimulus time, 266, 287
        for /ma/ and /ba/ synthetic stimuli, 294
    of auditory nerve fibers to single
        formant stimulus, 300

I

Implants, cochlear, 309–332
Inferior colliculus, neurotransmitters of,
    359–360
Inner ear, damage to, effect on mechanics
    of ear, 234–235
    differentiation of, 113–120, 114, 116–118,
        121
    function of, based on mechanical tuning
        of hair cells, 213–235
    functional development of, model of, 125
    mammalian, developmental mechanisms
        of, 49–103

congenital malformations and, 97–99,
    98, 100
effect of localized periotic
    mesenchyme deficiency on,
    68, 70
effect on otocyst on otic capsule
    formation, 68–71, 72, 73
effect on periotic mesenchyme and,
    62–68, 66, 67, 69
epitheliomesenchymal interactions in,
    61–76, 64, 66, 67, 69, 70,
    72, 73
fate mapping and, 86–89, 87, 88,
    90, 91(t)
in early stages, 49–52, 50–56
neural influence on, 52–61, 57, 59,
    60, 62, 63
neurotrophic interactions in, 77–85,
    78–80, 82–85
role of endolymphatic duct and sac
    anlage in, 89–97, 93–96
summary of, 99–103, 101
Interferometer, laser, measurement of
    mechanical response of basilar
    membrane by, 217–218
Interferometry, for measuring basilar
    membrane, 216–217
    speckle, 217
Interspike interval histograms, 266
Interspike intervals, time course of, in
    response to frequency-modulated
    tone, 285
Intrauterine environment, acoustic, factors
    influencing, 132

K

Kainate receptor type, in
    neurotransmission, 346–351, 350

L

Labyrinth, membranous. See Membranous
    labyrinth.
Laminar nucleus. See Nucleus laminaris.

Laser interferometer, measurement of
mechanical response of basilar
membrane by, 217–218
Lateral line organ, neurotransmitters of,
159–161, 163–164, 166–167, 170–171
Lateral superior olive. See *Superior olive,
lateral.*

M

Magnocellular nucleus. See *Nucleus
magnocellularis.*
Malformations, congenital, of mammalian
inner ear, mechanisms of, 97–99, *98,
100*
Mammals, inner ear of, developmental
mechanisms of, 49–103
Map, response. See *Response map.*
Mapping, fate. See *Fate mapping.*
Medial geniculate body, nucleus of,
neurotransmitters of, 360
Medial superior olive. See *Superior olive,
medial.*
Membranous labyrinth, development of,
114
Mesenchyme, interaction of with
epithelium, in development of inner
ear, 61–76, *64, 66, 67, 69, 70, 72, 73*
periotic, deficiency of, effect of on
cochlea, 68, *70*
influence of on otic development,
62–68, *66, 67, 69*
role of in early development of inner ear,
51, *54, 55*
N-Methyl-D-aspartate receptor type, in
neurotransmission, 346–351, *350*
Middle ear, development of conducting
elements of, 110–112
Monoamines, as transmitters in
acousticolateralis systems, 171–172
Mossbauer method, for measuring basilar
membrane, 215–216
Multipolar cells, of cochlear nucleus,
distribution of, 383, *385–387*
of ventral cochlear nucleus, efferent
projections of, 403

N

Nerve, auditory. See *Auditory nerve.*
Nerve fiber, tuning curve of, versus basilar
membrane tuning curve, 221, *222*
tuning of, in papilla of amphibians,
229–230, *230*
Neuroactive peptides, as neurotransmitters
of cochlear nucleus, 356–357
Neuroepithelium, in development of inner
ear, 51–52, *51, 54*
Neurons, cochlear, afferent and efferent,
and myelination, *245*
from nucleus magnocellularis, changes
in number and cross-sectional area
of following cochlea removal, *139*
from nucleus laminaris, of monaurally
deprived chicks, *149*
of cochlear nucleus, physiological
response types of, 425–437
response characteristics of, 423–453
unit types of, based on poststimulus
histograms, 430–433, *433*
based on response maps, 425–430,
426, 428
olivocochlear, large medial and small
lateral, projecting to inner and
outer hair cells, *244*
synaptic organization of, in cochlear
nucleus, 394–401
types of, in cochlear nucleus, 375–389
Neurotransmitters. See also specific
transmitters, such as *Acetylcholine;*
γ-Aminobutyrate.
criteria for, 160–161
of auditory nerve and central auditory
system, 341–362
model of synapse and, *350*
of cochlea, 159–163, 164–166, 167–170,
172–173
of lateral line organ, 159–161, 163–164,
166–167, 170–171
Noise, exposure to, effect of on energy
dispersive X-ray analysis of cochlea,
206–210, *209*
sinusoidally amplitude modulated, *20*
Nonlinearity, of basilar membrane and hair
cell responses, 221–223, *223*

Nucleus, angular. See *Nucleus angularis.*
auditory, in chick brain stem,
organization of, *135*
cochlear. See *Cochlear nucleus.*
laminar. See *Nucleus laminaris.*
magnocellular. See *Nucleus
magnocellularis.*
Nucleus angular, *135*
Nucleus laminaris, *135*
effect of partial deafferentation on,
142–144, *145, 146*
tonotopic organization of, in chick
embryos versus hatchlings, *131*
Nucleus magnocellularis, *135*
effect of cochlea removal on, 134–142,
138, 139, 141, 143
effect of otocyst ablation on, *137*
tonotopic organization of in chick
embryos versus hatchlings, *131*

O

Octopus cells, *377, 378, 384*
synaptic organization of, *397, 398*–399
efferent projections of, 403
Olivocochlear bundle, crossed, cell circuits
and relationships to signal processing
in, *405*
effect of on otoacoustic signal, *254*
Olivocochlear neurons, projecting to inner
and outer hair cells, *244*
Organ, lateral line. See *Lateral line organ.*
Organ of Corti, afferent pattern of
innervation, in cat, *242*
stages of differentiation of, in cat, *117*
in rabbit, *118*
uptake of amino acids by, 183–186, *184,
185*
Otic cup, 51, *52*
Otic placode, *50*
Otoacoustic distortion signal, effect
of crossed olivocochlear bundle on,
253, *254*
Otoconia, energy dispersive X-ray analysis
of, *203*
Otocyst. See also *Otocyst/rhombencephalon
interaction.*

ablation of, effects of on development of
magnocellular nucleus, *137*
abnormal, fate map of, 89, *90*
effect of on otic capsule formation,
69–71, *72, 73*
normal, fate map of, 86–89, *87, 88, 90*
Otocyst/rhombencephalon interaction, in
development of inner ear, 55–61, *57,
60, 62, 63,* 58(t)

P

Papilla, basal. See *Cochlea.*
Peptides, neuroactive, as neurotransmitters
of cochlear nucleus, 356–357
Perception, of biological signals,
comparative, 3–16
Perilymph, residue of, energy dispersive
X-ray analysis of, *202*
Period histograms, 266, *267*
Periphery, auditory, effect of on auditory
system development, 133
Pitch, representation of, in speech
encoding, 299–301, *302*
Place principle, development of, 120–132
Polypeptides, as neurotransmitters, in
cochlea, 172–173
Poststimulus time histograms, 266, *287*
and response types of cochlear neurons,
430–433, *433*
locations of types of in cochlear nucleus,
436(t)
types of, in cochlear nucleus, *433*
Prostaglandins, as neurotransmitters, in
cochlea, 172
Prostheses, cochlear, 309–332. See also
Cochlear implants.
Psychoacoustics, comparative, new
directions for, 1–38

Q

Quisqualate receptor type, in
neurotransmission, 346–351, *350*

R

Rate, normalized, smoothed, for /da/, 292
  versus characteristic frequency, for
    /ɛ/, 291
  versus characteristic frequency for low
    spontaneous rate units, 281
  normalized average, for vowels at three
    stimulus levels, 277, 278
  spontaneous, relationship of to relative
    threshold, 279
  synchronized, 273
    average localized, for stop consonant
      /da/, 289
    for vowels /ɛ/, /I/, and /a/, 282
    smoothed, 290
    temporal profile of, 272
    for /ɛ/ at seven levels, 273, 274
    versus stimulus level, for a two-tone
      stimulus, 271
Rate-place representation, 264–266, 265
  for vowels, 276, 277, 278, 281
Receptors, postsynaptic, of auditory nerve,
  346–349
  sensory. See Sensory receptors.
Rectifier distortion, 268
Response maps, correspondence with
    morphological cell types, 434–437
  distribution of among cochlear nucleus
    subdivisions, 431(t)
  of auditory neuron, 425–430, 426, 428
  of dorsal cochlear nucleus type II unit,
    446
  of dorsal cochlear nucleus type IV unit,
    426, 446
    with acoustic calibration, 449
  types of, and rate versus sound level
    functions, 428
Rhombencephalon, influence on
    development of inner ear, 52–61, 57,
    59, 60, 62, 63
  interaction of with otocyst, in
    development of inner ear, 55–61,
    57, 60, 62, 63, 58(t)

S

Sac, endolymphatic. See Endolymphatic duct.
Sensory receptors, trophic effect of, on
    statoacoustic ganglion, 81–85, 83–85
Serotonin, as neurotransmitter of cochlear
    nucleus, 355–356
Serotonin, as neurotransmitter of inferior
    colliculus, 360
Serotonin, as neurotransmitter of medial
    geniculate nucleus, 360
Sharp tuning response, of basilar
    membrane, and susceptibility to
    trauma, 218–220
Sharp tuning response, of basilar
    membrane, origin of, 220–229
Shifts, threshold. See Threshold shifts.
Signal coding, in cochlear nucleus, 404,
    405, 406–413
Signals, biological, comparative perception
    of, 3–16
Small cell cap, of dorsal cochlear nucleus,
    385–388, 387
Song themes, brown-headed cowbird,
    sonograms of, 9
  red-winged blackbird, sonograms of, 9
Sonograms, of bird calls, 9
  of Japanese monkey clear call, 12
  for monkey clear calls and harsh calls, 15
Sound, attenuation of, effect
    of on intrauterine acoustic
    environment, 132
Sound level, effect of on intrauterine
    acoustic environment, 132
Spectrum, and pitch cepstrum, of /da/, 302
  stimulus, for vowels /I/, /ɛ/, and /a/, 273,
    275
Speech encoding, in auditory nerve, of
    fricative consonants, 293–298
  in auditory nerve, of stop consonants,
    283–293
  of vowels, 264–283
  representation of pitch in, 299–301, 302
Speech sounds, synthetic, responses of
    chinchillas and humans to, 7
Spiral ganglion, uptake of amino acids by,
    186, 187
Spiral ligament, chemical spectra of, 208

Statoacoustic ganglion, origin of, 71–76, *74–76*
   trophic effect of, on sensory receptors, 77–81, *78–80, 82*
Stellate cells, in cochlear nucleus, *377*
   synaptic organization of, 396–398, *397*
   microstructure of, effect of trauma on, 232–233
      mechanical properties related to, 232
      tuning curves of, direct measurement of, 230–231
Stimuli, acoustic, representation of in central nervous system, *404, 405,* 406–413
Stimulus coding, structural basis for, in cochlear nucleus, 371–414
Stop consonants, poststimulus time histograms, for /da/, *287*
   representation of, in speech encoding, 283–293
Stria vascularis, chemical spectra of, *208*
   energy dispersive X-ray analysis of, *207*
Superior olive, lateral, cell circuits and relationships to signal processing in, *405*
   medial, cell circuits and relationships to signal processing, *404*
   neurotransmitters of, 358–359
Synapse, auditory nerve, model of, *350*
   of specific neuronal types, in cochlear nucleus, 394–401
Synchronization. See also *Rate, synchronized.*
   as a function of characteristic frequency, *269*

T

Tectorial membrane, fluid residue of, energy dispersive X-ray analysis of, *204*
Temporal modulation transfer function, 19, *20, 21*
   neural versus psychophysical, *27*
   obtained with sinusoidally amplitude modulated noise, *20*
Temporal-place representation, 264–266
   for vowels, 276, *282*

Threshold, relative, relationship of to spontaneous rate, *279*
Threshold shifts, absolute, in guinea pig treated with kanamycin, *35*
   intensity difference, in guinea pig treated with kanamycin, *35*
TMTF. See *Temporal modulation transfer function.*
Tones, combination, 268
   sinusoidally amplitude modulated, *20*
Transmitters. See *Neurotransmitters* and specific substances, such as *Acetycholine.*
Tuning, of hair cells, basis of, 231–232
   sharp, reversible loss in, 233–234
Tuning curve, basilar membrane, effect of trauma on, 221
   basilar membrane and hair cell, differences between, 225, *226*
   comparison of basilar membrane and nerve fiber, 221, *222*
   nerve fiber, effect of trauma on, 221
      of amphibian papilla, 229–230, *230*
   neural and psychophysical, for various species, *25*
   of basilar membrane, 218, *219*
   of stereocilia, direct measurement of, 230–231
   psychophysical, of fish, *18*

V

Vibration amplitude, ratio of, of basilar membrane and malleus, as function of frequency, *223*
Vowels, amplitude spectrum of, *265, 267*
   average localized synchronized rate, *274, 275, 282*
   normalized average rate profiles for, *277, 278*
   rate-place representation of, 264, *265, 276, 277, 278, 281*
   representation of, in speech encoding, 264–283
   temporal-place representation of, 276, *282*
   whispered, spectrum of electrical signal and acoustic signal, *297*
      temporal profile for, *298*